Cardiac Markers

Pathology and Laboratory Medicine

Series Editors: Stewart Sell and Alan H. B. Wu

Cardiac Markers

Second Edition

Edited by

Alan H. B. Wu, PhD

Department of Pathology and Laboratory Medicine
Hartford Hospital, Hartford, CT

Foreword by

William E. Boden, MD, FACC

Professor of Medicine
University of Connecticut School of Medicine
Director, Division of Cardiology
Program Director, The Henry Low Heart Center
Hartford Hospital
Hartford, Connecticut

Humana Press Totowa, New Jersey

© 2003 Humana Press Inc.
999 Riverview Drive, Suite 208
Totowa, New Jersey 07512

humanapress.com

For additional copies, pricing for bulk purchases, and/or information about other Humana titles, contact Humana at the above address or at any of the following numbers: Tel.: 973-256-1699; Fax: 973-256-8341; E-mail: humana@humanapr.com or visit our Website: http://humanapress.com.

This publication is printed on acid-free paper. ∞
ANSI Z39.48-1984 (American Standards Institute) Permanence of Paper for Printed Library Materials.

Cover illustration: *Cardiovascular Toxicology,* v1, n4. Used with permission.
Cover design by Patricia F. Cleary.

Printed in the United States of America. 10 9 8 7 6 5 4 3 2 1

Library of Congress Cataloging-in-Publication Data

Cardiac markers / edited by Alan H. B. Wu.–2nd ed.
     p.;cm.–(Pathology and laboratory medicine)
  Includes bibliographical references and index.
  ISBN 1-58829-036-0 (alk. paper)   eISBN 1-59259-385-2
  1. Coronary heart disease–Serodiagnosis. 2. Biochemical markers. I. Wu, Alan H. B. II. Pathology and laboratory medicine (Unnumbered)
  [DNLM: 1. Myocardial Infarction–diagnosis. 2. Angina, Unstable–physiopathology. 3. Biological Markers. 4. Heart Failure, Congestive–diagnosis. 5. Myocardial Ischemia–diagnosis. 6 Troponin–diagnostic use. WG 300 C2668 2003]
  RC685.C6 C265 2003
  616.1'23075–dc21   2002038720

Dedication

This book is dedicated to my parents, my loving wife, Pam, and to our children Ed, Marc, and Kim, whose career journals have only just begun.

Foreword

The management of patients with acute coronary syndromes (ACS) has evolved dramatically over the past decade and, in many respects, represents a rapidly moving target for the cardiologist, internist, emergency medicine specialist, intensivist, and clinical pathologist—all of whom seek to integrate these recent advances into contemporary clinical practice.

Unstable angina and non-ST-segment elevation myocardial infarction (MI) comprise a growing percentage of patients with ACS and is emerging as a major public health problem worldwide, especially in Western countries, despite significant improvements and refinements in management over the past 20 years. In the United States alone, over 2.3 million people are admitted to coronary care units annually with either unstable angina or acute MI, the great majority of whom now present with non-ST-segment elevation ACS. Consequently, much attention has been directed toward optimizing the diagnosis and management of such patients, where risk stratification remains a pivotal component to sound clinical decision-making. The clinical spectrum of ischemic heart disease is diverse, ranging from silent ischemia to acute MI to congestive heart failure. Fundamental initial components of assessing a patient with ischemic heart disease—and properly gauging risk—include the clinical history, physical examination, 12-lead electrocardiography, and, increasingly, the measurement of biochemical markers.

Over the past decade, however, there has been a progressive evolution of cardiac marker testing in patients with ACS, MI, and CHF. Not only has this resulted in a dramatic shift in how we view the diagnosis of these clinical conditions, but it has also extended the role of cardiac marker testing into risk stratification and guidance of treatment decisions. By the year 2000, the development of highly sensitive and cardiac-specific troponin assays had resulted in a consensus change in the definition of acute MI, placing increased emphasis on cardiac marker testing with troponins as the new "gold standard." Furthermore, and perhaps more importantly, the role of the troponins as superior markers of subsequent cardiac risk in acute coronary syndrome patients has now become firmly established.

But, with so much attention directed at troponin as the dominant cardiac marker, it has likewise become increasingly clear that, for both diagnostic and risk stratification purposes, cardiac troponin testing alone may only quantify risk incompletely for many subsets of ACS, MI, and CHF patients. For example, the use of high-sensitivity (hs) C-reactive protein (CRP) and other novel inflammatory markers may add significantly to our ability to correctly identify patients presenting with ACS who are at high risk for future cardiovascular events. The predictive value of CRP appears to be independent of, and additive to, troponin. Individuals with evidence of heightened inflammation may benefit most from aggressive life-style modification and intensification of proven preventive therapies such as aspirin and statins. Moreover, the benefits of an early invasive strategy may also be greatest among those with elevated levels of inflammatory biomarkers.

In addition, other novel cardiac markers, including B-type natriuretic peptide (BNP) and pro-BNP, have become important determinants of risk and prognosis in both patients with CHF and ACS. Thus, as increasingly more sophisticated biochemical testing modalities become available clinically, there will be an even greater ability to delineate various risk strata for patients with ACS, MI, and CHF who present to emergency departments and coronary care units and, equally importantly, to direct, or tailor, the magnitude and extent of therapy to the level or severity of risk. Such an approach holds great promise to optimize event-free survival among all subsets of patients by balancing the benefits and risks of various treatment strategies.

Against this swiftly evolving landscape, Dr. Alan Wu has once again assembled a distinguished cadre of opinion leaders and subject matter experts to update the expanding field of cardiac markers. In *Cardiac Markers, Second Edition*, Dr. Wu expands our applications of biomarkers beyond the general analytic and clinical use of troponins in ACS patients and provides a much-needed, lucid, and more comprehensive assessment of the role of early cardiac marker use in myocardial ischemia and risk stratification. Both the diagnostic and prognostic roles of troponins, as well as novel, emerging markers (such as BNP, ischemia-modified albumin, free fatty acids, glycogen phosphorylase BB, among others) as well as hs-CRP are discussed in detail for their application to patients with ACS, MI, and CHF.

As we seek ever-improving technologies and pharmacologic approaches to enhance clinical outcomes in patients with cardiac disease, so too, do we seek concomitant, sophisticated diagnostic modalities that provide clinicians with greater precision in delineating various strata of risk that will permit the more timely, efficient, and cost-effective application of event-reducing therapies. Without question, the future of diagnostic testing will evolve increasingly toward a more refined approach to using multiple cardiac markers to better and more reliably identify which patients with ACS, MI, and CHF will benefit from an increasingly wide array of aggressive or conservative treatment strategies, and Dr. Wu has helped significantly to elucidate the critical role such cardiac markers play today in arming physicians with the tools they need to achieve these goals.

Thus, *Cardiac Markers, Second Edition*, is a valuable resource for both clinicians and laboratory medicine specialists who require a thorough understanding of this exciting and important diagnostic area, and is must reading for all healthcare professionals who want to keep abreast of this rapidly evolving field in cardiovascular medicine.

William E. Boden, MD, FACC

Professor of Medicine
University of Connecticut School of Medicine
Director, Division of Cardiology
Program Director, The Henry Low Heart Center
Hartford Hospital
Hartford, Connecticut

Preface

The incidence of cardiovascular disease has decreased in the last several years with a better understanding of the pathophysiology of acute coronary syndromes (ACS), widespread implementation of lipid lowering drugs, improved surgical treatments such as stent placements, and new therapeutic regimens such as the statins, low molecular weight heparins, and platelet glycoprotein IIb/IIIa receptor inhibitors. Nevertheless, it remains today as the leading cause of morbidity and mortality in the Western world.

Serologic markers of cardiac disease continues to grow in importance in the diagnosis and management of patients with ACS, as witnessed by the recent incorporation of cardiac troponin into new international guidelines for patients with acute coronary syndromes *(1–5)*. Of paramount importance to the field of cardiac markers is the redefinition of myocardial infarction, putting emphasis on cardiac troponin *(4)*.

Cardiac troponin are not only useful for diagnosis and risk stratification of ACS patients, but also in the optimum selection of therapies. Technical advances continue to be developed at a rapid pace, especially in the implementation of point-of-care testing (POCT) devices. Evidence for the efficacy of POCT has accumulated in the last few years.

Despite the success of cardiac troponin, there is still a need for development of early markers that can reliably rule out acute cardiac disease from the emergency room at presentation. The American College of Emergency Physicians concluded that none of the existing markers are reliably in early rule out reversible coronary ischemia *(5)*. This second edition of *Cardiac Markers* documents the importance of early rule out, and the research markers that have been studies to date in this regard. With the population getting older, and more patients are surviving episodes of acute coronary disease, the incidence of congestive heart failure is growing at a dramatic rate. The second edition details discussion of cardiac markers for diagnosis and management of patients with heart failure, an area where biochemical tests have traditionally not played any role. With the characterization of the natriuretic peptides, this promises to be an emerging field of laboratory medicine.

As with the first edition, *Cardiac Markers* is intended for clinicians and laboratorians working in the fields of cardiology, pathology and laboratory medicine, and emergency medicine. With the emergence of the natriuretic peptides, this book also has relevance to critical care, geriatrics, and family practice medicine. This book is appropriate to clinical and research scientists, and sales, marketing and product support personnel who work in the in vitro worldwide diagnostics industry.

Alan H. B. Wu

REFERENCES

1. Antman et al. ACC/AHA Diagnosis and Management of UA. Am Heart J 2000;139:461–475.
2. Hamm et al. UA classification. Circulation 2000;102:118–122.
3. Aroney et al. Management of unstable angina. Guidelines—2000. Med J Aust 2000;173 Suppl:S65–S88.

4. Myocardial Infarction Redefined—A Consensus Document of The Joint European Society of Cardiology / American College of Cardiology Committee for the Redefinition of Myocardial Infarction. J Am Coll Cardiol 2000;36:959–969.
5. Fesmire et al. American College of Emergency Physicians. Clinical Policy for suspected AMI. Ann Emerg Med 2000;35:534–539.

Contents

Contributors

ANTONIO ABBATE • *Institute of Cardiology, Catholic University of Rome, Rome, Italy*

JESSE E. ADAMS, III • *Medical Center Cardiologists, Jewish Hospital Heart and Lung Institute, Louisville, KY*

FRED S. APPLE • *Department of Laboratory Medicine and Pathology, Hennepin County Medical Center, and University of Minnesota School of Medicine, Minneapolis, MN*

CONSTANTINE N. ARONEY • *Cardiology Department, Prince Charles Hospital, Brisbane, Australia*

D. KENT ARRELL • *Department of Physiology, Queen's University, Kingston, Ontario, Canada*

HASSAN M. E. AZZAZY • *Department of Pathology, University of Maryland School of Medicine, Baltimore, MD*

LUIGI M. BIASUCCI • *Institute of Cardiology, Catholic University of Rome, Rome, Italy*

GAVIN J. BLAKE • *Cardiovascular Division, Department of Medicine, Brigham and Women's Hospital, Harvard Medical School, Boston, MA*

ANDRA L. BLOMKALNS • *Department of Emergency Medicine, University of Cincinnati College of Medicine, Cincinnati, OH*

ROBERT H. CHRISTENSON • *Department of Pathology, University of Maryland School of Medicine, Baltimore, MD*

PAUL O. COLLINSON • *Department of Chemical Pathology, St. George's Hospital, London, UK*

PETER CROSBY • *Ischemia Technologies, Arvada, CO*

OLIVER DANNE • *Department of Medicine, University Hospital Charite/Campus Virchow-Klinikum, Humboldt Univesrsity, Berlin, Germany*

CHRISTOPHER R. DEFILIPPI • *Division of Cardiology, Department of Medicine, University of Maryland, Baltimore, MD*

GARY FAGAN • *Ischemia Technologies, Arvada, CO*

VICTOR J. FERRANS • *Department of Pathology, National Heart, Lung and Blood Institute, National Institutes of Health, Bethesda, MD*

ULRICH FREI • *Department of Medicine, University Hospital Charite/Campus Virchow-Klinikum, Humboldt University, Berlin, Germany*

W. BRIAN GIBLER • *Department of Emergency Medicine, University of Cincinnati College of Medicine, Cincinnati, OH*

JAN F. C. GLATZ • *Cardiovascular Research Institute Maastrict (CARIM), Masstricht University, Maastricht, The Netherlands*

EUGENE H. HERMAN • *Division of Applied Pharmacology Research, Food and Drug Administration, Laurel, MD*

WIM T. HERMENS • *Cardiovascular Research Institute Maastrict (CARIM), Masstricht University, Maastricht, The Netherlands*

DANIEL M. HOENFER • *Department of Pathology, Dartmouth Medical School and Dartmouth-Hitchcock Medical Center, Lebanon, NH*

PAUL HOLVOET • *Center for Experimental Surgery and Anesthesiology, Katholieke Universiteit Leuven, Belgium*

ROBERT JESSE • *Division of Cardiology, Virginia Commonwealth University Health System, Medical College of Virginia Hospitals, McGuire Veteran Affairs Medical Center, Richmond, VA*

ALEX KATRUKHA • *HyTest Limited, Turku, Finland*

JOSEPH KEFFER • *Department of Pathology, University of Texas Southwestern Medical School, Dallas, TX, and Spectral Diagnostics, Toronto, Ontario, Canada*

RALF LABUGGER • *Department of Physiology, Queen's University, Kingston, Ontario, Canada*

THOMAS B. LEDUE • *Foundation for Blood Research, Scarborough, ME*

JAMES A. DE LEMOS • *Donald W. Reynolds Cardiovascular Clinical Research Center and the University of Texas Southwestern Medical Center and Parkland Hospital, Dallas, TX*

GIOVANNA LIUZZO • *Institute of Cardiology, Catholic University of Rome, Rome, Italy*

STEVEN E. LIPSHULTZ • *Department of Pediatrics and Oncology, University of Rochester Medical Center and Children's Hospital at Strong, Rochester, NY*

JOHANNES MAIR • *Division of Cardiology, Department of Internal Medicine, Innsbruck, Austria*

ALAN MAISEL • *Division of Cardiology and Department of Medicine, San Diego VA Healthcare System and University of California, San Diego, CA*

LESLIE W. MILLER • *Cardiovascular Division, University of Minnesota, Minneapolis, MN*

EMIL MISSOV • *Cardiovascular Division, University of Minnesota, Minneapolis, MN*

MARTIN MÖCKEL • *Department of Cardiology, University Hospital Charite/Campus Virchow-Klinikum, Humboldt Univesrsity, Berlin, Germany*

DAVID MORROW • *Cardiovascular Division, Department of Medicine, Brigham and Women's Hospital and Harvard Medical School, Boston, MA*

TORBJØRN OMLAND • *Research Institute for Internal Medicine, The National Hospital, University of Oslo, Oslo, Norway*

MAURO PANTEGHINI • *Laboratorio Analisi Chimico Cliniche 1, Azienda Ospedaliera Spedali Civili, Brescia, Italy*

PAUL M. RIDKER • *Department of Medicine, Brigham and Women's Hospital, Harvard Medical School, Boston, MA*

NADER RIFAI • *Department of Pathology, Children's Hospital and Harvard Medical School, Boston, MA*

ALEXANDER S. RO • *Division of Cardiology, Department of Medicine, University of Maryland, Baltimore, MD*

ROY F.M. VAN DER PUTTEN • *Cardiovascular Research Institute Maastrict (CARIM), Masstricht University, Maastricht, The Netherlands*

RAMIN TABBIBIZAR • *Division of Cardiology and Department of Medicine, San Diego VA Healthcare System and University of California, San Diego, CA*

JENNIFER E. VAN EYK • *Department of Physiology, Queen's University, Kingston, Ontario, Canada*

ALAN H. B. WU • *Department of Pathology and Laboratory Medicine, Hartford Hospital, Hartford, CT*

KIANG-TECK J. YEO • *Department of Pathology, Dartmouth Medical School and Dartmouth-Hitchcock Medical Center, Lebanon, NH*

Part I
Cardiac Markers in Clinical Practice

Early Detection of Myocardial Necrosis in the Emergency Setting and Utility of Serum Biomarkers in Chest Pain Unit Protocols

Andra L. Blomkalns and W. Brian Gibler

INTRODUCTION

Chest pain accounts for nearly 8 million Emergency Department (ED) patient visits each year and represents the second most common emergency complaint (1). Although nearly half of these patients are admitted to inpatient units for further evaluation and treatment, only one third of these individuals are ultimately found to have the diagnosis of an acute coronary syndrome (ACS) (2). The cost to society is large, approx 3–6 billion dollars per year in the United States for admissions involving "noncardiac" chest pain 3–6 (3). With continued economic constraints discouraging unnecessary or preventable inpatient admissions, EDs and physicians have developed various strategies for identifying and "ruling out" low- to moderate-risk patients with chest pain. Emergency physicians are challenged with the task of sifting through this high cost, high volume, and high morbidity complaint to distill an appropriate evaluation of a dynamic process within the first few hours of symptom onset. Cardiac markers are an integral part of these strategies. They serve not only to identify patients with acute myocardial infarction (AMI), but also to provide risk stratification to help dictate initial patient treatment as well as in-hospital disposition.

Chest pain units (CPUs) and ED observation units using various cardiac marker protocols have been successful in identifying patients with or at risk for adverse cardiac events in a timely and cost-efficient manner. Point-of-care testing (POCT) or bedside testing of cardiac markers at the patient's bedside allows for even more timely determination.

This chapter outlines the use of cardiac markers in heterogeneous patients presenting to EDs with chest discomfort. Specific cardiac marker strategies are reviewed along with their contribution to CPU protocols. We discuss the impact of POCT on marker determination and briefly discuss ED treatment modalities based on marker results.

CARDIAC MARKER PROTOCOLS IN THE ED

Initial assessment of ED patients with chest pain begins with a careful history, physical examination, and initial electrocardiogram (ECG). Each of these components contributes to an initial chest pain risk stratification impression. A fourth component, cardiac

From: *Cardiac Markers, Second Edition*
Edited by: Alan H. B. Wu @ Humana Press Inc., Totowa, NJ

markers, helps to complete the picture and more appropriately identify patients at high risk. While the initial aim of the emergency physician is to "rule out MI," an equally important goal of ACS risk assessment is aided by these markers as well.

Low- to moderate-risk patients can now typically be evaluated in the ED setting or CPU. CPUs arose from the necessity for decreasing inpatient admissions to reduce costs and minimizing inappropriate ED discharge by providing efficient care to those patients presenting with chest pain. Early CPUs and other accelerated diagnostic protocols have proved to be efficient, safe, and cost effective for the evaluation of patients in the ED with low- to moderate-risk chest pain (4–6). Their popularity continues to grow in a variety of settings. Many CPUs and ED chest pain evaluation protocols utilize a system of cardiac marker determination combined with serial ECG determination, perfusion imaging, and/or provocative testing. These combination marker strategies include several variations over several different time courses ranging from 3 to 24 h. Ideally a CPU will evaluate patients for evolving myocardial necrosis and ongoing myocardial ischemia not detected initially on presentation to the hospital.

Cardiac markers have undergone an amazing transformation from aspartate aminotransferase (AST) and lactate dehydrogenase (LDH) to the three cardiac marker families available at present for routine use in ED for the evaluation of the chest discomfort: myoglobin, creatine kinase (CK) and the MB isoenzyme of CK (CK-MB), and the troponins I and T (cTnI and cTnT). Each of these has well known kinetics of release from dying myocardial cells and should be carefully applied to each patient as directed by timing of symptoms and presentation (7). Myoglobin has been touted as an early marker with a high negative predictive value but low specificity. CK and CK-MB represent the "gold standard" for the diagnosis of MI as defined by the World Health Organization criteria. The troponins are cardiac-specific proteins with high degrees of both sensitivity and specificity for myocardial necrosis. These serum markers of necrosis have been well studied in high-risk groups with a high prevalence of AMI. Promising research has also proven benefit in lower-risk patients in the CPU setting (8).

Inflammatory markers such as C-reactive protein (CRP) and markers of platelet activation such as P-selectin are currently being studied but have not yet been accepted for widespread use, particularly in the setting of CPUs.

CK-MB Protocols

Early myocardial necrosis "rule-out" protocols challenged the traditional notion of a 24-h period required to detect AMI. Lee and colleagues' multicenter trial validated a 12-h algorithm using CK and CK-MB in patients identified as "low risk" through assessment of clinical characteristics in the ED. "Low risk" was defined as the probability of AMI <7%. Among patients with CK-MB levels <5% of the total CK without recurrent chest pain after 12 h, there was a 0.5% missed AMI rate while 94% of AMI patients were identified (9). Farkouh et al. demonstrated the utility of a CPU protocol and CK-MB measurements for patients identified as intermediate risk for adverse cardiac events. In this study, patients underwent 6 h of observation followed by provocative testing. This protocol identified all patients with short- and long-term cardiac events while using fewer resources over a 6-mo time period (10).

Symptom onset to patient presentation is a crucial factor in the use of cardiac marker protocols. Marker release kinetics vary with time and as time to ED presentation may be as short as 90 min or as long as several days, no single marker determination is suitable for adequately "ruling out" ACS *(4,11,12)*. In one of the first studies with CPU protocols, Gibler et al. used a 9-h protocol with serial CK-MB at 0, 3, 6, and 9 h along with continuous ECG monitoring, echocardiography, and exercise testing. They found that serial markers alone had a sensitivity and specificity for AMI of 100% and 98%, respectively *(4)*. The American Heart Association currently recommends serial cardiac marker determinations to increase sensitivity for detecting necrosis, rather than a single determination on ED presentation.

Several other studies have examined the value of cardiac markers in the risk stratification of heterogeneous patients with chest pain presenting to the ED. In a multicenter study of more than 5000 patients in 53 EDs, the relative risk of ischemic complications and death for ED patients with positive CK-MB at 0 or 2 h was 16.1 and 25.4, respectively *(13)*. Serial CK-MB results have also proved to be sensitive in MI detection when collected at 0 and 3 h after ED presentation. Young et al. found a 93% and 95% sensitivity and specificity when combining 0, 3, and net change in CK-MB level. As expected, this sensitivity improved with increased time from symptom onset *(14)*. Serial marker measurements and comparison of marker elevation over 3–6 h also improved sensitivity for MI *(15–17)*. Even minor elevations of CK-MB as small as twice the upper limit of normal are associated with an increased 6-mo mortality when compared to those with normal levels *(18)*.

Serial CK/CK-MB protocols have largely become the diagnostic standard for AMI in the CPU setting. Almost all of the studied protocols use a specific threshold, levels above which are diagnostic for AMI or ACS. Fesmire et al. studied a promising novel approach of change in CK-MB levels within the normal range over the course of ED evaluation. In his population of 710 CPU patients, a CK-MB increase or delta of 1.6 ng/mL over 2 h was more sensitive for AMI than a second CK-MB drawn 2 h after patient arrival (93.8% vs 75.2%) *(17)*. Validation of these novel protocols will add to the utility of markers in the CPU setting.

CK-MB (CK-MB$_1$ and CK-MB$_2$) isoforms are additional markers with promising results in the CPU setting. A small study of 100 patients with AMI prevalence of 41% found that CK-MB isoform were equal or more sensitive than CK-MB and myoglobin when measured >2 h after symptom onset *(19)*. In the Diagnostic Marker Cooperative Study, 955 ED chest pain patients were evaluated using a 24-h marker protocol utilizing CK-MB isoform, CK-MB, myoglobin, cTnI, and cTnT. CK-MB isoforms were found to be most sensitive and specific (91% and 89%) for AMI within 6 h of symptom onset. In addition, CK-MB isoforms were elevated in 29.5% of unstable angina patients as compared to myoglobin (23.7%), cTnI (19.7%), and cTnT (14.8%). This study concluded that protocols utilizing CK-MB isoforms could reliably triage chest pain patients, thereby improving treatment and reducing costs *(20)*. Puleo et al. demonstrated CK-MB isoform sensitivity for AMI of 95.7% 6 h after symptom onset in a population whose prevalence of AMI was 18% as compared to 48% for the conventional CK-MB assay. The specificity of this marker protocol was 93.9% and 96.2% among hospitalized and discharged patients, respectively *(21)*.

Myoglobin Protocols

Myoglobin is a small cytosolic protein found in striated muscle. The diagnostic strength of myoglobin lies in its early release kinetics and sensitivity, while its primary weakness is a lack of specificity. Davis et al. showed that serial myoglobin levels were 93% sensitive and 79% specific in detecting MI in patients within 2 h of arrival *(22)*. Similarly, Tucker et al. showed a myoglobin sensitivity of 89% in patients with nondiagnostic ECGs within 2 h of ED presentation *(7)*. Myoglobin appears to achieve maximal diagnostic accuracy within 5 h of symptom onset *(23)*.

Therefore, it is reasonable and recommended that myoglobin should be combined with other more specific cardiac markers when used in CPU protocols. Brogan et al. found that a combination of carbonic anhydrase III and serum myoglobin was more sensitive and equally specific as CK-MB in patients presenting early, within 3 h of symptom onset *(24)*. Contrastingly, Kontos et al. reported less encouraging results from a study of 2093 patients combining CK, CK-MB, and myoglobin obtained at 0, 3, 6, and 8 h. A CK-MB level >8.0 ng/mL at 3 h was 93% sensitive and 98% specific for AMI, adding myoglobin decreased the sensitivity to 86% with no significant increase in sensitivity *(25)*.

Much like the other cardiac markers, myoglobin levels also increase in utility when used in a serial fashion. In a study of 133 consecutive admitted chest pain patients, myoglobin levels were obtained at 2, 3, 4, and 6 h after symptom onset. This regimen was found to be 86% sensitive for AMI at 6 h. The negative predictive value in patients with negative myoglobin levels during 6 h of evaluation and without doubling over any 2-h period was 97% *(26)*.

Data from protocols using myoglobin measurements in patients with lower risk for AMI are sometimes conflicting. In a study of 3075 low-risk CPU patients with AMI prevalence of 1.4%, a 4-h serial myoglobin protocol was reported as 100% sensitive for AMI *(27)*. Conversely, in a study of 368 patients whose MI prevalence was 11%, the sensitivity and specificity of myoglobin at 0 and 2–3 h were only 61% and 68%. Myoglobin change or increase did not improve diagnostic performance either *(16)*.

Myoglobin in the ED setting is probably best used in a serial fashion along with another cardiac marker of necrosis. It is most valuable when used in patients presenting very early in the time course of symptoms and less so for remote events.

Troponins Protocols

cTnI and cTnT are the newest commonly available highly specific cardiac markers that have been proven extremely valuable and sensitive in the diagnosis of myocardial necrosis *(28,29)*. In addition to diagnosis of myocardial necrosis in acute ischemic syndromes, the troponins are more valuable in risk stratification of both low- and high-risk patient populations. Troponin release begins about the same time as CK-MB, but persists for days to weeks after AMI.

The main issues surrounding the cardiac troponins include (1) cutoff values for cTnI and (2) appropriately defining the time of chest pain onset in the context of the ED presentation. Although exhaustive time and study have been performed to determine the more superior troponin, most large studies and analyses have determined that cTnI and cTnT can both identify patients at risk for adverse cardiac events *(30,31)*.

Cardiac TnT is detected at slightly lower serum levels than cTnI and has proved valuable in the emergency setting for early identification of myocardial necrosis. Recently, the Global Use of Strategies to Open Occluded Coronary Arteries in Acute Coronary Syndromes (GUSTO)-II investigators compared cTnI and cTnT in short-term risk stratification of ACS patients. This model compared troponins collected within 3.5 h of ischemic symptoms. Ohman and colleagues found that cTnT showed a greater association with 30-d mortality ($\chi^2 = 18.0$, $p < 0.0001$) than cTnI ($\chi^2 = 12.5$, $p = 0.0002$) *(32)*. These authors concluded that cTnT is a strong, independent predictor of short-term outcome in ACS patients, and serial levels were useful in determining the risk of adverse cardiac events *(33)*.

As with all new cardiac markers, initial studies on troponin risk stratification were initially performed on patients with known ACS. Studies using cTnI in ACS patients showed a statistically significant increase in mortality among those patients with levels >0.4 ng/ mL *(34)*. Stubbs and colleagues showed that patients with elevated baseline cTnT levels have up to four times higher mortality than ACS patients with normal values *(35,36)*.

Although the increased risk of troponin-positive patients is now well established, the degree of risk varies greatly between studies and patient populations. Meta-analyses have helped consolidate conclusions and clinically useful parameters when using troponins for the evaluation of patients. One such analysis in high-risk patients performed by Wu demonstrated a cumulative odds ratio of a positive cTnT for the development of AMI or death from hospital discharge to 34 mo was 4.3 (2.8–6.8 95% CI) *(37)*. The cumulative odds ratio of a positive cTnT for predicting need for cardiac revascularization within the same period was 4.4 (3.0–6.5 95% CI). Another analysis involving more than 18,000 patients in 21 ACS studies found that troponin-positive patients had an odds ratio of 3.44 for death or MI at 30 d. Troponin-positive patients with no ST-segment elevation and patients with unstable angina carried odds ratios of 4.93 and 9.39 for adverse cardiac outcomes *(31)*.

Benamer et al. compared the prognostic value of cTnI combined with CRP in patients with unstable angina. They found that whereas 23% of patients with elevated cTnI had major in-hospital cardiac events; there was no such prognostic significance associated with CRP *(38)*.

Troponin applications in low- to moderate-risk patients presenting to EDs have shown similar encouraging results. Tucker et al. used a comprehensive marker strategy including myoglobin, CK-MB, cTnI, and cTnT in ED patients over 24 h after arrival. As expected within the first 2 h of presentation, CK-MB and myoglobin maintained better sensitivity. The troponins were useful only when measured 6 h or more after arrival, exhibiting sensitivities and specificities of 82% and 97% for cTnI and 89% and 84% for cTnT *(7)*. Troponin use seems to be more beneficial in later or delayed patient presentations. In a study of 425 patients using serial cTnI and CK-MB over 16 h, Brogan et al. showed no increase in sensitivity or specificity between troponin and CK-MB in patients with symptoms <24 h. However, in patients presenting with >24 h of symptoms, troponin I had a sensitivity of 100% compared to CK-MB (56.5%) *(39)*.

Sayre et al. showed that patients with a cTnT level of 0.2 ng/mL or greater were 3.5 times more likely to have a cardiac complication within 60 d of ED presentation *(40)*. In a CPU population, Newby et al. determined that cTnT-positive patients had angiographically significant lesions (89% vs 49%) and positive stress testing (46% vs 14%) more frequently than cTnT-negative patients. Long-term mortality was also higher in cTnT-positive patients (27% vs 7%) *(41)*. Johnson et al. studied a heterogeneous patient population admitted from an urban teaching hospital and found that cTnT was elevated in 31% of patients without MI who had major short-term complications as compared to CK-MB activity and mass *(29)*.

Other authors have found that although patients with troponin positivity are at higher risk for adverse cardiac events, the test in isolation lacks sensitivity. Kontos et al. found that although cTnI-positive patients were more likely to have significant complications (43% vs 12%), the sensitivity for these end points was low (14%) *(42)*. Similarly, Polanczyk et al. demonstrated that peak cTnI >0.4 ng/mL was associated with only a 47% sensitivity and 80% specificity for a major cardiac event within 72 h of presentation *(43)*.

POINT-OF-CARE TESTING

As cardiac markers gain acceptance for diagnosis and risk stratification, the need to obtain these results in a timely and reliable manner becomes paramount. POCT at the patient's bedside could increase cardiac marker utility and promote more efficient use of pharmacologic and interventional therapies, particularly in institutions where central laboratory determination requires significant time.

Several generations of bedside testing for several cardiac markers have entered the clinical arena for evaluation. An earlier study evaluating a rapid assay for CK-MB isoforms concluded that the rapid assay had a sensitivity for detecting MI within 6 h of symptom onset of 95.7% as compared to only 48% in the conventional CK-MB analysis *(21)*. Bedside tests of cTnT and cTnI proved to be strong independent predictors of death or MI at 30 d in an ED population chest-pain cohort. Event rates for patients with negative tests were 1.1% for cTnT and 0.3% for cTnI *(44)*. Panteghini and colleagues determined that a bedside whole blood assay for CK-MB mass (CARDIAC STATus) was helpful in early detection of MI and hence implementation of various revascularization strategies *(45)*. However, in studying alternative uses of thrombolytic agents, the Serial Markers, Acute Myocardial Infarction, and Rapid Treatment Trial (SMARTT) trial found no benefit of bedside myoglobin and CK-MB results *(46)*.

A Thrombolysis in Myocardial Infarction (TIMI) 11A substudy found that 33.6% of patients with a positive bedside cTnT assay had an end point of death, nonfatal MI, or recurrent ischemia within 14 d as opposed to only 22.5% in patients with a negative cTnT ($p = 0.01$). Hospital stays were longer in the cTnT-positive group as well, 5 vs 3 d *(47)*. In a GUSTO-III substudy involving more than 12,000 patients receiving thrombolysis for acute ST-segment elevation MI, elevated bedside whole blood cTnT patients had two- to threefold higher 30-d mortality rates *(48)*.

Most recently, Newby et al. used a bedside multimarker strategy for risk stratification of CPU patients. Bedside myoglobin, CK-MB, and cTnI were measured serially over 24 h in 1005 patients and end points of 30-d death or infarction were compared with the local laboratory single marker method. Patients with positive and negative baseline triple multimarker status had an event rate of 18.8% and 3.0%, respectively, compared to 13.6% and 5.5% for the local laboratory. This study concluded that a bedside multimarker strategy could more efficiently identify patients at risk for adverse cardiac events.

POCT testing may improve test turnaround time and hence time to diagnosis and treatment, but it is also hampered by regulatory, logistical, and interpretive issues. Some institutions are unable or unwilling to invest the resources and commitment necessary to perform bedside testing. Further study in this area is therefore warranted that includes analyses for cost-effectiveness.

CARDIAC MARKERS
AND EMERGENCY DEPARTMENT TREATMENT

Recent investigation with cardiac markers suggests that not only are markers important for diagnosis and risk stratification, but they also identify patients with ACS that benefit from antiplatelet and antithrombotic pharmacologic management.

The Fragmin in Unstable Coronary Artery Disease (FRISC) study group found that patients with cTnT elevation had improved outcomes with prolonged dalteparin treatment. Dalteparin significantly reduced short-term incidence of death or MI in patients with a positive cTnT from 6.0% to 2.5% ($p < 0.05$) as compared to an insignificant decrease from 2.4% to 0% in patients with normal levels of cTnT ($p = 0.12$). The incidence of long-term death and MI in cTnT-positive patients at 40 d was 14.2% and 7.4% in placebo and dalteparin treatment groups, respectively. There was no difference in long-term outcome in the troponin-negative patients *(49)*.

Platelet glycoprotein IIb/IIIa (GP IIb/IIIa) receptor antagonists are used in patients with ACS and the subgroup of patients undergoing interventional procedures. Several landmark studies such as the Chimeric c7E3 AntiPlatelet Therapy in Unstable Angina Refractory to Standard Treatment Trial (CAPTURE), Platelet Glycoprotein IIb/IIIa in Unstable Angina Receptor Suppression Using Integrilin Therapy (PURSUIT), and Platelet Receptor Inhibition in Ischemic Syndrome Management (PRISM) collaboratives have demonstrated significant benefit of GP IIb/IIIa receptor antagonists in the setting of ACS by reducing death, MI, and refractory ischemia *(50–52)*. The cardiac troponins help identify ACS patients who may benefit from these agents. The PRISM study investigators showed that tirofiban lowered the risk of death (adjusted hazard ratio 0.25) and MI (0.37) at 30 d in cTnI-positive ACS patients undergoing medical management or coronary revascularization. No significant treatment effect was evident for cTnI-negative patients *(53)*. The CAPTURE investigators correlated angiographic findings such as visible thrombus, lesion severity, and TIMI flow with cTnT to determine which patients might benefit from abciximab therapy. In this study of 853 patients, cTnT was a more powerful predictor of cardiac risk and efficacy of abciximab treatment than either lesion characteristics or thrombus formation alone. The authors suggested that cTnT was a sensitive marker for identifying patients with unstable angina who benefit from antiplatelet therapy *(54)*. In another analysis of patients with refractory unstable angina, the relative risk of death or nonfatal MI in patients treated with abciximab and elevated cTnT levels was 0.32 (95% CI 0.14–0.62) when compared to cTnT-negative patients *(55)*.

CONCLUSIONS

The ideal cardiac marker evaluation protocol varies between institutions, laboratories, patient populations, and resource availability. Specific marker regimens should be tailored to meet the objectives of diagnosing MI and providing risk stratification. Cardiac markers have proved extremely valuable for diagnosis, risk stratification, and treatment of patients in the emergency setting. Further research will likely further clarify how myocardial necrosis markers can be combined with testing for rest ischemia and exercise-induced ischemia to identify and institute consistently and efficiently treatment for ED patients with ACS.

ABBREVIATIONS

ACS, Acute coronary syndrome(s); AMI, acute myocardial infarction; AST, aspartate aminotransferase; CAPTURE, Chimeric c7E3 AntiPlatelet Therapy in Unstable Angina Refractory to Standard Treatment Trial; CI, confidence interval; CK, creatine kinase; CPUs, chest pain units; CRP, C-reactive protein; cTnT and cTnI, cardiac troponins T and I; ECG, electrocardiogram; ED, emergency department; FRISC, Fragmin in Unstable Coronary Artery Disease; GP IIb/IIIa, glycoprotein IIb/IIIa; GUSTO, Global Use of Strategies to Open Occluded Coronary Arteries in Acute Coronary Syndromes; LDH, lactate dehydrogenase; POCT, point-of-care testing; PRISM, Platelet Receptor Inhibition in Ischemic Syndrome Management; PURSUIT, Platelet Glycoprotein IIb/IIIa in Unstable Angina: Receptor Suppression Using Integrilin Therapy; SMARTT, Serial Markers, Acute Myocardial Infarction, and Rapid Treatment Trial; TIMI, Thrombolysis in Myocardial Infarction.

REFERENCES

1. Nourjah P. National hospital ambulatory medical care survey: 1997 emergency department summary. Advance data from vital and health statistics. Hyattsville, MD: National Center for Health Statistics; 2001 Report No. 304.
2. Graff LG, Dallara J, Ross MA, et al. Impact on the care of the emergency department chest pain patient from the Chest Pain Evaluation Registry (CHEPER) Study. Am J Cardiol 1997; 80:563–568.
3. Weingarten SR, Ermann B, Riedinger MS, Shah PK, Ellrodt AG. Selecting the best triage rule for patients hospitalized with chest pain. Am J Med 1989;87:494–500.
4. Gibler WB, Runyon JP, Levy RC, et al. A rapid diagnostic and treatment center for patients with chest pain in the emergency department. Ann Emerg Med 1995;25:1–8.
5. Tatum JL, Jesse RL, Kontos MC, et al. Comprehensive strategy for the evaluation and triage of the chest pain patient. Ann Emerg Med 1997;29:116–125.
6. Roberts RR, Zalenski RJ, Mensah EK, et al. Costs of an emergency department-based accelerated diagnostic protocol vs hospitalization in patients with chest pain: a randomized controlled trial. JAMA 1997;278:1670–1676.
7. Tucker JF, Collins RA, Anderson AJ, Hauser J, Kalas J, Apple FS. Early diagnostic efficiency of cardiac troponin I and troponin T for acute myocardial infarction. Acad Emerg Med 1997;4:13–21.
8. O'Neil BJ, Ross MA. Cardiac markers protocols in a chest pain observation unit. Emerg Med Clin North Am 2001;19:67–86.
9. Lee TH, Juarez G, Cook EF, et al. Ruling out acute myocardial infarction: a prospective multicenter validation of a 12-hour strategy for patients at low risk. N Engl J Med 1991;324: 1239–1246.
10. Farkouh ME, Smars PA, Reeder GS, et al. A clinical trial of a chest-pain observation unit for patients with unstable angina chest pain evaluation in the Emergency Room (CHEER) Investigators. N Engl J Med 1998;339:1882–1888.
11. Newby LK, Rutsch WR, Califf RM, et al. Time from symptom onset to treatment and outcomes after thrombolytic therapy GUSTO-1 Investigators. J Am Coll Cardiol 1996;27:1646–1655.
12. Lambrew CT, Bowlby LJ, Rogers WJ, Chandra NC, Weaver WD. Factors influencing the time to thrombolysis in acute myocardial infarction. Time to thrombolysis substudy of the National Registry of Myocardial Infarction-1. Arch Intern Med 997;157:2577–2582.
13. Hoekstra JW, Hedges JR, Gibler WB, Rubison RM, Christensen RA. Emergency department CK-MB: a predictor of ischemic complications. National Cooperative CK-MB Project Group. Acad Emerg Med 1994;1:17–27.

14. Young GP, Gibler WB, Hedges JR, et al. Serial creatine kinase-MB results are a sensitive indicator of acute myocardial infarction in chest pain patients with nondiagnostic electrocardiograms: the Second Emergency Medicine Cardiac Research Group Study. Acad Emerg Med 1997;4:869–877.
15. Gibler WB, Young GP, Hedges JR, et al. Acute myocardial infarction in chest pain patients with nondiagnostic ECGs: serial CK-MB sampling in the emergency department. The Emergency Medicine Cardiac Research Group. Ann Emerg Med 1992;21:504–512.
16. Polanczyk CA, Lee TH, Cook EF, Walls R, Wybenga D, Johnson PA. Value of additional two-hour myoglobin for the diagnosis of myocardial infarction in the emergency department. Am J Cardiol 1999;83:525–529.
17. Fesmire FM, Percy RF, Bardoner JB, Wharton DR, Calhoun FB. Serial creatine kinase (CK) MB testing during the emergency department evaluation of chest pain: utility of a 2-hour deltaCK-MB of +1.6 ng/mL. Am Heart J 1998;136:237–244.
18. Alexander JH, Sparapani RA, Mahaffey KW, et al. Association between minor elevations of creatine kinase-MB level and mortality in patients with acute coronary syndromes without ST-segment elevation. PURSUIT Steering Committee Platelet Glycoprotein IIb/IIIa in Unstable Angina: Receptor Suppression Using Integrilin Therapy. JAMA 2000;283:347–353.
19. Laurino JP, Bender EW, Kessimian N, Chang J, Pelletier T, Usategui M. Comparative sensitivities and specificities of the mass measurements of CK-MB2, CK-MB, and myoglobin for diagnosing acute myocardial infarction. Clin Chem 1996;42:1454–1459.
20. Zimmerman J, Fromm R, Meyer D, et al. Diagnostic marker cooperative study for the diagnosis of myocardial infarction. Circulation 1999;99:1671–1677.
21. Puleo PR, Meyer D, Wathen C, et al. Use of a rapid assay of subforms of creatine kinase-MB to diagnose or rule out acute myocardial infarction. N Engl J Med 1994;331:561–566.
22. Davis CP, Barrett K, Torre P, Wacasey K. Serial myoglobin levels for patients with possible myocardial infarction. Acad Emerg Med 1996;3:590–597.
23. de Winter RJ, Lijmer JG, Koster RW, Hoek FJ, Sanders GT. Diagnostic accuracy of myoglobin concentration for the early diagnosis of acute myocardial infarction. Ann Emerg Med 2000;35:113–120.
24. Brogan GX Jr, Vuori J, Friedman S, et al. Improved specificity of myoglobin plus carbonic anhydrase assay versus that of creatine kinase-MB for early diagnosis of acute myocardial infarction. Ann Emerg Med 1996;27:22–28.
25. Kontos MC, Anderson FP, Schmidt KA, Ornato JP, Tatum JL, Jesse RL. Early diagnosis of acute myocardial infarction in patients without ST-segment elevation. Am J Cardiol 1999;83:155–158.
26. Tucker JF, Collins RA, Anderson AJ, et al. Value of serial myoglobin levels in the early diagnosis of patients admitted for acute myocardial infarction. Ann Emerg Med 1994;24:704–708.
27. Mikhail MG, Smith FA, Gray M, Britton C, Frederiksen SM. Cost-effectiveness of mandatory stress testing in chest pain center patients. Ann Emerg Med 1997;29:88–98.
28. Falahati A, Sharkey SW, Christensen D, et al. Implementation of serum cardiac troponin I as marker for detection of acute myocardial infarction. Am Heart J 1999;137:332–337.
29. Johnson PA, Goldman L, Sacks DB, et al. Cardiac troponin T as a marker for myocardial ischemia in patients seen at the emergency department for acute chest pain. Am Heart J 1999;137:1137–1144.
30. Ottani F, Galvani M, Ferrini D, et al. Direct comparison of early elevations of cardiac troponin T and I in patients with clinical unstable angina. Am Heart J 1999;137:284–291.
31. Ottani F, Galvani M, Nicolini FA, Ferrini D, Pozzati A, Di Pasquale G, Jaffe AS. Elevated cardiac troponin levels predict the risk of adverse outcome in patients with acute coronary syndromes. Am Heart J 2000;140:917–927.
32. Christenson RH, Duh SH, Newby LK, et al. Cardiac troponin T and cardiac troponin I: relative values in short-term risk stratification of patients with acute coronary syndromes. GUSTO-IIa Investigators. Clin Chem 1998;44:494–501.

33. Newby LK, Christenson RH, Ohman EM, et al. Value of serial troponin T measures for early and late risk stratification in patients with acute coronary syndromes. The GUSTO-IIa Investigators. Circulation 1998;98:1853–1859.
34. Antman EM, Tanasijevic MJ, Thompson B, et al. Cardiac-specific troponin I levels to predict the risk of mortality in patients with acute coronary syndromes. N Engl J Med 1996; 335:1342–1349.
35. Stubbs P, Collinson P , Moseley D, Greenwood T, Noble M. Prognostic significance of admission troponin T concentrations in patients with myocardial infarction. Circulation 1996; 94:1291–1297.
36. Ohman EM, Armstrong PW, Christenson RH, et al. Cardiac troponin T levels for risk stratification in acute myocardial ischemia. GUSTO IIA Investigators. N Engl J Med 1996;335: 1333–1341.
37. Wu AHB, Lane PL. Metaanalysis in clinical chemistry: validation of cardiac troponin T as a marker for ischemic heart diseases. Clin Chem 1995;41:1228–1233.
38. Benamer H, Steg PG, Benessiano J, et al. Comparison of the prognostic value of C-reactive protein and troponin I in patients with unstable angina pectoris. Am J Cardiol 1998;82: 845–850.
39. Brogan GX Jr, Hollander JE, McCuskey CF, et al. Evaluation of a new assay for cardiac troponin I vs creatine kinase-MB for the diagnosis of acute myocardial infarction. Biochemical Markers for Acute Myocardial Ischemia (BAMI) Study Group. Acad Emerg Med 1997; 4:6–12.
40. Sayre MR, Kaufmann KH, Chen IW, et al. Measurement of cardiac troponin T is an effective method for predicting complications among emergency department patients with chest pain. Ann Emerg Med 1998;31:539–549.
41. Newby LK, Kaplan AL, Granger BB, Sedor F, Califf RM, Ohman EM. Comparison of cardiac troponin T versus creatine kinase-MB for risk stratification in a chest pain evaluation unit. Am J Cardiol 2000;85:801–805.
42. Kontos MC, Anderson FP, Alimard R, Ornato JP, Tatum JL, Jesse RL. Ability of troponin I to predict cardiac events in patients admitted from the emergency department. J Am Coll Cardiol 2000;36:1818–1823.
43. Polanczyk CA, Lee TH, Cook EF, et al. Cardiac troponin I as a predictor of major cardiac events in emergency department patients with acute chest pain. J Am Coll Cardiol 1998;32: 8–14.
44. Hamm CW, Goldmann BU, Heeschen C, Kreymann G, Berger J, Meinertz T. Emergency room triage of patients with acute chest pain by means of rapid testing for cardiac troponin T or troponin I. N Engl J Med 1997;337:1648–1653.
45. Panteghini M, Cuccia C, Pagani F, Turla C. Comparison of the diagnostic performance of two rapid bedside biochemical assays in the early detection of acute myocardial infarction. Clin Cardiol 1998;21:394–398.
46. Gibler WB, Hoekstra JW, Weaver WD, et al. A randomized trial of the effects of early cardiac serum marker availability on reperfusion therapy in patients with acute myocardial infarction: the Serial Markers, Acute Myocardial Infarction and Rapid Treatment Trial (SMARTT). J Am Coll Cardiol 2000;36:1500–1506.
47. Antman EM, Sacks DB, Rifai N, McCabe CH, Cannon CP, Braunwald E. Time to positivity of a rapid bedside assay for cardiac-specific troponin T predicts prognosis in acute coronary syndromes: a Thrombolysis in Myocardial Infarction (TIMI) 11A Substudy. J Am Coll Cardiol 1998;31:326–330.
48. Ohman EM, Armstrong PW, White HD, et al. Risk stratification with a point-of-care cardiac troponin T test in acute myocardial infarction. GUSTOIII Investigators. Global Use of Strategies to Open Occluded Coronary Arteries. Am J Cardiol 1999;84:1281–1286.

49. Lindahl B, Venge P, Wallentin L. Troponin T identifies patients with unstable coronary artery disease who benefit from long-term antithrombotic protection. Fragmin in Unstable Coronary Artery Disease (FRISC) Study Group. J Am Coll Cardiol 1997;29:43–48.
50. Randomised placebo-controlled trial of abciximab before and during coronary intervention in refractory unstable angina: the CAPTURE Study. Lancet 1997;349:1429–1435.
51. Inhibition of platelet Glycoprotein IIb/IIIa with eptifibatide in patients with acute coronary syndromes. The PURSUIT Trial Investigators. Platelet Glycoprotein IIb/IIIa in Unstable Angina: receptor Suppression Using Integrilin Therapy. N Engl J Med 1998;339:436–443.
52. Comparison of Aspirin Plus Tirofiban With Aspirin Plus Heparin for Unstable Angina Platelet Receptor Inhibition in Ischemic Syndrome Management (PRISM) Study Investigators. N Engl J Med 5-21-1998;338(21):1498–1505.
53. Heeschen C, Hamm CW, Goldmann B, Deu A, Langenbrink L, White HD. Troponin concentrations for stratification of patients with acute coronary syndromes in relation to therapeutic efficacy of tirofiban. PRISM Study Investigators Platelet Receptor Inhibition in Ischemic Syndrome Management. Lancet 1999;354:1757–1562.
54. Heeschen C, van Den Brand MJ, Hamm CW, Simoons ML. Angiographic findings in patients with refractory unstable angina according to troponin T status. Circulation 1999;100:1509–1514.
55. Hamm CW, Heeschen C, Goldmann B, et al. Benefit of abciximab in patients with refractory unstable angina in relation to serum troponin T levels. C7E3 Fab Antiplatelet Therapy in Unstable Refractory Angina (CAPTURE) Study Investigators. N Engl J Med 1999;340:1623-1629.

2

Management of Acute Coronary Syndromes

Constantine N. Aroney and James A. de Lemos

CLINICAL SYNDROME AND PATHOPHYSIOLOGY

The term "acute coronary syndrome" (ACS) describes the spontaneous presentation of acute ischemic heart disease, and encompasses the diagnoses of unstable angina, non-ST elevation myocardial infarction (MI) (NSTEMI), and ST elevation MI (STEMI). Because Q waves can be detected only retrospectively, previous classification schemes based the presence or absence of Q waves are less useful than schemes that classify patients based on the presence or absence of ST-segment elevation.

Acute coronary syndromes represent a spectrum of disease, with a common pathophysiologic base (Fig. 1). The extracellular lipid core in the plaque is encapsulated by a collagen cap, which can be infiltrated by macrophages. Intracoronary ultrasound has demonstrated that atheromatous plaques that are vulnerable to plaque rupture and the development of acute coronary syndromes are more likely to be eccentric, with a shallow lipid-rich echolucent zone (1). Macrophages, T lymphocytes, and mast cells are found in high concentrations within the shoulder region of the vulnerable plaque. Rupture or erosion of the fibrous cap of the plaque exposes circulating platelets and coagulation factors to subendothelial collagen and von Willebrand factor, resulting in platelet aggregation and varying degrees of coronary thrombosis, coronary vasospasm, and distal platelet microembolization. Whether the patient develops non-ST or ST elevation MI is determined by the degree and duration of reduction in coronary flow, the quality of collateral flow to the jeopardized myocardium, and the nature of the thrombus forming at the site of plaque rupture. Patients with NSTEMI usually develop white (platelet) thrombi, whereas 80% of STEMIs are associated with red (fibrin with entrapped erythrocytes) thrombus (2). These differences in pathophysiology and presentation are also reflected by the effectiveness of platelet glycoprotein IIb/IIIa (GP IIb/IIIa) inhibitors and antithrombotic therapy (Table 1) in NSTEMI compared with the utility of fibrinolytic therapy for STEMI.

The platelet is now recognized as the first component of coronary thrombosis. With endothelial injury, platelets adhere via both integrin and non-integrin receptors to exposed connective tissue. Platelets then become activated, extruding filopodia (spiculation) and causing a release of the contents of storage granules, which include ADP, serotonin, and thromboxane A_2. These agonists lead to platelet aggregation (white thrombus) at the

From: *Cardiac Markers, Second Edition*
Edited by: Alan H. B. Wu @ Humana Press Inc., Totowa, NJ

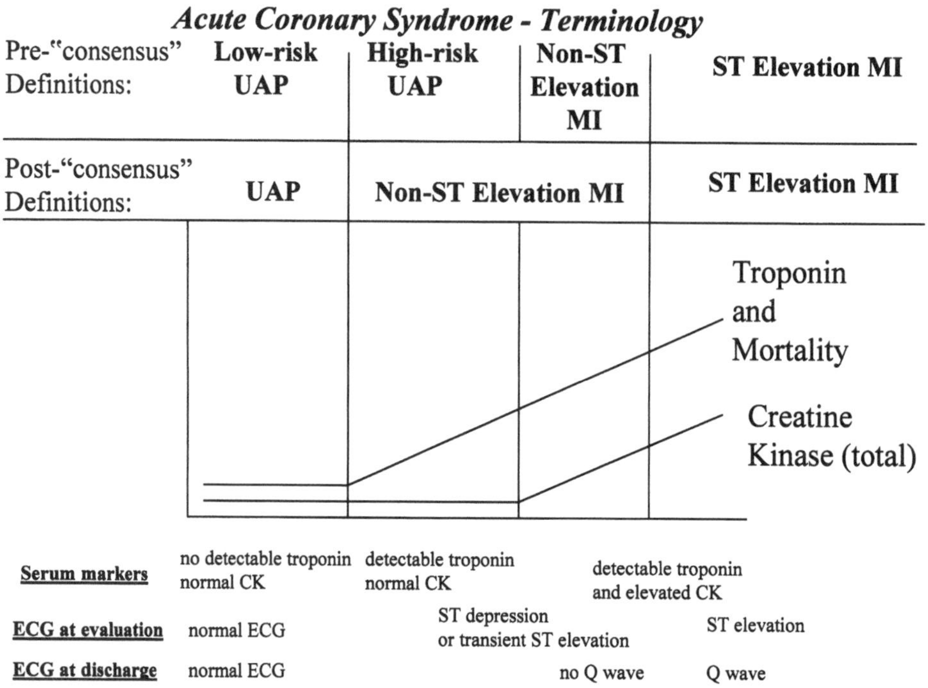

Acute Coronary Syndrome - Terminology

Pre-"consensus" Definitions:	Low-risk UAP	High-risk UAP	Non-ST Elevation MI	ST Elevation MI
Post-"consensus" Definitions:	UAP	Non-ST Elevation MI		ST Elevation MI

Troponin and Mortality

Creatine Kinase (total)

Serum markers	no detectable troponin normal CK	detectable troponin normal CK	detectable troponin and elevated CK
ECG at evaluation	normal ECG	ST depression or transient ST elevation	ST elevation
ECG at discharge	normal ECG	no Q wave	Q wave

Fig. 1. New terminology, diagnosis, and risk stratification of the ACS. (Adapted from Aroney et al., Management of Unstable Angina Guidelines—2000. Med J Aust; 173: S65-88, with consideration of the new consensus guidelines *[5]*.)

site of the injury, whereby platelets are bound together by crosslinking of GP IIb/IIIa receptors with fibrinogen. Thrombin may be generated, leading to a deposition of fibrin and the development of red thrombus, which may lead to total vessel occlusion.

With the advent of the cardiac troponins as preferred and specific markers of myocardial injury, a need arose to identify a new group of patients with an adverse prognosis who have a cardiac troponin elevation without an elevation of total creatine kinase (CK) (Fig. 1). The differentiation between the diagnosis of unstable angina and NSTEMI has become clouded, with a subgroup of patients with cardiac troponin elevation in the absence of CK or MB isoenzyme of CK (CK-MB) elevation being labeled as having "minor myocardial damage" *(3)*. These patients with minor myocardial damage have an adverse cardiac prognosis *(4)* and form a newly identified subgroup of patients with an acute coronary syndrome. The differentiation between minor myocardial damage and MI is necessarily an empiric one, and a new consensus document *(5)* recommends an MI diagnostic cutoff at the 99th percentile of the normal range for cardiac troponin. However, further changes to the definition are likely *(6)*. The diagnoses of unstable angina, minor myocardial damage, and NSTEMI may, however, be considered a continuum, with prognosis closely correlated with troponin concentration.

RISK STRATIFICATION OF ACSs

Clinical risk stratification *(7,8)* of the acute coronary syndrome has been well described. Several quantitative risk scores have been proposed and are described in Table 2. Markers

Table 1
Targets for Antiplatelet Inhibitors and Anticoagulant Therapy

a. Platelet Aggregation (white thrombus) mediated by:	
1. Thromboxane A$_2$	Aspirin
2. ADP receptor	Clopidogrel
	Ticlopidine
3. GP IIb/IIIa receptor	Abciximab
(platelet bridging via fibrinogen)	Tirofiban
	Eptifibatide
	Lamifiban
b. Fibrin Generation (red thrombus) mediated by:	
Factors VII, IX, Xa: high-concentration multiplier effect	
Factor IIa (thrombin): catalytic conversion of fibrinogen to fibrin	
1. Anti-Xa > anti-IIa effect	LMWHs
2. Anti-IIa > anti-Xa effect	UFH
(indirect effect via ATIII)	
3. Direct anti-IIa effect hirudin	Hirulog
	Inogatran
	Argatroban
4. Mixed effects (II, VII, IX, X)	Warfarin
(vitamin K dependent factors)	

that identify cardiac myocyte injury (cardiac troponins) and inflammation [C-reactive protein (CRP) and the total white cell count] are increasingly utilized for risk stratification.

Cardiac Troponins

The cardiac troponins are markers of myocyte injury caused by proximal thrombotic coronary occlusion or distal vascular microembolization of platelet aggregates. It is controversial whether cytosolic troponin is released with reversible myocardial ischemia, but accepted that, with myocyte necrosis, the structurally bound troponins are released. The concentration of troponin at the time of presentation to the hospital is used for the diagnosis and risk stratification of unstable angina and also identifies patients who benefit from aggressive medical or invasive therapy. Patients with increased troponin concentrations benefit from treatment with low-molecular-weight heparins, GP IIb/IIIa inhibitors, and early percutaneous coronary intervention (PCI). There is additional prognostic value in measuring a 6–8 h troponin concentration, particularly if the baseline concentration is normal. In the Global Use of Strategies to Open Occluded Coronary Arteries in Acute Coronary Syndromes (GUSTO) IIa study, 30-d mortality was 10% with a positive baseline cardiac troponin, 5% with a late positive concentration, and zero in those patients with both normal baseline and late troponin concentrations.

Patients with a positive troponin but a normal CK and CK-MB are at significantly increased risk for recurrent ischemic events. It has been suggested that with the advent of the troponins as the preferred markers of myocardial injury, CK-MB should be regarded as an obsolete assay. As it is not cost effective to measure both cardiac troponin and CK-MB, and because of the superior prognostic value of the troponins, many cardiac units have abandoned the use of CK-MB.

Table 2
Quantitative Risk Stratification Systems for the ACS

A. RUSH model *(89,90)*
   Mathematical algorithm that uses the following variables:
   • Admission following a MI in the past 14 d
   • Not receiving a β-blocker or rate-lowering calcium channel blocker at admission
   • ST depression on admission ECG
   • History of diabetes
   • Age

B. TIMI Risk Score *(91)*
   Age ≥65 yr
   Three or more coronary risk factors
   Prior coronary stenosis of 50% or more
   ST deviation on presenting ECG
   Two or more anginal episodes in prior 24 h
   Aspirin use in prior 7 d
   Increased serum cardiac markers

Score	Adverse cardiac event in 14 d
0/1	4.7%
2	8.3%
3	13.2%
4	19.9%
5	26.2%
6/7	40.9%

C. MGH Model *(92)*
   Age >65 yr
   Prior coronary bypass grafting
   Antecedent aspirin use
   Antecedent β-blocker use
   ST depression on ECG

Score	Adverse event in 7 d
0/1	6.5%
2	14.6%
3	22.7%
4/5	37.1%

C-Reactive Protein

Instability of coronary plaques is associated with macrophage accumulation *(9)*, inflammation, and an increase in acute phase proteins such as high-sensitivity CRP and serum amyloid A *(10)*. High concentration of both baseline *(11–16)* and discharge *(17)* high-sensitivity CRP are independent predictors of subsequent events *(11,12,18)*. CRP and cardiac troponin have been shown to be independent and additive in the prediction of cardiac death *(13,19)*. Although high-sensitivity commercial assays required to detect minimal increases of CRP have only recently been released, the concentrations of CRP

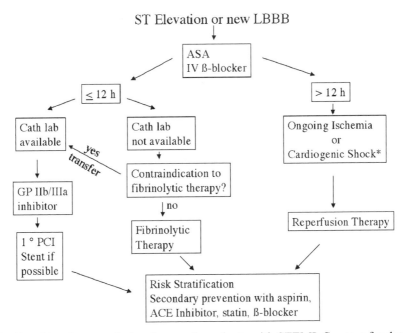

Fig. 2. Algorithm for reperfusion therapy in patients with STEMI. See text for details. *For patients < 75 yr old who present with cardiogenic shock, immediate percutaneous revascularization is the treatment strategy of choice.

associated with risk in the early period after presentation with ACS are approximately tenfold higher than the concentration associated with risk in a healthy population.

White Cell Count

Like CRP, the white cell count is a marker of inflammation. Two recent retrospective studies of the white cell count in the Platelet Glycoprotein IIb/IIIa in Unstable Angina Receptor Suppression Using Integrilin Therapy (PURSUIT) and Chimeric c7E3 AntiPlatelet Therapy in Unstable Angina Refractory to Standard Treatment (CAPTURE) studies (12,213 patients) *(20)* and the Orbofiban in Patients with Unstable Coronary Syndromes (OPUS) study (10,288 patients) *(21)* demonstrated a strong relationship between the total white cell count and mortality at 30 and 180 d.

MEDICAL MANAGEMENT
WITH ANTITHROMBOTIC AND ANTIPLATELET DRUGS

Reperfusion Therapy for STEMI

The pathophysiologic substrate for STEMI is complete thrombotic occlusion of an epicardial coronary artery. As a result, management centers on immediate restoration of epicardial blood flow (Fig. 2). Either fibrinolytic therapy or primary PCI are acceptable reperfusion options for patients presenting within 12 h of symptom onset with ST elevation or new left bundle branch block (LBBB) on the presenting electrocardiogram (ECG). Owing to concerns about suboptimal efficacy and increased risk for intracranial hemorrhage in elderly patients *(22,23)*, primary PCI is preferred in this population. Fibrinolytic therapy is not recommended routinely for patients presenting between 12 and 24 h after the onset of symptoms or for those who have a blood pressure above 180/110, and is contraindicated for patients presenting >24 hours after the onset of symptoms, and in those with only ST depression on the presenting ECG, unless a true posterior MI is suspected.

Primary percutaneous coronary intervention is considered an alternative to fibrinolytic therapy for patients with ST elevation or presumed new LBBB, if the following criteria are met: anticipated door-to-balloon time of 90 min or less; high-volume operators; and a collaborative environment that includes experienced support staff and close integration between the emergency room and the cardiac catheterization laboratory. Primary PCI is the treatment of choice for patients presenting with cardiogenic shock, provided they are <75 yr old, and can be treated within 18 h of the onset of shock and within 36 h of the onset of symptoms *(24)*. An algorithm for the management of STEMI is shown in Fig. 2.

Fibrinolytic Therapy for Non-ST Elevation ACS

In the TIMI IIIB study *(25)*, 1473 patients with unstable angina or non-Q MI were randomized to tissue plasminogen activator (tPA) or placebo, in addition to unfractionated heparin (UFH) and aspirin. It was found that fibrinolytic therapy did not lead to an improvement in clinical end points, but was associated with an increase in fatal and nonfatal MI at 6 wk and 1 yr (7.5% vs 4.9%, $p = 0.04$). Cerebral hemorrhage occurred in four patients with tPA and in no control patients ($p = 0.06$). As a result of this and other trials, fibrinolytic therapy is contraindicated for patients without ST elevation or new LBBB on the presenting ECG.

Aspirin and Dipyridamole

Aspirin irreversibly inhibits cyclooxygenase I, preventing platelet synthesis of thromboxane A_2, a potent vasoconstrictor and stimulator of platelet aggregation. It is indicated for all patients with ST elevation and non-ST elevation ACSs and it reduces the rate of death or MI by about 50% *(26)*. Despite clear evidence of benefit in all patient subgroups with acute coronary syndromes, aspirin is frequently underutilized. In the Global Unstable Angina Registry and Treatment Evaluation Study (GUARANTEE) Registry *(27)* of unstable angina patients, only 82% of patients received aspirin. In subjects without known cardiac disease enrolled in the Physicians' Health Study *(28)*, the benefits of aspirin were shown, particularly in those with higher serum concentrations of CRP. In this setting, CRP may be serving predominantly as a marker of those at the highest risk for adverse events. However, part of the benefit of aspirin could relate to its antiinflammatory properties, which could reduce plaque rupture and its sequelae. In patients with unstable angina, dipyridamole does not confer benefit when added to aspirin *(29)*.

Thienopyridines: Ticlopidine and Clopidogrel

Ticlopidine is an ADP-receptor antagonist that has been shown to be useful in patients intolerant to aspirin *(30)*. However, this agent is associated with frequent side effects, and, more important, is also associated with an increased risk for neutropenia and thrombotic thrombocytopenic purpura. Clopidogrel is another ADP-receptor antagonist that has replaced ticlopidine in clinical practice owing to a more favorable side effect profile and the fact that it is not associated with neutropenia. At steady state, this drug inhibits platelet aggregation by 40–60%. In patients with recent MI, stroke, or peripheral arterial disease, clopidogrel and aspirin appear to provide similar long-term secondary prevention benefits *(31)*. Thus, clopidogrel is indicated as secondary prevention for patients who have either allergy or intolerance to aspirin. In the Clopidogrel in Unstable Angina to Prevent Recurrent Events (CURE) trial, the *combination* of clopidogrel and aspirin was compared with aspirin alone in a population of patients with ACS *(32)*. Compared with aspirin alone, the combination of clopidogrel and aspirin led to a 20% relative reduction in the composite end point of cardiovascular death, MI, and stroke from 11.5% to 9.3% at a mean of 9 mo follow-up (RR: 0.80, CI: 0.72–0.89, $p < 0.00005$). The benefit was driven by a reduction in MI (6.7% to 5.2%; RR: 0.77, CI: 0.68–0.89, $p < 0.001$), but there were also trends to reduction in cardiovascular death (5.5% to 5.1%; RR: 0.92, CI: 0.79–1.07) and stroke (1.4% to 1.2%). Reduction in events began within 2 h of the administration of the 300-mg loading dose. These benefits were achieved at the cost of an increase in major bleeding events (2.7% to 3.6%, RR: 1.34, $p < 0.003$) and transfusions (2.2% to 2.8%, RR: 1.28, $p < 0.03$).

Unfractionated Heparin

Heparin binds with antithrombin, enhancing its ability to inactivate factor Xa and thrombin. Clinical data to support the use of UFH in addition to aspirin for patients with non-ST elevation ACS are surprisingly limited. A meta-analysis of six randomized short-term trials assessed the value of adding UFH to aspirin for the treatment of unstable angina in 1353 patients *(33)*. There was a trend toward reduced mortality and MI (RR: 0.67; 95% CI: 0.44–1.02, $p = 0.06$) in the patients receiving heparin. However, only four studies reported results to 12 wk, when much of the trend in benefit was attenuated (RR: 0.82, 95% CI: 0.56–1.20, $p = 0.76$).

Although it has not been definitively established that the combination of heparin and aspirin is superior to either aspirin or heparin alone, guidelines usually recommend their combined use in patients with unstable angina or NSTEMI. Rebound ischemia on cessation of treatment may occur, particularly in those patients not taking aspirin. The target activated partial thromboplastin time (aPTT) is recommended to be in the range of 45–60 s on the basis of evidence from randomized trials *(34)*. Control may be facilitated by the use of bedside monitoring and dosing indexed to patient weight.

A number of factors may contribute to limited efficacy of UFH. These include the need for antithrombin for its action, and reduced effectiveness of the heparin–antithrombin complex in the presence of fibrin monomers. The release of platelet factor 4 in response to heparin may also contribute to reactivating acute ischemia. Other limitations of UFH are the need for continuous infusions and difficulty in achieving target activated partial thromboplastin times, because of wide variation in antithrombotic response. Heparin-induced thrombocytopenia occurs in 1–3% of patients *(35)*.

Low-Molecular-Weight Heparins

Low-molecular-weight heparins (LMWHs) are derived from UFH by depolymerization. They have a number of practical advantages, including greater activity against factor Xa than thrombin, and greater bioavailability than UFH because of lower binding to plasma proteins and endothelial cells. This leads to a more predictable antithrombotic dose–response relationship, and eliminates the need for routine laboratory monitoring of the anticoagulant effect. The long half-life of about 4 h after subcutaneous injections enables once or twice daily subcutaneous injection. LMWHs have an increase in minor (cutaneous) bleeding compared to UFH, but have the distinct advantages of not requiring aPTT monitoring, have a reduced rate of heparin-induced thrombocytopenia *(35)*, and intravenous site infections are avoided. Because of the long half-life of LMWH, and difficulties in achieving rapid reversal of effect, UFH is often preferred in those patients in whom early or immediate intervention is planned, and in patients with marked obesity or renal failure. However, administration of protamine sulfate results in approx 60% reversal of the anti-factor Xa effects of LMWH and may result in decreased bleeding *(36,37)*.

The only clinical trial of a LMWH (dalteparin) compared with placebo in patients on aspirin (Fragmin in Unstable Coronary Artery Disease [FRISC]) *(38)* showed a benefit in death and MI (1.8% vs 4.8%) at 6 d, which persisted at 40 d. In this study, patients were required to have an unstable coronary syndrome and transient or persistent ECG changes (ST depression of 0.1 mV or more, or T-wave inversion of 0.1 mV in two adjacent leads). In FRISC, a positive troponin T ($\geq$0.1 ng/mL) differentiated between those patients who responded to dalteparin (48% lower incidence of death or MI at 40 d) from nonresponders *(39)* (Fig. 3). Similarly, in the Thrombolysis in Myocardial Infarction (TIMI) 11B study troponin I predicted response to enoxaparin *(40)* (Fig. 3).

Several major clinical studies of LMWHs have examined their efficacy compared with intravenous unfractionated heparin. Both the FRISC study *(41)* (dalteparin) and the Fraxiparine in Ischemic Syndrome (FRAXIS) study *(42)* (nadroparin) demonstrated equivalence but no advantage over UFH. Two studies of enoxaparin (Efficacy and Safety of Subcutaneous Enoxaparin in Non-Q-wave Coronary Events [ESSENCE] *[43]* and TIMI 11B *[44]*) demonstrated superiority over UFH with reduction in the composite end point of death, infarction, recurrent angina, or revascularization. A prospectively planned meta-analysis of the two trials of enoxaparin (ESSENCE and TIMI 11B *[45]*) demonstrated superiority with a 20% reduction in the combination of death and MI when compared with UFH ($p = 0.05$) at 8, 14, and 43 d. Benefit has been confirmed to persist at 1 yr *(46)*. Economic analyses of data from ESSENCE show cost savings both at 30 d *(47)* and 1 yr *(48)* in patients treated with enoxaparin.

The LMWHs differ in their ratio of anti-Xa/anti-IIa activity, with enoxaparin having relatively greater anti-Xa activity (3.5:1) than dalteparin (2.5:1) *(49)*. The LMWHs also vary in their pharmacologic effects *(50,51)*, including their rates of clearance, the amount of nonspecific binding, duration of effect, and effects on von Willebrand factor. In the absence of direct comparisons in clinical trials the relative effectiveness of the different LMWHs is uncertain. The current evidence, however, demonstrates the clinical benefit of enoxaparin over UFH, which is not proven with dalteparin or nadroparin.

It was hoped that the LMWHs might be particularly effective for prolonged therapy in patients at high risk for recurrent ischemic events. However, this has not been substantiated with a 3-mo study of twice daily dalteparin, compared with placebo (FRISC II) showing a reduction in the composite end point of death and MI at 1 mo, which was not sustained at 6-mo follow-up *(52)*. Another study (TIMI 11B) of prolonged enoxaparin for 35 d after initial stabilization demonstrated no incremental benefit for prolonged therapy, with an increased risk of major bleeding *(44)*.

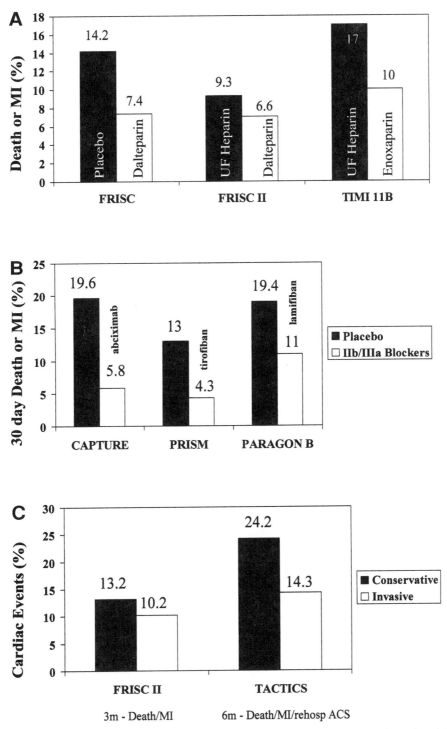

Fig. 3. Benefits of therapy in troponin-positive patients. (**A**) Efficacy of LMW heparins: dalteparin *(36,49)* and enoxaparin *(37)* in troponin-positive patients. (**B**) Efficacy of GP IIb/IIIa receptor blockers: abciximab *(71)*, tirofiban *(82)*, and lamifiban *(83)* in troponin-positive patients. (**C**) Efficacy of an invasive strategy *(66,67)* in troponin-positive patients. In each of these studies there was no significant benefit of these treatments in troponin-negative patients.

Direct Antithrombins

Hirudin, hirulog, inogatran, and argatroban are selective antithrombin agents that have been subjected to clinical trials. They differ from heparin in that they do not require inter-action with an intermediate enzyme and bind directly to the catalytic site of thrombin. Their proposed benefits over heparin include the ability to inactivate clot-bound thrombin, and reduction in thrombin-induced platelet activation, factor V and VIII activation, and endothelin release. The direct antithrombins are not inhibited by platelet factor 4, remain active in platelet-rich environments, and are not associated with thrombocytopenia.

Despite these theoretical advantages, large-scale trials of direct antithrombins have been disappointing. Only a small incremental benefit has been shown over standard UFH in large-scale studies. A meta-analysis (53) of the hirudin trials from the Organization to Assess Strategies for Ischemic Syndromes (OASIS) pilot, OASIS-2, and GUSTO-IIb of non-ST elevation ACS patients demonstrated a trend to risk reduction at 35 d (RR: 0.90, $p = 0.06$). Hirudin was associated with a higher rate of bleeding requiring transfusion than heparin. Similarly, a study of inogatran (54) showed no improvement in ischemic end points despite a clear dose-related improvement in activated partial thromboplastin time.

Early benefit at 7 d (53,55) may be attenuated by 30 d because of rebound activation of the coagulation system after termination of treatment (54,56). Owing to low event rates in these large trials, it has been difficult to demonstrate significant differences in out-comes, and apparent gains appear to be small. In addition, these agents are associated with an increase in major bleeding and are more expensive than heparin.

Warfarin

Warfarin antagonizes carboxylation of glutamate residues on vitamin K-dependent proteins, thereby inhibiting the biologic activity of coagulation factors II, VII, IX, and X. Warfarin monotherapy appears to be at least as effective as aspirin for secondary prevention in patients following MI (57). Owing to its improved safety profile and ease of use, however, aspirin is preferred for all patients except those with MI complicated by atrial fibrillation or severe left ventricular dysfunction (particularly following large anterior MI), as in these circumstances the risk for systemic embolization is markedly increased. Studies have also evaluated the *combination* of warfarin and aspirin post-MI. Neither fixed-dose warfarin nor low-dose warfarin titrated to an INR of approx 1.5–2.5 appears to be superior to monotherapy with either agent alone, and the combination is associated with excess bleeding risk (58–61). Thus, although warfarin is a suitable alter-native to aspirin following MI in selected patients, there is currently no evidence to sup-port a combination regimen of warfarin plus aspirin.

GP IIb/IIIa Inhibitors

By blocking the final common pathway of platelet aggregation, GP IIb/IIIa antago-nists potently inhibit platelet aggregation in response to all types of stimuli. The first GP IIb/IIIa antagonist to reach clinical practice was abciximab, a murine monoclonal Fab antibody fragment. Subsequently, both peptide (eptifibatide) and nonpeptide small mole-cules (tirofiban, lamifiban, sibrafiban, xemilofiban, and orbofiban) have been assessed in clinical trials. At their recommended doses, all three of the currently approved agents (abciximab, eptifibatide, and tirofiban) inhibit platelet aggregation by >80%.

In the Platelet Receptor Inhibition in Ischemic Syndrome Management in Patients Limited by Unstable Signs and Symptoms (PRISM-PLUS) study *(62)*, the combination of aspirin, heparin, and tirofiban, compared with aspirin and heparin alone, reduced the composite end point of death, nonfatal infarction, and refractory ischemia at 7 d (12.9% vs 17.9%, $p = 0.004$), 30 d (18.5% vs 22.3%, $p = 0.03$), and 6 mo (27.7% vs 32.1%, $p = 0.02$). Death and nonfatal infarction were reduced at 7 d (4.9% vs 8.3%, $p = 0.006$) and 30 d (8.7% vs 11.9%, $p = 0.03$), but not at 6 mo (12.3% vs 15.3%, $p = 0.06$). The combination of aspirin, heparin, and eptifibatide *(63)* similarly reduced the combination of death and MI from 15.7% to 14.2% ($p = 0.042$) at 30 d when compared to heparin and aspirin alone.

In the Platelet Receptor Inhibition in Ischemic Syndrome Management (PRISM) study *(64)* comparing tirofiban with heparin, 13% of patients who were troponin I positive had a cardiac event (death, MI) at 30 d, compared with 4.9% in troponin-negative patients ($p < 0.0001$). At 30 d, in cTnI-positive patients, tirofiban lowered the risk of death (adjusted RR: 0.25, 95% CI: 0.09–0.68, $p = 0.004$) and MI (RR: 0.37, CI: 0.16–0.84, $p = 0.01$) (Fig. 3). This benefit was seen in medically managed patients (RR: 0.30, CI: 0.10–0.84, $p = 0.004$) and in those undergoing revascularization (RR: 0.37, CI: 0.15–0.93, $p = 0.02$) after 48 h of infusion treatment. In contrast, no treatment effect was seen for cTnI-negative patients.

In the GUSTO IV-ACS study *(65)*, patients with non-ST elevation ACS were randomized to an abciximab bolus with a 24- or 48-h infusion, or to placebo. All patients received aspirin and either UFH or dalteparin. Patients were required to have chest pain lasting at least 5 min in the previous 24 h, with either 0.5-mm ST depression or positive cardiac troponin, but were excluded if revascularization was planned within 30 d. The trial enrolled 7800 patients and the primary end point (death or MI at 30 d) was reached in 8.0%, 8.2%, and 9.1% of the placebo, 24-h infusion, and 48-h infusion groups, respectively ($p = $ NS). There was no improvement in outcome in the troponin-positive or ST depression groups. Minor and major bleeding was increased, particularly in the 48-h infusion group.

The benefits of the small molecule GP IIb/IIIa inhibitors, tirofiban *(62)* and eptifibatide *(63)*, have been consistent in patients with ACSs: early reductions in death, MI, and refractory ischemia have been observed, but there has been some attenuation of benefit at 6 mo. The combination of GP IIb/IIIa receptor antagonists together with LMWHs has not yet been evaluated in large clinical trials, although large studies are currently underway. A small study *(66)* of tirofiban in combination with enoxaparin demonstrated more consistent inhibition of platelet aggregation than when combined with UFH. As yet, there are no head-to-head studies of GP IIb/IIIa inhibitors compared with LMWHs.

Some GP IIb/IIIa inhibitors may have other clinically important effects on long-term inflammation and hyperplasia. Abciximab binds the leukocyte Mac-1 receptor *(67)*, which may have long-term benefits in reducing inflammation, and also blocks the vitronectin receptor *(68)*, which integrin is involved in tissue proliferation. Despite hopes that oral GP IIb/IIIa inhibitors could provide prolonged receptor inhibition and prevent recurrent ischemic events, all studies to date have been disappointing and these agents have no role in contemporary practice (Table 3).

Antiischemic Therapy

β-Blockers exert their beneficial effect in ACS by decreasing myocardial contractility and heart rate, improving the balance between oxygen supply and demand. In patients

Table 3
Summary of Evidence for Antithrombotic and Antiplatelet Drugs in the ACS

- Aspirin reduces progression to MI and cardiac mortality by about 40%.
- When used with aspirin, clopidogrel leads to a significant reduction in the composite of cardiovascular death, MI, and stroke, and in particular reduces MI by 23%, but at a cost of increased major bleeds.
- Dipyridamole does not confer any additional reduction in coronary events when added to aspirin.
- UFH, when used with aspirin, only marginally reduces death and MI when compared with placebo.
- Dalteparin reduces death and MI when compared with placebo.
- Enoxaparin is superior to UFH in reducing death and MI, whereas dalteparin and nadroparin are not.
- Prolonged use of LMWHs shows no additional benefit over short-term use.
- Direct antithrombins appear to have a marginal advantage and have the risk of increased bleeding.
- Intravenous thrombolytic therapy is ineffective and may be harmful.
- Warfarin has minimal benefits over aspirin.
- In the ACS the intravenous administration of GP IIb/IIIa inhibitors (tirofiban and eptifibatide, but not abciximab) in combination with aspirin and UFH reduce death and MI in the first months after treatment, but with attenuation of effect at 6 mo.
- The benefits of GP IIb/IIIa inhibitors are additive to the use of revascularization.

with STEMI, β-blockers reduce infarct size and prevent short-term mortality. The reduction in early mortality is largely due to prevention of sudden cardiac death, which is caused predominantly by early ventricular arrhythmias and ventricular rupture *(69)*. In patients with normal left ventricle (LV) function, the primary benefit of long-term therapy with β-blockers is the prevention of recurrent infarction *(69)*, whereas in patients with LV dysfunction, long-term β-blocker therapy markedly reduces mortality *(70)*. In recent guidelines, the recommendations for β-blocker use have broadened to reflect a growing appreciation for the role of these agents in patients with LV dysfunction and mild-to-moderate congestive heart failure (CHF). Currently, early (intravenous followed by oral) β-blockers are recommended for all patients with ACS, unless moderate to severe heart failure, significant bradycardia, or severe bronchospasm is present. Long-term secondary prevention with β-blockers is indicated for most patients discharged with ACS.

Because they favorably affect both myocardial oxygen supply and demand, nitrates are of particular value in the early management of ACS. Current guidelines recommend that sublingual followed by intravenous nitroglycerin be given to patients for the immediate relief of ischemia and CHF symptoms. Clinical trial evidence does not support routine administration of nitrates after the first 24–48 h in patients without ongoing ischemic symptoms. Although effective at relieving symptoms, nitrates have not been shown to lower mortality.

The indications for angiotensin-converting-enzyme (ACE) inhibitors in patients with ACS have expanded rapidly in recent years. Previous guidelines focused on the role of ACE inhibitors following STEMI to prevent adverse ventricular remodeling, CHF, and death. With the publication of the Heart Outcomes Prevention Evaluation Study *(71)*, it is now clear that this class of agents also prevents ischemic complications in patients with established vascular disease and in patients at high risk for vascular disease. As a result, ACE inhibitors are now indicated for most patients with ACS who do not have hypotension (systolic blood pressure < 100) after initial treatment with β-blockers.

While recommendations for the use of β-blockers and ACE inhibitors have been extended in recent guidelines, the role of calcium channel blockers continues to diminish. In contrast to evidence for β-blockers and ACE inhibitors, clinical trials do not suggest that calcium channel blockers lower mortality. No clear indication exists for calcium channel antagonists in STEMI, and in non-ST elevation ACS, diltiazem or verapamil is recommended only in patients who meet the following criteria: (1) contraindication to β-blocker or ACE inhibitors, (2) persistent or frequently recurring ischemia, (3) absence of severe LV dysfunction, and (4) presence of refractory hypertension or tachycardia. It is also recommended that short-acting dihydropyridine calcium channel blockers be avoided altogether.

Lipid-Lowering Therapy

Long-term therapy with lipid-lowering agents (statins) is currently recommended for patients with ACS provided the concentration of LDL is > 100 mg/dL, based on results from a number of landmark secondary prevention trials *(72–74)*. Recently, several lines of clinical evidence have converged to suggest that initiation of statin therapy should be advanced from the discharge phase to the hospital phase in patients with ACS. First, patients initiated on statins in the hospital are much more likely to remain on therapy at long-term follow-up *(75)*. Second, in-hospital initiation of high-dose statins reduces recurrent ischemic events when compared with traditional strategies in which statins are initiated after several months of dietary intervention *(76)*. A variety of mechanisms likely explain the benefits of statins in the early phase following ACS, including low-density-lipoprotein (LDL) reduction, improved endothelial function, reduced inflammation, and inhibition of thrombin generation.

EARLY INVASIVE MANAGEMENT AND UPSTREAM MEDICAL THERAPY

It was hoped that intensive medical therapy of unstable angina with antiplatelet and antithrombin therapy might "passivate" the coronary plaque. Results have been disappointing, however: at 6–9 mo death or MI occurs in approx 12% of patients and 40% of patients undergo ischemia-driven revascularization *(77)*. Two recent studies comparing invasive and conservative strategies and using differing upstream therapies have clarified the role of invasive management. The FRISC II study *(77)* examined an early invasive strategy in 2457 patients with unstable angina who had ECG changes or positive serum markers. Patients first received dalteparin for at least 2 d before a randomized comparison of an early invasive strategy employing early PCI (stenting in 61–70%) or bypass surgery, which significantly reduced death and MI by 22% (the primary end point) from 12.1% to 9.4%, ($p = 0.03$) at 6 mo, compared with a conservative strategy in which revascularization was driven by recurrent or ongoing ischemia. The event curves continued to diverge at 6 mo after randomization. In addition, there was a trend to reduction (by 35%) in total mortality alone (from 2.9% to 1.9%, $p = 0.10$). Total mortality was significantly reduced in men but not in women treated with the invasive strategy. MI alone was significantly reduced from 10.1% to 7.8% ($p < 0.05$) at 6 mo. There were also highly significant reductions in angina (22% vs 39%, $p < 0.001$), class III–IV angina (3% vs 8%, $p < 0.001$), requirement for long-acting nitrates (17% vs 38%, $p < 0.001$), and hospital readmission rates (31% vs 49%, $p < 0.001$) in the invasive compared with the noninvasive group.

PCI was performed at a median of 4 d and coronary bypass surgery at a median of 7 d. Upstream medical therapy with dalteparin for an average of 4 d prior to angiography and intervention may have been synergistic in leading to an improved outcome. The benefits of an even earlier invasive strategy, which included upstream treatment with tirofiban and heparin, were examined in 2220 patients in the Treat Angina with Aggrastat and Determine Cost of Therapy with an Invasive or Conversative Strategy (TACTICS)–TIMI 18 study *(78)*. Patients with accelerating, recurrent, or prolonged (>20 min) angina within 24 h were entered in the study provided they had new ST depression of 0.5 mm or transitory ST elevation of 1 mm, T-wave inversion of 0.3 mV in two leads, increased cardiac markers, or a history of documented coronary disease. Patients received aspirin, IV tirofiban, and UFH and those randomized to an invasive strategy underwent coronary angiography between 4 and 48 h and revascularization in 61%. PCI was performed in 41% at a median of 25 h and bypass surgery in 20% at a median of 89 h. Conservatively managed patients underwent angiography if they had recurrent pain associated with ischemia on ECG or changes in cardiac markers, hemodynamic instability, a positive stress test, stress echocardiogram or myocardial perfusion study, rehospitalization with angina or infarction, or class III or IV angina.

An early hazard with intervention (which was found in FRISC II) was not found in TACTICS–TIMI 18, which employed upstream and postprocedural tirofiban and intracoronary stents in 83% of patients. The TACTICS–TIMI 18 study provided the lowest adverse event rate of an intervention study in patients with high-risk unstable angina. The primary end point (death, nonfatal MI, or rehospitalization with unstable angina at 6 mo) was reduced from 19.4% to 15.9% (OR: 0.78, CI: 0.62–0.97, $p = 0.025$). Death and nonfatal infarction were also reduced from 9.5% to 7.3% at 6 mo ($p < 0.05$). Benefit with an invasive strategy was particularly found in patients with ST changes, increased troponin concentration (Fig. 3), and high TIMI risk score. The TIMI IIIB *(25)* and Veterans Affairs Non-Q-Wave Infarction Strategies in Hospital (VANQWISH) studies *(79)*, two previous and smaller studies (1473 and 920 patients, respectively), which included the use of balloon angioplasty prior to the widespread availability of intracoronary stents and GP IIb/IIIa receptor antagonists, did not demonstrate an overall reduction in death or infarction from an early invasive approach.

In the PRISM-PLUS study *(62)* of IV heparin with tirofiban vs heparin, coronary angiography was encouraged at 2–4 d after randomization, leading to a 90% rate of early angiography. Consequently, there was a 54% rate of early revascularization overall (31% angioplasty and 23% bypass surgery). Although there was no randomization between invasive and medical strategies, the reduction in the composite end point with heparin/tirofiban was significant only in patients undergoing angioplasty (RR: 0.55, 95% CI: 0.32–0.94) and not in patients treated medically (RR: 0.87, 95% CI: 0.60–1.25). This suggests that the major benefits of this aggressive medical management accrue when it is used as complementary therapy with an early invasive strategy. An angiographic subgroup assessment *(80)* of patients treated with tirofiban and heparin in the PRISM-PLUS study demonstrated persistent thrombus in 45% of patients. Persistent thrombus was associated with an increase in both death (RR: 2.4, 95% CI: 1.3–4.3) and MI (RR: 2.0, 95% CI: 1.3–3.1) at 30 d. This problem raises the need for possible complementary mechanical revascularization, as well as the need for continued research to develop more effective medical regimens.

In conclusion, the complementary use of upstream medical and invasive approaches should be considered in all patients with high-risk features. Early coronary angiography and revascularization with either PCI or coronary bypass surgery is associated with significant and sustained reductions in death, infarction, recurrent angina, and readmission to hospital.

INVASIVE MANAGEMENT
AND DOWNSTREAM MEDICAL THERAPY

The platelet also plays a central role in complications *after* PCI or stenting. Use of the GP IIb/IIIa platelet receptor inhibitor abciximab has been shown to improve outcomes in patients undergoing PCI and stenting, particularly in patients with unstable angina or MI *(81)*. The troponin concentration can predict which patients will benefit from abciximab therapy with a risk ratio of MI at 6 mo of 0.23 (95% CI: 0.12–0.49, $p < 0.001$) for troponin-positive patients receiving abciximab compared with placebo *(82)*. Improved outcomes are maintained 3 yr following treatment. The GP IIb/IIIa platelet receptor inhibitor eptifibatide also reduces adverse events in patients undergoing PCI with a reduction in death or MI at 6 mo from 11.5% to 7.5% (RR: 0.63, 95% CI: 0.47–0.84, $p = 0.002$) *(83)*. The TARGET study *(84)* compared adjunctive treatment with abciximab compared with tirofiban in 4812 patients undergoing PCI. Patients receiving tirofiban had a higher adverse cardiac event rate at 30 d than those receiving abciximab (7.55% vs 6.01%, RR: 1.26, $p = 0.038$), with this difference greatest in those patients undergoing PCI for an ACS. However, by 6 mo this difference in event rates was less evident (14.4% vs 13.8%, RR: 1.04, $p = 0.51$).

After stent implantation, treatment with the combination of aspirin and clopidogrel for 2–4 wk has been shown to provide excellent protection against thrombotic complications (Tables 4 and 5) *(85,86)*.

COMPETING STRATEGIES AND GAPS IN KNOWLEDGE

There are currently many choices in managing high-risk ACS patients but directly comparable data between strategies is incomplete. Definitive recommendations for any specific strategy are therefore difficult. Aspirin should be administered to all patients unless there is a specific contraindication to its use. In addition, the following strategies are variably supported by clinical trial evidence, as detailed previously in this chapter.

- Administration of subcutaneous LMWH for at least 3–4 d followed by an invasive strategy *(77)*. (Breakthrough ischemia might be treated with the addition of intravenous tirofiban or eptifibatide before proceeding to an invasive strategy.)
- Immediate administration of tirofiban (but not abciximab) along with UFH, before proceeding to an invasive strategy *(62,78)*. (The infusion of tirofiban with heparin is continued during and after percutaneous coronary intervention.)

Table 4
Upstream Therapy and Early Invasive Management

o In high-risk patients managed with an early invasive strategy, the benefit from PCI is enhanced by upstream heparin/tirofiban.
o In addition to aspirin, either LMWH or IV tirofiban with UFH is recommended:
  • In high-risk patients.
  • In geographically isolated patients requiring transfer to a tertiary facility, or patients not suitable for an invasive approach (very elderly, severe comorbidities).
o IV tirofiban and UFH may be particularly useful where LMWH fails and in high-risk patients for whom an invasive strategy is planned.
o The complementary use of aggressive medical and invasive approaches should be considered in all patients with high-risk features.

Table 5
Indications for an Early Invasive Strategy

With the exception of patients of advanced age or with severe or multiple comorbidities, an early invasive approach should be considered in the following high-risk groups:
• Positive serum markers (troponin I or T).
• ECG changes (ST depression or T inversion in multiple leads).
• Pain or ischemia refractory to medical therapy.
• Associated heart failure or hemodynamic instability.
• High-risk features on early exercise testing.
• Recent MI or revascularization.

• A planned early invasive strategy, with use of IV heparin but avoiding GP IIb/IIIa receptor antagonists until cardiac catheterization is performed when a GP IIb/IIIa receptor antagonist is administered at the time of percutaneous coronary intervention *(83,87,88)*.
• Bolus and maintenance administration of clopidogrel at the time of presentation and continued long term, with or without the use of IV or LMWHs *(32)*. Although trial data on the concomitant administration of clopidogrel with tirofiban or eptifibatide are not available, the combination has frequently been used in patients undergoing PCI without adverse effects in this group.

Clearly, there is an ongoing need for further comparative studies including those testing the efficacy, synergism and safety of combinations of the antiplatelet and antithrombotic agents discussed in the preceding, and their role in association with the invasive approach.

ABBREVIATIONS

ACE, Angiotensin converting enzyme; ACS, acute coronary syndrome(s); aPTT, activated partial thromboplastin time; ATACS, Antithrombotic Therapy in Acute Coronary Syndromes Research Group; CAPTURE, Chimeric c7E3 AntiPlatelet Therapy in Unstable Angina Refractory to Standard Treatment; CHF, congestive heart failure; CK, creatine kinase; CK-MB, MB isoenzyme of CK; CPR, C-reactive protein; CURE, Clopidogrel in Unstable Angina to Prevent Recurrent Events Trial; ECG, electrocardiogram; ESSENCE, Efficacy and Safety of Subcutaneous Enoxaparin in Non-Q-wave Coronary

Events; FRAXIS, Fraxiparine in Ischemic Syndrome; FRISC, Fragmin in Unstable Coronary Artery Disease; GP IIb/IIIa, glycoprotein IIb/IIIa; GUARANTEE, Global Unstable Angina Registry and Treatment Evaluation Study; GUSTO, Global Use of Strategies to Open Occluded Coronary Arteries in Acute Coronary Syndromes; LBBB, left bundle branch block; LDL, low density lipoprotein; LMWH, low molecular weight heparin; LV, left ventricle; OASIS, Organization to Assess Strategies for Ischemic Syndromes; OPUS, Orbofiban in Patients with Unstable Coronary Syndromes; PCI, percutaneous coronary intervention; PRISM, Platelet Receptor Inhibition in Ischemic Syndrome Management; PRISM-PLUS, Platelet Receptor Inhibition in Ischemic Syndrome Management in Patients Limited by Unstable Signs and Symptoms; PURSUIT, Platelet Glycoprotein IIb/IIIa in Unstable Angina: Receptor Suppression Using Integrilin Therapy; STEMI, ST elevation myocardial infarction; TACTICS, Treat Angina with Aggrastat and determine Cost of Therapy with an Invasive or Conservative Strategy; TARGET, TIMI, Thrombolysis in Myocardial Infarction; tPA, tissue plasminogen activator; UFH, unfractionated heparin; VANQWISH, Veterans Affairs Non-Q-Wave Infarction Strategies in Hospital.

REFERENCES

1. Yamagishi M, Terashima M, Awano K, et al. Morphology of vulnerable coronary plaque: insights from follow-up of patients examined by intravascular ultrasound before an acute coronary syndrome. J Am Coll Cardiol 2000;35:106–111.
2. Sinapius D. Zur morphologie verschliessender koronarthromben. Dtsch Med Wochenschr 1972;97:544.
3. Gerhardt W, Katus H, Ravkilde J, et al. (1991) S-troponin T in suspected ischemic myocardial injury compared with mass and catalytic concentrations of S-creatine kinase isoenzyme MB. Clin Chem 1991;37:1405–1411.
4. Hamm CW, Ravkilde J, Gerhardt W, et al. The prognostic value of serum troponin T in unstable angina. N Engl J Med 1992;327:146–150.
5. Joint ESC/ACC Committee. Myocardial infarction redefined—a consensus document of The Joint European Society of Cardiology/American College of Cardiology Committee for the redefinition of myocardial infarction. J Am Coll Cardiol 2000;36:959–969.
6. Wagner GS, Bahit MC, Criger D, et al. Moving toward a new definition of acute myocardial infarction for the 21st century: status of the ESC/ACC consensus conference. European Society of Cardiology and American College of Cardiology. J Electrocardiol 2000;33: 57–59.
7. Braunwald E, Antman EM, Beasley JW, et al. ACC/AHA guidelines for the management of patients with unstable angina and non-ST-segment elevation myocardial infarction. A report of the American College of Cardiology/American Heart Association Task Force on Practice Guidelines (Committee on the Management of Patients With Unstable Angina). J Am Coll Cardiol 2000;36:970–1062.
8. Aroney CN, Boyden AN, Jelinek MV, Thompson P, Tonkin AM, White H. Management of unstable angina. Guidelines—2000. Med J Aust 2000;173(Suppl):S65–S88.
9. Moreno PR, Falk E, Palacios IF, Newell JB, Fuster V, Fallon JT. Macrophage infiltration in acute coronary syndromes. Implications for plaque rupture. Circulation 1994;90:775–778.
10. Fyfe AI, Rothenberg LS, DeBeer FC, Cantor RM, Rotter JI, Lusis AJ. Association between serum amyloid A proteins and coronary artery disease: evidence from two distinct arteriosclerotic processes. Circulation 1997;96:2914–2919.
11. Liuzzo G, Biasucci LM, Gallimore JR, et al. The prognostic value of C-reactive protein and serum amyloid a protein in severe unstable angina. N Engl J Med 1994;331:417–424.

12. Haverkate F, Thompson SG, Pyke SD, Gallimore JR, Pepys MB. Production of C-reactive protein and risk of coronary events in stable and unstable angina. European Concerted Action on Thrombosis and Disabilities Angina Pectoris Study Group. Lancet 1997;349: 462–466.

13. Morrow DA, Rifai N, Antman EM, et al. C-reactive protein is a potent predictor of mortality independently of and in combination with troponin T in acute coronary syndromes: a TIMI 11A substudy. Thrombolysis in Myocardial Infarction. J Am Coll Cardiol 1998;31: 1460–1465.

14. Rebuzzi AG, Quaranta G, Liuzzo G, et al. Incremental prognostic value of serum concentrations of troponin T and C-reactive protein on admission in patients with unstable angina pectoris. Am J Cardiol 1998;82:715–719.

15. Toss H, Lindahl B, Siegbahn A, Wallentin L. Prognostic influence of increased fibrinogen and C-reactive protein concentrations in unstable coronary artery disease. FRISC Study Group. Fragmin during Instability in Coronary Artery Disease. Circulation 1997;96:4204–4210.

16. de Winter RJ, Bholasingh R, Lijmer JG, et al. Independent prognostic value of C-reactive protein and troponin I in patients with unstable angina or non-Q-wave myocardial infarction. Cardiovasc Res 1999;42:240–245.

17. Biasucci LM, Liuzzo G, Grillo RL, et al. Increased concentrations of C-reactive protein at discharge in patients with unstable angina predict recurrent instability. Circulation 1999;99: 855–860.

18. Biasucci LM, Liuzzo G, Fantuzzi G, et al. Increasing concentrations of interleukin (IL)-1Ra and IL-6 during the first 2 days of hospitalization in unstable angina are associated with increased risk of in-hospital coronary events. Circulation 1999;99:2079–2084.

19. Lindahl B, Toss H, Siegbahn A, Venge P, Wallentin L. Markers of myocardial damage and inflammation in relation to long-term mortality in unstable coronary artery disease. FRISC Study Group. Fragmin during Instability in Coronary Artery Disease. N Engl J Med 343: 1139–1143.

20. Blatt DL, Chew DP, Simoons ML, et al. An increased white cell count is an independent predictor of mortality in patients with acute coronary syndromes. Circulation 2000;102(Suppl II):776.

21. Cannon CP, McCabe CH, Wilcox RG, Bentley JH, Braunwald E. Association of white blood cell count with increased mortality in acute myocardial infarction and unstable angina pectoris. OPUS-TIMI 16 Investigators. Am J Cardiol 2001;87:636–639.

22. Thiemann DR, Coresh J, Schulman SP, Gerstenblith G, Oetgen WJ, Powe NR. Lack of benefit for intravenous thrombolysis in patients with myocardial infarction who are older than 75 years. Circulation. 2000;101:2239–2246.

23. Brass LM, Lichtman JH, Wang Y, Gurwitz JH, Radford MJ, Krumholz HM. Intracranial hemorrhage associated with thrombolytic therapy for elderly patients with acute myocardial infarction: results from the Cooperative Cardiovascular Project. Stroke 2000;31: 1802–1811.

24. Hochman JS, Sleeper LA, White HD, et al. One-year survival following early revascularization for cardiogenic shock. JAMA 2001;285:190–192.

25. TIMI IIIB Investigators. Effects of tissue plasminogen activator and a comparison of early invasive and conservative strategies in unstable angina and non-Q-wave myocardial infarction. Results of the TIMI IIIB Trial. Thrombolysis in Myocardial Ischemia. Circulation 89: 1545–1556.

26. The RISC Group. (1990) Risk of myocardial infarction and death during treatment with low dose aspirin and intravenous heparin in men with unstable coronary artery disease. Lancet 1990;336:827–830.

27. Cannon CP, Moliterno DJ, Every N, et al. Implementation of AHCPR guidelines for unstable angina in 1996. Unfortunate differences between men and women. Results from the GUARANTEE registry. J Am Coll Cardiol 1997;29 (Suppl):217A.

28. Antiplatelet Trialists' Collaboration. Collaborative overview of randomised trials of anti-platelet therapy—I: prevention of death, myocardial infarction, and stroke by prolonged antiplatelet therapy in various categories of patients. Br Med J 308:81.

29. The Persantine–Aspirin Reinfarction Study Research Group. Persantine and aspirin in coronary heart disease. Circulation 1994;62:449–461.

30. Balsano F, Rizzon P, Violi F, et al. Antiplatelet treatment with ticlopidine in unstable angina. A controlled multicenter clinical trial. The Studio della Ticlopidina nell'Angina Instabile Group. Circulation 82:17–26.

31. CAPRIE Steering Committee. A randomised, blinded, trial of clopidogrel versus aspirin in patients at risk of ischemic events (CAPRIE). Lancet 348:1329–1339.

32. Yusuf S, Zhao F, Mehta SR, Chrolavicius S, Tognoni G, Fox KK. Effects of clopidogrel in addition to aspirin in patients with acute coronary syndromes without ST-segment elevation. N Engl J Med 2001;345:494–502.

33. Oler A, Whooley MA, Oler J, Grady D. Adding heparin to aspirin reduces the incidence of myocardial infarction and death in patients with unstable angina. A meta-analysis. JAMA 1996;276:811–815.

34. Becker RC, Cannon CP, Tracy RP, et al. Relation between systemic anticoagulation as determined by activated partial thromboplastin time and heparin measurements and in-hospital clinical events in unstable angina and non-Q wave myocardial infarction. Am Heart J 1996;131:421–433.

35. Chong BH. Heparin induced thrombocytopenia. Br J Haematol 89:431–439.

36. Massonnet-Castel S, Pelissier E, Bara L, et al. Partial reversal of low molecular weight heparin (PK 10169) anti-Xa activity by protamine sulfate: in vitro and in vivo study during cardiac surgery with extracorporeal circulation. Haemostasis 1986;16:139–146.

37. Van Ryn-McKenna J, Cai L, Ofosu FA, Hirsh J, Buchanan MR. Neutralization of enoxaparine-induced bleeding by protamine sulfate. Thromb Haemost 63:271–274.

38. FRISC Investigators. Low-molecular-weight heparin during instability in coronary artery disease, Fragmin during Instability in Coronary Artery Disease. Lancet 1996;347:561–568.

39. Lindahl B, Venge P, Wallentin L. Troponin T identifies patients with unstable coronary artery disease who benefit from long-term antithrombotic protection. Fragmin in Unstable Coronary Artery Disease (FRISC) Study Group. J Am Coll Cardiol 1997;29:43–48.

40. Morrow DA, Antman EM, Tanasijevic M, et al. Cardiac troponin I for stratification of early outcomes and the efficacy of enoxaparin in unstable angina: a TIMI-11B substudy. J Am Coll Cardiol 36:1812–1817.

41. Klein W, Buchwald A, Hillis SE, et al. Comparison of low-molecular-weight heparin with unfractionated heparin acutely and with placebo for 6 weeks in the management of unstable coronary artery disease. Fragmin in Unstable Coronary Artery Disease Study (FRISC). Circulation 1997;96:61–68.

42. FRAXIS Investigators. Comparison of two treatment durations (6 days and 14 days) of a low molecular weight heparin with a 6-day treatment of unfractionated heparin in the initial management of unstable angina or non-Q wave myocardial infarction: FRAXIS (FRAxiparine in Ischemic Syndrome). Eur Heart J 1999;20:1553–1562.

43. Cohen M, Demers C, Gurfinkel EP, et al. A comparison of low-molecular-weight heparin with unfractionated heparin for unstable coronary artery disease. Efficacy and Safety of Subcutaneous Enoxaparin in Non-Q-Wave Coronary Events Study Group. N Engl J Med 1997;337:447–452.

44. Antman EM, McCabe CH, Gurfinkel EP, et al. Enoxaparin prevents death and cardiac ischemic events in unstable angina/non-Q-wave myocardial infarction: results of the Thrombolysis in Myocardial Infarction (TIMI) 11B trial. Circulation 1999;100:1593–1601.

45. Antman EM, Cohen M, Radley D, et al. Assessment of the treatment effect of enoxaparin for unstable angina/non-Q-wave myocardial infarction. TIMI 11B-ESSENCE meta-analysis. Circulation 100:1602–1608.

46. Goodman S, Langer A, Demers C, et al. One year follow-up of the ESSENCE trial: sustained clinical benefit. Can J Cardiol 1998;14:122F.

47. Mark DB, Cowper PA, Berkowitz SD, et al. Economic assessment of low-molecular-weight heparin (enoxaparin) versus unfractionated heparin in acute coronary syndrome patients: results from the ESSENCE randomized trial. Efficacy and Safety of Subcutaneous Enoxaparin in Non-Q Wave Coronary Events (unstable angina or non-Q-Wave myocardial infarction). Circulation 1998;97:1702–1707.

48. O'Brien BJ, Willan A, Blackhouse G, Goeree R, Cohen M, Goodman S. Will the use of low-molecular-weight heparin (enoxaparin) in patients with acute coronary syndrome save costs in Canada? Am Heart J 2000;139:423–429.

49. Hirsh J. Low-molecular-weight heparin: a review of the results of recent studies of the treatment of venous thromboembolism and unstable angina. Circulation 1998;98:1575–1582.

50. Antman EA, Handin R. Low-molecular-weight heparins. An intriguing new twist with profound implications. Circulation 1998;98:287–289.

51. Montelescot G, Phillippe F, Ankri A, et al. Early increase of von Willebrand factor predicts adverse outcome in unstable coronary artery disease. Beneficial effects of enoxaparin. Circulation 1998;98:294–299.

52. FRISC II Investigators. Long-term low-molecular-mass heparin in unstable coronary-artery disease: FRISC II prospective randomised multicentre study. Lancet 1999;354:701–707.

53. OASIS-2 Investigators. Effects of recombinant hirudin (lepirudin) compared with heparin on death, myocardial infarction, refractory angina, and revascularisation procedures in patients with acute myocardial ischaemia without ST elevation: a randomised trial. Organisation to Assess Strategies for Ischemic Syndromes (OASIS-2). Lancet 1999;353:429–438.

54. Thrombin Inhibition in Myocardial Ischaemia (TRIM) study group. A low molecular weight, selective thrombin inhibitor, inogatran, vs heparin, in unstable coronary artery disease in 1209 patients. A double- blind, randomized, dose-finding study. Eur Heart J 1997; 18:1416–1625.

55. GUSTO IIb investigators. A comparison of recombinant hirudin with heparin for the treatment of acute coronary syndromes. The Global Use of Strategies to Open Occluded Coronary Arteries. N Engl J Med 1996;335:775–782.

56. Rao AK, Sun L, Chesebro JH, et al. Distinct effects of recombinant desulfatohirudin (Revasc) and heparin on plasma concentrations of fibrinopeptide A and prothrombin fragment F1.2 in unstable angina. A multicenter trial. Circulation 1996;94:2389–2395.

57. Anand SS, Yusuf S. Oral anticoagulant therapy in patients with coronary artery disease: a meta-analysis. JAMA 1999;282:2058–2067.

58. Cohen M, Adams PC, Parry G, et al. Combination antithrombotic therapy in unstable rest angina and non-Q-wave infarction in nonprior aspirin users. Primary end points analysis from the ATACS trial. Antithrombotic Therapy in Acute Coronary Syndromes Research Group. Circulation 1994;89:81–88.

59. Fiore LD, Ezekowitz MD, Brophy MT, Lu D, Sacco J, Peduzzi P. Department of Veterans Affairs Cooperative Studies Program Clinical Trial comparing combined warfarin and aspirin with aspirin alone in survivors of acute myocardial infarction: primary results of the CHAMP study. Circulation 2002;105:557–563.

60. Anand SS, Yusuf S, Pogue J, Weitz JI, Flather M. Long-term oral anticoagulant therapy in patients with unstable angina or suspected non-Q-wave myocardial infarction: organization to assess strategies for ischemic syndromes (OASIS) pilot study results. Circulation 98:1064–1070.

61. Huynh T, Theroux P, Bogaty P, Nasmith J, Solymoss S. Aspirin, warfarin, or the combination for secondary prevention of coronary events in patients with acute coronary syndromes and prior coronary artery bypass surgery. Circulation 2001;103:3069–3074.

62. PRISM-PLUS Study Investigators. Inhibition of the platelet glycoprotein IIb/IIIa receptor with tirofiban in unstable angina and non-Q-wave myocardial infarction. Platelet Receptor

Inhibition in Ischemic Syndrome Management in Patients Limited by Unstable Signs and Symptoms. N Engl J Med 1998;338:1488–1497.

63. The PURSUIT Trial Investigators. Inhibition of platelet glycoprotein IIb/IIIa with eptifibatide in patients with acute coronary syndromes. Platelet Glycoprotein IIb/IIIa in Unstable Angina: Receptor Suppression Using Integrilin Therapy. N Engl J Med 1998;339:436–443.

64. PRISM Study Investigators. A comparison of aspirin plus tirofiban with aspirin plus heparin for unstable angina. Platelet Receptor Inhibition in Ischemic Syndrome Management (PRISM). N Engl J Med 1998;338:1498–1505.

65. Simoons ML. Effect of glycoprotein IIb/IIIa receptor blocker abciximab on outcome in patients with acute coronary syndromes without early coronary revascularisation: the GUSTO IV-ACS randomised trial. Lancet 2001;357:1915–1924.

66. Cohen M, Theroux P, Weber S, et al. Combination therapy with tirofiban and enoxaparin in acute coronary syndromes. Int J Cardiol 1999;71:273–281.

67. Neumann FJ, Zohlnhofer D, Fakhoury L, Ott I, Gawaz M, Schomig A. Effect of glycoprotein IIb/IIIa receptor blockade on platelet–leukocyte interaction and surface expression of the leukocyte integrin Mac-1 in acute myocardial infarction. J Am Coll Cardiol 1999;34: 1420–1426.

68. Le Breton H, Plow EF, Topol EJ. Role of platelets in restenosis after percutaneous coronary revascularization. J Am Coll Cardiol 1996;28:1643–1651.

69. Yusuf S, Peto R, Lewis J, Collins R, Sleight P. Beta-blockade during and after myocardial infarction: an overview of the randomized trials. Prog Cardiovasc Dis 1985;27:335–371.

70. Gottlieb SS, McCarter RJ, Vogel RA. Effect of beta-blockade on mortality among high-risk and low-risk patients after myocardial infarction. N Engl J Med 1998;339:489–497.

71. Yusuf S, Sleight P, Pogue J, Bosch J, Davies R, Dagenais G. Effects of an angiotensin-converting-enzyme inhibitor, ramipril, on cardiovascular events in high-risk patients. The Heart Outcomes Prevention Evaluation Study Investigators. N Engl J Med 2000;342:145–153.

72. Scandinavian Simvastatin Survival Study Group. Randomised trial of cholesterol lowering in 4444 patients with coronary heart disease: the Scandinavian Simvastatin Survival Study (4S). Lancet 1994;344:1383–1389.

73. The Long-Term Intervention with Pravastatin in Ischaemic Disease (LIPID) Study Group. Prevention of cardiovascular events and death with pravastatin in patients with coronary heart disease and a broad range of initial cholesterol concentrations. N Engl J Med 1998; 339:1349–1357.

74. Sacks RM, Pfeffer MA, Moye LA, et al. for the Cholesterol and Recurrent Events Trial Investigators. The effect of pravastatin on coronary events after myocardial infarction in patients with average cholesterol concentrations. N Engl J Med 1996;335:1001–1009.

75. Fonarow GC, Gawlinski A, Moughrabi S, Tillisch JH. Improved treatment of coronary heart disease by implementation of a Cardiac Hospitalization Atherosclerosis Management Program (CHAMP). Am J Cardiol 2001;87:819–822.

76. Schwartz GG, Olsson AG, Ezekowitz MD, et al. Effects of atorvastatin on early recurrent ischemic events in acute coronary syndromes: the MIRACL study: a randomized controlled trial. JAMA 2001;285:1711–1718.

77. FRISC II Investigators. Invasive compared with non-invasive treatment in unstable coronary-artery disease: FRISC II prospective randomised multicentre study. Lancet 1999;354: 708–715.

78. Cannon CP, Weintraub WS, Demopoulos LA, et al. Comparison of early invasive and conservative strategies in patients with unstable coronary syndromes treated with the glycoprotein IIb/IIIa inhibitor tirofiban. N Engl J Med 2001;344:1879–1887.

79. Boden WE, O'Rourke RA, Crawford MH, et al. Outcomes in patients with acute non-Q-wave myocardial infarction randomly assigned to an invasive as compared with a conservative management strategy. Veterans Affairs Non-Q-Wave Infarction Strategies in Hospital (VANQWISH) Trial Investigators. N Engl J Med 1998;338:1785–1792.

80. Zhao XQ, Theroux P, Snapinn SM, Sax FL. Intracoronary thrombus and platelet glycoprotein IIb/IIIa receptor blockade with tirofiban in unstable angina or non-Q-wave myocardial infarction: angiographic results from the PRISM-PLUS trial (Platelet Receptor Inhibition for Ischemic Syndrome Management in Patients Limited by Unstable Signs and Symptoms). Circulation 1999;100:1609–1615.
81. Montalescot G, Barragan P, Wittenberg O, et al. Platelet glycoprotein IIb/IIIa inhibition with coronary stenting for acute myocardial infarction. N Engl J Med 344:1895–1903.
82. Hamm CW, Heeschen C, Goldmann B, et al. Benefit of abciximab in patients with refractory unstable angina in relation to serum troponin T concentrations. c7E3 Fab Antiplatelet Therapy in Unstable Refractory Angina (CAPTURE) Study Investigators. N Engl J Med 1999;340:1623–1629.
83. O'Shea JC, Hafley GE, Greenberg S, et al. Platelet glycoprotein IIb/IIIa integrin blockade with eptifibatide in coronary stent intervention: the ESPRIT trial: a randomized controlled trial. JAMA 2001;285:2468–2473.
84. Topol EJ, Moliterno DJ, Herrmann HC, et al. Comparison of two platelet glycoprotein IIb/IIIa inhibitors, tirofiban and abciximab, for the prevention of ischemic events with percutaneous coronary revascularization. N Engl J Med 2001;344:1888–1894.
85. Moussa I, Oetgen M, Roubin G, et al. Effectiveness of clopidogrel and aspirin versus ticlopidine and aspirin in preventing stent thrombosis after coronary stent implantation. Circulation 1999;99:2364–2366.
86. Berger PB, Bell MR, Hasdai D, Grill DE, Melby S, Holmes DR, Jr. Safety and efficacy of ticlopidine for only 2 weeks after successful intracoronary stent placement. Circulation 1999;99:248–253.
87. The EPIC Investigation. Use of a monoclonal antibody directed against the platelet glycoprotein IIb/IIIa receptor in high-risk coronary angioplasty. N Engl J Med 1994;330:956–261.
88. The EPISTENT Investigators. Randomised placebo-controlled and balloon-angioplasty-controlled trial to assess safety of coronary stenting with use of platelet glycoprotein-IIb/IIIa blockade. Evaluation of Platelet IIb/IIIa Inhibitor for Stenting. Lancet 1998;352:87–92.
89. Calvin JE, Klein LW, VandenBerg BJ, et al. Risk stratification in unstable angina. Prospective validation of the Braunwald classification. JAMA 1995;273:136–141.
90. Calvin JE, Klein LW, VandenBerg EJ, Meyer P, Parrillo JE. Validated risk stratification model accurately predicts low risk in patients with unstable angina. J Am Coll Cardiol 2000; 36:1803–1808.
91. Antman EM, Cohen M, Bernink PJ, et al. The TIMI risk score for unstable angina/non-ST elevation MI: a method for prognostication and therapeutic decision making. JAMA 2000; 284:835–842.
92. Sabatine MS, Januzzi JL, Snapinn S, Theroux P, Jang I. A risk score system for predicting adverse outcomes and magnitude of benefit with glycoprotein IIb/IIIa inhibitor therapy in patients with unstable angina pectoris. Am J Cardiol 88:488–492.

3

Evolution of Cardiac Markers in Clinical Trials

Alexander S. Ro and Christopher R. deFilippi

INTRODUCTION

The use of biochemical markers has long been one of the major parameters for detecting and stratifying risk in acute coronary syndromes (ACS). In the past, however, the value of biochemical markers was limited by their rather simplistic ability to categorize patients into one of two groups—those with myocardial infarctions (MI) and those without. Their initial place in clinical trials was therefore often confined to defining specific patient populations for further testing, or they were used to diagnose strict study end points based on a binary definition of ischemic heart disease. The current ability to detect smaller quantities of myocardial cell injury with serum markers in patients who would not previously have been diagnosed with MIs led to the realization that the past perspective of ACS was incomplete. With the development of more sensitive and specific assays for detecting myocardial injury, clinicians have come to appreciate the continuous, wider spectrum of ACS as well as the dynamic influence of plaque instability (1). With newer serum markers for ischemic heart disease come the possibilities of earlier diagnosis, better assessment of clinical risk, and a more complete fundamental knowledge of what truly constitutes unstable coronary artery disease.

At present, a better understanding of the pathogenesis of ACS, coupled with the constraint of limiting medical costs in the face of significant improvement in treatments, has led physicians to attempt to target the most aggressive and expensive therapies to those patients who would most benefit from them (2). Previous study methods, based on the binary principle of "rule-in"/"rule-out" MI, relied on the electrocardiogram (ECG), clinical features, and classic biomarkers of MI (creatine kinase [CK] and MB isoenzyme of CK [CK-MB]), were not sufficient to help physicians satisfactorily accomplish this goal beyond the realm of patients who had ST-segment elevations. It is clear now that various cardiac markers can be used as harbingers of adverse outcomes and can identify where patients lie on the ACS risk continuum (3). Clinical trials have made use of this knowledge prospectively and through *post hoc* analysis to test novel and more aggressive therapies. In these trials newer cardiac markers have proven their worth as an effective means for the risk stratification of individual patients. Their evolution in clinical trials has established them as powerful tools for defining a broader patient population at risk while focusing attention on a subset of patients for whom future targeted therapies can be tested

From: *Cardiac Markers, Second Edition*
Edited by: Alan H. B. Wu @ Humana Press Inc., Totowa, NJ

and applied *(4)*. This chapter reviews the clinical data that support the use of commercially available cardiac markers to guide the management of ACS patients and discusses their potential future applications.

EARLY ROLES OF CARDIAC MARKERS

Cardiac markers have played an important role in the diagnosis and treatment of ACS for more than four decades. From the introduction of aspartate aminotransferase (AST) in 1954 *(5)* to the establishment of CK as a marker of myocardial cell injury in 1965 *(6)*, markers have been vital in helping to risk stratify patients who may otherwise have been inappropriately diagnosed. It is clear that many MIs are "silent" and patients often present without the classic symptom of chest pain. The Framingham patient population verified this and demonstrated that 25% of MIs were initially unrecognized because of absence of chest pain or because of the presence of "atypical" symptoms *(7)*. For this very reason, serum myocardial markers of injury have taken on an important role. Measurement of serum protein levels remains one of the most accurate means of diagnosing acute myocardial infarction (AMI) *(8)*.

The importance of being able to establish a diagnosis of AMI with regard to clinical trials is clear. The World Health Organization (WHO) established a definition of MI that utilized biochemical markers as one of three major criteria used to establish this diagnosis *(9)*. It defined a specific subset of patients who were at increased risk for future cardiac events. Markers have also helped to determine infarct size, which has been proved to be an important determinant for predicting increased mortality *(10,11)*. These findings had important implications for past clinical trials that focused on the treatment of ACS. They helped to establish specific negative patient end points that could hopefully be avoided with therapy, and helped to define a patient population with increased risk for whom therapy could be specifically directed and tested.

The importance of platelet aggregation and thrombus formation in the pathogenesis of unstable coronary artery disease became increasingly evident throughout the 1980s and 1990s *(12,13)*. Experimental animal models suggested a major role for platelets and platelet-derived thromboxane A_2 in ACS *(14)*. To define further the clinical usefulness of therapies directed against these factors, numerous controlled clinical trials were required *(15–19)*. The primary and specific role that cardiac enzymes played during these earlier studies, which involved aspirin, heparin, and thrombolytics, was identifying MI as a negative study end point in the treatment of unstable coronary syndromes.

A more interesting observation is, however, the manner by which these markers were used to define specific patient populations for study. A minority of early studies actually used markers as exclusion criteria for patient selection *(15–17)*. By doing so, investigators attempted to focus solely on a group of patients who could be labeled as having unstable angina (UA). Separate studies were then required for patients who would eventually rule-in for MI from serial enzyme measurements. While attempting to determine which therapies would most benefit this subgroup of patients, investigators became increasingly aware that ACS were on a continuum rather than a binary phenomenon *(18,19)*.

In 1988, Theroux et al. published a study exemplifying the above points. They evaluated the usefulness of heparin and aspirin in the setting of UA *(17)*. Using a typical population of patients hospitalized with UA, the study set out to determine the efficacy of aspirin, intravenous heparin, or a combination of the two. Each patient was, however, required to have a CK level less than twice the upper limit of normal, which effectively eliminated those who might have ruled-in for MI at presentation. MI as a study end point was defined as a new doubling of CK levels from baseline in addition to having an abnormally elevated CK-MB fraction. Findings indicated reduced incidence of MI in all groups compared to placebo at 6 ± 3 d.

Because the diagnosis of AMI was usually made retrospectively, it was often necessary to lump patients with UA and non-ST elevation myocardial infarctions (NSTEMI) together at presentation. It is not surprising therefore that the literature was flooded with studies of patients with NSTEMI, UA, or a variable mixture of the two *(1)*. While these initial trials were underway, other investigators were slowly demonstrating that the pathogenic mechanisms of NSTEMI and UA were very similar *(12,13)*. Findings from angiographic studies looking at the morphology of suspected responsible lesions were similar for both groups *(20)*. It was subsequently suggested that plaque disruption was a common link between both syndromes *(21)*. Given the fact that aspirin and heparin had previously been shown to decrease the mortality of patients with UA *(15–17)*, it was logical that these therapies would eventually be applied directly to patients with NSTEMIs.

Two studies, the Research Group on Instability in Coronary Artery Disease (RISC) study *(18)* and the Antithrombotic Therapy in Acute Coronary Syndromes Research Group (ATACS) trial *(19)*, demonstrate this dynamic. In an effort to define further the role of heparin and aspirin in ACS, these studies were initiated with the intent of including both UA patients and NSTEMI patients. The RISC study eventually enrolled 796 patients, approx 50% of whom qualified as having a NSTEMI at enrollment based on the WHO criteria for AMI. Results showed the usefulness of 75 mg a day of aspirin for reducing adverse event rates at 3 mo *(18)*. The ATACS trial was initiated in the wake of trends seen in the RISC study, which suggested a positive benefit from treatment prolonged past the acute hospital phase. Again, UA patients and NSTEMI patients were included in the study. Large reductions in total ischemic events were revealed in the combination group of aspirin with long-term anticoagulation compared with the aspirin-alone group *(19)*.

The ultimate value of both of these studies was the *post hoc* analysis of their data to evaluate these treatments in the specific subgroups of UA and NSTEMI diagnosed at presentation. In the RISC study population, it was determined that aspirin was equally as effective in preventing events in UA patients and in NSTEMI patients. In the ATACS trial, 46 of the 214 patients enrolled qualified for the NSTEMI diagnosis retrospectively. Of the patients treated with aspirin alone, 32% had an event compared to 17% of patients treated with the combination of aspirin and anticoagulation at 14 d. This difference paralleled a trend seen in the UA group. On the basis of these findings it was becoming evident that the definition of NSTEMI relying on CK and CK-MB elevations had a limited ability to differentiate patients into high-risk groups who might ultimately benefit from therapy.

CARDIAC MARKERS IN TRIALS
OF NEWER TREATMENT MODALITIES

With substantial morbidity and mortality persistently associated with UA and NSTEMI, along with early invasive protocols under debate *(22,23)*, clinicians turned their attention to promising novel medical treatment modalities that might prove more useful than heparin or aspirin. In particular, low-molecular-weight heparin (LMWH) theoretically offered a targeted treatment against clot propagation that could prove useful for patients with ACS *(24)*. Promising results from a pilot study *(25)* prompted investigators to test further the usefulness of LMWH for patients spanning the continuum of unstable coronary disease. Cardiac markers were again used in the diagnosis of NSTEMI so as to enroll patients who were putatively at higher risk than traditional UA patients (Table 1).

The Fragmin during Instability in Coronary Artery Disease I (FRISC I) study *(26),* the Fragmin in Unstable Coronary Artery Disease (FRIC) study *(27)*, and the Efficacy and Safety of Subcutaneous Enoxaparin in Non-Q-Wave Coronary Events (ESSENCE) trial *(28)* helped to establish the effectiveness of LMWHs in the setting of ACS. Subgroup analysis of the FRISC I study revealed that the beneficial effects of dalteparin at 40 d seemed to be confined primarily to the 80% of the study population who were smokers and to those who qualified for the study with a diagnosis of NSTEMI. This was one of the first studies published to indicate that cardiac markers could effectively define a subgroup of ACS patients who could specifically benefit from a particular treatment *(26)*.

The development of platelet glycoprotein IIb/IIIa receptor inhibitors (GP IIb/IIIa inhibitors) offered the possibility of an even more directed means of stabilizing the unstable coronary plaques and thrombi that are the etiology of unstable coronary syndromes *(29)*. With hopes of expanding the clinical role of GP IIb/IIIa inhibitors, Theroux and colleagues tested the use of lamifiban, a synthetic low-molecular-weight nonpeptide compound *(30)*. Two important observations were made at the end of the study. For one, patients with NSTEMI at enrollment had poorer outcomes than those labeled with UA (death or MI/recurrent MI in 11.4% of 44 patients with NSTEMI vs 4.4% of 321 patients with UA). Second, although not statistically significant because of the small sample, patients with NSTEMI at admission appeared to receive a more beneficial effect from higher doses of lamifiban than patients in the UA subgroup (reduction from 18.8% to 4.8% for NSTEMI patients; reduction from 6.5% to 2.1% for UA patients).

UNSTABLE ANGINA REDEFINED

The WHO definition of MI, utilizing CK and CK-MB values, is prevalent throughout the literature described above. It has proved to be an effective means of stratifying patients into a high-risk group as well as defining specific end points for the testing of various treatments. The limitations of the WHO criteria for diagnosing MI become evident as greater insight into the pathophysiology of ACS became available *(12,13,20,21)*. Although the WHO definition clearly made the distinction between equivocal and unequivocal diagnoses of MI by delineating the required pattern of the rise and fall of serial serum levels *(9)*, how a rise and fall were defined varied between studies, limiting the aggregate meaningfulness of their findings. Furthermore, this early binary stratification failed to identify a gradient of risk among patients classified as having UA. It is not surprising therefore that for some time the literature remained confusing and often contradictory regarding the significance of detectable marker levels.

Various investigators have attempted to risk stratify patients into predefined subgroups, such as age, sex, characterization of pain, and other comorbidities. ST alterations on ECG at presentation have long been known to predict higher frequencies of future cardiac events *(31,32)*. Synthesizing years of clinical data, in 1989 Braunwald proposed a clinical classification for UA *(33)*. The Braunwald classification scheme depended on three factors: severity of symptoms, clinical circumstances, and ECG findings. In

Table 1
Cardiac Markers (CK, CK-MB) to Differentiate Patients at Risk and Define Outcomes in Trials of Newer Treatment modalities (LMWH)

Study—year	n	Treatment	Admission MI defined	Endpoint MI defined	Results	NSTEMI vs UA
Gurfinkel et al.—1995 (26)	219	Aspirin vs aspirin + heparin vs aspirin + nadroparin	N/A—acute MI excluded	1, MB > 50 IU/L	50% reduction of in-hospital recurrent angina for nadroparin	N/A
FRISC study group—1996 (27)	1506	Daltaparin vs placebo	Retrospective classification based on markers, $n = 572$	1, 2.	Reduction in composite endpoint of death/MI/ urgent revascularization at 6 and 40 d	Beneficial effect of daltaparin at 40 d primarily seen in patients with MI as qualifying event
ESSENCE—1997 (29)	3171	Enoxaparin vs UFH	1, CK > 2× normal, and elevated MB at least 3% total CK	Same as admit, post PCI MI defined as 1 or CK > 3× nl or > 50% previous nadir	Reduction in cumulative 14- and 30-d event rates of death/MI/ recurrent angina (16.6% vs 19.8%, $p = 0.019$)	N/A
FRIC study group—1997 (28)	1482	Daltaparin vs UFH	New Q waves excluded, patients with subsequent biochemical evidence remained eligible (16%)	1, 2 (CK-MB above nl or total CK > 2× nl)	No significant difference between either treatment group at 6 and 45 d	Event rates similar in both treatment groups regardless of Dx of UA or NSTEMI
TIMI 11B—1999 (60)	3910	Enoxaparin vs UFH	1 or Elevated MB (≥3% total CK) or total CK > 2× nl	1 or elevated MB (≥50% previous value) or ↑ CK (≥ 2× nl and ≥ 25% previous value) or ↑ CK ≥ 50% previous value. Post PCI MI defined as CK-MB ≥ 3× nl and > 50% previous value	Benefit from enoxaparin for reducing death/MI/ urgent revascularization through 43 d (17.3% vs 19.7%, $p = 0.048$)	UA showed more of a trend in favor of enoxaparin at 14 d than NSTEMI

1 = New Q waves on ECG; 2 = 2 of 3 (chest pain, ECG changes, rise in biochemical markers).

1994, national guidelines refined these definitions *(34)*, assigning patients to one of three appropriate risk groups (low, intermediate, and high) in an attempt to initiate targeted therapy as well as to determine appropriate follow-up care. A growing emphasis was placed on the need to suppress ischemia early and aggressively in high-risk groups and it was becoming increasingly important to determine which patients would be most appropriately targeted for therapy. Most pertinent to this discussion is that Braunwald's definition and subsequent guidelines provided a precise basis for enrolling patients into future clinical trials.

The Braunwald classification system has subsequently been validated in numerous clinical trials, including a high correlation with the severity of underlying disease as determined by angiography *(35)*. In addition, the concept of risk stratifying unstable coronary patients further was supported by growing evidence that UA, NSTEMI, and ST elevation MIs (STEMI) were all linked to abrupt reductions in coronary blood flow of varying degrees *(12,13,21)*. This reduction was likely caused by a dynamic and repetitive process of atherosclerotic plaque disruption leading to thrombus formation made up of varied amounts of erythrocytes, fibrin, and platelets *(12,13,21)*. These early guidelines placed only modest emphasis on the use of biomarkers to assist in the risk stratification of UA. This position reflected the limitations of technology and limitations in understanding the complexities of ACS at the time.

THE EVOLVING ROLE OF CK-MB

Until recently and since the 1960s, the CK-MB isoenzyme level has been considered to be the "gold standard" for making the diagnosis of AMI. Historically it has been measured by electrophoresis and enzymatic analysis with reference intervals dependent on the methods used. For activity-based assays (electrophoresis and column chromatography) the upper limit of normal (ULN) ranged between 10 and 20 U/L. For immunoassays (mass measurements) the ULN usually ranged between 5 and 10 ng/mL. Once the CK-MB assay was optimized via monoclonal antibodies, it became the standard for biochemical assessment of myocardial injury *(36)*. Typically, however, diagnosis of AMI required not only elevated CK-MB levels, but also elevated CK levels greater than one to two times the ULN *(8)*. These standards have been in place and have served physicians for nearly three decades.

Working from arguments in favor of developing better risk stratifying tools, investigators focused their attention on the clinical significance of elevated CK and CK-MB levels that fell outside the standard WHO criteria for defining MI. Minimal elevations of CK-MB in the setting of UA had been known to occur for years, but its pathogenesis and significance remained unknown. Investigators during the past 20 yr have thus evaluated the significance of CK-MB elevations in the absence of total CK elevation and in the setting of UA. These studies span the evolution of the assays' abilities to measure CK-MB and subsequent improvement in their accuracy for the detection of this marker *(37–43)*. The message is remarkably consistent: minor elevations of CK-MB in the setting of UA portend an increased risk of subsequent MI and death (Table 2).

The clinical usefulness of the above findings was tested most definitively in a subanalysis of the Platelet Glycoprotein IIb/IIIa in Unstable Angina: Receptor Suppression Using Integrilin Therapy (PURSUIT) trial *(43,44)*. The purpose of the original study was to evaluate prospectively the efficacy of eptifibatide (Integrilin) for up to 72 h for patients presenting with ACS. All enrolled patients either had ECG changes consistent with ischemia or serum CK-MB levels elevated above normal values. Results showed a 1.5% absolute reduction in the primary event of death or MI/recurrent MI at 96 h (14.2% vs 15.7%). The observed benefits persisted for 30 d. There was an even larger risk reduction for patients who eventually had angioplasty *(44)*.

Following this original publication came a retrospective analysis designed to determine if the prognostic significance of CK-MB elevation was comparable with results from the studies described above *(43)*. Eight hundred and twenty-five patients with ACS, but without ST elevations on ECG, were followed up for outcomes for 30 d and 6 mo, and the findings were that peak elevation of CK-MB strongly correlated with mortality. In addition, the data showed that the increased risk began when marker levels rose just above the ULN. This finding was based on the observation of a trend for worse outcomes even for those patients who exhibited levels just one to two times greater than normal values. Because increased risk was independent from pharmacologic treatment and was the same for patients who received eptifibatide or placebo, the implication was that CK-MB levels alone could not specifically define a subset of patients who would most benefit from eptifibatide treatment. This finding would prove to be consistent in future studies of treatment with GP IIb/IIIa inhibitors.

TROPONINS

Although the clinical usefulness of minor elevations of CK and CK-MB continued to be investigated in the setting of ACS, more questions were arising than answers supplied. For one, with the availability of more accurate assays, CK-MB demonstrated less specificity for myocardial injury than once believed. False-positives were caused by muscle disease, alcohol, diabetes mellitus, trauma, exercise, and convulsions. The number of false-positives could be effectively decreased by raising discriminator levels, but at the expense of identifying fewer patients with minor myocardial injuries. The ability of CK-MB to risk stratify patients further with UA thus hit a biologic ceiling. In efforts to overcome the limitations inherent in assessing CK-MB, the focus changed to newer serum biomarkers that were potentially more specific for myocardial injury.

To this end, in 1989 cardiac troponin T (cTnT) was introduced *(45)*, followed by cardiac troponin I (cTnI) in 1992 *(46)*, initially as a complementary biochemical means of detecting AMIs. The troponins are three distinct proteins that play an important role in the actin–myosin interaction of muscle contraction and relaxation. The cardiac isoforms for cTnT and cTnI are encoded on different genes than their skeletal muscle counterparts *(47)*. Combined with detection by sensitive and specific immunoassays, measurements of cTnT and cTnI provided the ability to differentiate myocardial injury from skeletal muscle injury, whereas CK and CK-MB measurement had fallen short of this goal *(48)*.

The significance of being able to detect smaller quantities of myocardial cell necrosis has challenged researchers and clinicians alike to rethink what truly constitutes an MI. Development of highly sensitive markers has shown that irreversible damage occurs beyond the parameters of an MI as defined by traditional WHO criteria *(47)*. This finding had previously been confirmed by pathologic studies of patients with UA who died suddenly *(49)*. The myriad of trials that followed confirmed the ability of the cardiac troponins to define a group of patients with increased risk for future cardiac events *(4)*.

Table 2
Studies of the Prognostic Significance of Minor Elevations of CK-MB in ACS Patients

Study—year	n	CK-MB criteria	Assay	Outcomes
White et al. —1985 (37)	244	Uncertain AMI defined as CK-MB range of 1–24 IU/L ($n = 22$)	Agarose gel electrophoresis	One-year cardiac mortality rate similar to those patients with AMI
Hong et al. —1986 (38)	347	Normal CK levels but elevated CK-MB% ≥ 5% total CK with typical enzyme curves ($n = 40$)	Agarose gel electrophoresis	Increased incidence of major CHF, in-hospital mortality, and longer hospitalizations
Markenvard et al. —1992 (39)	101	CK-MB between 10 and 20 ng/mL, "gray zone" ($n = 29$)	Enzyme immunoinhibition	Significantly higher risk of developing an AMI or requiring revascularization at 6 mo
Ravkilde et al. —1992 (40)	156	Negative MI by WHO criteria but "changing" CK-MB levels as determined by statistical variance of serial measurements ($n = 24$)	Enzyme immunoinhibiton	Significantly worse outcomes than for patients with stable CK-MB levels out to 30 mo
Pettersson —1992 (41)	102	No traditional evidence for AMI but increases in CK-MB defined as a 1.5- to 2.0-fold increase between 2 adjacent samples ($n = 14$)	Enzyme immunoinhibition	50% mortality rate at 1 yr
Lloyd Jones et al. —1999 (42)	595	Elevated MB relative index but normal CK levels ($n = 263$)	Monoclonal antibody based immunoassay	One-year mortality rate intermediate between NSTEMI and ST elevation MI
Alexander et al. —2000 (43)	8250	At least one CK-MB sample collected during index hospitalization	Enzyme immunoinhibition	Increased risk of mortality at 30 d begins with CK-MB levels just above normal—1–2 times upper limit of normal (1.8% vs 3.3%, $p < 0.001$)

By providing improved risk stratification, and helping effectively target therapy in ways that CK and CK-MB had failed to, it became clear that sensitive detection of minor myocardial necrosis was as, if not more, important than the ability to establish the traditional diagnosis of AMI.

Hamm and colleagues, in their landmark study in 1992, identified the prognostic ability of cardiac troponins to predict subsequent adverse cardiac events for patients with the diagnosis of UA *(50)*. Observing 109 patients, they showed that cTnT levels ≥ 0.2 ng/mL were associated with worse outcomes during hospitalization. Ten out of 33 of these patients (30%) had subsequent MIs, compared with 1 of 51 patients without cTnT elevations ($p < 0.001$). Four years after Hamm's initial publication, two large multicenter studies confirmed the observations of Hamm and those from earlier small trials of assessing cTnT for risk stratification *(51,52)*.

Blood samples taken within 2 h of enrollment from 855 patients, enrolled in the Global Use of Strategies to Open Occluded Coronary Arteries in Acute Coronary Syndromes (GUSTO IIA) study, were analyzed to evaluate the prognostic ability of early cTnT and CK-MB compared with results from the ECG *(51)*. This was a randomized trial of recombinant hirudin, the prototypical direct thrombin inhibitor, vs standard heparin. There was a significant difference in 30-d mortality for the 289 patients with cTnT levels > 0.1 ng/mL vs patients with lower cTnT values (11.8% vs 3.9%, $p < 0.001$). A multivariate analysis confirmed that a cTnT level could better differentiate the risk of cardiac death than CK-MB level or ECG findings.

The FRISC I study also compared the prognostic utility of cTnT with the clinical risk indicators available at that time *(52,53)*. For a subset of patients ($n = 976$) from the original FRISC I population, blood samples obtained at enrollment were analyzed and correlated with events at 5 and 36 mo follow-up. A cTnT level > 0.06 ng/mL remained an independent predictor of cardiac death during long-term follow-up (Fig. 1) *(53)*. cTnT remained an independent prognostic indicator.

Similar results were found by measuring cTnI levels. In a retrospective study of serum samples taken from patients on presentation in the Thrombolysis in Myocardial Infarction (TIMI) IIIB study, cTnI was identified as an excellent risk stratifier of adverse cardiac outcomes in ACS patients *(54)*. At 42 d, patients with cTnI levels ≥ 0.4 ng/mL had higher mortality rates than patients without levels ≥ 0.4 ng/mL (3.7% vs 1.0%, $p < 0.001$). As with cTnT levels, this result was independent from baseline clinical and ECG characteristics. The ability of both cTnT and cTnI levels to risk stratify patients with ACS has recently been summarized in a meta-analysis (Table 3) *(4)*.

Moving beyond the traditional ACS patient enrolled in clinical trials on the basis of clinical or ECG criteria, several studies extended the prognostic utility of troponins. One study includes a broad cohort of patients seen in the emergency department (ED) with chest pain and considered to be low risk by established clinical indicators. Hamm et al. found that rapid qualitative bedside testing of both cTnT and cTnI provided strong independent prognostication of 30-d cardiac events in this heterogeneous group *(55)*. Only one patient with a negative cTnT result at presentation and 4 h later had a cardiac event within 2 wk. No patient with an MI was inappropriately discharged home. This was one of the first studies that allowed troponin levels to be immediately available to practicing ED physicians. deFilippi et al. studied the prognostic role of cTnT for chest pain patients sent exclusively to "low-risk" chest pain observation units *(56)*. Patients

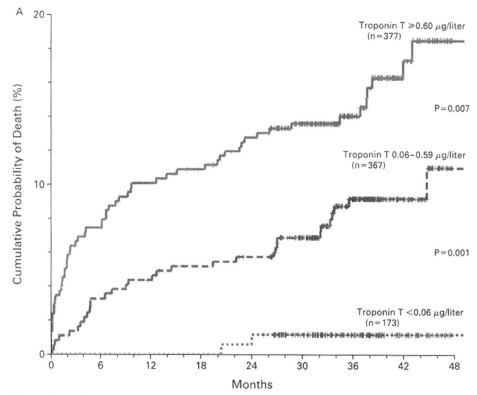

Fig. 1. Cumulative probability of death from cardiac causes in relation to maximal cTnT levels during the first 24 h after enrollment. The long-term results of the FRISC I study. (Reproduced with permission from the Massachusetts Medical Society, N Engl J Med 2000;343:1142.)

with cTnT > 0.1 ng/mL (9% of patients) had increased cardiac events (death, MI, re-presentation with UA) after as long as 1 yr (32.4% vs 12.8%). Furthermore, despite the initial low clinical risk, angiography, which was routinely performed in cTnT-positive patients, revealed multivessel disease in 63% and complex morphology in 51%. Kontos et al., using cTnI as part of a rapid 8-h protocol in the ED, found that a level >2.0 ng/mL indicated an increased incidence of future complications, including MI, at 1 wk and death at 5 wk *(57)*. This finding still held for patients without ischemic ECG changes.

ROLE OF TROPONINS FURTHER DEFINED

By the late 1990s, the prognostic abilities of cardiac troponin measurements in patients presenting with signs and symptoms suggestive of ACS were no longer debated. This change of attitude is reflected by the incorporation of troponin results into the original Braunwald UA classification scheme in the year 2000 *(58)*. Furthermore, angiographic data supported the concept that cardiac troponin elevation in this setting was associated with a high prevalence of high-risk angiographic features, including complex lesion morphology, visible thrombus, and multivessel coronary artery disease *(56,59)*. Troponins were therefore increasingly interpreted as downstream markers of unstable intracoronary atherosclerotic plaques, thrombus formation, distal embolization, and subsequent myocyte cell death.

Table 3
Summary Results for Troponin and Mortality

	Troponin T		Troponin I	
	Clinical trials	Cohort studies	Clinical trials	Cohort studies
Total patients	2904	2255	4912	1491
Mean age (yr)	64	60	63	63
Male (%)	68	66	69	69
Troponin-positive (%)	40	21	33	23
Death rate, troponin-positive (%)	3.8	11.6	4.8	8.4
Death rate troponin-negative (%)	1.3	1.7	2.1	0.7
Medial follow-up (wk)	4	18	4	8
Summary OR (95% CI)	3.0	5.1	2.6	8.5
	(1.6–5.50)	(3.2–8.4)	(1.8–3.6)[a]	(3.5–21.1)[a]
Study heterogeneity p value	0.28	0.11	0.28	0.16

[a]p = 0.01 for difference between trial and nontrial troponin I results; a p value < 0.05 indicates significant heterogeneity between trials in the mortality odds ratio for a positive troponin. CI, confidence interval; OR, odds ratio. (Adapted from ref. *4.*)

In the absence of persistent ST elevation, dichotomizing MI from non-MI patients using previous standards seemed less clinically meaningful. This led the professional societies of both laboratorians and cardiologists to incorporate cardiac troponin values into new definitions of AMI *(60,61)*. It was, however, the clinical studies leading up to these revisions as well as the trials that followed where the troponins would prove their value beyond risk stratification and triage of patients. To accomplish what biochemical cardiac markers had never effectively demonstrated, the troponins could target patients for increasingly specific and aggressive therapies. As a consequence, the standard of care for ACS would require revisions once again *(2)*.

In 1997 a retrospective analysis of the FRISC-I study of dalteparin vs placebo was published that created interest for using troponins to identify ACS patients who could benefit from a specific antithrombotic treatment *(62)*. Patients with cTnT levels < 0.1 ng/mL showed no difference in benefit from dalteparin compared to placebo with regard to cardiac death or MI during 40 d of active treatment (4.7% vs 5.7%). In contrast, patients with levels ≥ 0.1 ng/mL demonstrated a significant reduction in adverse events from dalteparin treatment (7.4% vs 14.2%, $p < 0.01$) (Fig. 2).

Attempting to examine further the usefulness of LMWHs for ACS on the basis of trends established by the FRISC I trial, the TIMI 11B trial tested the acute and long-term use of enoxaparin vs unfractionated heparin (UFH) in 3910 patients with UA or NSTEMI *(63)*. In a subanalysis of 359 CK-MB negative patients, elevated cTnI levels (>0.1 ng/mL) measured within 24 h of enrollment were predictive of a risk reduction for the combined end point of death/MI/urgent revascularization at 14 d for patients treated with enoxaparin vs UFH (21% vs 40%, $p = 0.007$). In contrast, for patients without cTnI elevation ($n = 179$) there was no difference in outcomes based on enoxaparin vs UFH (9% vs 6%, p = NS for death, MI, urgent revascularization) *(64)*.

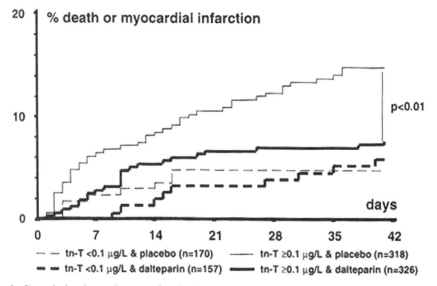

Fig. 2. Cumulative hazard curves for death or MI in patients with and without dalteparin treatment and with and without elevation of troponin T (tn-T). (Reproduced with permission from the American College of Cardiology 1997;29:47.)

In addition to LMWHs, GP IIb/IIIa platelet inhibitors were attracting considerable attention for the treatment of non-ST elevation ACS. The significance of findings in this heterogeneous population, although positive for the use of these agents, was at times less than overwhelming *(44,65–67)*. With considerable insight into the mechanism of troponin elevation in this setting, Hamm and Heeschen evaluated the role of troponins to potentially identify patients who would derive maximal efficacy with these potent platelet inhibitors. Their retrospective analysis of two major GP IIb/IIIa inhibitor ACS trials set the stage for routine use of cardiac troponins to direct early therapy in ACS *(68,69)*.

The c7E3 AntiPlatelet Therapy in Unstable Refractory Angina (CAPTURE) study was designed to determine the efficacy of abciximab (a monoclonal Fab fragment that binds to the activated GP IIb/IIIa platelet receptor) infusion before and during single-vessel angioplasty with a suitable culprit lesion in the setting of UA refractory to medical management *(65)*. Specifically, the study enrolled patients with evidence of recurrent myocardial ischemia despite appropriate initial treatment with heparin and nitrates. Each patient had a suitable target stenosis at angiography and was scheduled for coronary angioplasty 18–24 h after presentation. Patients were randomized to receive abciximab or placebo along with heparin after the initial diagnostic catheterization through 1 h after intervention. The primary difference seen for patients receiving abciximab vs placebo was the reduction of MI/death/urgent revascularization at 30 d (11.3% vs 15.9%, $p = 0.012$). At 6 mo follow-up, however, there was no difference in outcome.

A follow-up analysis evaluated the serum samples from 890 of the 1265 enrolled patients *(68)*. Patients with cTnT ≥ 0.1 ng/mL at the time of enrollment had a dramatic reduction in occurrence of MI or death when treated with abciximab vs placebo for as long as 6 mo posttreatment (9.5% vs 23.9%, $p = 0.002$). In contrast, patients with cTnT levels below this cutoff level showed no difference in outcomes based on assigned treat-

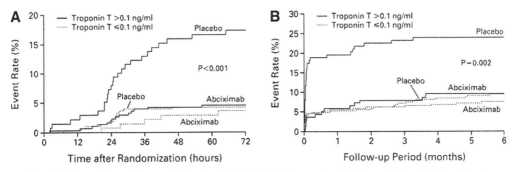

Fig. 3. Rates of cardiac events in the initial 72 h after randomization (**A**) and during the 6 mo of follow-up (**B**) among patients with serum cTnT levels above and those with levels below the diagnostic cutoff point. Cardiac events were death and nonfatal MI. Percutaneous transluminal coronary angioplasty was performed 18–24 h after randomization. (Reproduced with permission from the Massachusetts Medical Society, N Engl J Med 1999;340:1626.)

ment (Fig. 3). Of note, although an elevated CK-MB level did prove to be a significant predictor of events at all time periods, it did not distinguish the specific patients who derived benefit from abciximab.

A retrospective analysis of troponin values in the Platelet Receptor Inhibition in Ischemic Syndrome Management (PRISM) study *(69)* followed the lead of the CAPTURE study. This study investigated the role of tirofiban (a nonpeptide small molecule competitive inhibitor of the platelet GP IIb/IIIa receptor) vs UFH in a more diverse patient population presenting with probable signs and symptoms of ACS. In the overall study there was a modest, but significant, reduction in the risk of death at 30 d in those treated with tirofiban vs heparin (2.3% vs 3.6%, $p = 0.02$). Serum samples were available for 2200 of 3200 patients at the time of enrollment (a mean of 8 h after symptom onset). Both cTnI and cTnT samples were analyzed and an outcomes analysis similar to the CAPTURE study was performed. The investigators were able to confirm the prognostic abilities of troponins, and they also showed a significant reduction in the risk of death and MI in the troponin-positive patients treated with tirofiban. No such effect was seen in troponin-negative patients. Results were similar for both cTnT and cTnI. Finally, consistent with the CAPTURE study findings, CK-MB levels were unable to differentiate patients who would or would not benefit from treatment with tirofiban vs heparin.

PROSPECTIVE USE OF TROPONIN TO GUIDE THERAPY

The concept of detecting minimal myocardial damage as a harbinger of continued plaque instability appeared to be a legitimate argument for using troponins as a means of triaging patients and delivering care in the ACS population. Measurement of cardiac troponins provided accurate detection of minor amounts of irreversible myocardial injury, whereas previous serum markers and clinical risk factors had fallen short of this goal. As surrogates of plaque instability, they could also clearly define which patients benefited most from aggressive anticoagulant therapies. The next logical step was to validate these findings via large prospective clinical trials for which troponin levels could serve as inclusion criteria for enrollment.

FRISC II was one of the first large clinical trials to use this prospective approach *(70)*. Seeking to determine the optimum treatment duration for LMWH in a high-risk ACS population, investigators used cTnT level as a criterion for enrollment. They analyzed 2267 patients who had symptoms of ischemia that raised the suspicion of ACS. Ischemia had to be verified by ECG findings or by raised biochemical marker levels, either CK-MB or cTnT. Overall, approx 60% of the patients entered in the study had an elevated cTnT > 0.1 ng/mL.

A simultaneous arm of the FRISC II trial, using the same inclusion criteria, compared a routine invasive vs an initial noninvasive treatment strategy in ACS *(71)*. This was the first major study to identify that patients undergoing an invasive strategy (the majority having angiography within 7 d) had a decreased incidence of death and MI compared to those treated conservatively (angiography only for evidence of spontaneous or inducible ischemia). Whereas this alone was a remarkable finding, further stratification determined that only patients with cTnT levels > 0.03 ng/mL were those who benefited from an early invasive strategy *(72)*. FRISC II prospectively validated the concept that troponin measurements could be used to identify high-risk patients and demonstrated that cardiac troponin measurements could guide ACS patients to the most beneficial nonpharmacologic treatments.

This hypothesis was recently confirmed by the TIMI-18 (Treat Angina with Aggrastat and determine Cost of Therapy with an Invasive or Conservative Strategy [TACTICS]) trial *(73)*. For this prospective study of 2220 patients with non-ST elevation ACS, elevated cardiac troponin levels sufficed for study entry. All patients received tirofiban and heparin. In addition, patients were randomly assigned to receive an early invasive intervention (4–24 h to angiography) or to be treated more conservatively. Once again, patients assigned to an early invasive strategy had a lower incidence of death and MI at 6 mo compared with patients who were initially treated conservatively (7.3% vs 9.5%, $p < 0.05$).

Characteristics that further identified patients who benefited from this early invasive approach included ST-segment depression (16.4% vs 26.3%, $p = 0.006$) and a value for cTnT >0.01 ng/mL (14.3% vs 24.2%, $p < 0.001$). This latter finding was particularly intriguing, as it suggested clinical relevance for the detection of myocardial injury with cTnT levels 10 times lower than levels traditionally used for the cutoff to diagnose ACS. In addition, cTnI results (Bayer Diagnostics, Tarrytown, NY) based on a cutoff of 0.1 ng/mL (lower limit of detection 0.03 ng/mL) provided efficacy similar to that of cTnT (Fig. 4) *(74)*. Ultimately, even more sensitive means of detecting myocardial injury or plaque rupture will likely play important roles in the future treatment of ACS.

A prospective approach to the use of cardiac troponin measurement has also been applied in studies involving GP IIb/IIIa inhibitors. Newby et al. prospectively evaluated the role of cTnT for risk stratification in Platelet IIb/IIIa Antagonism for the Reduction of Acute Coronary Syndrome Events in a Global Organization Network (PARAGON B) *(75)*, a placebo-controlled trial to test the efficacy of the small-molecule GP IIb/IIIa inhibitor lamifiban in 1160 patients with non-ST elevation ACS. Their initial hypothesis, based on prior retrospective analyses of pharmacologic studies detailed above, was that patients with cTnT elevation would have a greater treatment effect with the study drug compared to placebo. Entry criteria were similar to FRISC II and TACTICS. For the 40.2% of patients who had cTnT levels ≥ 0.1 ng/mL, there was a significant reduc-

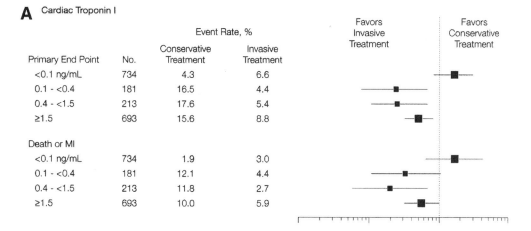

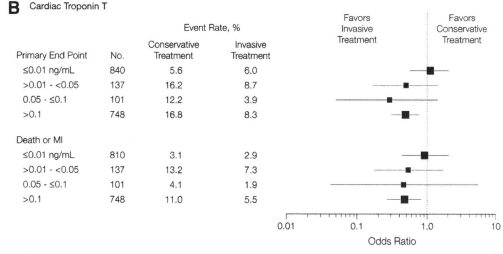

Fig. 4. Benefit of an early invasive vs conservative management strategy through 30 d strati-fied by baseline concentrations of cTnI and cTnT. (Reproduced with permission from the Ameri-can Medical Association, JAMA 2001;286:2419.)

tion in the primary end point of MI or death at 30 d (19.4% to 11.0%, $p = 0.01$) with lamifiban vs placebo. In contrast, this beneficial effect was not seen in cTnT-negative patients (11.2% to 10.8%, $p = 0.86$). Overall, combining the cTnT-positive and -nega-tive groups resulted in no overall benefit of lamifiban vs placebo.

It was evident that ACS studies incorporating either a retrospective or prospective analysis of troponins demonstrated remarkable consistency in identifying patients who would ultimately benefit from specific therapies. This was true whether the treatment was an antithrombotic therapy, an antiplatelet therapy, or a revascularization strategy. In 2001, however, publication of the GUSTO IV trial presented a challenge to the use-fulness of troponin measurement for guiding therapy for ACS patients *(76)*. Using a patient population that included selection on the basis of cTnT >0.1 ng/mL, patients were randomized to placebo, abciximab for 24 h, or abciximab for 48 h. Of the 7800 patients enrolled, 1000 qualified via elevated troponin levels alone. All patients received aspirin and either UFH or LMWH. Despite this aggressive treatment protocol, study results were unlike those in the CAPTURE trial with abciximab or with those from the other GP IIb/IIIa trials discussed earlier.

For both abciximab regimens, patients received no benefit above that seen in the placebo group for the risk of MI and death at 30 d. Furthermore, analysis using cTnT levels drawn from all patients at enrollment, showed no benefit from treatment in the subgroup with elevated levels. Several hypotheses have been proposed to explain the negative results of this trial. These include suboptimal dosing regimens, differences in local and core laboratory troponin measurements, infrequent use of coronary revascularization (2% vs 100% in the CAPTURE study), and selection of patients who were inherently at very low risk of a poor outcome. Regardless of the reasons for the negative results of this study, the GUSTO IV trial forced all clinicians to rethink how most appropriately to use troponins and GP IIb/IIIa inhibitors in the setting of ACS.

UNSTABLE ANGINA/MI REDEFINED

The role that cardiac markers played in the preceding studies helped redefine unstable coronary syndromes and the manner by which we approach them. In 2000, Braunwald revised his classification of UA to include the use of troponins, suggesting that these markers could act as surrogates for thrombus formation to effectively guide aggressive antiplatelet/antithrombotic therapy *(58)*. In conjunction with this recommendation, the American College of Cardiology/American Heart Association guidelines for unstable angina/NSTEMI made clear recommendations that biochemical markers of cardiac injury should be measured in all patients who present with chest discomfort consistent with ACS, and that cardiac-specific troponin is the preferred marker. In addition, they recommended that a platelet GP IIb/IIIa receptor antagonist should be administered, along with aspirin and UFH, to patients with continued ischemia or with high-risk features, which includes patients with elevated troponin levels *(2)*. The optimal cutoff for the various troponin assays remains to be defined.

Along similar lines, the profile of MI was also redefined to reflect the increased capacity of the cardiac troponins to detect accurately small quantities of myocardial necrosis. Both the National Academy of Clinical Biochemistry *(60)* and the European Society of Cardiology/American College of Cardiology *(61)* recently recommended that increased troponin concentrations become part of the accepted definition for AMI. The impact that these new definitions of MI will have on clinical trials is quite clear. As CK and CK-MB were often used in the past for defining clinical end points based on their ability to diagnose MIs, troponins will likely become the standard for defining the end points of future studies.

There are still obvious questions and debates about issues that need to be addressed. Many clinicians feel that although elevations in cardiac troponin values may indicate cardiac injury, they are not synonymous with MI *(77)*. Moreover, the definition proposed by the European and American societies of cardiology sets a standard (greater than the 99th percentile of normal) that is well below the current clinical cutoffs for all troponin assays and challenges the low-end accuracy of most commercial assays *(78)*. In addition, there are uncertainties regarding the appropriate timing for collecting samples, as well as a need for a standardization of cTnI assays *(79)*. This is extremely important from a clinical trials perspective. Ideally, data would be presented so that the patients included and the clinical end points obtained can be translated from one study to another, thus facilitating exchange of meaningful information *(61)*.

Finally, it should be noted that the absence of troponin elevations identifies a lower risk group, but not necessarily a low-risk group *(80)*. Although further refinements of commercial troponin assays will inevitably improve their low-end accuracy, there ultimately may be limitations to the clinical utility of identifying myocyte cell death. What the next direction will be for cardiac markers is not yet certain, but preliminary evidence for markers that can detect coronary artery plaque instability *(81)*, cardiac neurohormonal activation *(82)*, cardiac ischemia in the absence of myocyte cell death *(83)*, and clinically silent coronary artery disease *(84)* are exciting potential candidates. This implies that further testing of newer markers will inevitably be required, and it is clear that these markers will have to undergo the same scrutiny and evolution in clinical trials that has been described for currently available markers.

ABBREVIATIONS

ACS, acute coronary syndrome(s); AMI, acute myocardial infarction; AST, aspartate aminotransferase; ATACS, Antithrombotic herapy in Acute Coronary Syndromes Research Group; CAPTURE, Chimeric c7E3 AntiPlatelet Therapy in Unstable Angina Refractory to Standard Treatment Trial; CK, creatine kinase; CTnT, cTnI, cardiac troponins T and I; ECG, electrocardiogram; FRISC, Fragmin during Instability in Coronary Artery Disease; GP, glycoprotein; GUSTO, Global Use of Strategies to Open Occluded Coronary Arteries in Acute Coronary Syndromes; LWMH, low molecular weight heparin; MI, myocardial infarction; NSTEMI, non-ST elevation myocardial infarction; PARAGON, Platelet IIb/IIIa Antagonism for the Reduction of Acute Coronary Syndrome Events in a Global Organization Network; PRISM, Platelet Receptor Inhibition in Ischemic Syndrome Management; PURSUIT, Platelet Glycoprotein IIb/IIIa in Unstable Angina: Receptor Suppression Using Integrilin Therapy; RISC, Research Group on Instability in Coronary Artery Disease; STEMI, ST elevation myocardial infarction; TACTICS, Treat Angina with Aggrastat and determine Cost of Therapy with an Invasive or Conservative Strategy; TIMI, Thrombolysis in Myocardial Infarction; UA, unstable angina; UFH, unfractionated heparin; ULN, upper limit of normal; WHO, World Health Organization.

REFERENCES

1. Keffer JH. Myocardial markers of injury. Evolution and insights. Am J Clin Pathol 1996; 105:305–320.
2. Braunwald E, Antman EM, Beasley JW, et al. ACC/AHA guidelines for the management of patients with unstable angina and non-ST-segment elevation myocardial infarction. A report of the American College of Cardiology/American Heart Association Task Force on Practice Guidelines (Committee on the Management of Patients With Unstable Angina). J Am Coll Cardiol 2000;36:970–1062.
3. Christenson RH, Azzazy HM. Biochemical markers of the acute coronary syndromes. Clin Chem 1998;44:855–864.

4. Heidenreich PA, Alloggiamento T, Melsop K, McDonald KM, Go AS, Hlatky MA. The prognostic value of troponin in patients with non-ST elevation acute coronary syndromes: a meta-analysis. J Am Coll Cardiol 2001;38:478–485.

5. Karmen A, Wroblewski F, LaDue JS. Transaminase activity in human blood. J Clin Invest 1954;34:126–133.

6. Duma RJ, Seigel AL. Serum creatine phosphokinase in acute myocardial infarction. Arch Intern Med 1965;115:443–451.

7. Kannel WB, Abbott RD. Incidence and prognosis of unrecognized myocardial infarction. An update on the Framingham study. N Engl J Med 1984;311:1144–1147.

8. Ellis AK. Serum protein measurements and the diagnosis of acute myocardial infarction. Circulation 1991;83:1107–1109.

9. Nomenclature and criteria for diagnosis of ischemic heart disease. Report of the Joint International Society and Federation of Cardiology/World Health Organization task force on standardization of clinical nomenclature. Circulation 1979;59:607–616.

10. Geltman EM, Ehsani AA, Campbell MK, Schechtman K, Roberts R, Sobel BE. The influence of location and extent of myocardial infarction on long-term ventricular dysrhythmia and mortality. Circulation 1979;60:805–814.

11. Rogers WJ, McDaniel HG, Smith LR, Mantle JA, Russell RO, Rackley CE. Correlation of CPK-MB and angiographic estimates of infarct size in man. Circulation 1977;56:199–205.

12. Fuster V, Badimon L, Badimon JJ, Chesebro JH. The pathogenesis of coronary artery disease and the acute coronary syndromes (1). N Engl J Med 1992;326:242–250.

13. Fuster V, Badimon L, Badimon JJ, Chesebro JH. The pathogenesis of coronary artery disease and the acute coronary syndromes (2). N Engl J Med 1992;326:310–318.

14. Bush LR, Campbell WB, Buja LM, Tilton GD, Willerson JT. Effects of the selective thromboxane synthetase inhibitor dazoxiben on variations in cyclic blood flow in stenosed canine coronary arteries. Circulation 1984;69:1161–1170.

15. Lewis HD Jr, Davis JW, Archibald DG, et al. Protective effects of aspirin against acute myocardial infarction and death in men with unstable angina. Results of a Veterans Administration Cooperative Study. N Engl J Med 1983;309:396–403.

16. Cairns JA, Gent M, Singer J, et al. Aspirin, sulfinpyrazone, or both in unstable angina. Results of a Canadian multicenter trial. N Engl J Med 1985;313:1369–1375.

17. Theroux P, Ouimet H, McCans J, et al. Aspirin, heparin, or both to treat acute unstable angina. N Engl J Med 1988;319:1105–1111.

18. The RISC Study Group. Risk of myocardial infarction and death during treatment with low dose aspirin and intravenous heparin in men with unstable coronary artery disease. The RISC Group. Lancet 1990;336:827–830.

19. Cohen M, Adams PC, Parry G, et al. Combination antithrombotic therapy in unstable rest angina and non-Q-wave infarction in nonprior aspirin users. Primary end points analysis from the ATACS trial. Antithrombotic Therapy in Acute Coronary Syndromes Research Group. Circulation 1994;89:81–88.

20. Ambrose JA, Hjemdahl-Monsen CE, Borrico S, Gorlin R, Fuster V. Angiographic demonstration of a common link between unstable angina pectoris and non-Q-wave acute myocardial infarction. Am J Cardiol 1988;61:244–247.

21. Falk E, Shah PK, Fuster V. Coronary plaque disruption. Circulation 1995;92:657–671.

22. TIMI IIIB Investigators. Effects of tissue plasminogen activator and a comparison of early invasive and conservative strategies in unstable angina and non-Q-wave myocardial infarction. Results of the TIMI IIIB Trial. Thrombolysis in Myocardial Ischemia. Circulation 1994; 89:1545–1556.

23. Boden WE, O'Rourke RA, Crawford MH, et al. Outcomes in patients with acute non-Q-wave myocardial infarction randomly assigned to an invasive as compared with a conservative management strategy. Veterans Affairs Non-Q-Wave Infarction Strategies in Hospital (VANQWISH) Trial Investigators. N Engl J Med 1998;338:1785–1792.

24. Samama MM, Bara L, Gerotziafas GT. Mechanisms for the antithrombotic activity in man of low molecular weight heparins (LMWHs). Haemostasis 1994;24:105–117.
25. Gurfinkel EP, Manos EJ, Mejail RI, et al. Low molecular weight heparin vs. regular heparin or aspirin in the treatment of unstable angina and silent ischemia. (see comments). J Am Coll Cardiol 1995;26:313–318.
26. The FRISC Study Group. Low-molecular-weight heparin during instability in coronary artery disease, Fragmin during Instability in Coronary Artery Disease (FRISC) Study Group. Lancet 1996;347:561–568.
27. Klein W, Buchwald A, Hillis SE, et al. Comparison of low-molecular-weight heparin with unfractionated heparin acutely and with placebo for 6 weeks in the management of unstable coronary artery disease. Fragmin in Unstable Coronary Artery Disease Study (FRIC). Circulation 1997;96:61–68.
28. Cohen M, Demers C, Gurfinkel EP, et al. A comparison of low-molecular-weight heparin with unfractionated heparin for unstable coronary artery disease. Efficacy and Safety of Subcutaneous Enoxaparin in Non-Q-Wave Coronary Events Study Group. (see comments). N Engl J Med 1997;337:447–452.
29. Coller BS. Platelets and thrombolytic therapy. N Engl J Med 1990;322:33–42.
30. Theroux P, Kouz S, Roy L, et al. Platelet membrane receptor glycoprotein IIb/IIIa antagonism in unstable angina. The Canadian Lamifiban Study. Circulation 1996;94:899–905.
31. Sclarovsky S, Davidson E, Lewin RF, Strasberg B, Arditti A, Agmon J. Unstable angina pectoris evolving to acute myocardial infarction: significance of ECG changes during chest pain. Am Heart J 1986;112:459–462.
32. Sclarovsky S, Davidson E, Strasberg B, et al. Unstable angina: the significance of ST segment elevation or depression in patients without evidence of increased myocardial oxygen demand. Am Heart J 1986;112:463–467.
33. Braunwald E. Unstable angina. A classification. Circulation 1989;80:410–414.
34. Braunwald E, Jones RH, Mark DB, et al. Diagnosing and managing unstable angina. Agency for Health Care Policy and Research. Circulation 1994;90:613–622.
35. Ahmed WH, Bittl JA, Braunwald E. Relation between clinical presentation and angiographic findings in unstable angina pectoris, and comparison with that in stable angina. Am J Cardiol 1993;72:544–550.
36. Wu AH, Gornet TG, Harker CC, Chen HL. Role of rapid immunoassays for urgent ("stat") determinations of creatine kinase isoenzyme MB. Clin Chem 1989;35:1752–1756.
37. White RD, Grande P, Califf L, Palmeri ST, Califf RM, Wagner GS. Diagnostic and prognostic significance of minimally elevated creatine kinase-MB in suspected acute myocardial infarction. Am J Cardiol 1985;55:1478–1484.
38. Hong RA, Licht JD, Wei JY, Heller GV, Blaustein AS, Pasternak RC. Elevated CK-MB with normal total creatine kinase in suspected myocardial infarction: associated clinical findings and early prognosis. Am Heart J 1986;111:1041–1047.
39. Markenvard J, Dellborg M, Jagenburg R, Swedberg K. The predictive value of CKMB mass concentration in unstable angina pectoris: preliminary report. J Intern Med 1992;231:433–436.
40. Ravkilde J, Hansen AB, Horder M, Jorgensen PJ, Thygesen K. Risk stratification in suspected acute myocardial infarction based on a sensitive immunoassay for serum creatine kinase isoenzyme MB. A 2.5-year follow-up study in 156 consecutive patients. Cardiology 1992;80:143–151.
41. Pettersson T, Ohlsson O, Tryding N. Increased CKMB (mass concentration) in patients without traditional evidence of acute myocardial infarction. A risk indicator of coronary death. Eur Heart J 1992;13:1387–1392.
42. Lloyd-Jones DM, Camargo CA Jr, Giugliano RP, Walsh CR, O'Donnell CJ. Characteristics and prognosis of patients with suspected acute myocardial infarction and elevated MB relative index but normal total creatine kinase. Am J Cardiol 1999;84:957–962.

43. Alexander JH, Sparapani RA, Mahaffey KW, et al. Association between minor elevations of creatine kinase-MB level and mortality in patients with acute coronary syndromes without ST-segment elevation. PURSUIT Steering Committee. Platelet Glycoprotein IIb/IIIa in Unstable Angina: Receptor Suppression Using Integrilin Therapy. JAMA 2000;283:347–353.

44. The PURSUIT Trial Investigators. Inhibition of platelet glycoprotein IIb/IIIa with eptifibatide in patients with acute coronary syndromes. The PURSUIT Trial Investigators. Platelet Glycoprotein IIb/IIIa in Unstable Angina: Receptor Suppression Using Integrilin Therapy. N Engl J Med 1998;339:436–443.

45. Katus HA, Remppis A, Looser S, Hallermeier K, Scheffold T, Kubler W. Enzyme linked immuno assay of cardiac troponin T for the detection of acute myocardial infarction in patients. J Mol Cell Cardiol 1989;21:1349–1353.

46. Bodor GS, Porter S, Landt Y, Ladenson JH. Development of monoclonal antibodies for an assay of cardiac troponin-I and preliminary results in suspected cases of myocardial infarction. Clin Chem 1992;38:2203–2214.

47. Wu AHB. Introduction to coronary artery disease (CAD) and biochemical markers. In: Cardiac Markers. Wu AHB, ed. Totowa, NJ: Humana Press, 1998, pp. 8–10.

48. Adams JE, III, Abendschein DR, Jaffe AS. Biochemical markers of myocardial injury. Is MB creatine kinase the choice for the 1990s? Circulation 1993;88:750–763.

49. Falk E. Unstable angina with fatal outcome: dynamic coronary thrombosis leading to infarction and/or sudden death. Autopsy evidence of recurrent mural thrombosis with peripheral embolization culminating in total vascular occlusion. Circulation 1985;71:699–708.

50. Hamm CW, Ravkilde J, Gerhardt W, et al. The prognostic value of serum troponin T in unstable angina. N Engl J Med 1992;327:146–150.

51. Ohman EM, Armstrong PW, Christenson RH, et al. Cardiac troponin T levels for risk stratification in acute myocardial ischemia. GUSTO IIA Investigators. N Engl J Med 1996;335:1333–1341.

52. Lindahl B, Venge P, Wallentin L. Relation between troponin T and the risk of subsequent cardiac events in unstable coronary artery disease. The FRISC study group. Circulation 1996;93:1651–1657.

53. Lindahl B, Toss H, Siegbahn A, Venge P, Wallentin L. Markers of myocardial damage and inflammation in relation to long-term mortality in unstable coronary artery disease. FRISC Study Group. Fragmin during Instability in Coronary Artery Disease. N Engl J Med 2000;343:1139–1147.

54. Antman EM, Tanasijevic MJ, Thompson B, et al. Cardiac-specific troponin I levels to predict the risk of mortality in patients with acute coronary syndromes. N Engl J Med 1996;335:1342–1349.

55. Hamm CW, Goldmann BU, Heeschen C, Kreymann G, Berger J, Meinertz T. Emergency room triage of patients with acute chest pain by means of rapid testing for cardiac troponin T or troponin I. N Engl J Med 1997;337:1648–1653.

56. deFilippi CR, Tocchi M, Parmar RJ, et al. Cardiac troponin T in chest pain unit patients without ischemic electrocardiographic changes: angiographic correlates and long-term clinical outcomes. J Am Coll Cardiol 2000;35:1827–1834.

57. Kontos MC, Jesse RL, Anderson FP, Schmidt KL, Ornato JP, Tatum JL. Comparison of myocardial perfusion imaging and cardiac troponin I in patients admitted to the emergency department with chest pain. Circulation 1999;99:2073–2078.

58. Hamm CW, Braunwald E. A classification of unstable angina revisited. Circulation 2000;102:118–122.

59. Heeschen C, van den Brand MJ, Hamm CW, Simoons ML. Angiographic findings in patients with refractory unstable angina according to troponin T status. Circulation 1999;100:1509–1514.

60. Wu AH, Apple FS, Gibler WB, Jesse RL, Warshaw MM, Valdes R Jr. National Academy of Clinical Biochemistry Standards of Laboratory Practice: recommendations for the use of cardiac markers in coronary artery diseases. Clin Chem 1999;45:1104–1121.

61. Myocardial infarction redefined—a consensus document of The Joint European Society of Cardiology/American College of Cardiology Committee for the redefinition of myocardial infarction. J Am Coll Cardiol 2000;36:959–969.
62. Lindahl B, Venge P, Wallentin L. Troponin T identifies patients with unstable coronary artery disease who benefit from long-term antithrombotic protection. Fragmin in Unstable Coronary Artery Disease (FRISC) Study Group. J Am Coll Cardiol 1997;29:43–48.
63. Antman EM, McCabe CH, Gurfinkel EP, et al. Enoxaparin prevents death and cardiac ischemic events in unstable angina/non-Q-wave myocardial infarction. Results of the thrombolysis in myocardial infarction (TIMI) 11B trial. Circulation 1999;100:1593–1601.
64. Morrow DA, Antman EM, Tanasijevic M, et al. Cardiac troponin I for stratification of early outcomes and the efficacy of enoxaparin in unstable angina: a TIMI-11B substudy. J Am Coll Cardiol 2000;36:1812–1817.
65. The CAPTURE Investigators. Randomised placebo-controlled trial of abciximab before and during coronary intervention in refractory unstable angina: the CAPTURE Study. Lancet 1997;349:1429–1435.
66. The PRISM Study Investigators. A comparison of aspirin plus tirofiban with aspirin plus heparin for unstable angina. Platelet Receptor Inhibition in Ischemic Syndrome Management (PRISM) Study Investigators. N Engl J Med 1998;338:1498–1505.
67. The PRISM-PLUS Investigators. Inhibition of the platelet glycoprotein IIb/IIIa receptor with tirofiban in unstable angina and non-Q-wave myocardial infarction. Platelet Receptor Inhibition in Ischemic Syndrome Management in Patients Limited by Unstable Signs and Symptoms (PRISM-PLUS) Study Investigators. N Engl J Med 1998;338:1488–1497.
68. Hamm CW, Heeschen C, Goldmann B, et al. Benefit of abciximab in patients with refractory unstable angina in relation to serum troponin T levels. c7E3 Fab Antiplatelet Therapy in Unstable Refractory Angina (CAPTURE) Study Investigators. N Engl J Med 1999;340: 1623–1629.
69. Heeschen C, Hamm CW, Goldmann B, Deu A, Langenbrink L, White HD. Troponin concentrations for stratification of patients with acute coronary syndromes in relation to therapeutic efficacy of tirofiban. PRISM Study Investigators. Platelet Receptor Inhibition in Ischemic Syndrome Management. Lancet 1999;354:1757–1762.
70. The FRISC II Investigators. Long-term low-molecular-mass heparin in unstable coronary-artery disease: FRISC II prospective randomised multicentre study. FRagmin and Fast Revascularisation during InStability in Coronary artery disease. Lancet 1999;354:701–707.
71. The FRISC II Investigators. Invasive compared with non-invasive treatment in unstable coronary-artery disease: FRISC II prospective randomised multicentre study. FRagmin and Fast Revascularisation during InStability in Coronary artery disease Investigators. Lancet 1999;354:708–715.
72. Diderholm E, Lindahl B, Lagerqvist B, et al. Invasive vs noninvasive strategy in relation to troponin T level and ECG findings—a FRISC 2—substudy (abstract). Circulation 2000;102: 11–752.
73. Cannon CP, Weintraub WS, Demopoulos LA, et al. Comparison of early invasive and conservative strategies in patients with unstable coronary syndromes treated with the glycoprotein IIb/IIIa inhibitor tirofiban. N Engl J Med 2001;344:1879–1887.
74. Morrow DA, Cannon CP, Rifai N, et al. Ability of minor elevations of troponins I and T to predict benefit from an early invasive strategy in patients with unstable angina and non-ST elevation myocardial infarction: results from a randomized trial. JAMA 2001;286:2405–2412.
75. Newby LK, Ohman EM, Christenson RH, et al. Benefit of glycoprotein IIb/IIIa inhibition in patients with acute coronary syndromes and troponin t-positive status: the paragon-B troponin T substudy. Circulation 2001;103:2891–2896.
76. Simoons ML. Effect of glycoprotein IIb/IIIa receptor blocker abciximab on outcome in patients with acute coronary syndromes without early coronary revascularisation: the GUSTO IV-ACS randomised trial. Lancet 2001;357:1915–1924.

77. Apple FS, Wu AH. Myocardial infarction redefined: role of cardiac troponin testing. Clin Chem 2001;47:377–379.
78. Yeo KTJ, Quinn-Hall KS, Bateman SW, Fischer GA, Wieczorek S, Wu AHB. Functional sensitivity of cardiac troponin assays and it implication for risk stratification for patients with acute coronary syndromes. In: Markers in Cardiology: Current and Future Clinical Applications. American Heart Association Monograph Series. New York: Futura, 2001, pp. 23–29.
79. Jaffe AS, Ravkilde J, Roberts R, et al. It's time for a change to a troponin standard. Circulation 2000;102:1216–1220.
80. Lindahl B, Diderholm E, Lagerqvist B, Venge P, Wallentin L. Mechanisms behind the prognostic value of troponin T in unstable coronary artery disease: a FRISC II substudy. J Am Coll Cardiol 2001;38:979–986.
81. Bayes-Genis A, Conover CA, Overgaard MT, et al. Pregnancy-associated plasma protein A as a marker of acute coronary syndromes. N Engl J Med 2001;345:1022–1029.
82. de Lemos JA, Morrow DA, Bentley JH, et al. The prognostic value of B-type natriuretic peptide in patients with acute coronary syndromes. N Engl J Med 2001;345:1014–1021.
83. Christenson RH, Duh SH, Sanhai WR, et al. Characteristics of an Albumin Cobalt Binding Test for assessment of acute coronary syndrome patients: a multicenter study. Clin Chem 2001;47:464–470.
84. Zhang R, Brennan ML, Fu X, et al. Association between myeloperoxidase levels and risk of coronary artery disease. JAMA 2001;286:2136–2142.

4

Assessing Reperfusion and Prognostic Infarct Sizing with Biochemical Markers

Practice and Promise

Robert H. Christenson and Hassan M. E. Azzazy

INTRODUCTION

Pioneering work in the early 1970s initiated the "thrombolytic era" *(1)*. During this era the therapeutic approach to acute myocardial infarction (AMI) focused on treatments aimed at limiting infarct size by improving myocardial oxygen supply, lowering myocardial oxygen demand, and minimizing autolytic damage to myocytes *(2,3)*. The thrombus became the primary therapeutic target for reperfusion therapy and monitoring because it is a keystone pathophysiological feature of the "acute coronary syndromes" (ACS), a continuum of ischemic disease ranging from unstable angina, associated with reversible myocardial cell injury, to frank MI with large areas of necrosis. This approach was validated in large randomized clinical trials during the 1980s and 1990s that unequivocally demonstrated the benefit of thrombolytic therapy *(4,5)*. Thrombolytic therapy has become critically important for AMI patients having characteristic electrocardiographic (ECG) features for resolving the thrombotic occlusion, reestablishing patency to the infarct-related artery (IRA), and improving "downstream" tissue reperfusion *(6)*. This chapter focuses on the utilization of cardiac markers for noninvasively assessing the success of reperfusion therapies and use of biochemical marker release to determine "infarct size" and, more important, prognosis. Prognostic infarct sizing is based on the notion that as myocytes die, cardiac function is compromised proportionately, resulting in a worse clinical outcome. The bridge uniting reperfusion assessment and prognostic infarct sizing is that both utilize serial monitoring of biochemical marker release. The contrast is that the focus of reperfusion assessment is the early 90-min time frame after thrombolytic therapy, whereas prognostic infarct sizing involves examining the entire cardiac marker release curve.

PATHOPHYSIOLOGY AND THE "OPEN ARTERY" HYPOTHESIS

Using canine models of coronary occlusion, Reimer et al. and Baughman et al. showed that infarct size directly related to the duration of epicardial occlusion—a finding later termed the "wavefront phenomenon" of myocyte death *(7,8)*. In the ACS, the fundamental event leading to coronary thrombus is rupture of an atherogenic fibrous plaque. Plaque rupture occurs in a focal segment of an epicardial coronary artery, which exposes subendothelial proteins such as collagen and von Willebrand factor (vWF) to

From: *Cardiac Markers, Second Edition*
Edited by: Alan H. B. Wu @ Humana Press Inc., Totowa, NJ

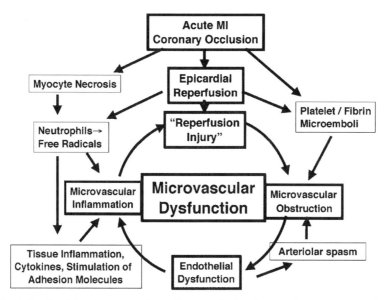

Fig. 1. Pathophysiological overview of events following acute coronary occlusion.

circulation, leading to adhesion of platelets having surface receptors for these proteins *(9)*. This interaction triggers platelet activation and a change in the platelet's shape from disk to stellate *(9)*. The membrane of activated platelets causes generation of the enzyme thrombin from prothrombin, its circulating precursor. Thrombin converts fibrinogen to fibrin that subsequently forms polymers that make up the framework of a thrombus. Because fibrinogen and vWF are multivalent, they bind to multiple activated platelets, leading to their aggregation, serving to magnify the activation-thrombus formation process. Shortly after plaque rupture and intracoronary thrombus formation, ischemia causes ultrastructural damage to myocytes and the microcirculation soon after coronary occlusion *(10)*. Evidence shows that the amount of tissue, or "size," of the MI is associated with left ventricular function and survival *(11,12)*.

The goal of reperfusion therapy for MI is to reestablish quickly the flow of nutritive, oxygenated blood to myocytes, whose function and survival are threatened by thrombotic occlusion of the IRA *(1,2)*. Correlations between sustained patency of the IRA and improved clinical outcomes culminated in the "open-artery hypothesis," the guiding principle and cornerstone of AMI therapeutic strategies in the modern reperfusion era for more than a decade *(13)*. This hypothesis suggests that reestablishing patency of the IRA with normal antegrade flow salvages stunned myocardial tissue, which, in turn, preserves left ventricular mechanical function and enhances clinical outcomes *(14)*.

It is important to note, however, that about 25% of patients show no reperfusion of the myocardial tissue despite restoration of normal flow in the epicardial IRA *(15,16)*. Figure 1 shows a diagram of the many complex interactions that, if blocked, may lead to disrupted myocardial tissue perfusion after fibrinolysis, despite having patent epicardial infarct vessels *(14–16)*. Even though prompt relief of epicardial occlusion was clearly shown to halt the wavefront of myocyte death, microvascular dysfunction in the infarct zone was identified as the limiting factor in the restoration of myocardial tissue perfusion

(6). In detailed histological studies, Kloner et al. showed that epicardial occlusion caused myocardial cellular damage first, followed by microvascular damage within 60–90 min of the onset of ischemia *(17)*. Despite restoration of normal epicardial flow, however, microvascular damage was shown to hinder perfusion of myocardial tissue in the canine model; this effect was coined the "no-reflow" phenomenon *(18)*. Reperfusion also was shown to exacerbate microvascular dysfunction, through generation of oxygen free radicals and stimulation of the tissue inflammatory response when blood flow was restored to the infarct region *(19,20)*. However, assessment of epicardial patency is not the whole story; there is less recovery of left ventricular ejection fraction, progressive left ventricular dilation, increased mortality, and increased congestive heart failure (CHF) in patients found to have impaired myocardial perfusion after epicardial reperfusion *(21–23)*. Therefore, historical observations defined the continuum of reperfusion—from upstream epicardial patency to downstream tissue perfusion—and emphasized that the ultimate goal of treatments for AMI should be the restoration of myocardial perfusion, smaller infarct size, and enhanced myocardial salvage *(24)*.

The (epicardial) open-artery hypothesis may be an oversimplification, because the goal of reperfusion therapy should be not only the restoration of upstream epicardial patency and flow but also downstream myocardial tissue perfusion. Markers for indicating this downstream myocardial perfusion both in terms of acute reperfusion monitoring and prognostic infarct sizing will become increasingly important *(6)*.

REFERENCE STANDARD FOR ASSESSING MYOCARDIAL PERFUSION

Coronary angiography was first established for identification of thrombotic occlusion and MI in 1980 *(25)* and remains the "gold standard" for evaluating patency in patients treated with reperfusion therapies *(6)*. To standardize angiographic characterization of reperfusion, the Thrombolysis in Myocardial Infarction (TIMI) investigators classified epicardial blood flow into four grades: TIMI 0, no flow past the occlusion; TIMI 1, partial flow past the occlusion; TIMI 2, coronary flow with abnormal filling past the obstruction; and TIMI 3, normal coronary flow *(26)*. The Global Utilization of Streptokinase and TPA (alteplase) for Occluded Coronary Arteries (GUSTO I) angiographic substudy, however, showed definitively that only restoration of TIMI grade 3 flow (normal epicardial flow) at 90 min is associated with improved short- and long-term survival and improved recovery of left ventricular function *(5)*. TIMI grade 0 or 1 flow was empirically considered to represent failed reperfusion, while TIMI grades 2 and 3 indicated epicardial patency and were initially considered to represent successful reperfusion *(27)*. This survival advantage closely matched the differences in mortality seen with the different fibrinolytic regimens tested in the overall GUSTO I trial *(5,27)*. These findings, which linked therapeutic efficacy to the early, complete restoration of normal flow in the epicardial infarct artery, redefined the goal of reperfusion therapy *(6)*.

Although restoration of TIMI grade 3 flow has since been used as the benchmark for reperfusion success, distal coronary flow varies considerably despite TIMI grade 3 grade flow in the epicardial vessel. Gibson developed the corrected TIMI frame count (CTFC) to quantify distal coronary flow based on the number of cineangiographic frames needed for contrast dye to reach distal coronary landmarks *(28,29)*. Recent evidence suggests that the CTFC can be used to further risk-stratify patients with TIMI grade 3 flow into

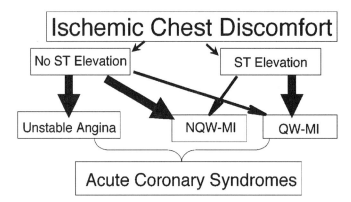

Fig. 2. Clinical classification of the ACS based on the electrocardiogram.

lower- and higher-risk subgroups after thrombolysis *(30)*. Refinement of the angiographic characterization of reperfusion over the last decade has emphasized the role of the microcirculation in the restoration of myocardial tissue perfusion *(6)*.

The spectrum of reperfusion defined by angiography should be considered a stepwise process that represents the pathophysiology of the coronary artery after occlusion. As indicated in Fig. 1, plaque rupture and thrombus formation initially lead to persistent epicardial occlusion (TIMI grade 0 or 1 flow) *(31)*. Initially, reperfusion therapy restores epicardial patency with disrupted epicardial flow (TIMI grade 2 flow), followed by normal epicardial flow with disrupted microvascular flow (TIMI grade 3 flow with a high CTFC). Successful reperfusion occurs only with restoration of normal epicardial and microvascular flow (TIMI grade 3 flow with a low CTFC) *(31)*.

FOCUS OF NONINVASIVE
REPERFUSION MONITORING AND INFARCT SIZING

As indicated above, the unstable coronary plaque represents the common pathophysiological feature of the ACS. Figure 2 shows that acute coronary syndrome patients can be classified according to their ECG findings. The full continuum of acute coronary syndromes consists of approx 19% ST elevation MI (STEMI), 22% non-ST elevation MI (NSTEMI), and approx 60% of patients with unstable angina (UA) *(32)*. It is of note that although some proportion of patients will shift from the UA to NSTEMI group because of the recent redefinition of MI *(33)*, this redefinition will have no effect on the STEMI group.

STEMI and patients with left bundle branch block are the primary focus for use of biochemical markers in assessing reperfusion. This is because evidence clearly shows that not all patients within the ACS continuum benefit from administration of thrombolytics, and in fact the therapy is contraindicated in NSTEMI and UA patients *(34)*. For this reason, the ECG is essential for targeting fibrinolytic therapy. ST elevation >2 mm appears to be important physiologically because such patients characteristically have thrombus that is rich in fibrin *(35),* and therefore responsive to early fibrinolytic therapy using intravenous streptokinase or tissue plasminogen activator. In contrast, patients with NSTEMI generally have clot that is platelet rich *(35);* therefore, fibrinolytic therapy in NSTEMI patients is contraindicated because they are subjected to risk of untoward side effects without a high probability of benefit. Furthermore, thrombolytic therapy is not applicable to approx 10–25% STEMI patients, because of contraindications including of age, bleeding diathesis, or drug allergies *(34)*. Guidelines for thrombolytic therapy include ST elevation >2 mm in contiguous ECG leads, age <75 yr, bundle branch block with a history suggestive of MI, and presentation <12 h after the onset of chest pain *(34)*.

Monitoring the success of reperfusion therapy is important because thrombolytic therapy does not result in successful reperfusion for all treated patients. Approximately 10–20% have TIMI 0, 1 flow; 20% achieve TIMI 2 flow; and 45–60% achieve successful, TIMI 3 grade flow *(36)*. Also, after thrombolysis approx 10–15% of TIMI 2 and 3 patients reocclude *(36)*. Timing of reperfusion assessment is important because both in-hospital mortality and 30–40-d mortality were shown to be statistically related to TIMI flow at 90 min post-initiation of thrombolytics *(5)*. Approximately 2–3% mortality was reported in TIMI 3 patients *(37)*.

As with reperfusion monitoring, the main focus of prognostic infarct sizing using biochemical markers has been ST elevation. In this group, biochemical markers including myoglobin, the MB isoenzyme of creatine kinase (CK-MB), cardiac troponin T (cTnT) or I (cTnI), and lactate dehydrogenase or its isoenzyme hydroxybutyrate dehydrogenase (HBDH) for assessing myocardial injury have been associated with important clinical outcomes such as death, (re)MI, and CHF. On the other hand, for NSTEMI patients there is a paucity of data associating important clinical outcomes with biochemical marker release. Although such relationships may be intuitive, there is at present little evidence from clinical trials. UA patients have reversible cell injury with ischemia, and therefore monitoring biochemical markers of necrosis will show no rise and limited prognostic information in these patients.

The general approach used for monitoring the success of reperfusion with biochemical markers involves monitoring the washout phenomenon after administration of thrombolytics. Successful reperfusion will involve lysis of the clot and robust washout of cardiac markers compared to the situation of persistent occlusion. The general approach for prognostic infarct sizing has been serial measurement of markers in blood in the hours and days following an index event. By mathematically modeling the time-release profile, and then examining fitted parameters such as the cumulative release or integrated curve area, it was possible to determine important clinical outcomes.

CLINICAL INDICATORS AND OTHER
TECHNOLOGIES FOR REPERFUSION ASSESSMENT

Simply observing and grading the rapid resolution of chest pain after thrombolytic therapy is associated with an increased probability of having a patent IRA *(38,39)* and TIMI 3 grade flow *(40)*. Data indicate, however, that clinical indicators alone are not sufficiently sensitive or specific to guide therapeutic or interventional decisions *(38)*. But in combination with other variables associated with reperfusion such as biochemical markers and time to treatment, resolution of chest pain adds significantly to the ability to predict patency by angiography *(41)*.

In addition to biochemical markers, a number of invasive and noninvasive technologies have been investigated and used for reperfusion assessment after thrombolytic therapy. Table 1 lists a number of these technologies, many of which are undergoing

Table 1
Technologies Other than Biochemical Markers
for Assessing Reperfusion After Thrombolytic Therapy

Diagnostic technology (references)	Description
Invasive technologies	
Coronary Doppler flow wires *(110,111)*	During angiography coronary flow can be measured to estimate the degree of microvascular dysfunction in the infarct zone. Appears to predict recovery of regional left ventricular function. Reproducibility has not been thoroughly studied.
Myocardial contrast echocardiography *(15)*	During angiography sonicated contrast solution is injected into the recanalized IRA to examine myocardial contrast enhancement, which reflects tissue perfusion in the infarct zone. New contrast agents are under development for bedside use.
Magnetic resonance imaging *(23,24)*	Comprehensive imaging technology that can be useful for assessment of coronary flow, myocardial tissue perfusion left ventricular volumes, and regional and left ventricular function. Although one of the most comprehensive techniques available, long procedure times and inability to accommodate unstable patients are significant limitations.
Noninvasive technologies	
Technetium-99m-sestamibi, single-photon emission computed tomography (SPECT) *(112)*	SPECT appears promising for cumulative infarct size measurements to determine left ventricular damage and myocardial salvage after reperfusion therapy. Performance is often difficult while treating MI; the ideal time for performance after reperfusion therapy is unclear.
Static ST-segment resolution *(45–48)*	Serial ECG assessment for evaluating ST resolution is a useful bedside marker of reperfusion success. The degree of ST-segment resolution is a reliable predictor of mortality that has been validated in multiple clinical studies.
Continuous ST-segment monitoring *(49,50)*	Continuous monitoring can be used to determine the exact timing of reperfusion; ST segment monitoring has been applied to estimate infarct size, left ventricular recovery, and clinical efficacy of new therapies.

substantial improvement and/or in combination with biochemical markers may enhance the ability of angiography for assessing reperfusion status and predicting outcome. The invasive technologies listed in Table 1 involve interventions such as cardiac catherization. Noninvasive perfusion imaging such as positron-emission tomography (PET) can be used directly to assess coronary vasodilatory function, and myocardial perfusion *(42)* allows direct assessment of tissue perfusion. Cardiac magnetic resonance imaging (MRI) appears to be the most comprehensive noninvasive technique to evaluate coronary flow, myocardial perfusion, left ventricular volume, and regional and global left ventricular function *(43,44)*. But the utility of noninvasive imaging is currently restricted by high costs, long procedure times, limited availability, and inability to accommodate unstable patients *(6)*.

Various formats of the ECG allow dynamic monitoring of IRA patency after thrombolytic therapy. ECG monitoring is predictive of clinical outcome and may add powerful independent information to biochemical markers for more accurately assessing reperfusion. Use of static electrocardiograms for assessing ST resolution was shown 25 yr ago to be a useful bedside marker of reperfusion success and interest in this tool has recently been rekindled *(6)*. Rapid ST-segment resolution within 30–60 min of successful primary angioplasty (a patent IRA with TIMI grade 3 flow) predicts greater improvement in ejection fraction, reduced infarct size, and improved survival compared with later ST-segment resolution *(45,46)*. The prognostic significance of ST resolution has been validated in GUSTO-III, TIMI-14, and a meta-analysis of almost 4000 patients *(47,48)*.

Rapid, intermittent events (such as cyclic flow in the IRA) that often are missed with static measures of reperfusion produce a highly characteristic appearance in continuous ST-segment recordings. Continuous monitoring of ST-segment resolution is advantageous as the only method that can precisely capture the timing, stability, and quality of reperfusion *(6,49,50)*. Quantitative variables derived from continuous ST-segment resolution analysis have been applied to estimate infarct size, left ventricular recovery, therapeutic effects of new drugs, and clinical efficacy *(6)*. In patients from the GUSTO-I trial, ST-segment reelevation within 24 h of fibrinolysis (after initial resolution) independently predicted 30-d and 1-yr mortality *(6,49,50)*. Continuous ST-segment monitoring is one of the most promising tools for evaluation of reperfusion efficacy and risk stratification in patients with AMI. However, further integration and application of this method remain dependent on the development of widely available, user-friendly ECG monitoring devices *(6)*.

BIOCHEMICAL MARKERS FOR CORONARY REPERFUSION ASSESSMENT

Overview and Background of Reperfusion Assessment

A simple model for noninvasive assessment of reperfusion begins with thrombus forming a sustained coronary occlusion resulting in downstream ischemia and myocyte death. The key assumption for reperfusion assessment using biochemical markers is that after thrombolytic therapy there is a detectable difference between the biochemical marker release pattern (washout) for patients with successful reperfusion compared to those for whom thrombolytic therapy has failed. For optimum performance, the ideal biochemical marker must demonstrate brisk washout with restoration of epicardial patency and myocardial tissue perfusion. The ideal marker has high specificity for cardiac tissue and the ability to differentiate TIMI 3 from TIMI 0–2 grade epicardial flow with 100% accuracy, reflect myocardial tissue perfusion, detect reocclusion, and have a strong association with important clinical outcomes.

An essential corollary involves timely reperfusion assessment, because if thrombolytic therapy is unsuccessful in restoring IRA patency, then strategies such as cardiac catheterization and percutaneous coronary intervention (PCI) or coronary artery bypass surgery can be quickly implemented to preserve myocardium *(36)*. Therefore, reperfusion assessment and decision within 60–120 min after thrombolytic therapy must be

Table 2
Characteristics of Cardiac Markers and their Suitability to Evaluate Reperfusion

Marker	Size (kDa)	Advantages as a reperfusion marker	Disadvantages as a reperfusion marker
Myoglobin	18.0	Abundant in myocytes Reaches a peak 6–9 h after necrosis	Not cardiac specific
FABP	15.0	Rapid release after opening of the artery Abundant in cardiomyocytes	Tests not widely available (performs equally well as myoglobin)
CK-MB	85.0	Predictable release profile Release completed in 24–30 h. Used for modeling prognostic infarct sizing	Some issues with cardiac specificity in skeletal injury patients
cTnT and	37.0	Excellent cardiac specificity	Unpredictable release pattern because release occurs up to 5–7 d after the index event often shows a bimodal pattern
cTnI	23.5	Excellent cardiac specificity	Unpredictable release pattern; many assays with different characteristics

the target because evidence *(5)* indicates that this time frame both allows time for clot lysis and marker washout and is soon enough to allow alternative reperfusion strategies for preserving myocardium if thrombolysis has failed. To meet this goal the marker must have rapid bedside or central laboratory availability at reasonable cost.

Table 2 shows various cardiac markers released into circulation after myocardial necrosis, including myoglobin, fatty acid binding protein (FABP), CK, CK-MB, and cTnI and cTnT. The rate at which these proteins are available for "washout" is determined by a number of factors including molecular size, cellular location (cytosolic vs structural), mechanism of clearance, and so on. Also, the characteristics of assay "measurement tools" play an important role. Unfortunately the ideal biochemical marker for reperfusion assessment has yet to be discovered. As a generalization, the characteristics of myoglobin appear to approximate most closely the ideal (re)perfusion marker. FABP, a small cytosolic protein that is abundant in myocytes, and myoglobin have been compared in several reports finding no difference in performance between these markers *(51–53)*. Until assays are commercially available, FABP use will be limited.

Figure 3 shows comparative CK-MB release patterns for two MI patients, one for whom thrombolytic therapy was successful and the other for whom thrombolysis failed at 90 min. As stated above, the importance of timely assessment requires that all noninvasive reperfusion strategies focus on the early, 0–120-min part of curve. Careful study of this portion of these washout curves reveals several possible strategies for discriminating successful from failed thrombolytic therapy. In fact, the strategies that have been utilized are relatively straightforward and include collecting blood samples shortly

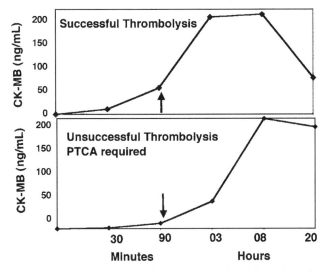

Fig. 3. CK-MB release curves for two patients who received thrombolytic therapy and coronary angiography at the times indicated (*arrow*). The **top panel** shows a patient who had successful thrombolysis and demonstrated TIMI 3 grade flow in the IRA. The **bottom panel** displays a patient for whom thrombolysis was unsuccessful and who had TIMI 0 grade flow. This patient's IRA was opened to TIMI 3 grade flow with angioplasty at the time indicated (*arrow*).

before thrombolytic therapy (pretreatment) and then at a later time(s) (posttreatment), usually at 60 and/or 90 min. With measurement of markers in these pre- and posttreatment samples, the slope (rate of release) can be determined, the posttreatment/pretreatment ratio can be calculated, or simply the raw marker values can be used. A few studies have used strategies that combine information from biochemical markers with other variables such as clinical indicators, ST resolution, and time to treatment.

It must be noted that the ACS include many complex and dynamic physiological processes and interactions involving disrupted plaque, coagulation cascade, platelet activation, other cellular responses, endothelial and vascular responses, hormonal release, as well as the effects of any medications administered. Other factors involve blood pressure, recent ischemic and nonischemic coronary events, myocardial tissue perfusion, and collateral flow in the region of the IRA. However, the context is that thrombolysis fails in 25% of patients (34,36), and there is no noninvasive tool for reliable perfusion assessment. Therefore, in spite of these physiological caveats, the use of biochemical markers can be a valuable clinical tool, and good performance for assessing reperfusion has been shown.

Association of Biochemical Markers of Reperfusion with Outcomes

Although the outcome goal on angiography for epicardial perfusion is TIMI 3 grade flow (37), studies have also defined successful thrombolysis as TIMI 2–3 grade flow (27,54). Table 3 shows a summary of data from a number of key studies that examined biochemical markers and combined strategies for noninvasively assessing reperfusion status. Association of important clinical outcomes such as death, (re)MI, and CHF with biochemical markers and perfusion status has also been examined.

TIMI 2–3 vs TIMI 0–1 Grade Coronary Flow as Outcome

Table 3 displays the operating characteristics from several studies. The receiver operator characteristic (ROC) curve area is perhaps the most important column in Table 3 because it allows direct comparison of the marker strategies in the same patient population. ROC areas are not dependent on use of a cutoff as are sensitivity, specificity, positive predictive value (PPV), and negative predictive value (NPV).

In addition to the data listed in Table 3, preliminary studies that examined myoglobin, CK-MB, and cTnI indicated that use of these markers was promising for assessing reperfusion status *(55,56)*. The ability of biochemical markers to predict spontaneous reperfusion, that is, reperfusion that occurs in MI patients prior to administration of thrombolysis, was examined in a study of 16 patients *(57)*. A ratio of myoglobin/total CK activity that was >5, measured in samples collected before administration, showed sensitivity 75%, specificity 96%, and accuracy of 92% in this small study *(57)*. The impact of infarct size on the ability of markers (myoglobin) to predict patency status has also been reported *(51,58)*. Including only patients with larger infarcts, the NPV of myoglobin for predicting reperfusion improved from 44% to 100% in a study of 49 patients *(58)*. In a separate study of 115 MI patients, the ROC curve area for myoglobin was improved to 0.86 when accounting for infarct size; the PPV improved from 87% to 95% and the NPV improved from 42% to 52% when combined with infarct size *(51)*. The larger the infarct, the better is the ability of biochemical markers to discriminate successful from failed thrombolysis.

Myoglobin strategies demonstrated the best performance across the studies in Table 3, showing ROC areas in the range of 0.80–0.90, with sensitivities at approx 90% and with relatively high specificity. The better performance of myoglobin is evidently due to its fundamental characteristic of robust washout. CK-MB and the troponins demonstrated ROC areas that were lower, in the range of 0.70–0.80; this performance is reflected in the comparatively lower sensitivities and specificities for discriminating TIMI 0–1 from TIMI 2–3 grade flow. Although similar ROC areas for myoglobin, CK-MB, and the troponins were demonstrated in one study *(59)*, coronary angiography was performed earlier than in other studies at 60 min, which may have diminished the performance of myoglobin. A comparison of CK-MB, cTnT, and myoglobin by logistic regression analysis showed that myoglobin was the only marker that was an independent predictor of IRA patency *(60)*. Consistent with this finding, a separate analysis showed that inclusion of myoglobin added significantly ($p < 0.04$) to a model that included CK-MB for predicting TIMI 2–3 patency *(61)*. Overall, the ROC areas for the various markers indicate that they have substantial potential for discriminating TIMI 0–1 from TIMI 2–3 grade coronary flow, perhaps permitting use as part of a rapid triage strategy by ruling out IRA occlusion *(59)*.

TIMI 3 vs TIMI 0–2 Grade Coronary Flow as Outcome

Several studies comparing the performance biochemical markers for predicting TIMI 3 grade coronary flow are displayed in Table 3. One study examined predictive performance of the markers using both 60-min and 90-min ratios *(62)*. Although ROC curve areas were not reported, there were no apparent differences in the ability of the ratios to predict TIMI 3 patency *(61)*. As expected, the ROC areas and performance characteristics for all biochemical marker strategies were decreased compared to the less restrictive

Table 3
Selected Clinical Studies Investigating the Use of Cardiac Markers for Detection of Reperfusion

Reference	Marker	Strategy[a]	TIMI 2,3 vs TIMI 0,1				ROC area	Comment
			Sensitivity	Specificity	PPV	NPV		
113	CK-MB	90/0 Ratio	91	100	100	75	—	n = 36; Ratios: ≥2.5 for LAD; ≥2.2 for RCA
60	Myo	0,90 Slope	94	88	94	82	0.89	n = 63
	CK-MB	0,90 Slope	87	71	89	67	0.79	
	cTnT	0,90 Slope	80	65	93	55	0.80	
51	Myo	0,90 Slope	67	71	88	42	—	n = 115; CAG at 120 min
	CK-MB	0,90 Slope	52	75	87	34	—	
59	Myo	60/0 Ratio	69	68	89	36	0.71	n = 422; CAG was performed at 60 min
	CK-MB	60/0 Ratio	62	68	87	34	0.70	
	cTnI	60/0 Ratio	68	62	88	31	0.71	
41	CK-MB	0,90 Slope	68	70	—	—	0.72	n = 97; CK-MB alone as the only predictive variable
61	Myo	90 Value	—	—	—	—	0.82	n = 96; Myo was only predictive variable (compare ROC value to that under combined analyses)

(Continued)

Table 3 (Continued)

Reference	Marker	Strategy	TIMI 3 vs TIMI 0,1,2					Comment
			Sensitivity	Specificity	PPV	NPV	ROC area	
62	Myo	90/0 Ratio	84	73	73	84	—	n = 105; ROC curve analysis performed but areas were were not reported. Visually, the ROC areas for myo and CK-MB curves appeared to be larger than for cTnT.
		60/0 Ratio	92	59	69	89	—	
	CK-MB	90/0 Ratio	91	49	61	87	—	
		60/0 Ratio	93	60	76	86	—	
	cTnT	90/0 Ratio	95	58	65	94	—	
		60/0 Ratio	97	43	63	94	—	
63	Myo	90/0 Ratio	75	63	62	75	0.72	n = 97; the ROC areas were 0.84 (myo) and 0.83 (cTnT) in a subset of 49 patients treated >3 hours after onset of symptoms.
	CK-MB	90/0 Ratio	45	68	56	69	0.62	
	cTnT	90/0 Ratio	70	66	62	73	0.66	
61	Myo	90 Value	—	—	—	—	0.71	n = 96; Myo was only predictive variable

70

Reference	Marker	Patency	Sensitivity	Combined variable analyses			ROC area	Comment
				Specificity	PPV	NPV		
41	CK-MB	TIMI 2–3	88	70	44	—	0.85	n = 97; Variables included chest pain intensity, time from symptoms onset to thrombolytic therapy, and CK-MB slope
		TIMI 3	—	—	—	—	0.73	
65	Myo, 60/0	TIMI 3	—	—	—	—	0.70	n = 169; Variables included ECG criteria, chest pain resolution, and myoglobin 60/0
		TIMI 0–1	—	—	—	—	0.84	
61	CK-MB	TIMI 2–3	88	78	—	—	0.88	n = 96; Variables included Myo 90 value, CK-MB slope, chest pain intensity, and time from symptoms onset to thrombolytic therapy
	& Myo	TIMI 3	—	—	—	—	0.74	

CAG, coronary artery graft; CK-MB, MB isoenzyme of creatine kinase; cTnT, cardiac troponin T; cTnI, cardiac troponin I; Myo, myoglobin; NPV, negative predictive value; PPV, positive predictive value.
[a]All numbers are in units of minutes.

patency goal of TIMI 2–3 flow. Only the ROC area for myoglobin exceeded 0.70 for discriminating TIMI 3 from TIMI 0–2 grade flow *(61,63)*.

Of interest, the importance of time to thrombolytic therapy was examined in a subset of 49 patients who were treated >3 h after symptom onset *(63)*. This examination found a very substantial improvement in the ability of myoglobin to discriminate TIMI 3 grade flow from TIMI 0–2 in these later presenting patients, as indicated by the ROC area increasing from 0.70 to 0.85 *(63)*. Furthermore, the ability of CK-MB, cTnT, and myoglobin to discriminate between TIMI 2 and TIMI 3 grade flow was examined in a later study, finding that time to treatment was important *(64)*. The difference between TIMI 2 and TIMI 3 grade flow was statistically significant for only the 90-min/pretreatment myoglobin ratio, and only among patients treated >3 h after onset of symptoms *(64)*. This finding, that of timing from symptom onset to treatment is important, is consistent with the significant contribution of time from symptom onset to thrombolytic therapy reported in studies of combined variables *(41,61)*.

Combining Biochemical Markers with Other Noninvasive Indicators of Reperfusion

It should not be surprising that combining noninvasive indicators of reperfusion status improves the ability to discriminate successful from failed thrombolysis. There is little doubt that the combined approach will be used clinically in the future for reperfusion assessment.

Variables including CK-MB slope, time from onset of symptoms to thrombolytic therapy, and chest pain intensity were combined in a model to predict reperfusion *(41)*. Although CK-MB slope added the most information to the model, Table 3 shows that use of the combined strategy significantly improved the ability to predict coronary patency as indicated by the ROC curve areas increasing from 0.72 for CK-MB slope alone to 0.85 for the combined model *(41)*. A separate analysis combined the 90-min myoglobin value, the CK-MB slope, time from onset of symptoms to thrombolytic therapy, and chest pain intensity *(61)*. Figure 4 shows the box plot and corresponding ROC curve for discriminating TIMI 0–1 from TIMI 2–3 coronary flow with this model (ROC area 0.88). As stated above, myoglobin added significantly to the model including CK-MB slope for the ability to predict IRA patency *(61)*. The ability of this model to predict TIMI 3 grade patency from TIMI 0–2 was 0.74, which is consistent with performance appropriate for clinical diagnostic utilization.

ST-segment resolution, chest pain resolution, and the (60-min/pretreatment) myoglobin ratio were combined in a model to predict TIMI 3 grade flow *(65)*. The ROC areas were similar to those in other studies; a value of 0.70 was reported for predicting <TIMI grade 3 flow, and an ROC area of 0.84 was reported for predicting TIMI 0–1 grade flow *(65)*. Importantly, these authors note that the use of combined markers can aid in the early noninvasive identification of candidates for rescue PCI *(65)*.

Risk Stratification and IRA Patency with Biochemical Markers

A logistic regression model incorporating baseline predictors of 30-d mortality showed that both ST resolution and a positive qualitative myoglobin result were independent predictors of mortality *(66)*. Table 4 shows data from this study indicating that patients

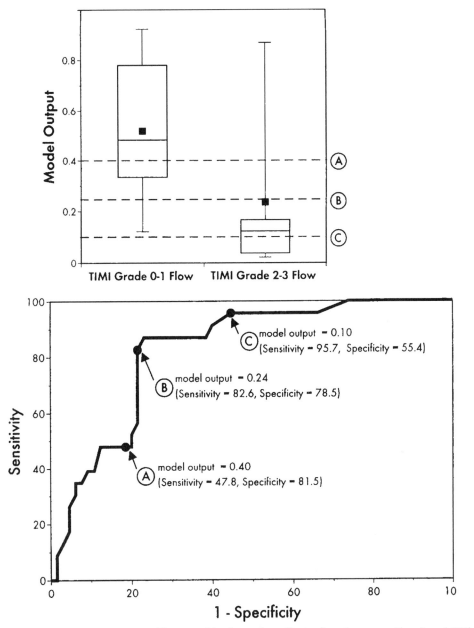

Fig. 4. (Top) Patency groups illustrated by box plots displaying the range (*bars*) and 25th/median/75th percentile (*box*) for values from the combined model that included myoglobin, CK-MB, time to treatment, and chest pain intensity in the TIMI 0-1 and TIMI 2-3 groups. The *broken lines* correspond to cutoff values displayed in the ROC curve (*bottom panel*). The ROC curve (**bottom**) area is 0.88.

having both positive myoglobin and ST resolution <70% are at high risk of in-hospital, 30-d, and 1-yr adverse events. This study suggested that within 90 min of thrombolytic therapy, clinicians can determine the risk for adverse events with a bedside myoglobin assay and 12-lead ECG, and facilitate triage after thrombolytic therapy (*66*).

Table 4
Clinical Outcomes for Combinations
of Baseline Qualitative Myoglobin (Myo) and ST Resolution

Combinations	Number of patients	In-hospital death	30-d death	1-Yr death	30-D death/CHF
Negative Myo and ST resolution ≥70%	242	0	0.4	7.0	0.8
Positive Myo or ST resolution <70%	538	4.3	4.8	15.6	6.5
Positive Myo and ST resolution <70%	239	7.9	9.6	21.8	12.6

$p < 0.001$ for trends in all variables.
Data from ref. *66*.

In 140 patients, cTnT ≥0.1 ng/mL on admission predicted lower rates of postprocedural TIMI 3 flow and more severely compromised myocardial perfusion as reflected by myoglobin washout, despite normal epicardial flow *(67)*. These findings may, in part, explain the clearly higher-risk profile of troponin-positive patients *(68)*. Because cTnT-positive patients are less likely to have TIMI 3 grade flow, this study suggested that they might require more aggressive adjunctive therapy when treated with PCI *(67)*. Although strategies involving myoglobin demonstrated the best performance, there is clearly a role for CK-MB and particularly troponin, as indicated by risk stratification and outcome-based studies *(61,67)*.

Interpretation, Insight, and Future Trends
for Reperfusion Assessment with Biochemical Markers

Although biochemical markers by themselves provide substantial information regarding epicardial patency, their performance is improved markedly by using a combined approach with time to treatment, clinical indicators, and ECG criteria (Table 3). The timing of decisions implicit with reperfusion assessment require rapid testing, a need best met by point-of-care testing. Of interest, myoglobin clearance was accepted as a surrogate for improved myocardial perfusion *(67)*. This is important because factors in addition to TIMI 3 epicardial perfusion must be the goal of reperfusion therapy *(6)*, and biochemical markers may better indicate microvascular flow and myocardial tissue perfusion. Biochemical markers will undoubtedly play a role in the downstream shift of the ACS treatment paradigm *(6)*.

BIOCHEMICAL MARKERS FOR PROGNOSTIC INFARCT SIZING

Overview and Background of Prognostic Infarct Sizing

The ideal marker for prognostic infarct sizing must be released only on death of myocytes. Specificity for cardiac tissue is highly desirable and, importantly, the release pattern must be predictable so that a minimum number of samples are required to characterize the curve fully. Furthermore, the marker's release must strike a balance between early rise and then completion of the curve in a "reasonable" time frame. On the one hand, markers having a very early and rapid rise and fall may not allow elucidation of the entire curve if there is any delay in patient presentation or sampling. On the other hand, markers having an extended lifetime in blood may require sampling for many days or even weeks for accurate characterization of the release curve. Measurements of CK total activity and CK-MB have been particularly well suited for determining infarct size *(69,70)*.

Since the 1970s investigators studied the use of markers for quantifying (sizing) myocardial necrosis *(71–74)*. In addition to total CK *(75)* and CK-MB *(76)*, markers including HBDH *(77)* and myoglobin *(78)* have been employed. Total CK and CK-MB remain the most practical markers because they are released only on cell death *(79)*; their release begins within 4–10 h after MI and is complete within approx 24 h *(80)*. Figure 3 shows CK-MB curves for sampling over 20 h for two patients after thrombolytic therapy. In contrast to reperfusion assessment in which the first 90-min samples are in the spotlight, the focus for prognostic infarct sizing includes the entire curve. Inspection of Fig. 3 reveals that one could compare variables such as curve area, peak time, peak concentration, or a variety of other parameters between the patients.

General Strategies for Reperfusion Assessment and Infarct Sizing and Prognosis

Approaches to prognostic infarct sizing have ranged from very simple strategies such as use of the highest value in a limited number of samples collected over a time period, that is, 24 h, to frequent sampling and use of rather complex equations for curve-fitting the data. Although simple, the "highest value" approach has been used to show valuable associations between outcomes *(81,82)* and interventions *(83,84)*. Early curve-fitting attempts involved determining the amount of a biochemical marker within myocardial cells and then serially measuring the marker in blood in the hours and days following the index event. By mathematically modeling the release profile and then integrating the area of the time-release curve it was possible to determine the quantity of myocardial tissue that was injured irreversibly. Curve-fitting the temporal pattern of cardiac marker release has been shown to be the most accurate method for prognostic infarct size using these markers. One of two curve-fitting approaches has been used extensively: 1. calculation of the cumulative release of HBDH or 2. assessment of area, peak, and so on from curve-fitting equations.

Quantifying the cumulative release of HBDH, first developed in the early 1980s *(85, 86)*, is a strategy for prognostic infarct sizing by estimating the gram-equivalents of myocardium per liter of plasma. To accomplish this estimation, cumulative HBDH activity between the onset of symptoms ($t = 0$) and time t is calculated according to the following equation *(85,86)*:

$$Q(t) = C(t) + TER \cdot \int exp^{ERR(\tau-1)} \cdot C(\tau)d\tau + FCR \cdot \int C(\tau)d\tau$$

where $C(t)$ = plasma activity of HBDH, TER = fractional transcapillary escape rate constant, exp = exponential function, ERR = fractional extravascular return rate constant, and FCR = fractional catabolic rate constant for elimination of HBDH.

The cumulative release of HBDH can be assessed over various time periods, represented by the t variable above, and may be 6 h, 12 h, or 72 h after the onset of symptoms ($t = 0$). In these cases Q(t) in the above equation is designated as $Q(6)$, $Q(12)$, or $Q(72)$. Various ratios of cumulative release over different time periods can be expressed by $Q(6)/Q(72)$, $Q(12)/Q(72)$, and so on. A possible issue with the cumulative HBDH strategy is that the nature of the marker used requires sampling over a 72-h period for reliable results.

A more straightforward approach is to utilize the log-normal function for curve-fitting. This approach aims at finding the best fit of the characteristic time-release curve, rather than attempting to explain complex physiological events such as clearance rates, transcapillary escape rates, and so on. Curve-fitting models have used numeric integration with the following functions: first-order kinetic model *(87)*, a two-compartment model *(88)*, the gamma function *(75)*, a validated exponential expediential function *(89)*, as well as the log-normal function *(90)*. These functions were compared using a standard data set *(91)*. Using criteria that included visual inspection, convergence of the data, and evaluation of the trend of residuals with time, the log-normal function demonstrated the best curve-fit properties *(91)*. The log-normal equation and its variables are listed below:

$$y\ (t) = a \cdot \exp\{-0.5 \cdot [(\ln t - b)/c]^2\}$$

where y = CKMB concentration predicted by the model , t = time from onset of infarct, a = peak CK-MB value of the fitted curve, b = natural logarithm of time from onset to peak, and c = a parameter reflecting the width of the curve.

Figure 5 shows a typical fitted curve for CK-MB, which illustrates the various parameters that can be determined from the log-normal model including curve area, peak height, and time of peak height. Figure 5 shows an additional parameter termed the falloff constant (k_f), which may be a new nonmortality end point valuable for both assessing treatment effects in clinical trials and for clinical prognosis of patients with acute coronary syndromes *(92)*. Logically, the value of (k_f) reflects the quality of reperfusion; the more rapid the falloff of the curve, the better the quality of reperfusion *(93)*. Mathematically, k_f is derived from the slope of the log-normal curve as described by the following equation:

$$dy/dt = a \cdot \exp(u)\ du$$

where $u = -0.5 \cdot [(\ln t - b)/c]^2$. This equation may be simplified to $dy/dt = y(t)\ du$, which represents the rate of change in CK-MB concentration. Because $dy/dt = y(t)\ du$ has the same form as a first-order rate equation, du may be viewed as a rate constant having its maximal value at the inflection point. As illustrated in Fig. 5, this rate constant, du at the inflection point, is defined as the falloff constant (k_f). k_f represents the balance between the rate of release of CK-MB from tissue into circulation and the protein's rate of elimination. Given normal CK-MB elimination, differences in k_f predominantly reflect variation in the rates of CK-MB release into the bloodstream, which in turn reflects the rate of CK-MB tissue clearance.

It is worth noting that models of marker release have been criticized in the past because the calculated quantity of biochemical markers often did not accurately relate to infarct size, commonly expressed in grams of infarcted tissue, in dogs with induced coronary occlusion *(94,95)*. Although the comparison of marker release and grams of infarcted tissue may be appropriate for use in animal models, in humans a semiquantitative pathological means is advocated for classifying myocardial cell death after prolonged ischemia according to the following four classifications: microscopic, with focal necrosis; small, <10% of the left ventricle; medium, 10–30% of the left ventricle; and large, >30% of the left ventricle *(33)*. However, estimating the infarct size in grams of myocardium should not be the goal, even though this is possible in theory. Instead,

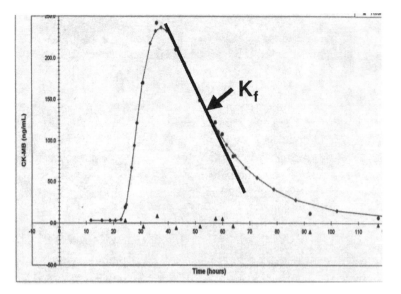

Fig. 5. Log-normal curve fitting for CK-MB measurements from an MI patient: the lognormal function is $y\ (t) = a \cdot \exp\{-0.5 \cdot [(\ln t - b)/c]^2\}$; where a = peak height; b = ln (peak time); c = curve width parameter; and k_f = fall off constant.

the focus for use of biochemical markers in living patients should be prognostic infarct sizing, relating marker release to patient outcomes and treatment differences. Anatomic infarct sizing should be left to the autopsy pathologist *(91)*.

Performance of Prognostic Infarct Sizing

Much of the clinical utilization of examining the shape of biochemical marker release and prognostic infarct sizing in individual patients has been semiquantitatively based on experience and anecdotal information. In particular, a bimodal shaped CK-MB curve has been associated with infarct extension for decades *(96)*. In addition, higher CK-MB peak values and larger CK-MB curve areas have been associated with more extensive cardiac necrosis and worse outcomes for individual patients. From a scientific perspective, the association between total CK, CK-MB, and HBDH with infarct size and prognosis and important outcomes has been well established when examining groups of patients, rather than individuals. In most studies, biochemical marker release is considered (or demonstrated) reflective of the quantity of myocardium infarcted and therefore prognosis.

The use of biochemical markers to indicate infarct size has been used to demonstrate the cardiac protective effect of preinfarction angina in a number of studies *(97–100)*. These studies have found that CK-MB is an important prognostic marker. A recent study of GUSTO I patients found that the measured peak CK-MB value was significantly correlated to 5-yr outcome, and was a more powerful predictor than time to treatment, preinfarction angina, and age *(101)*. In the setting of PCI, it has been shown that elevations in CK-MB that exceed twofold the upper limit of normal are at proportionate increased risk of death, MI, and urgent revascularization at both 30 d and 6 mo *(84)*. CK-MB has also been used as an indicator of infarct size when evaluating infarct sizing scoring systems

(102) and strategies that include rotablator artherectomy *(83)*. Although CK-MB measurements in these studies revealed important prognostic information, the *measured* peak value of the enzyme in the 24 h after the index event was used. Compared to mathematical modeling, this approach has limitations because information is lost in the assumption that the measured value captures the true peak. In addition, modeling allows objective estimation of the curve area, k_f, time to peak, and other parameters. Properties of the cardiac marker release pattern can be used to represent an overall measure of myocardial cellular injury and clinical outcome. Infarct sizing and prognosis have shown that the cumulative release of cardiac markers after AMI could be used to estimate infarct size, predict recovery of left ventricular function, and predict survival *(105–107)*. The term prognostic infarct sizing is used here to represent systematic strategies that have been associated to outcomes and treatments.

Cumulative release of HBDH has been used to indicate the extent of cell death and to predict recovery of left ventricular function and survival *(105–107)*. With regard to reperfusion therapy, cumulative HBDH release was used to compare fibrinolytic treatment with streptokinase (SK) or tissue plasminogen activator (tPA) *(105)*. This study showed a significant difference in median infarct size for tPA-treated patients ($p < 0.04$) by cumulative HBDH release, which was consistent with survival differences between treatments *(105)*. A comparison between thrombolytic treatment with SK and PCI also utilized HBDH cumulative release as a prognostic indicator of infarct size, finding that PCI resulted in smaller infarct size. Furthermore, cumulative HBDH release showed that despite successful thrombolysis, PCI was superior to thrombolytic therapy with regard to infarct size *(36)*. The results of prognostic infarct sizing were consistent with lower mortality and improved ejection fraction at discharge for the PCI-treated patients *(36,105)*.

Log-normal curve fitting was performed in a substudy of Thrombolysis and Angioplasty in Myocardial Infarction (TAMI) 7 patients to relate in-hospital outcomes and CK-MB parameters after thrombolysis *(108)*. Sampling for CK-MB mass measurements in TAMI 7 was performed at enrollment and 30 min, 90 min, 3 h, 8 h, and 20 h after thrombolysis. The calculated CK-MB maxima were significantly related to ejection fraction at 90 min ($p = 0.0004$) and at 5–7 d ($p = 0.0014$), as was curve area ($p = 0.0076$ and 0.030, respectively). Both CK-MB maxima and curve area predicted CHF ($p = 0.008$ and $p = 0.042$, respectively) and a composite of CHF or death ($p = 0.004$ and $p = 0.047$, respectively). In summary, this study showed that CK-MB maxima determined by log-normal curve fitting with a limited number of samples collected over only 20 h related well to infarct zone function, left ventricular function, and in-hospital outcomes after thrombolysis for MI *(108)*.

Clinical trials in which the incidence of short-term mortality and other outcomes is relatively low have need for nonmortality end points *(33)*. Prognostic infarct sizing with the log- normal equation was used to model CK-MB release in 581 MI patients enrolled in the Promotion of Reperfusion by Inhibition of Thrombin During Myocardial Infarction Evolution (PRIME) and Efegatran Sulfate as an Adjunct to Streptokinase versus Heparin as an Adjunt to Tissue Plasminogen Activator in Patients with Myocardial Infarction (ESCALAT) trials *(109)*. In these studies CK-MB mass measurements and log-normal curve fitting were performed in serum specimens collected at enrollment, and then at 1, 6, 12, 24, 36, and 72 h later. CK-MB maxima and area under the curve (AUC) from curve fitting CK-MB release were compared to infarct sizing by nuclear imaging at hospital discharge, finding a significant correlation (both $p < 0.0001$). Furthermore, CK-MB maxima and AUC demonstrated a significant relationship with discharge ejection fraction determined 5–7 d after MI ($p = 0.02$ and $p = 0.026$, respectively). The conclusion of this study was that parameters from quantitative CK-MB curve fitting provide a reasonable surrogate end point of infarct size and function in phase II clinical trials *(109)*.

Interpretation, Insight, and Future Trends for Reperfusion Assessment with Biochemical Markers

Nonmortality endpoints, including use of prognostic infarct sizing with biochemical markers and the technologies listed in Table 1, are currently being used in clinical trials of devices and therapies. Although, clearly troponin is important for risk stratification, the characteristic release of CK-MB, and to a lesser extent HBDH, are more predictable and there is far more evidence for their use in prognostic infarct sizing. Innovative strategies that employ combinations of technologies will become increasingly important as overall mortality from the acute coronary syndromes continues to decrease and therapies aimed at the non-ST elevation and UA are further developed *(6)*. Clinically, the anecdotal use of biochemical markers for prognosis should be standardized and automated so that systematic study is possible.

SUMMARY OF REPERFUSION MONITORING AND PROGNOSTIC INFARCT SIZING

Despite significant advances in the treatment of AMI, thrombolytic therapy is neither successful in, nor appropriate for patients in the entire spectrum of ACS. Many new therapies are emerging, which are designed to further improve reperfusion strategies, reduce infarct size, and improve outcome. Current tools for assessing the success of reperfusion therapies are invasive, expensive, and are not generally available 24 h a day, 7 d per week at all medical centers. Combinations of rather simple, widely available tools enhance the ability for evaluating reperfusion therapies (Table 3). Evaluation of microvascular dysfunction—the physiological "bottom line"—after epicardial reperfusion will increasingly become a focus *(6)*; myoglobin release has been accepted as a surrogate for microvascular perfusion *(67)*. Relationships between infarct size, the ability to predict IRA patency on angiography, and important clinical outcomes are compelling; it has been stated that all studies involving cardiac markers should include infarct sizing *(33,110)*. The information gained from quantitatively examining the shape and pattern of early and late marker release is currently limited, except for evaluating infarct extension. There is need for rapid turnaround of cardiac marker measurements to optimize many emerging applications. The serial measurements of cardiac markers that are routinely performed can add insight into early (re)perfusion monitoring and over the total coronary for prognosis.

ABBREVIATIONS

ACS, Acute coronary syndrome(s); AMI, acute myocardial infarction; AUC, area under the curve; CHF, congestive heart failure; CK, creatine kinase; CK-MB, MB isoenzyme of CK; CTFC, corrected TIMI frame count; cTnT and cTnI, cardiac troponins

T and I; ECG, Electrocardiogram; ESCALAT, Efegatran Sulfate as an Adjunct to Streptokinase versus Heparin as an Adjunct to Tissue Plasminogen Activator in Patients with
Myocardial Infarction; FABP, fatty acid binding protein; GUSTO, Global Use of Strategies to Open Occluded Coronary Arteries in Acute Coronary Syndromes; HBDH,
hydroxygutyrate dehydrogenase; IRA, infarct-related artery; MI, myocardial infarction; MRI, magnetic resonnance imaging; NPV, negative predictive value; NSTEMI,
non-ST elevation MI; PCI, percutaneous coronary intervention; PET, positive-emission
tomography; PPV, positive predictive value; PRIME, Promotion of Reperfusion by Inhibition of Thrombin During Myocardial Infarction Evolution; ROC, receiver operating
characteristic; STEMI, ST elevation MI; TAMI, Thrombolysis and Angioplasty in Myocardial Infarction; TIMI, Thrombolysis in Myocardial Infarction; tPA, tissue plasminogen activator; vWF, von Willegrand factor.

REFERENCES

1. Braunwald E, Maroko PR. The reduction of infarct size—an idea whose time (for testing)
has come. Circulation 1974;50:206–209.
2. Maroko PR, Kjekshus JK, Sobel BE, et al. Factors influencing infarct size following experimental coronary artery occlusions. Circulation 1971;43:67–82.
3. Maroko PR, Braunwald E. Effects of metabolic and pharmacologic interventions on myocardial infarct size following coronary occlusion. Circulation 1976;53:I-162–168.
4. Effectiveness of intravenous thrombolytic treatment in acute myocardial infarction. Gruppo
Italiano per lo Studio della Streptochinasi nell'Infarto Miocardico (GISSI). Lancet 1986;
1:397–402.
5. The GUSTO Angiographic Investigators. The effects of tissue plasminogen activator,
streptokinase, or both on coronary-artery patency, ventricular function, and survival after
acute myocardial infarction. (Erratum published N Engl J Med 1994;330:516). N Engl J
Med 1993;329:1615–1622.
6. Roe MT, Ohman EM, Maas AC, et al. Shifting the open-artery hypothesis downstream:
the quest for optimal reperfusion. J Am Coll Cardiol 2001;37:9–18.
7. Reimer KA, Lowe JE, Rasmussen MM, Jennings RB. The wave-front phenomenon of ischemic cell death: myocardial infarct size vs duration of coronary occlusion in dogs. Circulation 1977;56:786–794.
8. Baughman KL, Maroko PR, Vatner SF. Effects of coronary artery reperfusion on myocardial infarct size and survival in conscious dogs. Circulation 1981;63:317–323.
9. Weissberg PL. Arteriosclerosis involves more than just lipids: plaque dynamics. E Heart
J 1999;(Suppl):T13–T18.
10. Kloner RA, Rude RE, Carlson N, Maroko PR, DeBoer LW, Braunwald E. Ultrastructural
evidence of microvascular damage and myocardial cell injury after coronary artery occlusion: which comes first? Circulation 1980;62:945–952.
11. Collaborative Organization for RheothRx Evaluation (CORE). Effects of RheothRx on
mortality, morbidity, left ventricular function, and infarct size in patients with acute myocardial infarction. Circulation 1997;96:192–201.
12. Kim CB, Braunwald E. Potential benefits of late reperfusion of infarcted myocardium. The
open artery hypotesis. Circulation 1993;88:2426–2436.
13. Braunwald E. Myocardial reperfusion, limitation of infarct size, reduction of left ventricular dysfunction, and improved survival: should the paradigm be expanded? Circulation
1989;78:441–444.
14. Braunwald E. The open-artery theory is alive and well—again. N Engl J Med 1993;329:
1650–1652.

15. Ito H, Tomooka T, Sakai N, et al. Lack of myocardial perfusion immediately after successful thrombolysis: a predictor of poor recovery of left ventricular function in anterior myocardial infarction. Circulation 1992;85:1699–1705.
16. Ito H, Okamura A, Iwakura K, et al. Myocardial perfusion patterns related to thrombolysis in myocardial infarction perfusion grades after coronary angioplasty in patients with acute anterior wall myocardial infarction. Circulation 1996;93:1993–1999.
17. Kloner RA, Rude RE, Carlson N, Maroko PR, DeBoer LW, Braunwald E. Ultrastructural evidence of microvascular damage and myocardial cell injury after coronary artery occlusion: which comes first? Circulation 1980;62:945–952.
18. Kloner RA, Ganote CE, Jennings RB. The "no-reflow" phenomenon after temporary coronary occlusion in the dog. J Clin Invest 1974;54:1496–1508.
19. Braunwald E, Kloner RA. Myocardial reperfusion: a double-edged sword? J Clin Invest 1985;76:1713–1719.
20. Kloner RA. Does reperfusion injury exist in humans? J Am Coll Cardiol 1993;21:537–545.
21. Ito H, Maruyama A, Iwakura K, et al. Clinical implications of the 'no reflow' phenomenon. A predictor of complications and left ventricular remodeling in reperfused anterior wall myocardial infarction. Circulation 1996;93:223–228.
22. Sakuma T, Hayashi Y, Sumii K, Imazu M, Yamakido M. Prediction of short- and intermediate-term prognoses of patients with acute myocardial infarction using myocardial contrast echocardiography one day after recanalization. J Am Coll Cardiol 1998;32:890–897.
23. Wu KC, Zerhouni EA, Judd RM, et al. Prognostic significance of microvascular obstruction by magnetic resonance imaging in patients with acute myocardial infarction. Circulation 1998;97:765–772.
24. Gersh BJ, Anderson JL. Thrombolysis and myocardial salvage: results of clinical trials and the animal paradigm-paradoxic or predictable. Circulation 1993;88:296–306.
25. DeWood MA, Spores J, Notske R, et al. Prevalence of total coronary occlusion during the early hours of transmural myocardial infarction. N Engl J Med 1980;303:897–902.
26. The TIMI Study Group. Thrombolysis in Myocardial Infarction (TIMI) trial. Phase I findings. N Engl J Med 1985;312:932–936.
27. Ross AM, Coyne KS, Moreyra E, et al. Extended mortality benefit of early postinfarction reperfusion. Circulation 1998;97:1549–1556.
28. Gibson CM, Cannon CP, Daley WL, et al. TIMI frame count: a quantitative method of assessing coronary artery flow. Circulation 1996;93:879–888.
29. Gibson CM, Ryan KA, Kelley M, et al. Methodologic drift in the assessment of TIMI grade 3 flow and its implications with respect to the reporting of angiographic trial results. Am Heart J 1999;137:1179–1184.
30. Gibson CM, Murphy SA, Rizzo MJ, et al. Relationship between TIMI frame count and clinical outcomes after thrombolytic administration. Thrombolysis in Myocardial Infarction (TIMI) Study Group. Circulation 1999;99:1945–1950.
31. Davies CH, Ormerod OJM. Failed coronary thrombolysis. Lancet 1998;351:1191–1196.
32. Fesmire FM, Percy RF, Bardoner JB, Wharton DR, Calhoun FB. Usefulness of automated serial 12-lead ECG monitoring during the initial emergency department evaluation of patients with chest pain. Ann Emerg Med 1998;31:3–11.
33. Alpert JS, Thygesen K, Antman E, et al. Myocardial infarction redefined—a consensus doc-ument of The Joint European Society of Cardiology/American College of Cardiology Committee for the redefinition of myocardial infarction. J Am Coll Cardiol 2000;36:959–969.
34. Ryan TJ, Antman EM, Brooks NH, et al. 1999 Update: ACC/AHA guidelines for the management of patients with acute myocardial infarction: executive summary and recommendations. J Am Coll Cardiol 1999;34:890–911.
35. Mizuno K, Satomura K, Miyamoto A, et al. Angioscopic evaluation of coronary-artery thrombi in acute coronary syndromes. N Engl J Med 1992;326:287–291.

36. Keeley EC, Weaver WD. Infarct size: thrombolysis vs. PTCA. Am Heart J 1999;137: 1007–1009.
37. Anderson JL, Karagounis LA, Becker LC, Sorensen SG, Menlove RL. TIMI perfusion grade 3 but not grade 2 results in improved outcome after thrombolysis for myocardial infarction: ventriculographic, enzymatic, and electrocardiographic evidence from the TEAM-2 study. Circulation 1993;87:1829–1839.
38. Califf RM, O'Neil W, Stack RS, et al. Failure of simple clinical measurements to predict perfusion status after intravenous thrombolysis. Ann Intern Med 1988;108:658–662.
39. Doevendans PA, Gorgels AP, van der Zee R, Partouns J, Bar FW, Wellens HJ. Electrocardiographic diagnosis of reperfusion during thrombolytic therapy in acute myocardial infarction. Am J Cardiol 1995;75:1206–1210.
40. Shah PK, Cercek B, Lew AS, Ganz W. Angiographic validation of bedside markers of reperfusion. J Am Coll Cardiol 1993;21:55–61.
41. Ohman EM, Christenson RH, Califf RM, et al. Noninvasive detection of reperfusion after thrombolysis based on serum creatine kinase MB changes and clinical variables. TAMI 7 Study Group. Thrombolysis and Angioplasty in Myocardial Infarction. Am Heart J 1993; 126:819–826.
42. Stewart RE, Miller DD, Bowers TR, et al. PET perfusion and vasodilator function after angioplasty for acute myocardial infarction. J Nucl Med 1997;38:770–777.
43. Wu KC, Zerhouni EA, Judd RM, et al. Prognostic significance of microvascular obstruction by magnetic resonance imaging in patients with acute myocardial infarction. Circulation 1998;97:765–772.
44. Bremerich J, Wendland MF, Arheden H, et al. Microvascular injury in reperfused infarcted myocardium: noninvasive assessment with contrast-enhanced echoplanar magnetic resonance imaging. J Am Coll Cardiol 1998;32:787–793.
45. Matetzky S, Novikov M, Gruberg L, et al. The significance of persistent ST elevation vs. early resolution of ST segment elevation after primary PTCA. J Am Coll Cardiol 1999;34: 1932–1938.
46. Santoro GM, Valenti R, Buonamici P, et al. Relation between ST-segment changes and myocardial perfusion evaluated by myocardial contrast echocardiography in patients with acute myocardial infarction treated with direct angioplasty. Am J Cardiol 1998;82:932–937.
47. Langer A, Krucoff MW, Klootwijk P, et al. Prognostic significance of ST segment shift early after resolution of ST elevation in patients with myocardial infarction treated with thrombolytic therapy: the GUSTO-I ST Segment Monitoring Substudy. J Am Coll Cardiol 1998;31:783–789.
48. Neuhaus KL, Zeymer U, Tebbe U, Schroeder R. Resolution of ST segment elevation is an early predictor of mortality in patients with acute myocardial infarction. Meta analysis of three thrombolysis trials (Abstract). Circulation 1998;98:I-632.
49. Veldkamp RF, Green CL, Wilkins ML, et al. Comparison of continuous ST-segment recovery analysis with methods using static electrocardiograms for noninvasive patency assessment during acute myocardial infarction. Am J Cardiol 1994;73:1069–1074.
50. Moons KGM, Klootwijk P, Meij SH, et al. Continuous ST-segment monitoring associated with infarct size and left ventricular function in the GUSTO-I trial. Am Heart J 1999; 138:525–532.
51. De Groot MJ, Muijtjens AM, Simoons ML, Hermens WT, Glatz JF. Assessment of coronary reperfusion in patients with myocardial infarction using fatty acid binding protein concentrations in plasma. Heart 2001;85:278–285.
52. de Lemos JA, Antman EM, Morrow DA, et al. Heart-type fatty acid binding protein as a marker of reperfusion after thrombolytic therapy. Clin Chim Acta 2000;298:85–97.
53. Ishii J, Nagamura Y, Nomura M, et al. Early detection of successful coronary reperfusion based on serum concentration of human heart-type cytoplasmic fatty acid-binding protein. Clin Chim Acta 1997;262:13–27.

54. Wall TC, Califf RM, George BS, et al. Accelerated plasminogen activator dose regimens for coronary thrombolysis. The TAMI-7 Study Group. J Am Coll Cardiol 1992;19:482–489.

55. Apple FS, Henry TD, Berger CR, Landt YA. Early monitoring of serum cardiac troponin I for assessment of coronary reperfusion following thrombolytic therapy. Am J Clin Pathol 1996;105:6–10.

56. Tanasijevic M, Cannon CP, Wybenga DR, et al. Myoglobin, creatine kinase MB, and cardiac troponin-I to assess reperfusion after thrombolysis for acute myocardial infarction: results from TIMI 10A. Am Heart J 1997;134:622–630.

57. Abe J, Yamaguchi T, Isshiki T, et al. Myocardial reperfusion can be predicted by myoglobin/creatine kinase ratio of a single blood sample obtained at the time of admission. Am Heart J 1993;126:279–285.

58. Jurlander B, Clemmenson, Ohman EM, Christenson R, Wagner GS, Grande P. Serum myoglobin for the early non-invasive detection of coronary reperfusion in patients with acute myocardial infarction. Eur Heart J 1996;17:399–406.

59. Tanasijevic M, Cannon CP, Antman EM, et al. Myoglobin, creatine-kinase-MB and cardiac troponin-I 60-minute ratios predict infarct-related artery patency after thrombolysis for acute myocardial infarction: results from the Thrombolysis in Myocardial Infarction study (TIMI) 10B. J Am Coll Cardiol 1999;343:739–747.

60. Zabel M, Hohnloser SH, Koster W, Prinz M, Kasper W, Just H. Analysis of creatine kinase, CK-MB, myoglobin, and troponin T time-activity curves for early assessment of coronary artery reperfusion after intravenous thrombolysis. Circulation 1993;87:1542–1550.

61. Christenson RH, Ohman EM, Topol EJ, et al. Assessment of coronary reperfusion after thrombolysis with a model combining myoglobin, creatine kinase-MB, and clinical variables. Circulation 1997;96:1776–1782.

62. Stewart JT, French JK, Theroux P, et al. Early noninvasive identification of failed reperfusion after intravenous thrombolytic therapy in acute myocardial infarction. J Am Coll Cardiol 1998;31:1499–1505.

63. Laperche T, Steg PG, Dehoux M, et al. A study of biochemical markers of reperfusion early after thrombolysis for acute myocardial infarction. The PERM Study Group. Prospective Evaluation of Reperfusion Markers. Circulation 1995;92:2079–2086.

64. Laperche T, Golmar JL, Steg PG. Early behavior of biochemical markers in patients with thrombolysis in myocardial infarction grade 2 flow in the infarct artery as opposed to other flow grades after intravenous thrombolysis for acute myocardial infarction. Am Heart J 1997;134:1044–1051.

65. de Lemos JA, Morrow DA, Gibson CM, et al. Early noninvasive detection of failed epicardial reperfusion after fibrinolytic therapy. Am J Cardiol 2001;88:353–358.

66. de Lemos JA, Antman EM, Giugliano RP, et al. Very early risk stratification after thrombolytic therapy with a bedside myoglobin assay and the 12-lead electrocardiogram. Am Heart J 2000;140:373–378.

67. Giannitsis E, Muller-Bardorff M, Lehrke S, et al. Admission troponin T level predicts clinical outcomes, TIMI flow, and myocardial tissue perfusion after primary percutaneous intervention for acute ST-segment elevation myocardial infarction. Circulation 2001;104: 630–635.

68. Ottani F, Galvani M, Nicolini FA, et al. Elevated cardiac troponin levels predict the risk of adverse outcome in patients with acute coronary syndromes. Am Heart J 2000;140:917–927.

69. Hindman N, Grande P, Harrell FE Jr, et al. Relation between electrocardiographic and enzymatic methods of estimating acute myocardial infarct size. Am J Cardiol 1986;58:31–35.

70. Sobel BE, Roberts R, Larson KB. Estimation of infarct size from serum MB creatine phosphokinase activity: applications and limitations. Am J Cardiol 1976:37:474–485.

71. Witteveen SAGJ, Hermens WT, Hemker HC, Hollaar L. Quantitation of enzyme release from infarcted heart muscle. In: Ischemic Heart Disease. Haas JH, Hemker HC, Snellen HA, eds. Baltimore: Williams & Wilkins, 1970, pp. 36–42.

72. Shell WE, Kjekshus JK, Sobel BE. Quantitative assessment of the extent of myocardial infarction in the conscious dog by means of analysis of serial changes in serum creatine phosphokinase activity. J Clin Invest 1971;50:2614–2625.

73. Roberts R, Henry PD, Sobel BE. An improved basis for enzymatic estimation of infarct size. Circulation 1975;52:743–754.

74. Norris RM, Whitlock RML, Barratt-Boyes C, Small CW. Clinical measurement of myocardial infarct size: modification of a method for the estimation of total creatine phosphokinase release after myocardial infarction. Circulation 1975;51:614–620.

75. Ryan W, Karliner JS, Gilpin E, Covell JW, DeLuca M, Ross J. The creatine kinase curve area and peak of creatine kinase after acute myocardial infarction: usefulness and limitations. Am Heart J 1981;101:162–166.

76. Grande P, Hansen BF, Christiansen C, Naestoft J. Estimation of acute myocardial infarct size in man by serum CK-MB measurements. Circulation 1982;65:756–764.

77. Hermens WT, van der Veen FH, Willems GM. Complete recovery in plasma of enzymes lost from the heart after permanent coronary artery occlusion in the dog. Circulation 1990; 81:649–659.

78. Poliner LR, Buja LM, Parkey RW, et al. Comparison of different noninvasive methods of infarct sizing during experimental myocardial infarction. J Nucl Med 1977;18:517–523.

79. Ishikawa Y, Saffitz JE, Mealman RL, Grace AM, Roberts R. Reversible myocardial ischemic injury is not associated with increased creatine kinase activity in plasma. Clin Chem 1997;43:467–475.

80. Christenson RH, Azzazy HME. Biochemical markers of the acute coronary syndromes. Clin Chem 1999;43:2301–2311.

81. Haider AW, Andreotti F, Hackett DR, Tousoulis D, Kluft C, Maseri A, Davies GJ. Early spontaneous intermittent myocardial reperfusion during acute myocardial infarction is associated with augmented thrombogenic activity and less myocardial damage. J Am Coll Cardiol 1995;26:662–667.

82. Andreotti F, Pasceri V, Hackett DR, Davies GJ, Haider AW, Maseri A. Preinfarction angina as a predictor of more rapid coronary thrombolysis in patients with acute myocardial infarction. N Engl J Med 1996;334:7–12.

83. Whitlow PL, Bass TA, Kipperman RM, et al. Results of the study to determine rotablator and transluminal strategy (STRATAS). Am J Cardiol 2001;87:699–670.

84. Tardiff BE, Califf RM, Tcheng JE, et al. Clinical outcomes after detection of elevated cardiac enzymes in patients undergoing percutaneous intervention. IMPACT-II Investigators. Integrilin (eptifibatide) to Minimize Platelet Aggregation and Coronary Thrombosis-II. J Am Coll Cardiol 1999;33:88–96.

85. Willems GM, Muijtjens AM, Lambi FH, Hermens WT. Estimation of circulatory parameters in patients with acute myocardial infarction. Significance for calculation of enzymatic infarct size. Cardiovasc Res 1979;13:578–587.

86. Willems GM, Visser MP, Krill MT, Hermens WT. Quantitative analysis of plasma enzyme levels based upon simultaneous determination of different enzymes. Cardiovasc Res 1982; 16:120–131.

87. Witteveen SAGJ, Hermens WT, Hemker HC, Hollaar L. Quantitation of enzyme release from infarcted heart muscle. In: Ischemic Heart Disease. Haas JH, Hemker HC, Snellen HA, eds. Baltimore: Williams & Wilkins, 1970, pp. 36–42.

88. Shell WE, Kjekshus JK, Sobel BE. Quantitative assessment of the extent of myocardial infarction in the conscious dog by means of analysis of serial changes in serum creatine phosphokinase activity. J Clin Invest 1971;50:2614–2625.

89. Schwerdt H, Ozbek C, Frohlig G, Schieffer H, Bette L. Optimised function for determining time to peak creatine kinase and creatine kinase-MB as non-invasive reperfusion indicators after thrombolytic therapy in acute myocardial infarction. Cardiovasc Res 1990;24: 328–334.

90. Shell WE, Lavelle JF, Covell JW, Sobel BE. Early estimation of myocardial damage in conscious dogs and patients with evolving acute myocardial infarction. J Clin Invest 1973; 52:2579–2590.

91. Vollmer RT, Christenson RH, Reimer K, Ohman EM. Temporal creatine kinase curves in acute myocardial infarction: implications of a good empiric fit with the log-normal function. Am J Clin Pathol 1993;100:293–298.

92. Christenson RH, Duh SH, Roe MT, Ohman EM. Determination of the falloff constant (k_f) from modeling biochemical marker release: a new variable for discriminating therapies. Cardiovasc Toxicol 2001;1:171–176.

93. Puleo PR, Perryman MB, Bresser MA, Rokey R, Pratt CM, Roberts R. Creatine kinase isoform analysis in the detection and assessment of thrombolysis in man. Circulation 1987; 75:1162–1169.

94. Roe CR Validity of estimating myocardial infarct size from serial measurements of enzyme activity in the serum. Clin Chem 1977;23:1807–1812.

95. Horder M, Petersen PH, Thygesen K, Nielsen BL. Plasma enzymes in myocardial infarction. An appraisal of quantitative, clinical and pathophysiological information. Scand J Clin Lab Invest 1981;41:41–47.

96. Marmor A, Sobel BE, Roberts R. Factors presaging early recurrent myocardial infarction ("extension"). Am J Cardiol 1981;48:603–610.

97. Shiraki H, Yoshikawa T, Anzai T, et al. Association between preinfarction angina and a lower risk of right ventricular infarction. N Engl J Med 1998;338:941–947.

98. Ottani F, Galvani M, Ferrini D, Sorbello F, Limonetti P, Pantoli D, Rusticali F. Prodromal angina limits infarct size. A role for ischemic preconditioning. Circulation 1995;91:291–297.

99. Kloner RA, Shook T, Przyklenk K, et al. Previous angina alters in-hospital outcome in TIMI 4. A clinical correlate to preconditioning? Circulation 1995;91:37–45.

100. Anzai T, Yoshikawa T, Asakura Y, et al. Preinfarction angina as a major predictor of left ventricular function and long-term prognosis after a first Q wave myocardial infarction. J Am Coll Cardiol 1995;26:319–327.

101. Bahr RD, Leino EV, Christenson RH. Prodromal unstable angina in acute myocardial infarction: prognostic value of short- and long-term outcome and predictor of infarct size. Am Heart J 2000;140:126–133.

102. De Sutter J, Van de Wiele C, Gheeraert P, et al. The Selvester 32-point QRS score for evaluation of myocardial infarct sizeafter primary coronary angioplasty. Am J Cardiol 1999; 83:255–257.

103. Sobel BE, Bresnahan GF, Shell WE, Yoder RD. Estimation of infarct size in man and its relation to prognosis. Circulation 1972;46:640–648.

104. Moroko PR. Assessing myocardial damage in acute infarcts. N Engl J Med 1974;290: 158–159.

105. Baardman T, Hermens WT, Lenderink T, et al. Differential effects of tissue plasminogen activator and streptokinase on infarct size and on rate of enzyme release: influence of early infarct related artery patency. The GUSTO Enzyme Substudy. Eur Heart J 1996;17:237–246.

106. de Boer MJ, Suryapranata H, Hoorntje JC, et al. Limitation of infarct size and preservation of left ventricular function afterprimary coronary angioplasty compared with intravenous streptokinase in acute myocardial infarction. Circulation 1994;90:753–761.

107. Ottervanger JP, Liem A, de Boer MJ, et al. Limitation of myocardial infarct size after primary angioplasty: is a higher patency the only mechanism? Am Heart J 1999;137:1169–1172.

108. Christenson RH, Vollmer RT, Ohman EM, et al. Relation of temporal creatine kinase-MB release and outcome after thrombolytic therapy for acute myocardial infarction. TAMI Study Group. Am J Cardiol 2000;85:543–547.

109. Mahaffey KW, Bastros EM, Christenson RH, Every NR, Ohman EM. Peak creatine kinase and creatine kinase MB after myocardial infarction strongly correlate with ejection fraction and infarct size by nuclear imaging. Circulation 2000;102:796 (abstract 3844).

110. De Winter RJ, Koster RW, Sturk A, Sanders GT. Value of myoglobin, troponin T, and CK-MBmass in ruling out an acute myocardial infarction in the emergency room. Circulation 1995;92:3401–3407.
111. Suryapranata H, Zijlstra F, MacLeod DC, van den Brand M, De Feyter PJ, Serruys PW. Predictive value of reactive hyperemic response on reperfusion on recovery of regional myocardial function after coronary angioplasty in acute myocardial infarction. Circulation 1994; 89:1109–1117.
112. Gibbons RJ, Miller TD, Christian TF. Infarct size measurement by single photon emission computed tomographic imaging with ^{99m}Tm-sestamibi: a measure of the efficacy of therapy in acute myocardial infarction. Circulation 2000;101:101–108.
113. Garabedian HD, Gold HK, Yasuda T, et al. Detection of coronary artery reperfusion with creatine kinase-MB determinations during thrombolytic therapy: correlation with acute angiography. J Am Coll Cardiol 1988;11:729–734.

5

The Use of Cardiac Biomarkers to Detect Myocardial Damage Induced by Chemotherapeutic Agents

Eugene H. Herman, Steven E. Lipshultz, and Victor J. Ferrans

INTRODUCTION

The treatment of neoplastic diseases with chemotherapeutic agents was initiated more than 50 yr ago. Since then, antineoplastic agents have been derived from diverse sources, such as synthetic chemicals, antibiotics, plant products, antibodies, and enzymes. These agents have contributed to prolongation of disease-free intervals and an increase in overall survival. It was thought that the toxicity associated with chemotherapeutic agents would most likely occur in rapidly proliferating tissues, such as the bone marrow and gastrointestinal tract. However, since the report by Tan et al. *(1)* of delayed heart failure in children treated with the anthracycline daunorubicin, there has been an increased awareness of the potential for cardiovascular side effects during the course of cancer chemotherapy.

CARDIAC TOXICITY OF ANTINEOPLASTIC AGENTS: GENERAL CONSIDERATIONS

A wide variety of antineoplastic agents has been found to exert toxic effects on the cardiovascular system (Table 1). Five of these agents, 5-fluorouracil (5-FU), cyclophosphamide, anthracyclines, mitoxantrone, and Herceptin (trastuzumab), have been found to be frequent causes of cardiotoxicity when used clinically.

5-Fluorouracil

The myocardial alterations induced by 5-FU consist of anginal chest pain, which can progress to the clinical and pathological picture of myocardial infarction (MI) *(2)*. This toxicity develops acutely, soon after the administration of the drug, and has been attributed to drug-induced coronary arterial spasm. The chest pain induced by 5-FU can be evaluated by means of the techniques in current use for the diagnosis of ischemic chest pain resulting from coronary atherosclerosis.

Cyclophosphamide

Very acute cardiotoxicity also can be caused by cyclophosphamide, which has been used in very large doses, either alone or in combination with other chemotherapeutic agents, to ablate bone marrow in preparation for bone marrow transplantation *(3,4)*.

From: *Cardiac Markers, Second Edition*
Edited by: Alan H. B. Wu @ Humana Press Inc., Totowa, NJ

Table 1
Chemotherapeutic Agents with Cardiotoxic Effects

Class/agent	Toxic effect(s)
Anthracyclines	
Doxorubicin	Arrhythmias, CHF
Daunorubicin	Arrhythmias, CHF
Epirubicin	CHF
Idarubicin	Arrhythmias, angina, CHF
Mitoxantrone	Arrhythmias, CHF
Alkylating agents	
Cyclophosphamide	Myocarditis, pericarditis, CHF
Ifosfamide	Arrhythmias, CHF
Mitomycin	CHF
Antimetabolite	
5-FU	Angina, MI
Antimicrotubule agents	
Paclitaxel	Arrhythmias
Etoposide	MI, ECG changes
Teniposide	Arrhythmias
Vinca alkaloids	MI, ECG changes, arrhythmias
Antibody	
Trastuzumab (Herceptin)	Cardiomyopathy
Miscellaneous	
Tretinoin	Pleural—pericardial effusions, MI
Pentostatin	Angina, MI, CHF, arrhythmias

This toxicity is manifested by hemorrhagic myocarditis and pericarditis, both of which can occur within a few hours or days after the administration of the drug. These changes are associated with cardiac microthrombosis and cardiopulmonary failure.

Anthracyclines

In contrast to the preceding two drugs, the cardiotoxicity produced by anthracyclines (doxorubicin, daunorubicin, epirubicin, idarubicin) can show a wide spectrum of clinical and morphological variations, depending on how the drugs are administered in clinical practice and on the amount of time elapsed after the completion of therapy. The cardiotoxicity produced by anthracyclines can be classified into the following subtypes: acute, subacute, chronic, and greatly delayed (5). The first three of these subtypes can be reproduced in a consistent manner in experimental animal models (6). In addition, single, extremely large, lethal doses of anthracyclines have been given to experimental animals. Such doses cause death due to extensive ulceration of the gastrointestinal tract (with subsequent sepsis) within a few days, before the classic cardiac morphologic changes have had time to develop. It is necessary to emphasize that great caution is required in the interpretation of data obtained from these types of studies, which do not have a direct relevance to the clinical use of anthracyclines.

The acute toxicity (electrocardiographic [ECG] changes) produced by anthracyclines is evident within a few minutes to several hours after administration of the drug *(7)*. It is manifested by decreased QRS voltage, sinus tachycardia, ventricular and supraventricular arrhythmia, and prolongation of the QT interval. The subacute type is characterized by acute myocarditis and pericarditis, which develop after a relatively small cumulative dose of the drug and occur uncommonly *(8)*.

The most important manifestation of anthracycline cardiotoxicity is the chronic form, which is dose related (incidence, 7% in patients receiving cumulative doses of 550 mg/m^2 of body surface, 18% incidence at total dose of 700 mg/m^2), and can develop either during the course of therapy or several months after its completion *(7)*. It is manifested by the insidious onset of congestive heart failure (CHF), which eventually can be fatal and is associated with characteristic morphological changes in the cardiac myocytes. These cells show progressively increasing loss of myofibrils and cytoplasmic vacuolization *(9)*. The latter is due to dilation of the tubules and cisterns of the sarcoplasmic reticulum. These changes can be graded semiquantitatively, and there is a good correlation between their severity and that of the clinical manifestations of cardiomyopathy *(10)*. Because of the frequency and importance of this complication, it is highly desirable to employ techniques for its detection at the earliest possible time. As discussed below, the development of these techniques has become an area of very active research.

The greatly delayed type of cardiac toxicity of anthracyclines becomes evident several years after successful completion of the chemotherapy, and is also manifested by CHF. It is most frequently observed in children and adolescents, but also has been recently described in adults. The pathophysiology of this cardiotoxicity remains poorly understood.

Mitoxantrone

Mitoxantrone has pharmaceutical effects similar to those of anthracyclines, and it also produces cardiotoxicity that in many ways resembles that caused by the latter agents *(11)*. Therefore, noninvasive monitoring of the cardiac effects of mitoxantrone is also considered to be of great clinical importance, particularly as this agent is frequently used after a course of anthracyclines has been administered. Furthermore, mitoxantrone has been proposed for the treatment of multiple sclerosis *(12)*.

Herceptin

Cardiac toxicity has been recently reported to occur following treatment with the recombinant human anti-HER2/neu (c-Erb-B2) antibody trastuzumab (Herceptin), in women with breast cancer. The *HER2* proto-oncogene is a transmembrane receptor tyrosine kinase that belongs to the epidermal growth factor family. This receptor is overexpressed in 10–35% of patients with cancer and is associated with decreased disease-free and overall survival in women with breast cancer. Decreases in cardiac function (>10% reduction in ejection fraction) or cardiomyopathy has been observed in approx 5% of patients receiving Herceptin alone *(13)* and 13% of women receiving Herceptin in combination with other chemotherapeutic agents *(14)*. Herceptin has been found to increase both the therapeutic and toxic effect of doxorubicin *(15)*.

THE USE OF BIOMARKERS FOR THE DETECTION OF DRUG-INDUCED MYOCARDIAL INJURY

A number of noninvasive methods (ECG, echocardiography, radionuclide ventriculography, and various other forms of myocardial imaging) have been used to detect and evaluate the extent of chemotherapy-induced myocardial damage *(16,17)*. These techniques have not been able to detect the early stages of doxorubicin cardiotoxicity, in which deterioration of cardiac function has not yet developed *(16,17)*. As a result, there has been interest in identifying other types of noninvasive methods that can be used, either alone or in conjunction with cardiac functional studies, to detect the initial stages and the progression of the cardiotoxicity to optimize the chemotherapeutic dose.

A more recent and promising approach for the detection of myocardial injury involves monitoring the serum concentrations of cytoplasmic enzymes (creatine kinase [CK], MB isoenzymes of CK [CK-MB], lactic dehydrogenase [LDH], LDH isozymes) or other cellular components (cardiac troponin T [cTnT] and cardiac troponin I [cTnI]) that are released from damaged myocytes into the circulating blood *(18)*. Most of the initial observations that detected increases in serum levels of these substances were associated with the cardiac damage produced by MI. These potential biomarkers can be classified into two categories, according to whether they are normally present in small concentrations in serum. The natriuretic peptides represent an exception to this generalization, as increases in their plasma levels indicate a response to cardiac dysfunction rather than a direct expression of myocyte damage.

LDH and CK

LDH is a cytoplasmic enzyme with a high activity in heart, skeletal muscle, liver, kidney, and red blood cells. At least five isozymes of LDH have been identified. The clinical usefulness of the assay for LDH was improved by electrophoretic separation of the isozymes, which found that the LDH1 isozyme was the predominant form found in serum after acute MI *(19)*. The LDH1 isozyme is also found in high concentration in the renal cortex and red blood cells. Other LDH isozymes (2, 3, and 4) also are found in the heart, kidneys, red blood cells, and several other tissues. Because LDH is not tissue-specific, increases in serum levels also may occur in a wide variety of noncardiac disorders, other than cardiac damage.

CK is another cytosolic enzyme that shows increased serum activity after acute MI. The sensitivity of this assay was also improved by monitoring CK-MB or CK mass *(20, 21)*. CK and CK-MB have been used in clinical and nonclinical studies to detect myocardial damage induced by various drugs and toxic agents. The specificity of such determinations is limited because significant amounts of CK-MB are present in skeletal muscle *(22)*. In addition, drugs such as benzodiazepines, tricyclic antidepressants, pyridoxine, and high doses of acetylsalicylic acid can cause elevations of CK-MB *(23)*. The usefulness of these enzymes as biomarkers for detecting drug-induced myocyte damage is limited because the amount of acute muscle injury produced by most drugs is considerably lower than that which occurs after MI. In addition, the timing of the release of these enzymes also may differ markedly in acute or chronic myocardial injury, thus making it more difficult to evaluate these types of data accurately.

Studies in Mice

The mouse has been utilized in many experiments involving acute anthracycline cardiotoxicity. Single high doses of doxorubicin or other anthracylines, ranging from 5 to 20 mg/kg, have caused significant increases in the serum levels of CK and/or LDH. Many investigators have attempted to utilize changes in the activities of these two enzymes as a means to identify potential cardioprotective agents.

Early protection studies in the mouse showed that the increases in CK, CK-MB, and LDH following treatment with daunorubicin were attenuated when the drug was incorporated into a synthetic biodegradable polymer or liposomes *(24,25)*. Electron microscopic evaluation also indicated that the lesions induced by 35 mg/kg of liposomal daunorubicin were less severe than those caused by the free form of the drug (25 mg/kg) *(24)*.

Other studies in mice have examined the potential protective activity of a variety of antioxidant compounds. Serum levels of CK and LDH increased following treatment with 12–20 mg/kg of doxorubicin *(26–31)*. Administration of WR-1065 (the dephosphorylated metabolite of WR-2721 [*S*-(3-aminopropylamino) ethylphosphorothiocic acid]) *(26)*, PZ-51 (Ebselen) *(27)*, 5,6,7,8-tetrahydroneopterin *(28)*, flavonoids *(29)*, thymoquinone *(30)*, or *S*-allylcysteine *(31)* significantly attenuated the increases in serum activity of these two enzymes. In the study of Al-Shabanah et al. *(30)* the maximal CK and LDH levels were 1300 IU and 1100 IU, respectively, 24 h after doxorubicin compared to 800 IU and 600 IU, respectively, at the same time in animals pretreated with thymoquinone. Morphologic confirmation of reduced doxorubicin-induced myocardial lesions was obtained by light microscopy *(30,31)* and electron microscopy *(28)*.

A transgenic mouse model in which metallothionein is overexpressed only in the heart was studied to determine whether elevation of this substance alters doxorubicin cardiotoxicity *(32)*. Administration of 20 mg/kg of doxorubicin caused significant increases in serum CK activity and myocardial lesions in nontransgenic controls, effects that were significantly attenuated in the metallothionein transgenic animals *(32)*. Increases in serum CK associated with buthionine sulfoxine-enhanced doxorubicin toxicity in nontransgenic mice were also significantly reduced in the myocardium in the transgenic mouse model of metallothionein overexpression *(33)*. Doxorubicin-induced increases in serum CK activity were prevented when mice were pretreated with zinc, an inducer of metallothioneins *(34)*. Lack of protective activity has also been detected. Mice treated with a single 10 mg/kg dose of doxorubicin had significantly increased LDH (1.8 times), CK (2.5 times), and CK-MB (7.5 times) serum activity within 24 h *(35)*. Neither the mortality nor the levels of these enzymes were affected by pretreatment with L-histidinol *(35)*.

Studies in Rats

New Zealand black rats were used by Olson and Capen *(36)* as models of doxorubicin toxicity. These investigators found that high doses of doxorubicin (5–20 mg/kg) caused significant elevations in serum LDH, LDH1, LDH2, and LDH3, and the LDH1/LDH2 ratio. Maximal levels were observed 48 h after dosing. Because of widespread tissue damage, these findings were thought to be too nonspecific to imply a cardiac source for the increases of these enzyme levels.

Monitoring the levels of CK and LDH following the administration of high doses of doxorubicin has been utilized in a number of acute cardioprotection studies. Increasing doses of doxorubicin (4–30 mg/kg) in rats caused a dose-related increase in serum CK *(37,38)*. A 29% and 41% decline in peak CK levels was observed in animals given 10 mg/kg of butylated hydroxyanisole plus 10 mg/kg of doxorubicin, or 30 mg/kg of butylated hydroxyanisole plus 30 mg/kg of doxorubicin, respectively, compared to animals receiving 10 or 30 mg/kg of doxorubicin alone *(37,38)*. Increased levels of CK and LDH developed within 24–48 h in rats given a single 6 or 10 mg/kg dose of doxorubicin *(39–41)*. Pretreatment with >25 IU/kg of vitamin A *(39)*, 50 and 100 mg/kg of propolis *(42)*, 300 mg/kg of WR-2721, and/or 1.6 mg/kg of sodium selenite *(40)* or 100 mg/kg/d × 3 d of phenobarbital *(41)* significantly lowered the serum levels of CK and LDH to values that were close to those observed in control animals. The lower values of the two enzymes in animals pretreated with propolis correlated with a reduction in cardiomyopathy scores from 2.5–3.0 (doxorubicin alone) to 1–1.5 (propolis + doxorubicin) *(42)*.

Wistar rats developed sarcoplasmic and mitochondrial alterations 96 h after treatment with a single 15 mg/kg dose of doxorubicin *(43)*. At 24 h after treatment, the levels of CK in these animals were comparable with those in control animals; however, they were significantly elevated (twofold) at 96 h *(43)*. The potential protective effects of desferrioxamine *(44)*, captopril *(45)*, and thymoquinone *(46)* were examined in adult Wistar and Swiss albino rats. Pretreatment with 250 mg/kg of desferrioxamine or 60 mg/kg of captopril just prior to treatment with 15 mg/kg of doxorubicin attenuated the increases in serum CK, CK-MB, LDH, and LDH isozyme activities seen 24 and 48 h after treatment with doxorubicin alone *(44,45)*. The cardiac isozymes of LDH and CK increased 194% and 68%, respectively, 48 h after treatment with doxorubicin alone, but the increases were significantly lower in rats pretreated with desferrioxamine prior to doxorubicin (56% and 17%, respectively) *(44)*. Thymoquinone, given in the drinking water starting 5 d before doxorubicin, also exerted protective activity, as shown by 30.5% and 62.3% decreases in LDH and CK activities, respectively, over the increases observed in rats given doxorubicin alone *(46)*. Changes in serum CK activity were monitored in normal and streptozoticin-diabetic hamsters and rats following treatment with 15 mg/kg of doxorubicin *(47)*. Serum CK activity peaked 6 h post-dosing in both groups of rats; however, doxorubicin appeared to be more toxic in diabetic rats. Maximal levels of CK were significantly higher in the diabetic animals *(47)*.

Several recent pretreatment studies in rats have utilized single doses of doxorubicin that ranged from 20 to 30 mg/kg. Animals pretreated with 200 mg/kg/d of curcumin for 10 d *(48)*, 5 mmol/kg/d of glutathione for 10 d *(49)*, or 25–200 mg/kg of desferrioxamine *(50)* all had significantly attenuated increases in LDH and CK levels compared to those observed in rats that received doxorubicin alone. The levels of CK-MB and LDH were increased 4.8- to 5.35-fold over control values in animals given 25 mg/kg of doxorubicin *(50)*. Pretreatment with various doses of desferrioxamine significantly reduced, but did not completely eliminate, the increases in serum enzyme activity. Cardiomyopathy scores were reduced from 3 (doxorubicin alone) to 1 in desferrioxamine-treated animals (125–500 mg/kg) *(50)*.

Few studies have been reported in which serum enzymes were monitored in rats after chronic treatment with doxorubicin. One such investigation sought to evaluate the potential protective activity of tetracycline *(51)*. Male Sprague–Dawley rats were treated with 2 mg/kg/wk of doxorubicin (weekly) and 10 mg/kg/d of tetracycline for 8 wk. At the end of the experiment, the mean CK activity in doxorubicin-treated animals was 104

IU, compared with 96 IU in animals pretreated with tetracycline and 59 IU in saline-treated control animals *(51)*. Based on the level of CK activity, the study concluded that tetracycline did not prevent doxorubicin cardiotoxicity.

Experiments in rats also have utilized changes in serum enzyme levels to assess the cardiotoxic potential of anthracyclines other than doxorubicin. Serum CK and CK-MB activities were monitored 3–6 d after the fourth daily treatment with 2.5 mg/kg of epirubicin *(52)*. CK-MB activity in control rats was 16% of the total CK activity. Three days after treatment with epirubicin, CK-MB isozyme activity increased approximately fivefold and amounted to 60% of the total CK activity *(52,53)*. The level of CK-MB returned to near predosing levels by d 6. Total CK activity increased to 160% of predosing levels and declined toward control activity in parallel with CK-MB. A single 10 mg/kg dose of epirubicin was given to a separate group of rats. The level of CK-MB activity observed was higher after the 10 mg/kg cumulative dose regimen than after the single 10 mg/kg high dose of epirubicin. Vitamin E (0.1 mg/kg), given orally prior to each of the 2.5 mg/kg doses of epirubicin, suppressed the increase in serum CK activity. Doxorubicin was not included for comparison nor was histopathological information reported in this study. The cardiotoxic potential of epirubicin was compared with that of seven other antitumor agents in a study that utilized serum enzyme activity to evaluate cardiotoxicity. Wistar rats were treated with 5 mg/kg of epirubicin, 5 mg/kg of chlorambucil, 5 mg/kg of cisplatin, or 3 mg/kg of methotrexate daily for 5 d *(54)*. Serum enzyme activity was increased by all four agents. However, epirubicin caused the most profound changes and was the only agent that increased levels of all enzymes monitored (CK, CK-MB, and LDH) *(54)*. The study concluded that epirubicin was considerably more cardiotoxic than cisplatin, chlorambucil, and methotrexate.

Studies in Rabbits

Although the rabbit was the first animal in which the chronic cardiotoxicity of doxorubicin and daunorubicin was detected, very few studies include monitoring serum enzymes in the analysis. In an early study, 0.7 mg/kg of doxorubicin was given to New Zealand rabbits every other day until reaching cumulative doses of 18–36 mg/kg *(55)*. Mean terminal serum LDH and CK levels of rabbits with cardiomyopathy were increased 2.5- and 2.8-fold over control values, respectively, in animals with significant cardiac lesions. No elevations in the activity of either enzyme were seen in rabbits with little or no cardiac changes. The protective effects of vitamin E (200 mg/d for 4 d) was evaluated in New Zealand rabbits treated with a single 7 mg/kg dose of doxorubicin *(56)*. Within 24 h serum CK increased two times over pretreatment levels and all rabbits died within 7 d. Treatment with vitamin E for 4 or more days prevented the elevation in CK activity and increased survival. The myocardial lesions observed by light and electron microscopy reflected the attenuation in CK activity and were less severe in the animals that had been given vitamin E and doxorubicin than in those given doxorubicin alone.

Studies in Dogs

The dog has been used primarily in chronic studies in which attempts have been made to mimic clinical treatment regimens. Very few of these studies included serum enzyme analyses. In a safety assessment study beagle dogs were given a single dose of 1.75 mg/kg of doxorubicin or 0.125 or 0.25 mg/kg of mitoxantrone once every 3 wk for a total of

eight or nine cycles *(57)*. A significant increase in CK-MB was detected 1 d after the
ninth dosing (24 wk) in four of six doxorubicin-treated dogs *(57)*. CK-MB levels remained
normal in the mitoxantrone-treated dogs. It was concluded that, at the doses utilized,
mitoxantrone was not cardiotoxic *(57)*. A comparison was made of the sensitivity of
various modes {electrocardiogram, cardiac ultrastructure and serum enzymes (CK-MB,
α-hydroxybutyrate dehydrogenase [α-HBDH])} to detect cardiotoxicity in beagle dogs
given 1.5 mg/kg of doxorubicin once a week for 3 wk *(58)*. Electrocardiographic abnormalities (progressive decrease in QT intervals, reduction in T-wave amplitude and sinus
tachycardia) and ultrastructural changes in the myocardium (dilation of sarcoplasmic
reticulum, alterations of T tubules) were detected by the fourth week of the study. However, the levels of both CK-MB and α-HBDH were comparable to pretreatment values
(58). These investigators concluded that CK-MB and α-HBH are not reliable markers
of slowly developing myocardial damage, such as that caused by anthracyclines.

Studies in Humans

The use of serum enzymes for monitoring anthracycline cardiotoxicity during treatment regimes has also been very limited. Neri et al. *(59,60)* monitored CK-MB prior to
and 15 h after anthracycline dosing. They determined that elevations of 8 IU or more
after treatment are indicative of acute cardiac toxicity. In a group of nine patients that
were tested with doxorubicin for a total of 66 therapeutic cycles (maximum cumulative
dose, 540 mg/m^2), CK-MB increased by more than 8 IU in 31 (57%) of the 66 cycles.
In comparison, patients treated with 121 cycles of epirubicin (maximum dose of 720 mg/
m^2) experienced increases in CK-MB in only 16 cycles of the 121 (13%) *(60)*. Based on
CK-MB data and echocardiographic analysis the study concluded that epirubicin was
40% less cardiotoxic than doxorubicin. Both CK-MB and myoglobin were monitored
in 15 patients 3, 5, 12, 24, and 36 h following administration of 25–50 mg/m^2 of doxorubicin *(61)*. No significant change in CK-MB levels was observed up to 36 h after treatment. Significantly elevated myoglobin values were found in eight patients. The highest
concentrations were observed 24 h after treatment. Because doxorubicin was administered with other drugs, it was not clear to what extent the other drugs may have been
responsible for the increases in myoglobin levels.

Evaluation of serum enzymes has been reported only in very few patients with 5-FU
cardiotoxicity. A young man without heart disease received 5-FU (25 mg/kg every 24 h
by continuous infusion over a period of 5 d) *(62)*. He experienced severe chest pain on
the second day of treatment. During the periods of pain both the ECG and serum CK
levels were normal *(62)*. A group of 104 patients received 24–30 mg/kg of 5-FU/d by
8-h infusion *(63)*. Cardiotoxic effects (ECG changes, palpitations, or cardiac distress)
were observed during 25 of 192 treatment cycles. However, no consistent changes
in serum enzyme activity were detected *(63)*. The serum CK levels in a patient who had
received 4 wk of 5-FU and levamisole therapy rose to >1000 U/L. In this instance, the
patient did not experience cardiac symptoms and the source of the enzyme was determined to be skeletal muscle *(64)*.

Three cases of acute cardiopulmonary toxicity that mimicked acute cardiac ischemia
were reported following treatment with vinorelbine *(65)*. However, neither elevations
in CK activity nor ECG changes were observed.

Cardiac Troponins

Measurement of serum levels of cTnT and cTnI are used clinically for the detection of myocardial damage in various conditions *(18)*. The troponins are localized in at least two intracellular compartments. Small quantities of cTnT and cTnI (3–7%) are found in the cytoplasm, and the remainder is complexed with actin *(18)* in the myofibrils. These proteins are products of different and unrelated genes. Both cTnT and cTnI are expressed in different isoforms in slow and fast-twitch skeletal muscle and cardiac muscle *(66,67)*. cTnI contains 31 amino acid residues at the amino terminus that differ from that of the fast or slow skeletal muscle isoforms *(66)*. As a result, there is a 40% difference between the structure of cTnI and that of the other isoforms. cTnI is expressed only in myocardium, even with ongoing chronic disease processes. These properties are favorable for a specific marker of myocardial injury. There are several commercially available immunoassays for the quantitative determination of cTnI in blood. These assays give varying measures of cTnI because of differences in calibration and epitopes recognized by the corresponding monoclonal antibodies *(68)*.

cTnT differs by only 6–11 amino acid residues from skeletal muscle isoforms *(67)*. The skeletal muscle form can be reexpressed in human myocardium under certain stressful conditions *(69)*. cTnT is expressed in a "fetal form" in embryonic skeletal muscle, but is not normally found in adult skeletal muscle. Nevertheless, this fetal form can be reexpressed in skeletal muscle of patients who have certain skeletal muscle diseases and in renal failure *(68)*. However, Ricchiuti et al. *(70)* have determined that the second-generation commercial assay will not detect the cTnT isoforms that are reexpressed in patients with renal or skeletal disease. An improved third-generation assay for cTnT retains specificity and requires less time to perform *(71)*. The increased specificity and sensitivity of these new assays have served to extend their clinical usefulness for diagnosing subtle myocardial injury related to exposure to cardiotoxic agents and for determining the efficiency of cardioprotective procedures in both preclinical and clinical situations.

The antibodies used in the first- and second-generation immunoassays for human cTnT also have been shown to recognize cTnT epitopes in a variety of animals *(72)*. Rat hearts had the highest cross-reactivity, and chicken and fish hearts, the lowest *(72)*. Skeletal muscle from rats, pigs, and goats had 10% of the reactivity of cTnT as determined by the first-generation cTnT assay but only 1% of the cTnT with the second-generation assay *(72)*. It appears that the second-generation assay for cTnT has sufficient reactivity and selectivity to distinguish between cardiac and skeletal muscle damage. In a recent study, Fredericks et al. *(73)* measured the cardiac troponins and CK isoenzymes (using commercially available assays) in cardiac and skeletal muscle samples from rats, dogs, pigs, and monkeys. In all four species, the content of cTnI and cTnT detected in skeletal muscle was <0.6% of that found in the myocardium. In all species, the amount of CK was greater in skeletal muscle than in cardiac tissue, and the CK-MB/total CK ratio was lower in skeletal muscle than in myocardium. The differences in CK-MB content between skeletal and heart muscle were considerably less than the tissue differences in the amounts of the two cardiac troponins in the same tissues. These findings provide additional support for the specificity of cardiac troponins as biomarkers of experimentally induced myocardial damage.

Only a single commercial cTnT assay (which is standardized) is currently available, in contrast to several cTnI immunoassays (with no standardization consensus). At present, it has not been determined whether all the antibodies developed for the various cTnI assays, which are directed against different epitopes of the human cTnI protein, would also be appropriate for monitoring cTnI in animals. Immunoassays for cTnT have been used to detect myocardial injury induced by a variety of means, such as ischemia (rats and dogs) *(74,75)*, rejection of transplanted hearts in rats *(76)*, viral myocarditis (mice) *(77,78)*, and drug toxicity (rats and mice) *(75,79)*. cTnT was monitored in all the studies except that of Smith et al. *(78)*, which utilized one of the cTnI immunoassays. The findings derived from these studies also tend to support the notion that monitoring serum levels of cTnT, and possibly of cTnI, can provide a sensitive means to detect and monitor myocardial injury in experimental studies.

The quantity of cTnT that reaches the blood varies according to the type of myocardial injury. The serum concentration of cTnT can reach levels of several nanograms per milliliter after acute MI *(18)*. In experimental ischemia–reperfusion studies, the serum concentrations of cTnT increased to 13 ng/mL after 4.5 h of reperfusion in dogs and 10 ng/mL after 130 min of reperfusion in rats *(75)*. Rats given two doses of isoproterenol developed myocardial necrosis and had high serum concentrations of cTnT (3.75 ng/mL) *(79)*. In contrast, considerably less cTnT is released from the myocardium damaged by anthracyclines. The highest concentration of cTnT detected by Herman et al. *(80)* was 0.66 ng/mL in a spontaneously hypertensive rat (SHR) given a total cumulative dose of 12 mg/kg of doxorubicin, with a maximal cardiomyopathy score of 3. Other SHRs with doxorubicin-induced cardiac lesions had serum levels of 0.30 ng/mL or less *(80)*. The terminal sampling in a study of daunorubicin-treated rabbits found a mean serum cTnT concentration of 0.13 ng/mL *(81)*. In children treated with doxorubicin, cTnT concentrations increased from 0.01 ng/mL to between 0.03 and 0.09 ng/mL. This increase in cTnT concentration was found to be clinically meaningful as a predictor of subsequent cardiotoxicity *(82,83)*. Thus, the small changes in cTnT detected after anthracycline therapy can provide useful diagnostic information.

Studies in Mice

A study was initiated to determine whether cTnT levels would increase after various types of experimentally induced myocardial damage *(75)*. As part of this study, mice were treated with 10 mg/kg of doxorubicin daily for 5 d. cTnT levels of 10 ng/mL were detected in the blood of these animals at the conclusion of doxorubicin treatment *(75)*. No information regarding cardiac morphology was reported.

Studies in Rats

Evidence for the usefulness of cTnT as a biomarker of doxorubicin cardiotoxicity in SHR was initially reported by Seino et al. *(84)*. These investigators found increased serum cTnT levels in SHR that were treated once a week with 1.5 mg/kg of doxorubicin for 8 wk. More recently, Herman et al. *(80,85)* detected increases in serum levels of cTnT in SHRs given cumulative doses of 2–12 mg/kg of doxorubicin. The magnitude of the increase in serum cTnT concentrations correlated with the total cumulative dose of doxorubicin and with the severity of the cardiomyopathy scores. An important finding was the small increase in serum concentrations of cTnT found after treatment with low cumulative doses of doxorubicin. Seven of 10 SHRs treated with either 2 or 4 mg/kg of doxorubicin had neither observable morphologic alterations nor changes in serum cTnT levels *(80)*. However, three other SHRs in these treatment groups had lesion scores of 1 or 1.5 and minimal increases in the serum concentration of cTnT (0.03 in one animal and 0.05 ng/mL in two animals). Each of these concentrations was above the limit of the assay (0.0123 ng/mL) and the highest nontreatment control level (0.02 ng/mL) *(79)*. In SHR, the 6 mg/kg cumulative dose of doxorubicin was the threshold dose that induced cardiac lesions (score of 1.5) and increased serum concentrations of cTnT (average = 0.13 ng/mL) in all animals. These findings strongly suggest that monitoring the levels of cTnT provides important information concerning both the incidence and the extent of doxorubicin-induced cardiotoxicity.

The cTnT released from damaged cells can arise from two separate troponin pools in the myocyte (a soluble cytosolic pool and a major pool bound to the contractile apparatus) *(18)*. It seems likely that both the cytosolic and the myofibrillar forms of cTnT contribute to the increased serum levels of this protein detected in doxorubicin-treated SHRs. Some of the cytosolic pool of cTnT could leak from the cardiac myocytes as a result of doxorubicin-induced oxidative damage to the cell membrane *(86)*. Myofibril-bound cTnT could also be released when myofibrillar loss occurs as a result of exposure to doxorubicin. Herman et al. *(80,85)* found evidence for the release of cTnT from myofibrils. The antibody used in the commercial cTnT assay was found to stain specifically myofibrillar-associated cTnT in myocytes of SHRs. The intensity of this staining was diminished in the myocytes of SHRs that had been treated chronically with doxorubicin and had elevated serum levels of cTnT *(80,85)*.

The usefulness of serum levels of cTnT to detect myocardial damage from other chemotherapeutic agents, such as mitoxantrone, was evaluated by Herman et al. *(11)*. Both doxorubicin (10 mg/kg cumulative dose) and mitoxantrone (6 mg/kg cumulative dose) were given chronically to SHRs. The degree of cardiotoxicity induced by doxorubicin in this study was similar to that reported previously at comparable cumulative doses *(80,85)*. The study also confirmed that the serum concentrations of cTnT are increased (0.79 ± 0.3 ng/mL) in SHRs given cumulative doses of 10 mg/kg of doxorubicin *(80, 85)*. This study also provided evidence that serum levels of cTnT are decreased (0.79 ± 0.3 to 0.24 ± 0.13 ng/mL) in association with reduced cardiomyopathy scores (mean of 2.5 and 1.5) in SHRs given the cardioprotectant agent, dexrazoxane prior to doxorubicin. The myocardial lesions observed after a cumulative dose of 6 mg/kg of mitoxantrone were similar to those found in an earlier study *(87)*. As in the case of doxorubicin-induced cardiac lesions, this cardiomyopathy was also accompanied by an increase in the serum levels of cTnT (mean 0.20 ± 0.12 ng/mL). This represents the first report showing that the cardiotoxicity of mitoxantrone can be detected by monitoring serum concentrations of cTnT. This study also assessed the cardioprotection provided by pretreatment with dexrazoxane, which clearly attenuated mitoxantrone cardiotoxicity. Cardioprotection was detected by both the reduction in cardiac lesion scores (2.1 vs 1.3) and the reduction in serum levels of cTnT (0.20 vs 0.04 ng/mL). This observation constitutes the first report of amelioration of mitoxantrone-induced cardiomyopathy by dexrazoxane in the SHR model.

Studies in Rabbits

Adamcova et al. *(81)* evaluated the usefulness of cTnT as a biomarker of cardiac damage caused by daunorubicin and Oracin (a new chemotherapeutic agent of the iso-quinoline type). They administered 3 mg/kg of daunorubicin/wk (for 9 wk) or 10 mg/kg of Oracin/wk (for 10 wk). cTnT levels were within the normal range (i.e., <0.1 ng/mL) through the fifth week of dosing. The initial (pretreatment) concentrations of cTnT were nearly zero, but showed small but significant elevations prior to the fifth dosing. Mean cTnT levels of 0.22 ± 0.08 ng/mL were detected in the three animals that had severe cardiac lesions and died after the eighth dose of daunorubicin. No increase in cTnT concentration occurred after 10 doses of Oracin, and this finding correlated with the lack of changes in cardiac function and cardiac morphology after treatment with this agent.

Studies in Humans

The results of the animal experiments have provided the impetus for evaluating the potential utility of monitoring the serum levels of the cardiac troponins to detect anthracycline cardiotoxicity in patients. In an early report, Genser et al. *(88)* monitored the plasma concentrations of cTnT and CK-MB mass in children 0, 6, 12, 24, and 72 h after receiving chemotherapy with doxorubicin ($n = 13$) or daunorubicin ($n = 4$). Plasma concentrations of both cTnT and CK-MB mass remained within the normal range at all time points up to 72 h post-dosing. None of the children showed any overt clinical or ECG signs of myocardial damage. These investigators concluded that the dosage regimen of anthracyclines used in this study did not cause acute myocardial damage. A subsequent clinical study also found no change in cTnT levels in children who had received three to five doses of doxorubicin, daunorubicin, or idarubicin chemotherapy *(89)*. These investigators may not have been able to detect small increases of cTnT because the criterion for elevation was established at a level of 0.2 ng/mL or greater. Raderer et al. *(90)* monitored serum cTnT concentrations for up to 48 h in adult patients after initial doses of 50 mg/m^2 doxorubicin or 100 mg/m^2 epirubicin. As in the previous studies, no elevation in cTnT levels was detected. They interpreted these observations as indicating that anthracycline-induced cardiotoxicity does not develop from acute myocardial damage. In contrast, Ottinger et al. *(82)* found that serum concentrations of cTnT increased from nonmeasurable to low concentrations in children undergoing treatment with doxorubicin. Subsequently, using the second-generation commercial assay, Lipshultz et al. *(83)* found that the low-level increases in serum cTnT (0.03–0.09 ng/mL) observed after the initial induction dose of doxorubicin or succeeding intensification doses (45–222 mg/m^2) were indicative of risk for left ventricular abnormalities (dilation and wall thinning) in children.

cTnI concentrations have also been monitored in patients undergoing chemotherapy with anthracyclines. Increases in serum levels of cTnI were reported by Missov et al. *(91)*, who found mean cTnI concentrations of 71.3 ± 29.2 pg/mL in adults treated with intermediate cumulative doses of doxorubicin (240–300 mg/m^2) compared to 35.8 ± 17.5 pg/mL found in patients with cancer but not receiving anthracyclines. It should be noted that for some undetermined reason, cTnI concentrations were above baseline (17.5 ± 17.9 ng/mL), even in some of the normal control subjects. Cardinale et al. *(92)* evaluated the value of monitoring serum levels of cTnI, CK, and CK-MB in a subgroup of 204 adults with aggressive neoplasms undergoing different combinations of high-dose chemotherapy (three or four cycles) containing potentially cardiotoxic drugs (200 mg/m^2 of epirubicin, 4–7 g/m^2 of cyclophosphamide, 10 g/m^2 of ifosfamide, 85 mg/m^2 of taxotere, and 45 mg/m^2 of idarubicin). Plasma cTnI, CK, CK-MB, and CK-MB mass were monitored prior to and 12, 24, 36, and 72 h after each cycle of chemotherapy. No change in CK levels was observed, whereas CK-MB levels were elevated in three patients who also had increases in cTnI levels. Patients were divided into cTnI– ($n = 139$) or cTnI+ ($n = 65$) subgroups depending on the maximal cTnI levels detected after chemotherapy. A patient was included in the cTnI+ group (range 0.5–2 ng/mL) if a cTnI concentration ≥0.5 ng/mL was detected at any time point after a cycle of chemotherapy, whereas patients in the cTnI– group had cTnI concentrations of <0.5 ng/mL in every determination. A progressive decline in left ventricular (LV) ejection fraction that was maximal 3 mo after completion of therapy was observed in the cTnI– patients. By 6 mo posttreatment this functional alteration had returned to normal values. By comparison, the decline of LV ejection fraction in the cTnI+ patients was more severe and was still apparent 6 mo after chemotherapy was terminated. These authors concluded that the increase in cTnI detected in patients subjected to high-dose chemotherapy serves as an accurate biomarker for the subsequent development of irreversible depression of myocardial function.

We have recently studied *(93)* cTnT in nearly 4000 serum samples obtained from more than 200 children newly diagnosed as having high-risk acute lymphoblastic leukemia. Approximately 10% of these patients have low-level elevations of cTnT, indicating the presence of active myocardial injury. These findings are very useful, as they identify a patient subpopulation that may be at high risk of developing doxorubicin-induced myocardial toxicity due to the fact that they have preexisting active cardiac injury prior to receiving this drug. This may reflect the fact that some children with newly diagnosed cancer can be in acutely poor health due to myocardial leukemic infiltrates, shock, anemia, acidosis, or other disorders leading to acute cardiac injury. Such patients are appropriate targets for individualized cardioprotective strategies to be used in conjunction with doxorubicin therapy. This study also showed that the maximal cTnT elevations in these children were below those found in adults with acute MI or unstable angina, and that there was a correlation between the cumulative dose of doxorubicin and the duration and degree of elevation of cTnT. Some children receiving doxorubicin had single isolated elevations of cTnT; however, other children had chronic elevations in cTnT for months, suggesting continuing myocardial injury. These findings also may serve to guide cardioprotective therapy in these patients.

In a randomized, blinded study of children with newly diagnosed leukemia, Lipshultz et al. (unpublished observations) found that both the duration and the magnitude of the elevation in serum cTnT levels were reduced by half in patients receiving the combination of doxorubicin and dexrazoxane compared to those in patients receiving doxorubicin alone. This suggests that continuing cardioprotection with dexrazoxane may be advisable in such cases (i.e., beyond the period of treatment with doxorubicin). However, the additional benefit of such therapy remains to be demonstrated.

Natriuretic Peptides

Both atrial natriuretic peptide (ANP) and brain natriuretic peptide (BNP) are normally detectable in blood *(94,95)*. They are secreted by the cardiac myocytes as a result of increases in atrial or ventricular wall stretch. Elevated levels of ANP and BNP occur in patients with various types of myocardial diseases *(94)*, associated with CHF. It has been suggested that the natriuretic peptides and their N-terminal propeptides (NT-proANP and NT-proBNP) may be useful biomarkers for evaluating the severity of cardiac dysfunction *(94,96–98)*. In this regard, BNP and NT-proBNP are thought to be superior to ANP or NT-proANP *(99)*.

There is interest in determining whether changes in plasma levels of the natriuretic peptides could be useful in assessing cardiac function during chemotherapy with cardiotoxic drugs such as the anthracyclines. Both ANP and BNP exert natriuretic, diuretic, and vasodilating activity and are released in response to increases in systemic arterial pressure and plasma volume *(100)*. They are therefore indicators of cardiac homeostatic responses and dysfunction and not of cardiac damage, per se.

Studies in Rats

Yokota et al. *(101,102)* compared the plasma levels of BNP in normal Wistar rats and in rats that developed a nephrotic syndrome after treatment with a single 7 mg/kg dose of doxorubicin. Plasma levels of BNP rose with time and more than doubled by 3 wk after dosing (2.3 ± 0.6 vs 0.8 ± 0.2 pmol/mL). Parallel increases in ANP were also observed. Examination of cardiac structure and function was not included in this study, and the rise in peptide levels was attributed to decreased renal elimination of sodium and water. In a cardiac-oriented study, Bernardini et al. *(103)* treated female Wistar rats with either a single 10 mg/kg dose of doxorubicin or 3 mg/kg doses once a week for 3 wk. Plasma ANP levels were significantly decreased 3 h (12.5 ± 2.9 compared to the untreated control mean value of 35.1 ± 5.7 pg/mL) and 6 h (19.4 ± 1.2 compared to the untreated control mean value of 37.9 ± 4.1 pg/mL) in animals following a single 10 mg/kg dose of doxorubicin. Rats given multiple doses of doxorubicin had significantly elevated plasma ANP levels 21 d (88.3 ± 7.7 pg/mL compared to 41.8 ± 8.0 pg/mL in control rats) and 31 d (61.00 ± 14.3 pg/mL compared to 26.5 ± 7.2 pg/mL in saline control animals) after the third dose of doxorubicin. However, ANP levels in these rats returned to control values by 42 d post-dosing. Thus, changes in plasma ANP levels observed in the rats were considered to represent an indication of a doxorubicin-induced myocardial damage. However, no direct evidence of myocardial damage was presented.

Studies in Rabbits

The rabbit was used as a model to study the effect of chronic doxorubicin treatment on cardiac β-adrenergic receptors *(104)*. Cardiovascular alterations characteristic of chronic heart failure (pulmonary congestion, hydrothorax, and ascites) were seen to varying degrees in male rabbits that were treated with 1 mg/kg of doxorubicin twice a week for 9 wk. Down-regulation of cardiac β-adrenergic receptors was detected in doxorubicin-treated rabbits. This down-regulation correlated with the severity of the heart failure. A fourfold increase in plasma ANP levels was found at the end of the study (68.8 ± 14.3 vs 17.1 ± 3.0 fmol/mL in saline control animals). As the hearts were used for determining the density of β-adrenergic receptors, no cardiac morphological information was obtained.

Studies in Dogs

Toyoda et al. *(105)* gave intracoronary doxorubicin (0.7 mg/kg once a week for 5 wk) to induce experimental cardiomyopathy in dogs. Significant alterations in myocardial structure and function were observed 3 mo after the final infusion. During this same period, plasma ANP concentrations increased from 33.8 ± 7.0 to 76.5 ± 14.8 pg/mL. These investigators concluded that doxorubicin-induced depression of left ventricular function is accompanied by alterations in plasma ANP, in accord with observations made in patients with heart failure.

Studies in Humans

Studies in patients have produced conflicting results regarding the use of ANP in evaluating anthracycline-induced cardiotoxicity. Neri et al. *(106)* monitored changes in myocardial function (radionuclide ventriculography) and ANP levels in 26 female patients who had received between 3 and 10 cycles of epirubicin (120 mg/m^2/cycle). The administration of epirubicin was limited to cumulative doses of 840 and 1200 mg/ m^2 because of a 25% decrease in LV ejection fraction and a progressive increase in plasma ANP levels. Two patients who developed symptoms of CHF had significantly elevated ANP concentrations (49% and 56%). The study indicated that monitoring plasma ANP is useful in detecting the severity of hemodynamic compromise in patients with anthracycline-impaired cardiac function. Bauch et al. *(107)* also reported changes in ANP associated with doxorubicin chemotherapy. Plasma levels of ANP were increased in 6 of 16 children (136.2 ± 23.3 pg/mL vs 33.3 ± 4.1 pg/mL in the 10 other patients). Significant increases occurred within 3 wk after the last dosing. Five of the six patients with elevated ANP levels were treated with 160–370 mg/m^2 of doxorubicin and subsequently developed CHF. Yamashita et al. *(108)* reported that plasma endothelin-1 levels progressively increased in two women who were treated with doxorubicin and ultimately developed CHF. They then carried out a prospective study with 30 patients treated with doxorubicin in whom plasma endothelin-1, plasma ANP, and M-mode echocardiography were monitored serially. The plasma concentrations of endothelin-1 increased progressively in five of the patients, two of whom ultimately developed CHF. In contrast, plasma ANP levels and measures of cardiac function remained stable until the development of CHF. This study concluded that monitoring plasma endothelin-1 would be more useful than plasma ANP for predicting the risk of doxorubicin-induced cardiotoxicity.

Tikanoja et al. *(109)* monitored serum levels of N-terminal ANP (NT-ANP) in 43 children during treatment and in 45 children after treatment with doxorubicin. During chemotherapy, the mean serum NT-ANP level was elevated over that in age-matched controls (0.26 vs 0.14 nmol/L), but the increase did not correlate with the cumulative doxorubicin dose. Blood collection times were not standardized and as a result the NT-ANP levels could have been influenced by diurnal variation. In a second group of patients who had previously completed chemotherapy (median of 5 yr) serum levels of NT-ANP were higher than those in age-matched controls (0.22 vs 0.14 nmol/L). The highest NT-ANP concentrations (0.30 nmol/L) were found in patients who had received bone marrow transplantation or cardiac irradiation or both. These investigators concluded that monitoring serum NT-ANP levels during chemotherapy was of relatively minor diagnostic utility but might be helpful in the overall long-term assessment of cardiac function in patients who have finished chemotherapy. Hayakawa et al. *(110)* monitored echocardiography and plasma levels of ANP and BNP in 34 children who were in remission after being treated with cumulative doxorubicin doses between 142 and 696 mg/m^2. Eight patients (23.5%) had echocardiographically detected left ventricular dysfunction. Both ANP and BNP levels in these patients were significantly increased over those in healthy age-matched controls (28.8 ± 14.6 pg/mL vs 14.8 ± 5.8 pg/mL and 29.0 ± 31.2 pg/mL vs 5.6 ± 3.8 pg/mL, respectively). Three of the eight patients with cardiac dysfunction had normal ANP and BNP levels. The increased ANP and BNP levels correlated significantly with systolic function but not with diastolic function. Thus, serial measurements of natriuretic peptide levels may provide an early identification of children at risk for late decompensation as a result of anthracycline therapy. However, there are indications that monitoring changes in diastolic function might provide better information than systolic function concerning the long-term cardiac status of patients who have received doxorubicin chemotherapy *(17)*. Nousiainen et al. *(111)* also conducted a study to determine the value of serial monitoring of the serum levels of natriuretic peptides for detecting LV dysfunction in patients receiving doxorubicin. Plasma levels of ANP increased from 16.4 ± 1.3 pmol/L to 22.7 ± 2.4 pmol/L, NT-proANP from 288 ± 22 to 380 ± 42 pmol/L, and BNP from 3.3 ± 0.4 to 8.5 ± 2.0 pmol/L 4 wk after the last dose of chemotherapy. LV ejection fraction declined from 58.0 ± 1.3% to 49.6 ± 1.7% during this time. The decrease in LV ejection fraction was already apparent after a 200 mg/m^2 cumulative dose of doxorubicin, while the increase in plasma natriuretic peptide levels was not detected until a 400 mg/m^2 cumulative dose of doxorubicin had been attained. These results suggest that serial natriuretic peptide measurements cannot be used in predicting impairment of LV function, but may be useful in the detection of subclinical LV dysfunction in patients treated with doxorubicin. These investigators had previously evaluated the acute neurohumoral and cardiovascular effects of idarubicin in 10 patients with the measurement of plasma levels of ANP, echocardiography, and ECG *(112)*. Patients were dosed with 12 mg/m^2 idarubircin on d 1, 3, and 5 as part of induction chemotherapy. Plasma concentrations of ANP increased from 18.2 ± 1.5 pmol/L to 27.8 ± 3.5 pmol/L, to 30.2 ± 3.0 pmol/L, and to 40.8 ± 6.0 pmol/L after the first, second, and third doses, respectively. Likewise increases in plasma BNP from 6.2 ± 1.9 to 9.0 ± 1.0 pmol/L and 17.5 ± 8.1 pmol/L were observed after the first and third doses of idarubicin. At the same time there was a trend toward an increase in LV end-diastolic diameter ($p < 0.07$). The elevated serum levels of BNP correlated significantly with the increase in LV dilatation. These investigators were not certain whether the changes observed in natriuretic protein levels or cardiac dimensions were predictive of late clinical cardiomyopathy. They did suggest that monitoring BNP was superior to ANP. BNP has been reported to be more stable as well as more sensitive and specific than ANP in the detection of LV dysfunction *(113)*.

Suzuki et al. *(114)* examined the potential diagnostic value of BNP in 27 adults who had received an average cumulative dose of 221 ± 54 mg/m^2 of doxorubicin. In 24 patients, transient BNP increases were maximal within 3–7 d after treatment and then returned to baseline levels over 2 wk. Two of three patients with persistently elevated BNP levels eventually died of cardiac failure. It should be noted that circulating levels of other hormones (ANP, renin, aldosterone, norepinephine, and epinephrine) and myocardial markers (CK-MB, myosin light chain) did not become abnormal.

Okumura et al. *(115)* monitored serum levels of ANP and BNP in 13 patients with acute leukemia who received chemotherapy that included daunorubicin (up to 700 mg/m^2 cumulative dose). Cardiac function was evaluated in all patients prior to initiation of chemotherapy. Three patients developed overt CHF and 15 patients were diagnosed as having subclinical heart failure following completion of treatment. The plasma levels of BNP in these 18 patients increased above the normal limit (40 pg/mL) prior to the detection of clinical or subclinical heart failure by radionuclide venticulography. In contrast, plasma concentrations of ANP did not always increase in these same patients. BNP levels did not increase above control values in patients who had no evidence of heart failure. This study concluded that BNP is superior to ANP in predicting early anthracycline-induced cardiotoxicity. A recent study included monitoring plasma natriuretic peptides as one means of assessing the cardiotoxic effects of epirubicin-containing adjuvant chemotherapy in 40 patients with breast cancer *(116)*. The treatment regimens, included five cycles of fluorouracil, epirubicin (90 mg/m^2), and cyclosphosphamide (group 1) or four cycles of these drugs followed by high-dose chemotherapy consisting of cyclophosphamide, thiotepa, and carboplatin (group 2). The cumulative dose of epirubicin was 450 mg/m^2 in group 1 and 360 mg/m^2 in group 2. Cardiac evaluation was performed up to 1 yr after the initiation of chemotherapy. Although the mean LV ejection fractions remained within the normal range, 17% of the patients had a LV ejection fraction below 0.5 and 28% of the patients experienced a decrease in the LV ejection fraction of more than 0.1. Plasma NT-ANP levels increased gradually from 237 ± 76 pmol to 347 ± 106 pmol/L after 1 yr. During the same period the concentration of BNP increased from 2.9 ± 2.8 pmol/L to 5.1 ± 4.3 pmol/L. The decline in LV ejection fraction and increased natriuretic peptide levels indicates that the relatively low doses of epirubicin used in this study as adjuvant chemotherapy for breast cancer induce mild subclinical myocardial damage. However, the increased level of natriuretic peptides was not associated with a decrease in LV ejection fraction, and as none of the patients developed CHF, the predictive value of the increased NT-ANP and BNP levels remains uncertain.

Snowden et al. *(117)* examined the use of plasma BNP as a marker of ventricular dysfunction in 15 patients treated with high-dose preparative chemotherapeutic regimens (including cyclophosphamide) and hematopoietic stem cell transplantation. The BNP was monitored prior to treatment and weekly up to 5 wk posttreatment. Seven patients had a significant elevation in BNP (above a previously established threshold of 43 pmol/L) associated with myocardial failure, which occurred from 1 to 4 wk after the initiation of therapy. In three of these patients, clinical evidence of cardiac failure was subsequently detected 3, 9, and 23 d after a BNP concentration of 43 pmol/L had been reached. These three patients had the highest peak BNP concentrations, which were sustained for a week or longer. The four patients in which the high level of BNP was not sustained were considered to have experienced a transient period of cardiac damage that was not sufficient to cause decompensation. Patients with BNP >43 pmol/L appeared more likely to have received high-dose cyclophosphamide in the preparative regimen. These investigators concluded that plasma BNP (particularly if concentrations are elevated for a week or more) could be used as biomarkers, in conjunction with other methods of patient monitoring, for early detection of myocardial dysfunction in patients undergoing therapy prior to stem cell transplantation.

ABBREVIATIONS

ANP, BNP, Atrial and brain naturietic peptides; CHF, congestive heart failure; CK, creatine kinase; CK-MB, MB isoenzyme of creatine kinase; cTnI and T, cardiac troponins I and T; ECG, electrocardiogram; 5-FU, 5-fluorouracil; HER2/neu, trastuzumab, Herceptin; LDH lactic dehydrogenase; LV, left ventricular; MI, myocardial infarction; NT-ANP and -BNP, N-terminal atrial and brain natriuretic peptides; NT-proANP and -proBNP, N-terminal atrial and brain natriuretic propeptides; PZ-51, Ebselen; SHR, spontaneously hypertensive rat; WR-1065, dephosphorylated metabolite of WR-2721; WR-2721, *S*-(3-aminopropylamino)ethylphosphorothiocic acid.

REFERENCES

1. Tan C, Tasaka H, Yu KP, Murphy ML, Karnofsky DA. Daunomycin, an antitumor antibiotic, in the treatment of neoplastic disease. Clinical evaluation with special reference to childhood leukemia. Cancer 1967;20:333–353.
2. Labianca R, Beretta G, Clerici M, Fraschini P, Luporini G. Cardiac toxicity of 5-fluorouracil: a study on 1083 patients. Tumori 1982;68:505–510.
3. Buja LM, Ferrans VJ, Graw RG Jr. Cardiac pathologic findings in patients treated with bone marrow transplantation. Hum Pathol 1976;7:17–45.
4. Braverman AC, Antin JH, Plappert MT, Cook EF, Lee RT. Cyclophosphamide cardiotoxicity in bone marrow transplantation: a prospective evaluation of new dosing regimens. J Clin Oncol 1991;9:1215–1223.
5. Grenier MA, Lipshultz SE. Epidemiology of anthracycline cardiotoxicity in children and adults. Semin Oncol 1998;25:72–85.
6. Herman EH, Ferrans VJ. Preclinical animal models of cardiac protection from anthracycline-induced cardiotoxicity. Semin Oncol 1998;25:15–21.
7. Von Hoff DD, Rozencweig M, Piccart M. The cardiotoxicity of anticancer agents. Semin Oncol 1982;9:23–33.
8. Shan K, Lincoff AM, Young JB. Anthracycline-induced cardiotoxicity. Ann Intern Med 1996;125:47–58.
9. Ferrans VJ. Overview of cardiac pathology in relation to anthracycline cardiotoxicity. Cancer Treat Rep 1978;62:955–961.
10. Billingham ME. Role of endomyocardial biopsy in diagnosis and treatment of heart disease. In: Cardiovascular Pathology. Silver MD, ed. New York: Churchill Livingstone, 1991, pp. 465–1486.
11. Herman EH, Zhang J, Rifai N, et al. The use of serum levels of cardiac troponin T to compare the protective activity of dexrazoxane against doxorubicin- and mitoxantrone-induced cardiotoxicity. Cancer Chemother Pharmacol 2001;48:297–304.
12. Millefiorini E, Gasperini C, Pozzilli C, et al. Randomized placebo-controlled trial of mitoxantrone in relapsing-remitting multiple sclerosis: 24-month clinical and MRI outcome. J Neurol 1997;244:153–159.
13. Cobleigh MA, Vogel CL, Tripathy D, et al. Multinational study of the efficacy and safety of humanized anti-HER2 monoclonal antibody in women who have HER2-overexpressing metastatic breast cancer that has progressed after chemotherapy for metastatic disease. J Clin Oncol 1999;17:2639–2648.
14. Sparano JA. Cardiac toxicity of trastuzumab (Herceptin): implications for the design of adjuvant trials. Semin Oncol 2001;28:20–27.
15. Stebbing J, Copson E, O'Reilly S. Herceptin (trastuzumab) in advanced breast cancer. Cancer Treat Rev 2000;26:287–290.
16. Carrio I, Estorch M, Lopez-Pousa A. Assessing anthracycline cardiotoxicity in the 1990s. Eur J Nucl Med 1996;23:359–364.
17. Ganz WI, Sridhar KS, Ganz SS, Gonzalez R, Chakko S, Serafini A. Review of tests for monitoring doxorubicin-induced cardiomyopathy. Oncology 1996;53:461–470.
18. Mair J. Progress in myocardial damage detection: new biochemical markers for clinicians. Crit Rev Clin Lab Sci 1997;34:1–66.

19. Vasudenvan G, Mercer DW, Varat MA. Lactic dehydrogenase isoenzyme determination in the diagnosis of acute myocardial infarction. Am J Cardiol 1978;57:1055–1057.

20. Robert R, Gowda KS, Ludbrook PA. Specificity of elevated serum MB creatine phosphokinase activity in the diagnosis of acute myocardial infarction. Am J Cardiol 1975;36: 433–437.

21. Apple FS, Presse LM. Creatine kinase-MB: detection of myocardial infarction and monitoring reperfusion. J Clin Immunoassay 1994;17:24–29.

22. Tsung JS, Tsung SS. Creatine kinase isoenzymes in extracts of various human skeletal muscles. Clin Chem 1986;32:1568–1570.

23. Chesebro MJ. Using serum markers in the early diagnosis of myocardial infarction. Am Fam Physician 1997;55:2667–2674.

24. Fichtner I, Arndt D, Elbe B, Reszka R. Cardiotoxicity of free and liposomally encapsulated rubomycin (daunorubicin) in mice. Oncology 1984;41:363–369.

25. Hrdina R, Bogusova TA, Kunova A, Kvetina J. Changes in the toxicity and therapeutic efficacy of daunorubicin linked with a biodegradable carrier. Neoplasma 1991;38:265–273.

26. Bhanumathi P, Saleesh EB, Vasudevan DM. Creatine phosphokinase and cardiotoxicity in adriamycin chemotherapy and its modification by WR-1065. Biochem Arch 1992;8: 335–338.

27. Pritsos CA, Sokoloff M, Gustafson DL. PZ-51 (Ebselen) in vivo protection against adriamycin-induced mouse cardiac and hepatic lipid peroxidation and toxicity. Biochem Pharmacol 1992;44:839–841.

28. Kojima S, Hayashi M, Kajiwara Y, Kitabatake K, Kubota K, Icho T. Inhibitory effect of 5,6,7,8-tetrahydroneopterin on adriamycin-induced cardiotoxicity. J Pharmacol Exp Ther 1993;266:1699–1704.

29. Sadzuka Y, Sugiyama T, Shimoi K, Kinae N, Hirota S. Protective effect of flavonoids on doxorubicin-induced cardiotoxicity. Toxicol Lett 1997;92:1–7.

30. Al-Shabanah OA, Badary OA, Nagi MN, Al-Gharably NM, al-Rikabi AC, al-Bekairi AM. Thymoquinone protects against doxorubicin-induced cardiotoxicity without compromising its antitumor activity. J Exp Clin Cancer Res 1998;17:193–198.

31. Mostafa MG, Mima T, Ohnishi ST, Mori K. S-Allylcysteine ameliorates doxorubicin toxicity in the heart and liver in mice. Planta Med 2000;66:148–151.

32. Kang YJ, Chen Y, Yu A, Voss-McCowan M, Epstein PN. Overexpression of metallothionein in the heart of transgenic mice suppresses doxorubicin cardiotoxicity. J Clin Invest 1997;100:1501–1506.

33. Wu HY, Kang YJ. Inhibition of buthionine sulfoximine-enhanced doxorubicin toxicity in metallothionein overexpressing transgenic mouse heart. J Pharmacol Exp Ther 1998;287: 515–520.

34. Kimura T, Fujita I, Itoh N, et al. Metallothionein acts as a cytoprotectant against doxorubicin toxicity. J Pharmacol Exp Ther 2000;291:299–302.

35. Al-Shabanah OA, Badary OA, Al-Gharably NM, Al-Sawaf HA. Effects of L-histidinol on the antitumour activity and acute cardiotoxicity of doxorubicin in mice. Pharmacol Res 1998;38:225–230.

36. Olson HM, Capen CC. Subacute cardiotoxicity of adriamycin in the rat: biochemical and ultrastructural investigations. Lab Invest 1977;37:386–394.

37. Vora J, Boroujerdi M. Pharmacokinetic-toxicodynamic relationships of adriamycin in rat: prediction of butylated hydroxyanisole-mediated reduction in anthracycline cardiotoxicity. J Pharm Pharmacol 1996;48:1264–1269.

38. Vora J, Khaw BA, Narula J, Boroujerdi M. Protective effect of butylated hydroxyanisole on adriamycin-induced cardiotoxicity. J Pharm Pharmacol 1996;48:940–944.

39. Tesoriere L, Ciaccio M, Valenza M, et al. Effect of vitamin A administration on resistance of rat heart against doxorubicin-induced cardiotoxicity and lethality. J Pharmacol Exp Ther 1994;269:430–436.

40. Dobric S, Dragojevic-Simic V, Bokonjic D, Milovanovic S, Marincic D, Jovic P. The efficacy of selenium, WR-2721, and their combination in the prevention of adriamycin-induced cardiotoxicity in rats. J Environ Pathol Toxicol Oncol 1998;17:291–299.

41. Behnia K, Boroujerdi M. Inhibition of aldo-keto reductases by phenobarbital alters metabolism, pharmacokinetics and toxicity of doxorubicin in rats. J Pharm Pharmacol 1999;51: 1275–1282.

42. Chopra S, Pillai KK, Husain SZ, Giri DK. Propolis protects against doxorubicin-induced myocardiopathy in rats. Exp Mol Pathol 1995;62:190–198.

43. Porta EA, Joun NS, Matsumura B, Sablan H. Acute adriamycin toxicity in rats. Res Common Chem Pathol Pharmacol 1993;41:125–137.

44. Al-Harni MM, al-Gharably NM, al-Shabanah OA, al-Bekairi AM, Osman AM, Tawfik HN. Prevention of doxorubicin-induced myocardial and hematological toxicities in rats by the iron chelates desferrioxamine. Cancer Chemother Pharmacol 1992;31:200–204.

45. Al-Shabanah O, Mansour M, El-Kashef H, Al-Bekairi A. Captopril ameliorates myocardial and hematological toxicities induced by adriamycin. Biochem Mol Biol Int 1998;45: 419–427.

46. Nagi MN, Mansour MA. Protective effect of thymoquinone against doxorubicin-induced cardiotoxicity in rats: a possible mechanism of protection. Pharmacol Res 2000;41:283–289.

47. Al-Shabanah OA, El-Kashef HA, Badary OA, al-Bekairi AM, Elmazar MM. Effect of streptozotocin-induced hyperglycaemia on intravenous pharmacokinetics and acute cardiotoxicity of doxorubicin in rats. Pharmacol Res 2000;41:31–37.

48. Venkatesan N. Curcumin attenuation of acute adriamycin myocardial toxicity in rats. Br J Pharmacol 1998;124:425–427.

49. Mohamed HE, El-Swefy SE, Hagar HH. The protective effect of glutathione administration on adriamycin-induced acute cardiac toxicity in rats. Pharmacol Res 2000;42:115–121.

50. Saad SY, Najjar TA, al-Rikabi AC. The preventive role of deferoxamine against acute doxorubicin-induced cardiac, renal and hepatic toxicity in rats. Pharmacol Res 2001;43:211–218.

51. Pour A, Cady W, Modrak J. Effect of tetracycline on adriamycin cardiotoxicity. Toxicol Lett 1981;7:379–382.

52. Przybyszewski WM, Widel M. Activity of creatine kinase MB-isoenzyme in rat serum after heart irradiation and/or farmorubicin (4'-epidoxorubicin) treatment. Cancer Lett 1996;100: 145–150.

53. Przybyszewski WM, Widel M, Koterbicka A. Early peroxidizing effects of myocardial damage in rats after gamma-irradiation and farmorubicin (4'-epidoxorubicin) treatment. Cancer Lett 1994;81:185–192.

54. Pispirigos K, Paradelis AG, Karakiulakis G. Evaluation of cardiac subacute toxicity of epirubicin, chlorambucil, cisplatin, methotrexate and a homo-aza-steroid ester with anti-tumor activity in rats using serum biochemical parameters. Arzneimittelforschung Drug Res 1997;47:92–96.

55. Olson HM, Young DM, Prieur DJ, LeRoy AF, Reagan RL. Electrolyte and morphologic alterations of myocardium in adriamycin-treated rabbits. Am J Pathol 1974;77:439–454.

56. Wang YM, Madanat FF, Kimball JC, et al. Effect of vitamin E against adriamycin-induced toxicity in rabbits. Cancer Res 1980;40:1022–1027.

57. Henderson BM, Dougherty WJ, James VC, Tilley LP, Noble JF. Safety assessment of a new anticancer compound, mitoxantrone, in beagle dogs: comparison with doxorubicin. I. Clinical observations. Cancer Treat Rep 1982;66:1139–1143.

58. Danesi R, Del Tacca M, Bernardini N, Cardini G, Bellini O. Evaluation of the JT and corrected JT intervals as a new ECG method for monitoring doxorubicin cardiotoxicity in the dog. J Pharmacol Methods 1989;21:317–327.

59. Neri B, Torcia MG, Comparini T, Guidi S, Miliari A, Ciapini A. Creatine kinase-MB: a noninvasive test monitoring acute adriamycin and daunomycin cardiotoxicity. J Exp Clin Cancer Res 1938;2:41–45.

60. Neri B, Cini-Neri G, Bandinelli M, Pacini P, Bartalucci S, Ciapini A. Doxorubicin and epirubicin cardiotoxicity: experimental and clinical aspects. Int J Clin Pharmacol Ther Toxicol 1989;22:217–221.

61. Clerico A, Marini A, Del Chicca MG, et al. Modifications in the concentrations of circulating myoglobin after treatment with low doses of adriamycin. Tumori 1985;71:463–468.

62. Braumann D, Mainzer K, Gunzl C, Lewerenz B. [Myocardial infarcts within the scope of 5-fluorouracil therapy]. Onkologie 1990;13:465–467.

63. Pan L, Yang X, Song H. [Cardiotoxicity of 5-fluorouracil]. Chung Hua Fu Chan Ko Tsa Chih 1996;31:86–89.

64. Cersosimo RS, Lee JM. Creatine kinase elevation associated with 5-fluorouracil and levamisole therapy for carcinoma of the colon. A case report. Cancer 1996;77:1250–1253.

65. Karminsky N, Merimsky O, Kovner F, Inbar M. Vinorelbine-related acute cardiopulmonary toxicity. Cancer Chemother Pharmacol 1999;43:180–182.

66. Wilkinson JM, Grand RJ. Comparison of amino acid sequence of troponin I from different striated muscles. Nature 1978;271:31–35.

67. Pearlstone JR, Carpenter MR, Smillie LB. Amino acid sequence of rabbit cardiac troponin T. J Biol Chem 1986;261:16795–16810.

68. Apple FS. Tissue specificity of cardiac troponin I, cardiac troponin T and creatine kinase-MB. Clin Chim Acta 1999;284:151–159.

69. Anderson PAW, Maloue NN, Oakley AE. Troponin T isoform expression in humans: a comparison among normal and failing heart. Circ Res 1991;69:122–123.

70. Ricchiuti V, Voss EM, Ney A, Odland M, Anderson PA, Apple FS. Cardiac troponin T isoforms expressed in renal diseased skeletal muscle will not cause false-positive results by the second generation cardiac troponin T assay by Boehringer Mannheim. Clin Chem 1998;44:1919–1924.

71. Kam PM, Raucher T, Mueller BM. Clinical evaluation of the cardiac markers troponin T and CK-MB on the elecsys 2010 system. Clin Chem 1997;43:S159.

72. O'Brien PJ, Dameron GW, Beck ML, Brandt M. Differential reactivity of cardiac and skeletal muscle from various species in two generations of cardiac troponin-T immunoassays. Res Vet Sci 1998;65:135–137.

73. Fredericks S, Merton GK, Lerena MJ, Heining P, Carter ND, Holt DW. Cardiac troponins and creatine kinase content of striated muscle in common laboratory animals. Clin Chim Acta 2001;304:65–74.

74. Voss EM, Sharkey SW, Gernert AE, et al. Human and canine cardiac troponin T and creatine kinase-MB distribution in normal and diseased myocardium. Infarct sizing using serum profiles. Arch Pathol Lab Med 1995;119:799–806.

75. O'Brien PJ, Dameron GW, Beck ML, et al. Cardiac troponin T is a sensitive, specific biomarker of cardiac injury in laboratory animals. Lab Anim Sci 1997;47:486–495.

76. Walpoth BH, Tschopp A, Peheim E, Schaffner T, Althaus U. Assessment of troponin-T for detection of cardiac rejection in a rat model. Transplant Proc 1995;27:2084–2087.

77. Bachmaier K, Mair J, Offner F, Pummerer C, Neu N. Serum cardiac troponin T and creatine kinase-MB elevations in murine autoimmune myocarditis. Circulation 1995;92:1927–1932.

78. Smith SC, Ladenson JH, Mason JW, Jaffe AS. Elevations of cardiac troponin I associated with myocarditis. Experimental and clinical correlates. Circulation 1997;95:163–168.

79. Bleuel H, Deschl U, Bertsch T, Bolz G, Rebel W. Diagnostic efficiency of troponin T measurements in rats with experimental myocardial cell damage. Exp Toxicol Pathol 1995; 47:121–127.

80. Herman EH, Zhang J, Lipshultz SE, et al. Correlation between serum levels of cardiac troponin-T and the severity of the chronic cardiomyopathy induced by doxorubicin. J Clin Oncol 1999;17:2237–2243.

81. Adamcova M, Gersl V, Hrdina R, et al. Cardiac troponin T as a marker of myocardial damage caused by antineoplastic drugs in rabbits. J Cancer Res Clin Oncol 1999;125:268–274.

82. Ottinger ME, Sallan S, Rikzi N, Sacks DG, Lipshultz SE. Myocardial damage in doxoru-
    bicin-treated children: a study of serum cardiac troponin T (abstract). Proc Am Soc Clin
    Oncol 1995;14:345.

83. Lipshultz SE, Rifai N, Sallan SE, et al. Predictive value of cardiac troponin T in pediatric
    patients at risk for myocardial injury. Circulation 1997;96:2641–2648.

84. Seino Y, Tomita Y, Nagai Y, et al. Cardioprotective effects of ACE-inhibitor (Cilazapril)
    on adriamycin cardiotoxicity in spontaneously hypertensive rats (abstract). Circulation
    1993;88:I–633.

85. Herman EH, Lipshultz SE, Rifai N, et al. Use of cardiac troponin T levels as an indicator
    of doxorubicin-induced cardiotoxicity. Cancer Res 1998;58:195–197.

86. Myers CE, Gianni L, Simone CB, Klecker R, Greene R. Oxidative destruction of erythro-
    cyte ghost membranes catalyzed by the doxorubicin–iron complex. Biochemistry 1982;21:
    1707–1712.

87. Herman EH, Zhang J, Hasinoff BB, Clark JR Jr, Ferrans VJ. Comparison of the structural
    changes induced by doxorubicin and mitoxantrone in the heart, kidney and intestine
    and characterization of the Fe(III)–mitoxantrone complex. J Mol Cell Cardiol 1997;29:
    2415–2430.

88. Genser N, Fink FM, Mair J, Dengg K, Ellenmuter H, Puschendorf B. Plasma concentra-
    tion of creatine kinase MB mass and troponin T in children receiving anthracycline che-
    motherapy (abstract). Clin Chem 1993;39:1170.

89. Fink FM, Genser N, Fink C, et al. Cardiac troponin T and creatine kinase MB mass con-
    centrations in children receiving anthracycline chemotherapy. Med Pediatr Oncol 1995;
    25:185–189.

90. Raderer M, Kornek G, Weinlander G, Kastner J. Serum troponin T levels in adults under-
    going anthracycline therapy. J Natl Cancer Inst 1997;89:171.

91. Missov E, Calzolari C, Davy JM, Leclercq F, Rossi M, Pau B. Cardiac troponin I in patients
    with hematologic malignancies. Cor Artery Dis 1997;8:537–541.

92. Cardinale D, Sandri MT, Martinoni A, et al. Left ventricular dysfunction predicted by early
    troponin I release after high-dose chemotherapy. J Am Coll Cardiol 2000;36:517–522.

93. Lipshultz SE, Sallan S, Dalton V, et al. Elevated serum cardiac troponin-T as a marker for
    active cardiac injury during therapy for childhood acute lymphoblastic leukemia (ALL)
    (abstract). Proc ASCO 18:568a.

94. Sagnella GA. Measurement and significance of circulating natriuretic peptides in cardio-
    vascular disease. Clin Sci (Colch) 1998;95:519–529.

95. Holmes SJ, Espiner EA, Richards AM, Yandle TG, Frampton C. Renal, endocrine, and
    hemodynamic effects of human brain natriuretic peptide in normal man. J Clin Endocrinol
    Metab 1993;76:91–96.

96. Mukoyama M, Nakao K, Hosoda K, et al. Brain natriuretic peptide as a novel cardiac hor-
    mone in humans. Evidence for an exquisite dual natriuretic peptide system, atrial natri-
    uretic peptide and brain natriuretic peptide. J Clin Invest 1991;87:1402–1412.

97. Omland T, Aakvaag A, Vik-Mo H. Plasma cardiac natriuretic peptide determination as a
    screening test for the detection of patients with mild left ventricular impairment. Heart
    1996;76:232–237.

98. Morita E, Yasue H, Yoshimura M, Okumura K, Ogawa H, Kagiyama K. Increased plasma
    level of BNP in patients with acute myocardial infarction. J Am Coll Cardiol 1993;88:82–91.

99. McDonagh TA, Robb SD, Murdoch DR, et al. Biochemical detection of left-ventricular
    systolic dysfunction. Lancet 1998;351:9–13.

100. Levin ER, Gardner DG, Samson WK. Natriuretic peptides. N Engl J Med 1998;339:321–328.

101. Yokota N, Yamamoto Y, Aburaya M, et al. Increased secretion of brain natriuretic peptide
     and atrial natriuretic peptide, but not sufficient to induce natriuresis in rats with nephrotic
     syndrome. Biochem Biophys Res Commun 1991;174:128–135.

102. Yokota N, Yamamoto Y, Iemura F, et al. Increased plasma levels and effects of brain natriuretic peptide in experimental nephrosis. Nephron 1993;65:454–459.

103. Bernardini N, Agen C, Favilla S, Danesi R, Del Tacca M. Doxorubicin cardiotoxicity is associated with alterations of plasma levels of atrial natriuretic factor. J Endocrinol Invest 1992;15:79–84.

104. Bocherens-Gadient SA, Quast U, Nussberger J, Brunner HR, Hof RP. Chronic adriamycin treatment and its effect on the cardiac beta-adrenergic system in the rabbit. J Cardiovasc Pharmacol 1992;9:770–778.

105. Toyoda Y, Okada M, Kashem MA. A canine model of dilated cardiomyopathy induced by repetitive intracoronary doxorubicin administration. J Thorac Cardiovasc Surg 1998; 115:1367–1373.

106. Neri B, De Scalzi M, De Leonardis V, Gemelli MT, Ghezzi P, Pacini P. Preliminary study on behaviour of atrial natriuretic factor in anthracycline-related cardiac toxicity. Int J Clin Pharmacol Res 1991;11:75–81.

107. Bauch M, Ester A, Kimura B, Victorica BE, Kedar A, Phillips MI. Atrial natriuretic peptide as a marker for doxorubicin-induced cardiotoxic effects. Cancer 1992;69:1492–1497.

108. Yamashita J, Ogawa M, Shirakusa T. Plasma endothelin-1 as a marker for doxorubicin cardiotoxicity. Int J Cancer 1995;62:542–547.

109. Tikanoja T, Riikonen P, Perkkio M, Helenius T. Serum N-terminal atrial natriuretic peptide (NT-ANP) in the cardiac follow-up in children with cancer. Med Pediatr Oncol 1998; 31:73–78.

110. Hayakawa H, Komada Y, Hirayama M, Hori H, Ito M, Sakurai M. Plasma levels of natriuretic peptides in relation to doxorubicin-induced cardiotoxicity and cardiac function in children with cancer. Med Pediatr Oncol 2001;37:4–9.

111. Nousiainen T, Jantunen E, Vanninen E, et al. Natriuretic peptides as markers of cardiotoxicity during doxorubicin treatment for non-Hodgkin's lymphoma. Eur J Haematol 1999; 62:135–141.

112. Nousiainen T, Jantunen E, Vanninen E, et al. Acute neurohumoral and cardiovascular effects of idarubicin in leukemia patients. Eur J Haematol 1998;61:347–353.

113. Cowie MR, Struthers AD, Wood DA, et al. Value of natriuretic peptides in assessment of patients with possible new heart failure in primary care. Lancet 1997;350:1349–1353.

114. Suzuki T, Hayashi D, Yamazaki T, et al. Elevated B-type natriuretic peptide levels after anthracycline administration. Am Heart J 1998;136:362–363.

115. Okumura H, Iuchi K, Yoshida T, Nakamura S, Takeshima M, Takamatsu H. Brain natriuretic peptide is a predictor of anthracycline-induced cardiotoxicity. Acta Haematol 2000; 104:158–163.

116. Meinardi MT, van Veldhuisen DJ, Gietema JA, et al. Prospective evaluation of early cardiac damage induced by epirubicin-containing adjuvant chemotherapy and locoregional radiotherapy in breast cancer patients. J Clin Oncol 2001;19:2746–2753.

117. Snowden JA, Hill GR, Hunt P, et al. Assessment of cardiotoxicity during haemopoietic stem cell transplantation with plasma brain natriuretic peptide. Bone Marrow Transplant 2000;26:309–313.

6

The Use of Biomarkers to Provide Diagnostic and Prognostic Information Following Cardiac Surgery

Jesse E. Adams, III

INTRODUCTION

Coronary artery bypass grafting (CABG) is utilized as a treatment for patients with multivessel coronary artery disease. More than 500,000 patients in the United States, Canada, and Europe undergo coronary artery bypass grafting each year, with an annual cost has been estimated to be at least 15 billion dollars per year *(1)*. While it has been estimated that cardiac morbidity and mortality may occur in up to 20% of patients who undergo this procedure, the accurate detection of those patients who suffer perioperative cardiac injury remains difficult, owing to the lack of a readily available gold standard for the detection of cardiac injury. It would be expected that detection of significant cardiac injury would be clinically and prognostically important, as the presence of myocardial cellular necrosis identifies patients at increased cardiovascular risk in situations as diverse as acute coronary syndromes (ACS), catheter-based interventions, pulmonary embolism, and severe medical illness. Thus, accurate detection of myocardial cellular necrosis in the setting of cardiac surgery should allow for the identification of patients who are at increased short-term risk. In addition, the ability to identify accurately the presence and degree of myocardial cellular necrosis after cardiopulmonary bypass would allow for improvement of the techniques utilized for myocardial protection utilized during cardiac surgery and cardiopulmonary bypass. Many of the techniques utilized during cardiac surgery are designed to minimize cellular trauma during the surgery itself. Without a sensitive and reliable gold standard, it is very difficult to compare alternative therapeutic techniques to determine the preferred method.

Many aspects of cardiac surgery, however, have made detection of cardiac injury that occurs during or immediately after cardiac surgery more difficult. This issue is clinically important; clinicians must often consider the possibility of myocardial ischemia and necrosis in the perioperative setting. While uncommon, some patients will have myocardial infarctions (MIs) that occur at the time of the cardiac surgery. These MIs can be due to technical problems during the surgery itself, inadequate cardioplegic solution, downstream emboli, and acute occlusion of a coronary bypass graft. However, discrimination of these patients in the immediate postoperative setting is extremely problematic. Episodes of hypotension, tachycardia, arrhythmia, or hypoxia are not uncommon,

From: *Cardiac Markers, Second Edition*
Edited by: Alan H. B. Wu @ Humana Press Inc., Totowa, NJ

Table 1
Factors Contributing to Cardiac Cell Death After Cardiac Surgery

Occlusion of a graft
Inadequate cardioplegia
Direct injury by the cardioplegic solution
Activation of platelets
Activation of cytokines and chemokines
Platelet–leukocyte conjugates
Activation of complement
Plaque rupture/thrombosis
Increased duration of cardiopulmonary bypass
Direct trauma (including necessary dissection during the procedure)
Spasm of bypass grafts (most commonly arterial grafts)
Valves in inappropriately placed venous grafts
Embolization of material into coronary arteries
Embolization of air into coronary arteries
New occlusion of native coronaries post-operatively
Aortic dissection (type A)

and typical symptoms of angina (such as shortness of breath, chest discomfort, and nausea) are universal in the first few days after cardiac surgery. Patients with perioperative cardiac injury may manifest themselves only via hemodynamic instability. Electrocardiograms (ECGs) often do not demonstrate diagnostic changes in the setting of potential ischemia, and this is especially true in the postoperative setting when nondiagnostic alterations in the ECG tracing are common. Because there is usually a low pretest likelihood that a particular patient will have suffered a perioperative MI, exclusion of a perioperative MI is more often the clinically important diagnostic need.

PATHOPHYSIOLOGY AND PROBLEMS OF DIAGNOSIS

The use of cardiopulmonary bypass, as well as the presence of associated disease processes, contribute to the nearly universal presence of myocardial cellular injury that is present after cardiac surgery (*see* Table 1). The use of the cardiopulmonary bypass is associated with a direct toxic effect, manifest in part by a systemic inflammatory response. A diverse number of chemokines and cytokines are released, such as interleukin-1β (IL-1β), IL-6, IL-8, IL-10, tumor necrosis factor, and complement activation (both the alternative pathway and the classical immune pathway). These mediators can be directly toxic to myocardial cells, can trigger cascades that are secondarily injurious, and can contribute to reperfusion injury. Cardiopulmonary bypass has been found to stimulate leukocyte–platelet adhesion, as well as stimulate the release of proinflammatory molecules such as endotoxin (which among other actions stimulate the complement system) *(2,3)*. In addition, there is a generalized inflammatory response to any operative procedure (and thus "off-pump" bypass procedures do not completely avoid inflammatory activity and subsequent cellular injury). Cardiac injury can occur during the operation due to inadequate myocardial protection during aortic cross-clamping, an unduly long period of time on the heart–lung machine (during which time the myocardium is not perfused), post-bypass reperfusion injury, spasm of the internal mammary artery (or other vascular conduits), and direct injury during surgical manipulation. Postoperatively, cardiac injury and necrosis can occur due to occlusion a grafted conduit, occlusion at the anastomotic site from the graft to the native coronary artery, occlusion in native arteries distal to the insertion of the graft, or other processes that result in a sufficiently severe and prolonged supply–demand mismatch. Cardiac morbidity and mortality can occur secondary to acute or chronic ventricular dysfunction, acute or preexisting coronary artery disease that was not remedied by the surgery, incomplete coronary revascularization, MI, renal insufficiency, cerebrovascular events, infections, and hemodynamically significant dysrhythmias. For all of these situations, optimum patient care would require accurate and prompt detection of the cardiac injury.

Thus, every patient who undergoes cardiac bypass will have some degree of myocardial cell death. We must separate those patients with an "expected" degree of cardiac cellular injury from those whose injury is greater and representative of undesirable additional myocardial injury. It is necessary to discriminate those patients who have had a larger amount of myocardial cellular injury (which can potentially affect patient care) from those with less. There is a spectrum of cardiac cellular injury therefore that is present in this cohort of patients in which all patients have had sufficient cardiac injury that they would otherwise be classified as having cardiac injury. Indeed, it is somewhat difficult to know the degree of perioperative cardiac injury that should be labeled as an MI. The question will be whether a "clinically significant" degree of myocardial cell injury has occurred; one must also be careful and cognizant of the precise definition of "clinically significant" that is utilized. The reference levels used to detect perioperative myocardial injury will be substantially higher than those thresholds utilized in other clinical situations and must be defined for this particular postcardiac surgery population.

In addition to the above issues, different assay formats for markers of myocardial necrosis (pertaining especially to measures of cardiac troponin I [cTnI]) also complicate establishing the diagnosis of cardiac injury following cardiac surgery. Differences among assay formats are a problem with many analytes but are currently a particular issue with cTnI. Approximately 15 different assays for cTnI are currently available, and they possess different antibodies (which recognize different portions of the troponin molecule), different reference values, lower levels of detectability, and coefficients of variation at the lower level of detectability *(4–6)*. It has been found that uncorrected values for levels of cTnI can vary up to 60-fold *(5,7)*. This disparity precludes direct comparison of the levels of troponin between different assay formats. All of these assays have been best analyzed in studies involving patients without cardiac disease and in those with ACS. Unfortunately, there is not yet sufficient information on the various assays to allow for correlation between cut points derived in studies utilizing various assays. Thus, at this time any studies performed in post-bypass patients utilizing cTnI will result in recommendations that will be assay-dependent due to the large number of assays for cTnI that are clinically available. It is not currently possible to correlate an abnormal troponin value determined with one assay with another. Recent work has demonstrated that profound degradation of troponin proteins occurs rapidly in the setting of ischemia, with the initial alterations occurring intracellularly (i.e., prior to release from the cell) and then continuing once the troponin protein or complex has been released from the cell *(8)*. This observation has implications for comparison of various troponin assays, as different antibodies demonstrate alterations in binding parameters to troponin degradation products. Much work, both by the manufacturers as well as the research community, remains to be done to resolve this lack of standardization of troponin assay systems *(6)*. This is not an issue for cardiac troponin T (cTnT), as there is only one manufacturer and assay available and the assays for the MB isoenzyme of creatine kinase (CK-MB) mass have been largely standardized to allow reasonable comparison between the various manufacturer's assay platforms.

While part of the problems of application of troponin proteins in this situation are due to analytical issues, use of CK-MB in the postoperative state has substantial potential complicating factors. Measurement of CK-MB has been utilized for <20 yr for the diagnosis of myocardial necrosis. Although there are some limitations of CK-MB in terms of both sensitivity and specificity, these issues have been of particular concern for the use of this marker in patients after surgery *(7,11,12)*. CK-MB is present in low amounts in skeletal muscle (1–5%) and can occur in significantly increased amounts in individuals with acute or chronic muscle disease or renal insufficiency. Cellular injury to skeletal muscle is associated with many operative procedures. This cellular injury will result in the release of skeletal muscle cell contents and will therefore often result in increased concentrations of total CK and CK-MB. Utilization of an absolute cutoff for CK-MB (as is often used in patients with ACS) in the perioperative period will result in impaired specificity. Although calculation of the ratio of CK-MB to total CK has been tried, this strategy results in unacceptable problems in both sensitivity and specificity *(11)*. Despite these limitations, studies have demonstrated that measurement of levels of CK-MB can be utilized successfully in populations studied following cardiac surgery.

Yet another complicating factor when one seeks to utilize markers of necrosis to detect myocardial injury after cardiac surgery is the use of various gold standards for "MI" utilized in the various trials. Given the lack of a readily available gold standard for the detection of perioperative myocardial ischemia, investigators have utilized various definitions. Because the responsible pathobiology of cardiac injury in the setting of cardiac surgery is different than in patients with ACS, the term "MI" is anatomically accurate but perhaps not the best term to use, given the connotations associated with the diagnosis. While patients with ACS typically have plaque rupture and occlusion of an epicardial coronary artery as the responsible lesion, as noted above there are a multitude of factors that can contribute to perioperative cardiac injury (Table 1). Potentially only those patients with occlusion of a coronary artery graft in the perioperative setting have a similar constellation of biologic factors that are active. In addition, this would be the only situation that would have cardiac injury with a "low-flow" state in the postoperative period. This could have important implications for the release ratio and rate of appearance and disappearance of protein markers *(7)*. Thus, application of diagnostic tests whose use was refined in the setting of ACS will often result in less that optimum diagnostic performance during and immediately after cardiac surgery. Utilization of the development of new Q waves as the criteria for MI in the postoperative setting, for example, will be highly specific but have severely compromised sensitivity. Conversely, utilization of a blood-based marker of necrosis and an end point utilized in typical situation of MI (such as reference levels of CK-MB or troponin derived from studies in patients with ACS) will result in an extremely high (and one can only hope falsely high) incidence of perioperative injury. In addition, although it is always important to evaluate results of blood-based markers of necrosis in the context of the time of the onset of the event (due to the rising and falling nature of their release), it becomes even more important when using or evaluating biomarkers in the postcardiac surgery population. Markers of necrosis (specifically troponins and CK-MB) typically rise and fall rapidly following surgery. The curve of release is usually different than that observed in patients with ACS and MI. Patients with marker elevations following cardiac surgery will often have a significant elevation that then falls rapidly within the first 24–36 h (in other words, we do not typically see the more gradual decline with troponin proteins that we observe in patients with MIs). Thus, it is important to define the time from cardiac surgery (usually defined from the aortic cross-clamp time, which generally corresponds to the onset of the cessation of cardiac circulation) when relating marker results and proposing abnormal reference values. The release of proteins form the heart after cardiac surgery and cardiopulmonary bypass is extremely rapid, presumably due to the high flow and hyperemic arterial flow that is present. Thus, levels of cardiac troponins and other markers tend to rise and fall rapidly in the first 24 h after cardiovascular surgery, and any reported level of a protein marker must be viewed in the context of it relationship to the surgery. This is reflected in the high levels of cut points recommended in the following studies. It is not currently possible to utilize the peak level of any marker in the postoperative situation and calculate the size of myocardial injury with any degree of reliability. Finally, cardiac surgery is understandably performed on individuals who have significant underlying cardiac disease, and some of these individuals will have abnormal levels of the protein of interest prior to the cardiac surgery. Any elevations present after surgery must be related to the level of the analyte present prior to the surgical procedure.

Thus, although detection of cardiac injury can be a challenge in diverse clinical situations, the difficulty in detecting potential myocardial ischemia or necrosis is far greater in individuals who are undergoing a cardiac operation, owing to factors related to the surgery as well as limitations of available diagnostic tests. We routinely evaluate patients in other clinical situations (most commonly those patients who present with a complaint of chest discomfort) for the presence or absence of myocardial necrosis, and the robust detection of patients in this situation is reasonably handled by serial testing for markers released following cellular necrosis. However, the detection of cardiac cellular necrosis after cardiac surgery is conceptually different from diagnostic strategies in patients with ACS or after noncardiac surgery. In these other clinical situations physicians can theoretically separate patients into two groups: those who have had and those who have not had any degree of myocardial cellular necrosis. Numerous trials have shown that this differentiation is prognostically important; patients who have detectable levels of cardiac troponins in the setting of chest pain, congestive heart failure, and the like have substantially worsened prognosis when compared to patients without detectable levels of troponin. These findings led, in part, to the recent consensus document by the European Society of Cardiology (ESC)/American College of Cardiology (ACC) that redefined a MI as a detectable rise and fall of cardiac troponin when symptoms attributable to ischemia were present *(9)*. Although this guideline stated that diagnostic levels would be different in patients after cardiac surgery, specific guidelines were not recommended owing to the difficulties expounded on in this chapter. Current guidelines, specifically in those patients with unstable angina and non-ST-segment elevation MI, have recommended treatment strategies predicated on the results of troponin testing (10).

CLINICAL APPLICATIONS

Past studies attempting to define the incidence of postcardiac surgery MIs have reported rates of 5% to 80%, with mortality rates ranging from 0.5% to 14% (13). This wide range is due to differing criteria for MI. Use of an increase in the level of CK-MB as the definition of a post-CABG MI will result in a relatively high incidence of perioperative cardiac complications. Conversely, defining a perioperative MI by the development of new Q waves on the postoperative ECG will miss all but those patients with transmural necrosis. In general, the diagnostic techniques most commonly utilized for the detection of MI after cardiac surgery are relatively insensitive, and there have been no clearly accepted criteria for the detection of perioperative myocardial injury. A recent consensus document from the joint committees of the ACC/ESC noted the reference criteria for the detection of post-CABG MI must be different and higher than those utilized in the routine acute coronary syndrome, but did not recommend specific criteria (9). This uncertainty in the diagnostic criteria for perioperative MI not only hinders routine patient care but deleteriously affects cardiac surgery research as well.

Accordingly, there has been interest in the utilization of blood-based markers of cardiac injury to diagnose perioperative MIs. Although many analytes have been studied, there has been the interest especially in CK-MB and cardiac troponins. Mair et al. first reported on the use of cTnT in 1991 for the detection of perioperative MI in 21 patients undergoing CABG (14). MI was defined as an abnormal ECG associated with increases in CK-MB lasting >12–18 h. Fourteen patients did not meet these criteria, and levels of cTnT were <1.6 ng/mL (upper limit of normal 0.1 ng/mL). Two patients had postoperative cardiac injury; levels of cTnT were elevated in both of these patients, and one died from cardiogenic shock. The authors proposed that a peak concentration of cTnT <2.5 ng/mL excluded clinically relevant cardiac injury. This report was followed by reports by others substantiating that the measurement of cTnT could be used to exclude perioperative MI with a reference level of 2.5–3.0 ng/mL (15,16). Patients with increased concentrations of cTnT present before cardiac surgery had a higher event rate, consistent with previous studies that found that individuals who undergo surgery shortly after MI are at increased perioperative risk.

Mair also evaluated the use of measurements of cTnI in 28 individuals who underwent coronary artery bypass grafting (17). The criteria for a perioperative MI was new persistent Q waves or CK-MB activity >50 IU/L on the first postoperative day in conjunction with new persistent wall motion abnormalities detected by echocardiography. Non-Q-wave MI was diagnosed in this study by new ST-segment deviation in conjunction with CK-MB activity >20 IU on the first postoperative day. Levels of cTnI up to 2 ng/mL (upper reference limit = 0.1 ng/mL) occurred routinely in patients with no postoperative complications. Patients with perioperative MI (n = 6) had peak cTnI concentrations >4.5 ng/mL and had peaks occurring approx 24 h after aortic cross-clamping. Another investigation using the same cTnI assay found that peak cTnI levels occur at approx 6 h after surgery and are usually absent by d 5 in patients without evidence of perioperative cardiac injury *(18)*. A correlation between total aortic cross-clamp time and levels of cTnI has been seen in most but not all trials.

Hirsch et al. measured levels of cTnI in pediatric cardiac surgery patients after the repair of congenital (mostly cyanotic) cardiac lesions *(17,18)*. All patients had increased concentrations, and there was a correlation between aortic cross-clamp time, total cardiac bypass time, and levels of cTnI *(19,20)*. Levels of cTnI at 12 and 24 h correlated with outcome (intraoperative support, duration of endotracheal intubation, hospital stay, and the duration of the ICU stay). Another study involving open heart surgery in children and infants found similar results; levels of cTnI obtained 4 h after admission to the ICU correlated strongly with the severity of renal dysfunction, the duration of intubation, and the need for inotropic support *(21)*.

Levels of cTnI (using the first-generation Dade assay) were found to correlate with the development of new wall motion abnormalities on postoperative echocardiograms in a study of 124 adult patients with both coronary artery bypass grafting as well as valve replacement surgery *(18,22)*. The gold standard for the presence of a "significant" perioperative MI was the detection of a new wall motion abnormality on serial echocardiograms. Patients with new wall motion abnormalities indicative of perioperative myocardial injury had significantly higher levels of cTnI than those who did not. A cutoff level of 11 ng/mL (again, using the first-generation Dade assay [URL = 1.5 ng/mL]) had a negative predictive value of 97%.

It is intuitively attractive that the detection of cardiac injury after cardiac surgery would be important. In a diverse number of clinical situations, those patients who possess elevations of cardiac biomarkers demonstrate an increased incidence of cardiac events when compared to those patients without increased concentrations. This has been true in patients with ACS, MI, catheter-based intervention (such as angioplasty, stent placement, rotoblade therapy, and the like), blunt chest wall trauma, and severe medical illness. Thus, it would not be surprising that elevations of cardiac biomarkers would be prognostically important in patients after surgery. Recent studies have shed some light on this important question. A recent study involving the use of cTnI in patients undergoing general surgery is useful for our purposes. In this trial, 304 patients who underwent diverse general surgical operations were enrolled in a retrospective study *(23)*. Of the 304 patients identified, 167 had at least one documented elevation of cTnI defined as a level >0.1 ng/mL; patients with elevations >2.5 ng/mL were excluded from the trial (the assumption was that patients with greater elevations of cTnI had sufficiently great cardiac necrosis that there was not any question as to the prognostic significance). In this study, patients with elevations of cTnI were much more likely to have a MI, congestive heart failure, and/or death when compared to those patients who did not manifest elevations of cardiac troponin in the postoperative period, when evaluated in the first 3 mo. Thus, even "lesser" elevations of cTnI conferred powerful prognostic significance akin to that seen in patients with ACS. CK was also recently evaluated and has been found to have prognostic importance in two recent trials. In the first evaluation, data accrued on a series of 2332 patients who underwent cardiac surgery were compared to patients with acute coronary syndromes enrolled in the Guard during Ischemia Against Necrosis (GUARDIAN) trial; these data were utilized to compare cardiac event rates in patients with and without increased concentrations of CK-MB after cardiac surgery *(24)*. Patients with elevations of CK-MB had increased 6-mo event rates (especially death) that were comparable or greater when compared to the rates seen with patients with ACS (enrolled in GUARDIAN). In another investigation, elevations of CK-MB present after cardiac surgery were found to demonstrate prognostic importance out to 5 yr *(25)*.

Given the superior cardiac specificity of cardiac troponins when compared to that of CK-MB, especially in patients with surgery and concomitant skeletal muscular injury, it would be anticipated that cardiac troponins would provide superior prognostic information, just as they provide superior diagnostic information *(7)*. A recent study has provided a direct comparison of use of cTnT and CK-MB in patients following cardiac surgery *(26)*. In this investigation, samples were obtained every 8 h after cardiac surgery in 224 serial patients. While the results of both CK-MB and cTnT provided prognostic information, that provided by cTnT was superior; levels of cTnT allowed improved detection of those patients who subsequently suffered MI, shock, or death. Measurment of CK-MB did not confer any additional prognostic information in this trial when combined with the results of cTnT. The cut point for this trial was a level of cTnT >1.58 ng/mL (which is approx 15-fold greater than the usual reference level).

Thus, it appears that increased concentrations of both troponins and CK-MB are indicative of cardiac injury after cardiac surgery and postoperative prognosis, although much more work needs to be done before this is defined. In addition, most would accept the contention that lesser amounts of myocardial cell death are desirable and should translate to lesser cardiac event rates. Thus, strategies that diminish release of markers of cardiac cell necrosis should be preferred.

Accordingly, measurements of levels of cardiac troponins have been used to assess therapies provided at the time of coronary artery bypass grafting. Hannes et al. used serial measurements of cTnT to assess the use of diltiazem to prevent spasm of internal mammary artery grafts *(27)*. Patients who received intravenous diltiazem had lower peak levels of cTnT. Serial measurements of cTnT were used in another trial to assess the application of intermittent aortic cross-clamp, on bypass pump, and off-pump with a beating heart *(28)*. Patients who had coronary artery bypass grafting without aortic cross-clamping and without cardiopulmonary bypass had less frequent elevations of cTnT after surgery, which the authors felt should indicate superior myocardial protection. Wendel et al. have used measurements of cTnT to assess the administration of aprotinin during aortic cross-clamping *(16)*. Pelletier used levels of cTnT in 120 patients undergoing cardiac surgery to compare the myocardial protection provided by intermittent antegrade warm vs cold blood cardioplegia *(29)*. As noted earlier, a number of deleterious pathways are activated during cardiopulmonary bypass, especially the activation of inflammatory cytokines. Measurement of levels of cTnT have been shown to be elevated but to a lesser extent in patients who undergo revascularization via beating heart surgery when compared to standard cardioplegic solution *(30)*. Recently, it has been noted that levels of cTnI correlate with levels of IL-8 after cardiopulmonary bypass, and that the use of heparin- coated tubing in the bypass circuits resulted in decreased levels of both IL-8 and cardiac troponin I. Administration of pexelizumab, a humanized scFv antibody fragment directed against the C5 complement component, during coronary artery bypass grafting, has been shown to result in lesser degrees of elevation of elevations of CK-MB, and data that have been presented but not yet published indicate that those patients with the greatest levels of CK-MB have the highest rate of cardiac mortality *(31,32)*. This correlation was independent of any abnormalities documented on the ECG.

CONCLUSIONS

The measurement of serial levels of markers of necrosis can be used to detect cardiac injury in the postoperative patient. Because of superior cardiac specificity, levels of troponin should be superior to those of CK-MB for detection of cardiac injury after cardiac surgery in individual patients. In applying measurements of troponins to patients after cardiac surgery, however, all patients have some degree of cardiac cell death, and thus reference levels will be higher and must be defined for this specific patient population. Unfortunately, recommendations dervied from clinical studies will necessarily be assay dependent, and currently we cannot compare recommended cut points with studies using different cTnI assays. Utilization of cTnT does not have this limitation at present (as there is only one manufacturer of cTnT), and thus utilization cTnT may be preferred in this situation. Thus, several conclusions can be derived from a review of current studies (*see* Table 1): (1) levels of troponin are increased in essentially all patients after cardiac surgery, (2) those patients who manifest the greatest levels of troponin are at the greatest risk, (3) reference cut points for the detection of significant perioperative MIs will be much higher than those derived in pateints with ACS—each indiviual assay for cTnI will have to be evaluated individually, and (4) it is not yet known what is the desired maximal level of troponin in the postoperative situation. Further studies will be necessary for defining the proper application of measurement of levels of troponin or other markers in this discrete population.

ABBREVIATIONS

ACC, American College of Cardiology; ACS, Acute coronary syndrome(s); CABG, coronary artery bypass grafting; CK, creatine kinase; CK-MB, MB isoenzye of CK; cTnT, cTnI, cardiac troponins T and I; ECG, electrocardiogram; ESC, European Society of Cardiology; GUARDIAN, GUARD during Ischemia Against Necrosis Trial; IL, interleukin.

REFERENCES

1. Mangano DT. Perioperative cardiac morbidity—epidemiology, costs, problems, and solutions (editorial). West Med J 1994;161:87–89.
2. Jansen NJG, van Oeveren W, Gu YJ, van Vliet MH, Eijsman L, Wildevuur CRH. Endotoxin release and tumor necrosis factor formation during cardiopulmonary bypass. Ann Thorac Surg 1992;54:744–748.
3. Rinder CS, Bonan JL, Rinder HM, Mathew J, Hines R, Smith BR. Cardiopulmonary bypass induces leukocyte-platelet adhesion. Blood 1992;79:1201–1205.
4. Apple FS, Adams JE, Wu AHB, Jaffe AS. Report on survey of analytical and clinical characteristics of commercial cardiac troponin assays. In: Markers in Cardiology; Current and Future Clinical Applications. Adams JE, Apple F, Jaffe A, Wu A, eds. Armonk, NY: Futura, 2000, pp. 31–34.
5. Tate JR, Heathcote D, Rayfield J, Hickman PE. The lack of standardization of cardiac troponin I assay systems. Clin Chim Acta 1999;284:141–149.
6. Valdes R, Jortani SA. Standardizing utilization of biomarkers in diagnosis and management of acute cardiac syndromes. Clin Chim Acta 1999;284:135–140.

7. Adams JE, Abendschein DR, Jaffe AS. Biochemical markers of myocardial injury: is MB creatine kinase the choice of the 1990s? Circulation 1993;88:750–763.

8. McDonough JL, Labugger R, Pickett W, et al. Cardiac troponin I is modified in the myocardium of bypass patients. Circulation 2001;103:58–64.

9. Alpert JS, Thygesen K, Antman E, Bassand JP. Myocardial infarction redefined—a consensus document of The Joint European Society of Cardiology/American College of Cardiology Committee for the redefinition of myocardial infarction. J Am Coll Cardiol 2000;36: 959–969.

10. Braunwald E, Antman EM, Beasley JW, et al. ACC/AHA Guideline Update for the Management of Patients with Unstable Angina and Non-ST-Segment Elevation Myocardial Infarction: a report of the American College of Cardiology/American Heart Association Task Force on practice Guidelines (Committee on the Management of Patients with Unstable Angina). 2002. Available at: http://www.acc.org/clinical/guidelines/unstable/unstable.pdf.

11. Adams JE, Sicard GA, Allen BT, et al. Diagnosis of perioperative myocardial infarction with measurement of cardiac troponin I. N Engl J Med 1994;330:670–674.

12. Badner NH, Knill RL, Brown JE, Novick TV, Gelb AW. Myocardial infarction after noncardiac surgery. Anesthesiology 1998:88:572–578.

13. Mangano DT, Siliciano D, Hollenberg M, et al. The Study of Perioperative Ischemia Research Group: postoperative myocardial ischemia-therapeutic trials using intensive analgesia following surgery. Anesthesiology 1992:76:342–353.

14. Mair J, Weiser C, Seibt I, et al. Troponin T to diagnose myocardial infarction in bypass surgery. Lancet 1991;337:434–435.

15. Triggiani M, Dolci A, Donatelli F, et al. Cardiac troponin T and peri-opertive myocardial damage in coronary surgery. J Cardiothor Vasc Anesthesiol 1995;9:484–488.

16. Wendel HP, Heller W, Michel J, et al. Lower cardiac troponin T levels in patients undergoing cardiopulmonary bypass and receiving high-dose aprotinin therapy indicate reduction of perioperative myocardial damage. J Thorac Cardiovasc Surg 1995;109:1164–1172.

17. Mair J, Larue C, Mair P, Balogh D, Calzolari C, Puschendorf B. Use of cardiac troponin I to diagnose perioperative myocardial infarction in coronary artery bypass grafting. Clin Chem 1994;40:2066–2070.

18. Etievent JP, Chocron S, Toubin G, et al. Use of cardiac troponin I as a marker of perioperative myocardial infarction. Ann Thorac Surg 1995;59:1192–1194.

19. Hirsch R, Dent C, Wood MK, et al. Patterns and predictive value of cardiac troponin I after cardiothoracic surgery in children. Circulation 1996;94(Suppl I):I–480.

20. Bodor GS, Porter S, Landt Y, Ladenson JH. Development of monoclonal antibodies for an assay of cardiac troponin-I and preliminary results in suspected cases of myocardial infarction. Clin Chem 1992;38:2203–2214.

21. Immer FF, Stocker F, Seiler A, Pfammatter JP, Bachman D, Prinzen G, Carrel T. Troponin I for prediction of early postoperative course after pediatric cardiac surgery. J Am Coll Cardiol 1999;33:1719–1723.

22. Adams JE III, Jeavens AW, Gray LA. Use of cardiac troponin I to detect cardiac injury after cardiac surgery. Circulation 1998:99:I–93.

23. Porter MJ, Moran JF, Leder D, Malinowsky K. Are minimal elevations of postoperative cardic troponin I levels following general surgery prognostically important? J Am Coll Cardiol 2002;39:438A.

24. Gavard JA, Chaitman BR, Sakai S, Stocke K, Boyce S, Theroux P. Does elevated CK-MB after coronary artery bypass surgery have the same prognostic significance as after an acute coronary syndrome? Circulation 2001;104:II–597.

25. Tleyieh I, Ziada KM, Almahameed A, et al. Perioperative creatine kinase elevation is a strong predictor of early and late mortality after coronary bypass grafting. J Am Coll Cardiol 2002; 39:436A.

26. Januzzi J, Lewandrowski K, Macgillivray T, Kathiresan S, Servoss S, Lewandrowski E. Troponin T is superior to CK-MB for patient evaluation and risk stratification following cardiac surgery. J Am Coll Cardiol 2001;104:II–597.
27. Hannes W, Seitelberger R, Christoph M, et al. Effect of peri-operative diltiazem on myocardial ischaemia and function in patients receiving mammary artery grafts. Eur Heart J 1995; 16:87–93.
28. Krejca M, Skiba J, Szmagala P, Gburek T, Bachenek A. Cardiac troponin T release during coronary surgery using intermittent cross-clamp with fibrillation, on-pump, and off-pump beating heart. Eur J CardioThor Surg 1999;16:337–341.
29. Pelletier LC, Carrier M, Leclerc Y, et al. Intermittent antegrade warm versus cold blood cardioplegia: a prospective, randomized study. Ann Thorac Surg 1994;58:41–48.
30. Nussmeier N, Fitch JCK, Malloy KJ, Shernan SK. C5-complement supression by pexelizumab in CABG patients is associated with reduction of postoperative myocardial infarction. Circulation 2002;104:II–150.
31. Shernan SK, Nussmeier N, Rollins SA, Mojik CF, Fitch JCK. Pexelizumab reduces death and myocardial infarction in CABG patients requiring CPB: results of the 914 patient phase II trial. Circulation 2002;104:II–474.
32. Fitch JC, Shernan SK, Todaro TG, Filloon TG, Nussmeier N. Mortality in CABG patients correlated with post-operative CK-MB independent of new Q waves of ECG. Presented at the Annual Meeting of the Society of Cardiothoracic Anesthesiologists, April 2002.

Part II
Clinical Use for Cardiac Troponins

7

Cardiac Troponins: Exploiting the Diagnostic Potential of Disease-Induced Protein Modifications

Ralf Labugger, D. Kent Arrell, and Jennifer E. Van Eyk

INTRODUCTION

The race to sequence the human genome, culminating with two ground-breaking publications in 2001 *(1,2)*, drew enormous attention to the possibility of using genetic information for diagnostic purposes, to guide therapy, for development of new therapeutics, or even for disease prevention. Despite the unquestioned importance of an organism's genes, it is the products of gene expression, the proteins, that will manifest health or disease. Furthering our understanding of how proteins are involved in the development or manifestation of diseases will increase our knowledge about the underlying pathological processes on the cellular level. Instead of simply "observing and analyzing pathological alterations; proteomics will permit the dissection of pathological pathways *(3)*." It should therefore become possible to explain why subgroups of patients have a better prognosis than others or respond differently to certain therapies. This will not only influence therapies through development of new therapeutic agents, but will also improve existing diagnostics. Furthermore, this may lead to the development of both new diagnostics and therapies, individually tailored to specific proteome phenotypes.

The cardiac myocyte proteome is susceptible to disease-induced changes, whether due to acute injury such as myocardial infarction (MI) or to chronic conditions such as congestive heart failure (CHF) and dilated cardiomyopathy *(4–7)*. Disease-induced protein changes may result from posttranslational modifications (including proteolysis, covalent crosslinking, phosphorylation, oxidation, and glycosylation, just to name a few), or through altered gene expression (including up- or down-regulation and/or isoform switching). The myocardial proteome of any given patient at any given time thus consists of a spectrum of various protein modifications. In addition, the myocardial protein modification profile of an individual patient will change over time, which may be complicated further as a result of multiple overlapping disease processes.

Intracellular proteins, modified by disease, may be released from the myocardium and detected in a patient's blood. Many ischemic conditions, including acute coronary syndromes (ACS) and chronic cardiovascular diseases, result in such a release of intracellular proteins. Currently used diagnostics for myocardial injury are based on the detection of such intracellular proteins, including cardiac troponins I and T (cTnI and cTnT), myoglobin, creatine kinase (CK), the MB isoenzyme of CK (CK-MB), lactate dehydrogenase

From: *Cardiac Markers, Second Edition*
Edited by: Alan H. B. Wu @ Humana Press Inc., Totowa, NJ

(LDH), and aspartate aminotransferase (AST). Of all these biomarkers, recently published consensus documents by the European Society of Cardiology (ESC), the American College of Cardiology (ACC), and the American Heart Association (AHA) *(8–10)* specifically recommend cardiac troponins to be the new laboratory standard for MI diagnosis as well as for diagnosis and management of unstable angina. There are several reasons for this consensus. First and foremost is the superior tissue specificity of cardiac troponins over conventionally used markers such as LDH, AST, CK, CK-MB, or myoglobin, combined with the improved diagnostic sensitivity of troponins since their first introduction as biomarkers for ACS. Additional factors include the prolonged time window of troponin elevation after onset of ACS *(11,12)*, the association of detectable troponin with a risk of adverse clinical events *(13–17)*, and, finally, the increasing international acceptance for the use of troponins as cardiac markers in the last five years *(18)*.

In theory, any myocardial protein (including its posttranslationally modified forms) has the potential to serve as a biomarker, provided that it can be detected in the blood, and this detection correlates with a disease. No longer must diagnostic assays simply give a yes/no answer. It is now possible for them to provide additional information about a patient's disease status as well as the condition of his or her remaining viable myocardium. Thus, understanding the changes in the myocardial proteome with progression of disease becomes imperative.

TROPONIN MODIFICATIONS
AND THEIR FUNCTIONAL SIGNIFICANCE

Serum levels of cardiac troponins, as well as total CK and CK-MB, have been used to determine infarct size in both ACS patients and animal models *(19–21)*. Unlike the other cardiac biomarkers, however, the troponins provide additional information about the functional consequences of an infarction. This relates to the essential role of the troponin complex (Tn) in the Ca^{2+}-dependent regulation of cardiac muscle contraction. Tn consists of three proteins: TnT, which interacts with tropomyosin; TnI, the inhibitory protein; and TnC, which binds Ca^{2+} and thereby triggers a conformational change leading to myofilament contraction. Troponin, in concert with tropomyosin, regulates cardiac muscle contraction through numerous tightly controlled Ca^{2+}-dependent interactions *(22–24)*. Troponin–tropomyosin binds to filamentous actin to form the thin filament and controls actin–myosin interactions through the intricate interplay of both steric and allosteric mechanisms *(25–30)*. Given the structural complexity of the thin filament assembly, as well as the allosteric and cooperative components of the mechanism, the cardiac myofilament constitutes a finely tuned system for regulation of force production. Therefore, myofilament protein modifications, including those that are disease induced, can alter cardiac contraction. This is seen in transgenic animal models expressing genetically altered cTnI *(31)* or cTnT *(32,33)*, in which low expression levels of modified troponins (mimicking disease-induced modifications) have dramatic functional consequences. The extent of contractile dysfunction is very much dependent on both the regions of the troponins that are modified as well as the forms of the modifications themselves. Various animal models have revealed that cTnI is specifically and selectively modified in the tissue of diseased hearts *(34–37)*. Of particular importance for the detection of ACS are the progressive, severity-dependent posttranslational modifications demonstrated to occur to cTnI in ischemia/reperfusion injury of Langendorff perfused rat hearts, including proteolysis *(38–40),* formation of covalent crosslinks *(39,40),* and changes in phosphorylation *(40,41).* Furthermore, these various disease-induced cTnI modifications, including the human equivalent of the carboxy-terminal truncation (cTnI$_{1-192}$) that is proposed to cause the stunned phenotype in a transgenic mouse model *(31),* were also found in the viable parts of the myocardium from patients undergoing coronary artery bypass surgery *(42).* Importantly, this demonstrates that such modifications are formed in the myocytes prior to, or even in complete absence of, subsequent necrosis. If the troponin modification products are finally released from the myocardium, a distinct troponin profile will be generated in the blood. Over time, this profile will reflect the progression of the disease, including both the severity and the time from onset of injury. From a diagnostic perspective, one can thus further appreciate the functional consequences of troponin modifications, as their detection in a patient's blood may allow us to then predict the functional status of the remaining viable myocardium. Of course, this will be possible only once diagnostic assays are developed that can distinguish between the different disease-induced forms of the analyte. Such information has the potential to improve patient triage, help physicians to decide between conventional or invasive therapy, and may even provide more precise and individualized long-term prognosis.

CARDIAC TROPONINS
AS BLOOD-BORNE DIAGNOSTIC MARKERS

To serve as biochemical markers, troponins must be released into the bloodstream. Apart from MI, elevated troponin levels have been found in cases of minor myocardial damage *(12)* with nonelevated CK-MB levels, CHF *(43,44),* unstable angina *(14),* pulmonary embolism *(45),* myocarditis *(46),* sepsis and septic shock *(47,48),* as well as in patients undergoing percutaneous intervention *(49),* cardiopulmonary bypass graft (CABG) surgery *(42),* or implantable cardioverter defibrillator shock application *(50).* The release of cardiac troponins does not automatically indicate myocardial necrosis (such as in MI), and must not necessarily reflect irreversible or necrotic damage to the myocardium *(48,51,52).* The possibility of non-necrotic release due to a reversible change in membrane permeability is under debate, but if confirmed, will change the view on cardiac troponins by widening their diagnostic potential beyond that of simple markers of necrosis. With increasing analytical sensitivity of troponin assays, detection of extremely low levels of troponin is pushing toward this point.

Of course, one must not overlook that processes involved in the different pathophysiological stages of cardiac disease can lead to different protein modifications, thus altering the myocardial proteome. Parameters that affect the quantity and forms of intracellular proteins (such as troponins) present in blood include both disease-induced processing of the protein in the myocardium, as well as any further processing in the blood following the release from the myocardium. The time course of appearance for each protein (or its modified products) in the blood will depend on its molecular mass, its affinity for other proteins, and its localization in the cell *(53,54).* In addition, their disappearance from the blood is influenced by other factors, including their susceptibility to proteolysis and filtration by the renal and lymphatic systems, further contributing (together with specificity and sensitivity) to the merits and shortcomings of the different diagnostic markers.

A lack of standardization remains as a major drawback of existing cTnI diagnostics. Apple et al. *(55)* recently discussed the analytical and clinical characteristics of 16 troponin assays from 10 different manufacturers, finding substantial variability in specific parameters (e.g., lower limit of detection [LLD], reference limits, concentration at 10% coefficient of variance [CV], receiver operating characteristic [ROC] cutpoints). This is in accordance with an earlier report *(56)* that showed up to 60-fold differences in absolute values for patient samples when tested with four different assay systems. Interestingly, results from these four cTnI assays were internally consistent (median CV between 3.3% and 8.3%), as neither false-positive nor false-negative samples were found *(56)*. What could explain the enormous differences in absolute values between these assays? Different calibration materials for the various assays will contribute to, but are very unlikely solely responsible for, such variations in the numeric values. It is known that cTnI degradation (as observed in MI patients) leads to detection difficulties if antibodies against proteolytically cleaved regions of cTnI are used in diagnostic assays *(57,58)*. Even so, degradation is not the only modification to cardiac troponins found after MI *(59)*. The reason for the variable performance of the different assays lies therefore in the potential incapability of anti-cTnI antibodies to recognize all of the possible cTnI modification products that may be present in the blood, let alone distinguish between these various forms. Thus, it is in fact the antibodies themselves that cause detection difficulties, rather than the cTnI modification. This is important, as certain cTnI modification products may be formed at specific times during the development of a disease and subsequently be present in a patient's blood at a distinct pattern of release over time *(59)*. What exact forms of cardiac troponins are actually circulating in a patient's blood is still under evaluation *(60–64)*, as well as if they differ with various heart diseases.

To address this issue we developed a method (Western Blot–Direct Serum Analysis [WB-DSA]) to separate serum proteins electrophoretically under denaturing conditions, allowing the visualization of intact as well as degraded forms of serum cTnI and cTnT from patients with MI *(59)*. Intact cTnI was the predominant form found in serum, while cTnT was predominantly cleaved, forming a 26-kDa product *(59)*. In addition, in a subset of patients intact cTnI as well as additional degradation products were also present. cTnI has been proposed to be proteolyzed in blood after the release from the myocardium *(57,65)*. Such proteolysis would further complicate the serum profile of troponin, as changes could originate both from the myocardium and due to processing in the blood after their release from the myocardium. Thus, the stability of the analyte in blood is critical for every diagnostic assay and essential for the accuracy and value of the assay result. Using WB-DSA, we monitored, over a time course of 48 h, proteolytic degradation of recombinant human cTnI and cTnT spiked in normal serum at a concentration of 100 ng/mL. Unlike previous reports in which up to 30-fold higher concentrations of recombinant cTnI were used *(57,65)*, we found only minimal serum proteolysis to troponins *(59)*. This suggests that cardiac troponin in serum at concentrations observed in pathophysiological conditions is protected from proteolysis, perhaps through binding to other troponin subunits or serum proteins. Only at excessive concentrations *(57,65)* at which it is not completely protected by these other proteins does cTnI become susceptible to serum proteases.

The lack of troponin proteolysis in serum indicates that troponin degradation products observed in the serum of acute MI (AMI) patients originated in the myocardium prior to release into the blood. These forms of cardiac troponins (intact as well as modified) display a characteristic "rising and falling" pattern after the onset of symptoms, producing a continuum of changing troponin profiles. The ability to distinguish between different forms of circulating troponins would offer more precise information about severity of damage, time of onset, or even type of disease, assisting in the triage of individual patients. This is not possible with the currently available diagnostic assays.

In addition to the advantage of providing information about certain modification states of the analyte, WB-DSA has a high analytical sensitivity. In fact, it enabled us to detect serum cTnI in patients undergoing CABG surgery at levels below the LLD of a routinely used commercial assay (0.1 ng/mL) *(42)*. This enhanced sensitivity most likely is due to the denaturing conditions used in WB-DSA, which would result in the complete exposure of linear epitopes, thereby increasing the probability of detection by various antibodies. cTnI in serum may be "hidden" owing to its ternary structure and/or the formation of three-dimensional complexes with other proteins. To test this method for its clinical application, serum from patients presenting at the emergency department early after onset of symptoms of ACS ($\leq$4 h) was analyzed by WB-DSA and the results compared to routine clinical testing *(66)*. A subset of the patients enrolled in this study with nondiagnostic electrocardiogram for ACS and nonsignificantly elevated routine biochemical markers (cTnI, CK, and CK-MB) showed detectable amounts of cTnI when retrospectively analyzed by WB-DSA ($n = 6/10$). These patients were diagnosed for unstable angina ($n = 3$), second-degree heart block ($n = 1$), or discharged from the ED as "chest pain not yet diagnosed" ($n = 2$). Three of the six patients revisited the ED within 3 mo complaining about chest pain.

ONE ANALYTE = ONE DISEASE = ONE ASSAY?

The exact release pattern of the various forms of cTnI (whether free or complexed with other proteins) after an ischemic insult and the correlation between the severity of the insult and the released forms in humans remains unknown, although it has been shown in Langendorff perfused rat hearts that cTnI undergoes selective and progressive modification with increased severity of ischemia/reperfusion injury *(38,40)*. Complex formation between cTnI and other troponin subunits influences its three-dimensional structure, having various consequences for the susceptibility of cTnI to enzymatic and chemical modification *(61)*. Certainly the same will apply to cTnI bound to any serum protein. cTnI is highly charged and insoluble in its free form at neutral pH. It has been proposed that only a small amount of free cTnI is detectable in blood of MI patients *(61)*, although the proportions of free cTnI varied among the patients analyzed and the severity of MI.

By comparing data from the three studies undertaken in our laboratory applying WB-DSA to identify serum cTnI *(42,59,66)*, the differences in the modification states of the analyte become apparent (Fig. 1). This is by no means surprising, as three very different cohorts of patients were enrolled in these studies, representing different stages of myocardial disease. While degradation seems preferably to occur in cases of MI, patients presenting with unstable angina show only intact cTnI. Patients undergoing thrombolytic therapy showed only intact cTnI before, but a variety of degradation products shortly after thrombolysis, again indicating that cTnI modifications occur prior to release from the myocardium (*unpublished data*). Extensive proteolytic degradation of

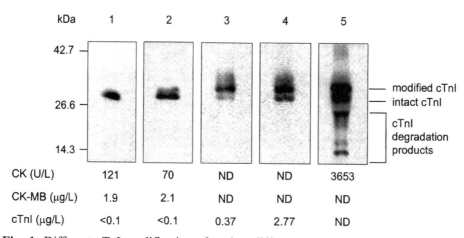

Fig. 1. Different cTnI modifications found at different stages of ischemic heart disease. WB-DSA using mAb 8I-7 (Spectral Diagnostics) on serum from four patients with the corresponding values for total CK (Beckman CX7), CK-MB, and cTnI (both Bayer Immuno1) indicated underneath and the relative molecular mass to the left. ND, Not determined. *Lane 1*: Patient with history of CHF and symptoms of chest pain, sample drawn 2 h after admission, discharged from the ED with "chest pain not yet diagnosed". *Lane 2*: Patient with history of myocardial infarction (6 mo prior) and symptoms of chest pain, sample drawn 2 h after admission, discharged from the hospital with unstable angina. *Lanes 3 and 4*: Patient undergoing CABG surgery with samples drawn 30 min and 24 h after removal of cross-clap respectively. *Lane 5*: Patient with AMI, sample drawn at admission.

cTnI and prolonged detectability in blood indicate longer ischemic periods and therefore cellular necrosis with disintegration of the troponin complex. On the other hand, intact cTnI as the only detectable form in angina patients, with faster clearance from the blood, may represent unassembled cytosolic troponin and resemble the first phase of a biphasic release as shown for cTnT on revascularization after MI *(67)*.

In their consensus document ESC and ACC suggest the use of a cutoff concentration for cardiac troponins at the 99th percentile (CV $\leq$ 10%) for the diagnosis of MI *(8,9)*. An increase in sensitivity of troponin assays can principally be appreciated because elevated troponins are associated with a risk of adverse clinical events *(13–17)*, even though the majority of manufacturers cannot yet meet these recommendations *(68)*. Automatically labeling an increase of cardiac troponin above this level as MI, in cases in which other causes of cardiac damage cannot be found, could be misleading. For example, a possible non-necrotic release (or a potential release with apoptosis) of troponins from the myocardium does not meet the criteria for MI. This leads to an important question. Is a single diagnostic assay adequate to diagnose all forms of cardiac disease that involve the release of troponins, or is it necessary to design specific assays for different patient cohorts to ensure precise diagnosis? The three studies mentioned above *(42,59,66)* must be confirmed for larger cohorts and other forms of cardiac disease. Regardless of the small groups of patients enrolled in these studies, our findings indicate significant variability of cTnI in patients with cardiac diseases. Different diseases or disease states may lead to different troponin modifications, creating disease-specific "troponin fingerprints" for MI, unstable angina, heart failure, and so on, as well as for damage caused by interventional procedures or cardiac surgery. Consequently, the use of antibodies raised against specific disease-induced troponin modification products would provide greater qualitative information than the simple determination of elevated troponin levels, and would in turn lead to the development of disease-specific diagnostic assays.

Although WB-DSA, for the first time, allows us to visualize modifications to serum troponins without any concentration or extraction step prior to analysis, it is still limited in scope. It can separate the analyte only by relative molecular mass, and the number of identified modification products depends on the antibodies used for western blotting *(59)*. This method is therefore inherently biased in the same manner as other immunoassays, and thus care in the selection of antibodies is paramount. To think that avoiding antibodies binding to epitopes within the very N- as well as C-terminus of cTnI, regions known to be proteolytically cleaved after MI *(57–61,65)*, would be enough to guarantee the detection of all cTnI modification products is far too simplistic. Katrukha et al. *(61)* very thoroughly listed possible modifications to cTnI that can influence immunogenicity and as a consequence detectability by a diagnostic assay. Within the region of cTnI that is supposed to be relatively resistant to proteolysis (between amino acids 30 and 110) there are at least two protein kinase C phosphorylation sites *(69)* and two Cys residues *(61)* that may be oxidized. Western blot analysis on native as well as on dephosphorylated human cardiac tissue *(42)* and serum from MI patients *(59)* showed that the affinity of some antibodies to cTnI is indeed altered by phosphorylation. The same may hold true for other posttranslational modifications (such as Cys oxidation) and might explain the differing performance of various commercial diagnostic cTnI assays. The impact of disease-induced posttranslational modifications to cTnT *(59)* on the two existing cTnT assays is more difficult to assess. There is no reason to believe that antibody binding to cTnT and, consequently, assay performance would be unaffected by such modifications. Standardization issues surrounding cTnI assays are not applicable to the currently marketed cTnT assays, as both use the same pair of antibodies *(70)*. Of course, similar issues undoubtedly will arise when additional assays using different antibodies are introduced in the future.

The identification and characterization of all myocardial-derived disease-induced forms of the analyte, be it cTnI, cTnT, or any other protein, must be the first step in the development of diagnostic assays capable of specifically detecting one or more of these modification products present in a particular patient's blood. To achieve this, we are well advised to endorse the tools of proteomics to investigate disease-induced protein modifications, elucidating the potential of these modifications to serve as diagnostic markers.

APPLICATION OF PROTEOMICS TO DIAGNOSTIC MARKER DEVELOPMENT

In one way or another, as the cause or a symptom, proteins are involved in virtually every disease, with cardiac diseases being no exception. It is therefore inevitable that a disease or disease state will manifest itself as a change to the proteome. Whether these changes are restricted to posttranslational modifications or also involve genetic alterations in protein levels depends on the particular disease state. For example, during ACS one will primarily observe the first group of modifications, whereas a subsequent development of CHF will also likely be accompanied by the latter. Therefore, various stages in the progression of a disease will be expected to reflect unique protein profiles. Not every protein change will automatically, but very well may, result in an altered physiological function. Understanding the functional consequences, if any, of a certain modification increases the value of an assay specific for this very modification. Thus, when a particular protein modification can be correlated with a certain disease or disease state and this modification is detectable, it serves as an invaluable diagnostic marker. It is in this venue that proteomics has the potential to revolutionize the development and application of future diagnostics.

The power of proteomics to identify disease-induced protein change is widely recognized, with an ever burgeoning number of publications dealing with this approach as a means to unravel the importance of protein modifications in the development, progression, treatment, and diagnosis of disease. Thus far, the majority of this work has focused on neurological and infectious diseases, cancer, and, to a lesser degree, cardiovascular diseases (for reviews *see 6,71–76)*. Collections of detailed proteomic techniques have extensively been described elsewhere *(77–79),* and we focus instead on the application of these techniques to the development of diagnostics.

A systematic use of the full armamentarium of proteomics will facilitate a much more detailed description of pathological processes in terms of protein modifications. The rapid development of proteomics, in both methods of protein separation and identification, now has the potential to guide the development of diagnostic assays as well as therapeutics in a number of ways. First, it may be used to identify and characterize specific disease-induced protein modifications associated with current biomarkers. Second, it may facilitate the identification of useful new biomarkers, which may stand alone for diagnostic purposes, or perhaps be used in combination with additional proteins to provide greater confidence in diagnosis or risk stratification. Finally, there is the possibility of the direct incorporation of proteomic techniques into diagnostic assays themselves.

The current tools of proteomics already allow us to improve the design of diagnostics through the identification and characterization of specific protein modifications. Unlike in cancer diagnosis, where biopsies and smears from patients are taken on a regular basis (and can be used for basic research purposes), proteomic analysis of human cardiac material at stages of onset or disease development is more difficult because of limited access. This is often possible only with samples from cadaveric donors or explanted hearts from end-stage heart failure patients, but such hearts will show overlapping disease- or drug-induced and postmortem changes to the proteome. Biopsies taken during heart surgery do provide a viable source of human myocardial material for determination of specific cardiac disease-induced protein modifications, but only recent technological advances in analytical proteomics are capable of the reproducible analysis of such minuscule samples.

Unfortunately, the dearth of available tissue samples, as well as a lack of immortalized cell lines (as are available for cancer research), has led to the widespread use of animal models to study cardiac/cardiovascular diseases. The majority of broad screening studies for proteome changes associated with these animal models employed the traditional proteomic separation method, two-dimensional gel electrophoresis (2-DE). While a number of proteins showed disease-induced changes (mainly in expression levels; for reviews *see 71,76),* few have the potential to serve as specific biomarkers due to their ubiquitous distribution in the body.

One recent development in the field of proteomics is the concept of simplifying the task of identifying protein modifications through a subproteomic approach, whereby only a fraction of the proteome is studied at any one time. Unlike the broad-based screening method mentioned above, partitioning the proteome into manageable portions facilitates identification of modifications to many proteins that would not otherwise be identified, by increasing the ability to detect both lower abundance proteins and protein modifications that are very subtle in nature, such as a shift in the extent of a protein posttranslational modification.

Using a subproteomic approach, we recently identified two ventricular myosin light chain 1 (vMLC1) posttranslational modifications. An analysis of isolated rabbit ventricular myocytes revealed that vMLC1 was phosphorylated at one serine and one threonine residue, which was quite remarkable considering that vMLC1 has also been called the unphosphorylatable light chain. Furthermore, we found that the extent of vMLC1 phosphorylation increased significantly following treatment with adenosine *(7)*, at levels previously demonstrated to be sufficient to precondition the cells, thereby protecting the heart from further ischemic injury *(80)*. Mass spectrometry was used not only to identify the presence of phosphorylated vMLC1 peptides, but also to map the actual modified amino acids. This is the type of information that is vital for the design of antibodies capable of binding and specifically detecting a modified protein.

While vMLC1 posttranslational modification is associated with early ischemic damage, vMLC1 was also found to be specifically degraded at its N-terminus in a rat model of extreme ischemia *(39)*. Therefore, differentiating between intact vMLC1 and its phosphorylated and its degraded forms may yield insights into the duration of an ischemic insult. To detect a specific modification and observe its change over time, rather than simply to look at the presence or absence of a protein, also offers the possibility of using marker proteins as surrogates for the progression of a disease or the success of a therapy. Species differences in protein sequences and, consequently, the possibility of different changes due to disease, make it difficult to draw direct conclusions from animal models for the identification of biomarkers in humans. These animal studies do, however, narrow down candidate proteins for a targeted approach using human tissue specimens. In parallel, the search for such proteins could be extended to blood and urine, sample sources more suitable for routine clinical testing. Ideally, the disease-induced modification will result in a change to a certain characteristic of the protein, that enables the modified and native forms to be easily distinguished by means such as specific antibodies or chromatographic and electrophoretic separation techniques.

In some instances it might be necessary to use more than one biomarker for a definitive diagnosis of a disease, or to distinguish between different diseases of the same organ or organ system. This is already routinely practiced when elevated CK or CK-MB levels are confirmed by an elevated troponin level to diagnose MI, or in the case of non-elevated troponin to rule out MI. A traditional proteomic approach may allow the identification of multiple proteins that show a specific pattern that can be correlated with a certain disease or disease state, while only a single one of these proteins might be non-indicative for disease. This is reiterating the concept of a "protein fingerprint" for a certain disease (as proposed for cardiac troponins earlier in this text), and the possibility that a specific protein can be used in the diagnosis of different diseases when combined with other proteins. An example of such an approach is mentioned below.

Protein separation by 2-DE followed by mass spectrometric identification and characterization of proteins and their disease-induced modifications are the main tools in identifying these "protein fingerprints." Despite this, the application of 2-DE to routine diagnosis is limited, for it is both labor intensive and time consuming. Ideally, it is desirable to incorporate information obtained from proteomic analysis on a platform suitable for routine diagnosis. This can be done by raising antibodies against specific disease-induced modifications, that can then be used on immunoassay platforms. This concept can even be extended to the design of antibody arrays for high-throughput screening of multiple proteins at the same time, as demonstrated by de Wildt et al. *(81)*.

Taken one step further, proteomic techniques may directly be used as future diagnostic tools. The development of methods such as laser capture microdissection (LCM), ProteinChip technology, and surface-enhanced laser desorption/ionization (SELDI) mass spectrometry may allow high-throughput analysis of very small samples to compare the entire protein profile between control and patient samples. Wright et al. applied ProteinChip proteomics to search for prostate cancer biomarkers *(82)*. The authors analyzed tissue and body fluid, and found expression level changes to a number of proteins. Interestingly, a combination of several proteins, and no single protein alone, was required to distinguish between cancer and non-cancer patient groups. Once again, the identification of one specific marker protein may well be insufficient, and instead the "protein fingerprint" concept may be required for accurate diagnoses. Furthermore, in combination, ProteinChip and SELDI technologies may also allow the development of quantitative immunoassays *(83)*. To our knowledge, however, LCM, ProteinChip, and SELDI have not yet been used to investigate cardiovascular diseases. As for any immunoassay, care has to be taken in antibody selection to guarantee that all forms of the analyte can be captured. This closes the loop to the initial determination of disease-induced protein modification as the key step in the improvement of diagnostic assays. How applicable these methods will be to the everyday routine in a clinical laboratory has to be evaluated, but their usefulness in the search for potential markers is unparalleled.

Because cardiac troponins are essential components of the contractile apparatus— the force generating part of the cardiomyocytes—it is no surprise that they outperform other biomarkers in sensitivity and specificity for the diagnosis of ACS, but we have not yet taken full advantage of their multiple forms that can exist in a patient. The moment we know the exact nature of the analyte we are really looking for, sensitivity and specificity of diagnostic assays will no doubt increase and differentiate potential diagnoses. On the other hand, like their predecessors, cTnI and cTnT may eventually be replaced by a better biomarker for certain cardiac conditions, or be used in combination with other proteins to provide superior diagnostic capability.

ACKNOWLEDGMENT

This work was supported by funding from the Canadian Institutes of Heatlh Research (grant-in-aid 49843) and the Ontario Heart and Stroke Foundation (grant-in-aid T-3759).

ABBREVIATIONS

ACC, American College of Cardiology; ACS, acute coronary syndromes; AHA, American Heart Association; AST, aspartate aminotransferase; CABG, cardiopulmonary bypass graft; CHF, congestive heart failure; CK, creatine kinase; CK-MB, MB isoenzyme of CK; cTnT and cTnI, cardiac troponin T and I; CV, coefficient of variance;

2-DE; two dimensional gel electrophoresis; ESC, European Society of Cardiology; LCM, laser capture microdissection; LDH, lactate dehydrogenase; LLD, lower limit of detection; MI, myocardial infarction; ROC, receiver operating characteristic; SELDI, surface-enhanced laser desoprtion/ionization; vMLC1, ventricular myosin light chain 1; WB-DSA, Western Blot–Direct Serum Analysis.

REFERENCES

1. International Human Genome Sequencing Consortium. Initial sequencing and analysis of the human genome. Nature 2001;409:860–921.
2. Venter JC, Adams MD, Myers EW. The sequence of the human genome. Science 2001;291: 1304–1351.
3. Lenfant C. Cardiovascular research: a look into tomorrow. Circ Res 2001;88:253–255.
4. Pleissner KP, Soding P, Sander S, et al. Dilated cardiomyopathy-associated proteins and their presentation in a WWW-accessible two-dimensional gel protein database. Electrophoresis 1997;18:802–808.
5. Weekes J, Wheeler CH, Yan JX, et al. Bovine dilated cardiomyopathy: proteomic analysis of an animal model of human dilated cardiomyopathy. Electrophoresis 1999;20:898–906.
6. Dunn MJ. Studying heart disease using the proteomic approach. Drug Discov Today 2000; 5:76–84.
7. Arrell DK, Neverova I, Fraser H, et al. Proteomic analysis of pharmacologically preconditioned cardiomyocytes reveals novel phosphorylation of myosin light chain 1. Circ Res 2001; 89:480–487.
8. Alpert JS, Thygesen K, Antman E, et al. Myocardial infarction redefined—a consensus document of the Joint European Society of Cardiology/American College of Cardiology Committee for the Redefinition of Myocardial Infarction. J Am Coll Cardiol 2000;36:959–969.
9. Joint European Society of Cardiology/American College of Cardiology Committee. Myocardial infarction redefined—a consensus document of the Joint European Society of Cardiology/American College of Cardiology Committee for the Redefinition of Myocardial Infarction. Eur Heart J 2000;21:1502–1513.
10. Braunwald E, Antman EM, Beasley JW, et al. ACC/AHA guidelines for the management of patients with unstable angina and non-ST segment elevation myocardial infarction: executive summary and recommendations. A report of the American College of Cardiology/ American Heart Association Task Force on Practice Guidelines (Committee on the Management of Patients with Unstable Angina). Circulation 2000;102:1193–1209.
11. Storrow AB, Gibler WB. The role of cardiac markers in the emergency department. Clin Chim Acta 1999;284:187–196.
12. Hudson MP, Cristenson RH, Newby LK, et al. Cardiac markers: point of care testing. Clin Chim Acta 1999;284:223–237.
13. Stubbs P, Collinson P, Moseley D, et al. Prognostic significance of admission troponin T concentrations in patients with myocardial infarction. Circulation 1996;94:1291–1297.
14. Hamm CW, Goldmann BU, Heeschen C, et al. Emergency room triage of patients with acute chest pain by means of rapid testing for cardiac troponin T or troponin I. N Engl J Med 1997;337:1648–1653.
15. Ottani F, Galvani M, Ferrini D, et al. Direct comparison of early elevations of cardiac troponin T and I in patients with clinical unstable angina. Am Heart J 1999;137:284–291.
16. Hamm CW, Heeschen C, Goldmann B, et al. Benefit of abciximab in patients with refractory unstable angina in relation to serum troponin T levels: c7E3 Fab Antiplatelet Therapy in Unstable Refractory Angina (CAPTURE) study investigators. N Engl J Med 1999;340: 1623–1629.

17. Lindahl B, Diderhohn E, Lagerqvist B, et al. Troponin T 0.1 µg/L is an inappropriate cut-off value for risk stratification in unstable coronary artery disease using the new third generation troponin T assay (abstract). Circulation 2000;102(Suppl II):S22.

18. Apple FS, Murakami M, Panteghini M, et al. International survey on the use of cardiac markers. Clin Chem 2001;47:587–588.

19. Voss EM, Sharkey SW, Gernert AE, et al. Human and canine cardiac troponin T and creatine kinase-MB distribution in normal and diseased myocardium: infarct sizing using serum profiles. Arch Pathol Lab Med 1995;119:799–806.

20. Ricchiuti V, Sharkey SW, Murakami MM, et al. Cardiac troponin I and T alterations in dog hearts with myocardial infarction: correlation with infarct size. Am J Clin Pathol 1998; 110:241–247.

21. Remppis A, Ehlermann P, Giannitsis E, et al. Cardiac troponin T levels at 96 hours reflect myocardial infarct size: a pathoanatomical study. Cardiology 2000;93:249–253.

22. Solaro RJ, Rarick HM. Troponin and tropomyosin: proteins that switch on and tune in the activity of cardiac myofilaments. Circ Res 1998;83:471–480.

23. Filatov VL, Katrukha AG, Bulargina TV, et al. Troponin: structure, properties, and mechanism of functioning. Biochemistry (Moscow) 1999;64:969–985.

24. Perry SV. Troponin I: inhibitor or facilitator. Mol Cell Biochem 1999;190:9–32.

25. Chalovich JM. Actin mediated regulation of muscle contraction. Pharmacol Ther 1992;55: 95–148.

26. Van Eyk JE, Hodges RS. The use of synthetic peptides to unravel the mechanism of muscle regulation. Methods: A Companion to Methods in Enzymology 1993;5:264–280.

27. Lehrer SS. The regulatory switch of the muscle thin filament: Ca^{2+} or myosin heads? J Muscle Res Cell Motility 1994;15:232–236.

28. Tobacman LS. Thin filament-mediated regulation of cardiac contraction. Annu Rev Physiol 1996;58:447–481.

29. Solaro RJ, Van Eyk JE. Altered interactions among thin filament proteins modulate cardiac function. J Mol Cell Cardiol 1996;28:217–230.

30. Lehrer SS, Geeves MA. The muscle thin filament as a classical cooperative/allosteric regulatory system. J Mol Biol 1998;277:1081–1089.

31. Murphy AM, Kogler H, Georgakopolous D, et al. Transgenic mouse model of stunned myocardium. Science 2000;287:488–491.

32. Tardiff JC, Factor SM, Tompkins BD, et al. A truncated cardiac troponin T molecule in transgenic mice suggests multiple cellular mechanisms for familial hypertrophic cardiomyopathy. J Clin Invest 1998;101:2800–2811.

33. Tardiff JC, Hewett TE, Palmer BM, et al. Cardiac troponin T mutations result in allele-specific phenotypes in a mouse model for hypertrophic cardiomyopathy. J Clin Invest 1999; 104:469–481.

34. Bolli R, Marban E. Molecular and cellular mechanisms of myocardial stunning. Physiol Rev 1999;79:609–634.

35. Lamers JM. Preconditioning and limitation of stunning: one step closer to the protected protein(s)? Cardiovasc Res 1999;42:571–575.

36. Solaro RJ. Troponin I, stunning, hypertrophy, and failure of the heart. Circ Res 1999;84: 122–124.

37. Foster DB, Van Eyk JE. In search of the proteins that cause myocardial stunning. Circ Res 1999;85:470–472.

38. Gao WD, Atar D, Liu Y, et al. Role of troponin I proteolysis in the pathogenesis of stunned myocardium. Circ Res 1997;80:393–399.

39. Van Eyk JE, Powers F, Law W, et al. Breakdown and release of myofilament proteins during ischemia and ischemia/reperfusion in rat hearts: identification of degradation products and effects on the pCa-force relation. Circ Res 1998;82:261–271.

40. McDonough JL, Arrell DK, Van Eyk JE. Troponin I degradation and covalent complex formation accompanies myocardial ischemia/reperfusion injury. Circ Res 1999;84:9–20.

41. Van Eyk JE, Organ LR, Buscemi N, et al. Cardiac disease-induced post-translational modifications of troponin I: differential proteolysis, phosphorylation and covalent complex formation. Biophys J 2000;78:107A.

42. McDonough JL, Labugger R, Pickett W, et al. Cardiac troponin I is modified in the myocardium of bypass patients. Circulation 2001;103:58–64.

43. Missov ED, Calzolari C, Pau B. Circulating cardiac troponin I in severe congestive heart failure. Circulation 1997;96:2953–2958.

44. Missov ED, Mair J. A novel biochemical approach to congestive heart failure: cardiac troponin T. Am Heart J 1999;138:95–99.

45. Giannitsis E, Muller-Bardorff M, Kurowski V, et al. Independent prognostic value of cardiac troponin T in patients with confirmed pulmonary embolism. Circulation 2000;102:211–217.

46. Lauer B, Niederau C, Kuhl U, et al. Cardiac troponin T in patients with clinically suspected myocarditis. J Am Coll Cardiol 1997;30:1354–1359.

47. ver Elst KM, Spapen HD, Nam Nguyen D, et al. Cardiac troponins I and T are biological markers of left ventricular dysfunction in septic shock. Clin Chem 2000;46:650–657.

48. Ammann P, Fehr T, Minder EI, et al. Elevation of troponin I in sepsis and septic shock. Intensive Care Med 2001;27:965–969.

49. Tardiff BE, Califf RM, Tcheng JE, et al. for the IMPACT-II Investigators. Clinical outcomes after detection of elevated enzymes in patients undergoing percutaneous intervention: IMPACT-II trial (Integrilin [eptifibatide] to Minimize Platelet Aggregation and Coronary Thrombosis-II). J Am Coll Cardiol 1999;33:88–96.

50. Schluter T, Baum H, Plewan A, et al. Effects of implantable cardioverter defibrillator implantation and shock application on biochemical markers of myocardial damage. Clin Chem 2001;47:459–463.

51. Wu AHB, Ford L. Release of cardiac troponin in acute coronary syndromes: ischemia or necrosis? Clin Chim Acta 1999;284:161–171.

52. Wu AHB. Increased troponin in patients with sepsis and septic shock: myocardial necrosis or reversible myocardial depression? Inten Care Med 2001;27:959–961.

53. Adams JE. Clinical application of markers of cardiac injury: basic concepts and new considerations. Clin Chim Acta 1999;284:127–134.

54. Mair J. Tissue release of cardiac markers: from physiology to clinical application. Clin Chem Lab Med 1999;37:1077–1084.

55. Apple FS, Adams JE, Wu AHB, et al. Report on a survey of analytical and clinical characteristics of commercial cardiac troponin assays. In: Markers in Cardiology: Current and Future Clinical Applications. Adams JE III, Apple FS, Jaffe AS, Wu AHB, eds. Armonk, NY: Futura, 2001, pp. 31–34.

56. Tate JR, Heathcote D, Rayfield J, et al. The lack of standardization of cardiac troponin I assay systems. Clin Chim Acta 1999;284:141–149.

57. Katrukha AG, Bereznikova AV, Filatov VL, et al. Degradation of cardiac troponin I: implication for reliable immunodetection. Clin Chem 1998;44:2433–2440.

58. Shi Q, Ling M, Zhang X, et al. Degradation of cardiac troponin I in serum complicates comparisons of cardiac troponin I assays. Clin Chem 1999;45:1018–1025.

59. Labugger R, Organ L, Collier C, et al. Extensive troponin I and T modification detected in serum from patients with acute myocardial infarction. Circulation 2000;102:1221–1226.

60. Katus HA, Remppis A, Neumann FJ, et al. Diagnostic efficiency of troponin T measurements in acute myocardial infarction. Circulation 1991;83:902–912.

61. Katrukha AG, Bereznikova AV, Esakova TV, et al. Troponin I is released in blood stream of patients with acute myocardial infarction not in free form but as a complex. Clin Chem 1997;43:1379–1385.

62. Wu AHB, Feng YJ, Moore R, et al. Characterization of cardiac troponin subunit release into serum after acute myocardial infarction and comparison of assays for troponin T and I. American Association for Clinical Chemistry Subcommittee on cTnI Standardization. Clin Chem 1998;44:1198–1208.

63. Wu AHB, Feng YJ. Biochemical differences between cTnT and cTnI and its significance for the diagnosis of acute coronary syndromes. Eur Heart J 1998;19(Suppl N):25–29.

64. Giuliani I, Bertinchant JP, Granier C, et al. Determination of cardiac troponin I forms in the blood of patients with acute myocardial infarction and patients receiving crystalloid or cold blood cardioplegia. Clin Chem 1999;45:213–222.

65. Morjana NA. Degradation of human cardiac troponin I after myocardial infarction. Biotechnol Appl Biochem 1998;8:105–111.

66. Colantonio DA, Pickett W, Brison RJ, et al. Detection of cardiac troponin I early after onset of symptoms in patients with acute coronary syndromes. Clin Chem 2002;48:668–671.

67. Katus HA, Remppis A, Scheffold T, et al. Intracellular compartmentation of cardiac troponin T and its release kinetics in patients with reperfused and nonreperfused myocardial infarction. Am J Cardiol 1991;67:1360–1367.

68. Apple FS, Wu AHB. Myocardial infarction redefined: role of cardiac troponin testing. Clin Chem 2001;47:377–379.

69. Noland TS Jr, Gao X, Raynor AL, et al. Cardiac troponin I mutants. Phosphorylation by protein kinases C and A and regulation of Ca^{2+}-stimulated MgATPase of reconstituted actomyosin S-1. J Biol Chem 1995;43:25445–25454.

70. Giannitsis E, Weidtmann B, Muller-Bardorff M, et al. Cardiac troponin T in coronary artery disease: where do we stand? In: Markers in Cardiology: Current and Future Clinical Applications. Adams JE III, Apple FS, Jaffe AS, Wu AHB, eds. Armonk, NY: Futura, 2001, pp. 117–130.

71. Jungblut PR, Zimny-Arndt U, Zeindl-Eberhart E, et al. Proteomics in human disease: cancer, heart and infectious diseases. Electrophoresis 1999;20:2100–2110.

72. Fung ET, Wright GL, Dalmasso EA. Proteomic strategies for biomarker identification: progress and challenges. Curr Opin Mol Ther 2000;2:643–650.

73. Rohlff C. Proteomics in molecular medicine: applications in central nervous systems disorders. Electrophoresis 2000;21:1227–1234.

74. Jain KK. Applications of proteomics in oncology. Pharmacogen 2000;1:385–393.

75. Banks RE, Dunn MJ, Hochstrasser DF, et al. Proteomics: new perspectives, new biomedical opportunities. Lancet 2000;356:1749–1756.

76. Arrell DK, Neverova I, Van Eyk JE. Cardiovascular proteomics: evolution and potential. Circ Res 2001;88:763–773.

77. Wilkins MR, Williams KL, Appel RD, Hochstrasser DF, eds. Proteome Research: New Frontiers in Functional Genomics. New York: Springer, 1998.

78. Link AJ, ed. Methods in Molecular Biology: 2-D Proteome Analysis Protocols. Totowa, NJ: Humana Press, 1999.

79. Rabilloud T, ed. Proteome Research: Two-Dimensional Gel Electrophoresis and Identification Methods. New York: Springer, 2000.

80. Sato T, Sasaki N, O'Rourke B, et al. Adenosine primes the opening of mitochondrial ATP-sensitive potassium channels: a key step in ischemic preconditioning? Circulation 2000;102:800–805.

81. de Wildt RM, Mundy CR, Gorick BD, Tomlinson IM. Antibody arrays for high-throughput screening of antibody–antigen interactions. Nat Biotechnol 2000;18:989–994.

82. Wright GL, Cazares LH, Leung S-M, et al. ProteinChip surface enhanced laser desorption/ionization (SELDI) mass spectrometry: a novel protein biochip technology for detection of prostate cancer biomarkers in complex protein mixtures. Prostate Cancer Prostate Dis 2000;2:264–276.

83. Xiao Z, Jiang X, Beckett ML, et al. Generation of a baculovirus recombinant prostate-specific membrane antigen and its use in the development of a novel protein biochip quantitative immunoassay. Protein Exp Purif 2000;19:12–21.

8

Cardiac Troponin Testing in Renal Failure and Skeletal Muscle Disease Patients

Fred S. Apple

INTRODUCTION

Cardiac disease is a major cause of death in patients with end-stage renal disease (ESRD), responsible for up to 45% of overall mortality *(1,2)*. Approximately 25% of deaths from cardiac causes are due to acute myocardial infarction (AMI). The overall mortality after AMI among 34,000 patients on long-term hemodialysis, identified form the US Renal Data System database, was 59% at 1 yr, 73% at 2 yr, and 89% at 5 yr *(1)*. Furthermore, the mortality rate after AMI was substantially greater for patients on long-term dialysis than for renal transplant recipients. Thus, sudden death and cardiac death are common occurrences in chronic hemodialysis patients. Based on data for approx 325,000 deaths from 1977 through 1997 recorded by the US Renal Data System database, Mondays and Tuesdays were the most common days for sudden and cardiac death for hemodialysis patients *(3)*. Approximately 20% of deaths occurred on Mondays and Tuesdays, compared to 14% on Wednesdays through Saturdays. The intermittent nature of hemodialysis, accompanied by large weight gains, increased potassium concentrations, and post-dialysis hypotension on Mondays and Tuesdays likely contributed to the differences in cardiac death rates. These data support the hypothesis that more aggressive strategies may be beneficial for the prevention of AMI in patients on dialysis.

Cardiac symptoms are seldom the presenting complaint in patients with muscular skeletal diseases, such as dermatomyositis (DM), polymyositis (PM), and muscular dystrophy (MD). However, 30–50% of DM/PM patients have cardiac manifestations coincident with the degenerative and inflammatory changes present in skeletal muscle in postmortem examination *(4)*. The diagnosis of Duchenne's muscular dystrophy is usually uncomplicated; the affected patient is usually a boy with proximal muscle weakness and has serum creatine kinase (CK) levels >20-fold the upper reference limit, and a muscle biopsy finding typical of the disease. The clinical criteria for the diagnosis of the less severe form of Duchenne's dystrophy, Becker's dystrophy, tend to vary. Furthermore, there are cases of intermediate severity that are difficult to assign to either category. Cardiac involvement occurs in the large majority of all dystrophy patients. Electrocardiogram (ECG) abnormalities may occur, tachycardia is common, and sudden death from myocardial failure occurs. However, distinguishing patients with severe serum CK and the MB isoenzyme of CK (CK-MB) increases between heart and skeletal muscle

From: *Cardiac Markers, Second Edition*
Edited by: Alan H. B. Wu @ Humana Press Inc., Totowa, NJ

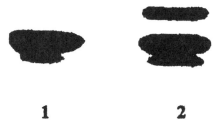

1   **2**

Fig. 1. Western blot of (1) failing human heart and (2) fetal human heart probed with monoclonal anti-cTnT antibody detecting 3 cTnT isoforms. (Adapted from ref. 5.)

etiology early in the course of the disease without clinical features of myocardial involvement can be challenging.

The purpose of this chapter is to review (1) cardiac troponin T (cTnT) and I (cTnI) expression in diseased myocardial and skeletal muscle, (2) the role of cardiac troponin testing for detecting myocardial injury in ESRD and diseases of skeletal muscle, and (3) the role of cardiac troponin testing in the assessment of long-term mortality in ESRD.

cTNT AND cTNI EXPRESSION
IN MYOCARDIAL AND SKELETAL MUSCLE

Three to four isoforms of cTnT, as shown in Fig. 1, have been shown to be expressed in developing cardiac muscle as well as in human fetal skeletal muscle and diseased human skeletal muscle *(5)*. A developmental down-regulation of cTnT and up-regulation of skeletal isoforms of TnT occurs in normal developing skeletal muscle, which leads to the absence of cTnT in nondiseased adult skeletal muscle. For cTnI, however, human cardiac muscle contains a single cTnI, and healthy and diseased human fetal and adult skeletal muscle have never been shown to express cTnI *(6,7)*.

One proposed explanation for the increase of cTnT in the blood of patients with ESRD (and patients with diseases of skeletal muscle) was the possibility of extracardiac expression of cTnT observed in diseased skeletal muscle. Several studies have now addressed cTnT expression in noncardiac tissues, specifically skeletal muscle tissues obtained from patients with varied underlying pathologies. Utilizing the cTnT-specific antibodies (M7, M11.7) used in the Roche cTnT immunoassay, no studies to date have demonstrated a cTnT isoform that would cause a false-positive cTnT circulating in serum, plasma, or whole blood. Skeletal muscle specimens obtained from patients with ESRD, Duchenne muscular dystrophy, polymyositis, and dermatomyositis as well as in kidney specimens from patients with varied renal diseases showed no expression of the cTnT isoform found in human hearts *(8–14)*. In a preliminary report, cTnT expression by Western blot analysis in skeletal muscles from ESRD patients was postulated *(15)*. However, the antibodies utilized in this study were not as cardiac specific as those found in the second- or third-generation cTnT immunoassay kit marketed by Roche. This initial report contrasted with a second report that showed no evidence of the expression of either cTnT mRNA or protein in truncal skeletal muscle from five ESRD patients *(16)*. Again, the antibodies used in the immunoblot experiments were not the same as those found in the cTnT Roche assay kit. In a more definite report, the expression of

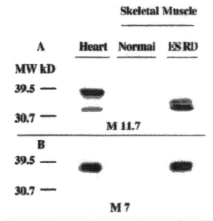

Fig. 2. Western blots of normal human heart and normal and ESRD skeletal muscle detecting cTnT and non-cTnT proteins using the cardiac-specific M11.7 and M7 antibodies. (Adapted from ref. *9*.)

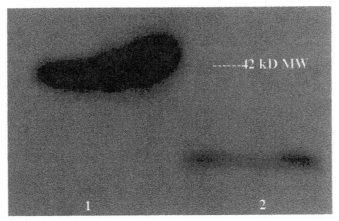

Fig. 3. Western blot of (1) normal human heart and (2) skeletal muscle from dermatomyositis patient using the Roche anti-cTnT monoclonal M7 antibody demonstrating lack of expression of cardiac specific troponin T in diseased skeletal muscle.

cTnT isoforms in ESRD skeletal muscles using both the capture antibody (M11.7) and detection antibody (M7) from the Roche cTnT assay kit was addressed *(8,9)*. As shown in Fig. 2, the M7 antibody detected a 39-kDa cTnT isoform similar to that expressed in human heart tissue, in 2 of 45 skeletal muscle biopsies. In contrast, the M11.7 antibody detected two or three cTnT isoforms at 34–36 kDa, and no cTnT at 39 kDa in 20 of 45 skeletal muscle biopsies. Given the differences in epitopes recognized by the M7 and M11.7 antibodies, it was concluded that the cTnT isoforms expressed in ESRD muscle would not be detected by the Roche cTnT assay if released into the circulation and were not the heart isoform of cTnT. Similar findings have been demonstrated in Western blots of skeletal muscle tissues obtained from DM, PM, and MD patients as shown in Fig. 3 *(9–14)*. These data support the claim that the tissue source of circulating cTnT in these patients is from the heart and are indicative of myocardial damage. Furthermore, Western blot analysis of skeletal muscle has never demonstrated expression of cTnI *(7,8)*.

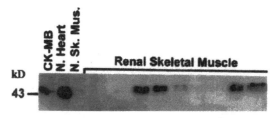

Fig. 4. Western blot of CK-MB standard, normal (N) human heart, normal human skeletal muscle, and nine skeletal muscle samples from ESRD patients probed with monoclonal anti-CK-B monoclonal antibody detecting substantial CK-MB expression in diseased skeletal muscles. (Adapted from ref. *37*.)

ROLE OF CARDIAC TROPONIN TESTING
FOR DETECTING MYOCARDIAL INJURY IN ESRD

Numerous studies have shown that both cTnI and cTnT are increased in serum and plasma in ESRD patients without clinical evidence of myocardial damage. From 1993 through 1998 a review of studies that measured cTnI involving more than 350 ESRD patients and studies which measured cTnT involving more than 500 ESRD patients showed 2–10% and 10–30% of patients had increased cTnI and cTnT values, respectively *(17–34)*. Explanations for these substantial differences are not clear at present. Both cTnI and cTnT assay manufacturers show data in their package inserts regarding the low percentage of ESRD patients who were found to have increased cardiac troponins. It should be noted that the studies reviewed in this chapter for cTnT involved only the second- or third-generation cTnT assays, which have eliminated any interference by skeletal muscle troponins. Explanations put forth for the cause of these increased troponin concentrations include expression of cTnT in skeletal muscle (without evidence), as well as detection of subclinical myocardial damage. The cause of the differences in positive rates between cTnT and cTnI also is not known. Possible mechanisms have been proposed for differences between cTnI and cTnT increases. First, circulating cTnT may reflect left ventricular hypertrophy with a different release pattern vs cTnI *(35)*. Second, a longer circulating half-life for cTnT may occur, possibly due to advanced glycosylated end products of cTnT known to accumulate in diabetics with ESRD *(36)*. Third, cTnT may be more sensitive due to accumulation in the circulation from lack of removal during the dialysis process compared to cTnI. Studies have emphasized the problems of using CK-MB as a marker for myocardial damage in ESRD. Falsely increased concentrations of CK-MB in up to 75% of ESRD patients have been demonstrated *(17, 18)*, likely due to the reexpression of CK-MB in myopathic skeletal muscles (Fig. 4) *(37)* in ESRD patients *(38)*. In one study addressing the role of biomarkers for ruling out AMI, serum cTnI monitoring was performed in 84 patients with renal insufficiency hospitalized to rule out AMI *(39)*. Clinical parameters (echocardiography, ECG) were used to diagnose AMI. The clinical sensitivity of cTnI was 77%, which was significantly better than CK-MB at 68%. Both markers showed >90% specificities. However, both sensitivity and specificity were lower in the renal diseased patients than observed in nonrenal disease ACS patients presenting to rule in/rule out AMI. No mechanisms are provided to explain this variance. Thus, the evidence supports cTnI and cTnT as markers with high specificity for cardiac damage, and can be used to distinguish whether increases in CK-MB are due to myocardial or skeletal muscle injury.

ROLE OF CARDIAC TROPONIN TESTING IN THE ASSESSMENT OF MORTALITY IN ESRD

The presence of increased cTnI and cTnT concentrations identify acute coronary syndrome patients at significantly higher risk of developing cardiac events, such as cardiac death and nonfatal AMI, both during hospitalization and at long-term follow-up *(40,41)*. Several studies have now also demonstrated that ESRD patients with increases in cTnI and cTnT concentrations tend to have a poor prognostic outcome. First, in a preliminary 1 yr follow-up study of 16 randomly selected ESRD patients, the cardiac event rate (*n* = 4 fatal AMIs) was correlated to patients who displayed the higher increases of serum cTnT and cTnI *(23)*. Second, serum cTnT concentrations measured in 49 ESRD patients who presented with no complaints of chest pain and in 83 renal insufficiency patients (serum creatinine >2 mg/dL and not on dialysis) were clinically followed for 6 mo after entry into the study *(42)*. Of the 25 ESRD patients with increased cTnT concentrations at entry, six had cardiac events. Thus, cTnT demonstrated 100% sensitivity and 56% specificity. In comparison, all three patients with an increased cTnI had cardiac events, demonstrating a 50% sensitivity and a 100% specificity for cTnI. Patients with diabetes were more likely to have increased cardiac troponin concentrations. In contrast, only three patients in the entire renal insufficiency group had an increased cTnI or cTnT. In the 6-mo follow-up, two patients suffered an AMI, but neither of these patients had increased troponins. These data suggest that cardiac troponin testing may be effective in elucidating cardiac risks of patients undergoing chronic dialysis.

Third, measurement of cTnT in the blood of 97 ESRD patients showed that cTnT was detectable in 29% of patients *(16)*. The prevalence of increased cTnT concentrations correlated with cardiac risk. Fifty percent (11 of 22) of known coronary artery disease (CAD) patients had an increased cTnT concentration (median 1.6 ng/mL), compared to 31% (15 of 33) of patients with ≥2 risk factors (median 0.1 ng/mL) and 11% (3 of 28) of patients with 0 or 1 risk factors; $p < 0.05$ vs known CAD patients. Thus, a positive relationship existed between increased risk of CAD and increases in cTnT concentrations. A fourth study investigated the use of monitoring cTnT and cTnI concentrations for predicting cardiac outcomes by 6 mo in patients presenting with suspected acute coronary syndromes (ACS) and renal insufficiency (creatinine >2.0 mg/dL) (*n* = 51) relative to ACS patients without renal disease (*n* = 102) *(43)*. Thirty-five percent of patients in the renal group and 45% in the nonrenal group experienced an adverse outcome during initial hospitalization. However, at 6 mos, both groups had experienced >50% adverse outcomes. The areas under the receiver operating characteristic (ROC) curves for both cTnT and cTnI, used as predictors of initial and long-term outcomes, were significantly lower in the renal group than the nonrenal group (0.56, 0.75, respectively). No mechanisms were given to explain these findings.

In addition to these studies, four recent studies now clearly demonstrate the prognostic power of cardiac troponin for predicting mortality in patients with ESRD. First, in 30 hemodialysis patients followed over 2 yr, cTnI (Dade Stratus II and Abbott AxSYM)

Table 1
Risk Associated with Cardiac Troponin in ESRD Patients

Study A (ref. *45*, n = 102)

cTnT (ng/mL)	n	Deaths	%
<0.01	17	0	0
0.01–0.04	45	10	22
>0.04–0.1	28	8	28
>0.1	12	10	83

Study B (ref. *46*, n = 244)

cTnT (ng/mL)	Deaths (%)	Cardiac deaths (%)
<0.01	6	0
0.01–0.09	43	14
≥0.1	59	24

Study C (ref. *47*, n = 441)

	cTnT (ng/mL)		cTnI,ng/mL	
	<0.04	≥0.04	<0.1	≥0.1
n	193	248	417	24
(%)	(44)	(56)	(94.5)	(5.5)
% Mortality	13	26	19	41

and cTnT (second- and third-generation Roche assay) concentrations were measured at baseline *(44)*. At 2 yr, an increased cTnT demonstrated 90% mortality vs 11% in patients with a normal cTnT. In comparison, both increased and normal cTnI patients had 40% mortality. Second (Study A, Table 1), in 102 ESRD patients with a baseline cTnT (Elecsys) measured 24-mo outcomes were assessed *(45)*. cTnT was a strong predictor of mortality, with 7-fold greater risk of death at cTnT >0.1 ng/mL. An increased cTnT resulted in a 3.6-fold greater hazard ratio for overall mortality. Even at the low cutoff concentration of 0.01 ng/mL, 22% of patients died at 24 mo. Third (Study B, Table 1), 244 ESRD patients with baseline cTnT (Elecsys) values were followed for 34 mo *(46)*. A significant correlation between increasing cTnT, all causes of death, and cardiac death was found. In addition, increasing cTnT over a 6-mo period showed an increasing death rate; risk ratio = 2.0. Fourth (Study C, Table 1), a preliminary study from the author's institution examined 18-mo mortality in 441 ESRD based on baseline cTnT (Elecsys) and cTnI (Dade Dimension RxL) values *(47)*. Both cardiac troponins demonstrated significant increases in mortality in the troponin-positive vs negative groups: cTnT 26% vs 13%; cTnI 41% vs 19%, respectively ($p < 0.01$). However, there were a substantially greater number of patients with increased cTnT (n = 238) compared to cTnI (n = 24).

CLINICAL IMPLICATIONS

The clinical chore for predicting the role of cardiac troponin testing in the ESRD population will be (1) to distinguish the mechanistic type of increase an individual patient has and (2) to determine whether it is best to (i) detect a larger number of patients with increased troponin T with the possibility of confounding increases with fewer outcomes, (ii) detect fewer increased troponins I with a possible higher predictive mortality rate (assay dependent), with the higher probability of missing patients who go on to have a poor outcome. As is generally true for all diagnostic tests, the price of higher sensitivity will usually be lower specificity.

The rationale for cardiac troponin testing in the management of ACS has been clearly established. The ultimate role of cardiac troponin testing for risk stratification in the outpatient dialysis unit is speculative, but attractive. The initiation of dialysis is temporally associated with the occurrence of AMI, as about half of myocardial infarcts occurring in these ESRD patients are clustered within the first 2 yr after dialysis initiation. There are a host of conceivable strategies for the identification of the highest cardiac risk dialysis patients after initiation of renal replacement therapy, but one plausible, potentially cost-effective scenario is the developing role of outpatient cardiac troponin testing.

In conclusion, the use of cardiac tissue specific cTnT and cTnI testing in blood to assist in ruling in and ruling out AMI in patients with renal disease and skeletal muscle pathologies, and as a tool for cardiac risk assessment in ESRD patients now appears to be evidence based. However, larger trial studies would be useful to increase the evidence base to determine the overall incidences and differences between cTnT and cTnI monitoring in ESRD patients for cardiac risk assessment. Incorporation of cardiac troponin testing in ESRD patients may assist in initiating more aggressive treatment of coronary artery disease, detection of subclinical myocardial injury, and correlate increases in cardiac troponin testing with increased cardiac risk. Further, monitoring blood cardiac troponin concentrations should assist in the detection and treatment of CAD before renal transplantation, potentially reducing the risk of adverse cardiac events. However, each cardiac troponin assay will need to be validated independently, as not all cardiac troponin assays are equivalent *(48)*.

ABBREVIATIONS

ACS, acute coronary syndrome(s); AMI, acute myocardial infarction; CAD, coronary artery disease; CK, creatine kinase; CK-MB, MB isoenzyme of CK; cTnT, cTnI, cardiac troponins T and I; DM, dermatomyositis; ECG, electrocardiogram; ERSD, end-stage renal disease; MD, muscular dystrophy; PM, polymyositis; ROC, receiver operating characteristic.

REFERENCES

1. Herzog CA, Ma JZ, Collins AJ. Poor long-term survival after acute myocardial infraction among patients on long-term dialysis. N Engl J Med 1998;339:799–805.
2. Herzog CA. Diagnosis and treatment of ischemic heart disease in dialysis patients. Curr Opin Neph Hyper 1997;6:558–565.
3. Bleyer AJ, Russell GB, Satko SG. Sudden and cardiac death rates in hemodialysis patients. Kid Int 1999;55:1553–1559.
4. Hoffman EP, Fishbeck KH, Brown RH, et al. Characterization of dystrophy in muscle biopsy specimens from patient's with Duchenne's or Becker's muscular dystrophy. N Engl J Med 1988;318:1363–1368.
5. Anderson PAW, Malouf NN, Oakley AE, Pagani ED, Allen PD. Troponin T isoform expression in humans: a comparison among normal and failing adult heart, fetal heart, and adult and fetal skeletal muscle. Circ Res 1991;69:1226–1233.

6. Wilkinson JM, Grand JA. Comparison of amino acid sequence of troponin I from different striated muscles. Nature 1978;271:31–35.

7. Bodor GS, Porterfield D, Voss EM, Smith S, Apple FS. Cardiac troponin I is not expressed in fetal and healthy or diseased adult human skeletal tissue. Clin Chem 1995;41:1710–1715.

8. Ricchiuti V, Voss EM, Ney A, Odland M, Anderson PAW, Apple FS. Cardiac troponin T isoforms expressed in renal diseased skeletal muscle will not cause false-positive results by the second generation cardiac troponin T assay by Boehringer Mannheim. Clin Chem 1998; 44:1919–1924.

9. Ricchiuti V, Apple FS. RNA expression of cardiac troponin T isoforms in diseased human skeletal muscle. Clin Chem 1999;45:2129–2135.

10. Hammer-Lercher A, Erlacher P, Bittner R, et al. Clinical and experimental results on cardiac troponin expression in Duchenne muscular dystrophy. Clin Chem 2001;47:451–458.

11. Erlacher P, Lercher A, Falkensammer J, et al. Cardiac troponin and beta-type myosin heavy chain concentrations in patients with polymyositis or dermatomyositis. Clin Chim Acta 2001;306:27–33.

12. Fredricks S, Murray JF, Bewick M, et al. Cardiac troponin T and creatine kinase MB are not increased in exterior oblique muscle of patients with renal failure. Clin Chem 2001;47: 1023–1030.

13. Davis GK, Labugger R, Van Eyk JE, Apple FS. Cardiac troponin T is not detected in Western blots of diseased renal disease. Clin Chem 2001;47:782–784.

14. Davis GK, Labugger R, Van Eyk JE, Apple FS. Cardiac troponin T is not detected in Western blot of diseased renal tissue. Clin Chem 2001;47:782–784.

15. Bodor GS, Survant L, Voss EM, Smith S, Porterfield D, Apple FS. Cardiac troponin T composition in normal and regenerating skeletal muscle. Clin Chem 1997;43:476–484.

16. Haller C, Zehelein J, Remppis A, Muller-Bardorff M, Katus HA. Cardiac troponin T in patients with end-stage renal disease: absence of expression in truncal skeletal muscle. Clin Chem 1998;44:930–938.

17. McLaurin MD, Apple FS, Voss EM, Herzog CA, Sharkey SW. Cardiac troponin I, cardiac troponin T, and creatine kinase MB in dialysis patients without ischemic heart disease: evidence of cardiac troponin T expression in skeletal muscle. Clin Chem 1997;43:976–982.

18. Adams J, Bodor G, Davila-Roman V, et al. Cardiac troponin I: a marker with high specificity for cardiac injury. Circulation 1993;88:101–106.

19. Trinquier S, Flecheux O, Bullenger M, Castex F. Highly specific immunoassay for cardiac troponin I assessed in noninfarct patients with chronic renal failure or severe polytrauma. Clin Chem 1995;41:1675–1676.

20. Li D, Jialal I, Keffer J. Greater frequency of increased cardiac troponin T than increased cardiac troponin I in patients with chronic renal failure. Clin Chem 1996;42:114–115.

21. Porter GA, Norton T, Bennett WB. Troponin T, a predictor of death in chronic haemodialysis patients. Eur Heart J 1998;19(Suppl):N34–37.

22. Bhayana V, Gougoulias T, Cohee S. Discordance between results for serum troponin T and I in renal disease. Clin Chem 1995;41:312–317.

23. Apple FS, Sharkey SW, Hoeft P, et al. Prognostic value of serum cardiac troponin I and T in chronic dialysis patients: a one year outcomes analysis. Am J Kidney Dis 1997;29:399–403.

24. Hafner G, Thome-Kromer B, Schaube J, Kupferwasser I, Ehrenthal W, Cummins P. Cardiac troponins in serum in chronic renal failure. Clin Chem 1994;40:1790–1791.

25. Ishii J, Ishikawa T, Yukitake J. Clinical specificity of a second generation cardiac troponin T assay in patients with chronic renal failure. Clin Chim Acta 1998;270:183–188.

26. Akagi M, Nagake Y, Makino H, Ota Z. A comparative study of myocardial troponin T levels in patients undergoing hemodialysis. Jpn J Nephrol 1995;37:639–643.

27. Frankel WL, Herold DA, Zregler TW, Fitzgerald RL. Cardiac troponin T is elevated in asymptomatic patients with chronic renal failure. Am J Clin Pathol 1996;106:118–123.

28. Ooi DS, House AA. Cardiac troponin T in hemodialyzed patients. Clin Chem 1998;44: 1410–1416.
29. Bhayana V, Gougoulias T, Cohoe S, Henderson AR. Discordance between results for serum troponin T and troponin I in renal disease. Clin Chem 1995;41:312–317.
30. Haller C, Stevanovich A, Katus HA. Are cardiac troponins reliable serodiagnostic markers of cardiac ischemia in end-stage renal disease? Nephrol Dial Transplant 1996;11:941–944.
31. Katus HA, Haller C, Müller-Bardorff M, Scheffold T, Remppis A. Cardiac troponin T in end-stage renal disease patients undergoing chronic maintenance hemodialysis. Clin Chem 1995;41:1201–1202.
32. Haller C, Katus HA. Cardiac troponin T in dialysis patients. Clin Chem 1998;44:358.
33. McNeil AR, Marshall M, Ellis CJ, Hawkins RC. Why is troponin T increased in the serum of patients with end-stage renal disease? Clin Chem 1998;44:2377–2378.
34. Collinson PO, Stubbs PJ, Rosalki SB. Cardiac troponin T in renal disease. Clin Chem 1995; 41:1671–1673.
35. Lowbeer C, Deeberger AO, Gustafsson SA, Norrman R, Hulting J, Gutierrez A. Increased cardiac T and endothelin-1 concentrations in dialysis patients may indicate heart disease. Nephrol Dial Transplant 1999;14:1948–1955.
36. Kinchi K, Nejima J, Takano T, Ohta M, Hashimoto H. Increased serum concentrations of advanced glycation end products: a marker of coronary artery disease activity in type 2 diabetic patients. Heart 2001;85:87–91.
37. Ricchiuti V, Apple FS. Regulation of muscle gene and protein expression of creatine kinase B in chronic renal disease (abstract). Clin Chem 2000;46:A90.
38. Diesel W, Emms M, Knight B, Noakes TD, Swanepoel CR, Smit R. Morphology features on the myopathy associated with chronic renal failure. Am J Kidney Dis 1993;22:677–684.
39. McLaurin MD, Apple FS, Falahati A, Murakami M, Miller EA, Sharkey SW. Cardiac troponin I and creatine kinase MB mass to rule out myocardial injury in hospitalized patients with renal insufficiency. Am J Cardiol 1998;82:973–975.
40. Ottani F, Galvani M, Nicolini FA, Ferrini D, Pozzati A, DiPasquale G, Jaffe AS. Elevated cardiac troponin levels predict the risk of adverse outcome in patients with acute coronary syndromes. Am Heart J 2000;40:917–927.
41. Heidenreich PA, Alloggiamento T, Melsop K, McDonald KM, Go AS, Hlatky MA. The prognostic value of troponin in patients with non-ST-elevation acute coronary syndromes: a meta-analysis. J Am Coll Cardiol 2001;38:478–488.
42. Roppolo LP, Fitzgerald R, Dillow J, Ziegler T, Rice M, Maisel A. A comparison of troponin T and troponin I as predictors of cardiac events in patients undergoing chronic dialysis at a Veteran's hospital: a pilot study. J Am Coll Cardiol 1999;34:448–454.
43. VanLente F, McErlean ES, DeLuca SA, Rao JS, Nissen SE. Ability of troponins to predict adverse outcomes in patients with renal insufficiency and suspected acute coronary syndromes: a case matched study. J Am Coll Cardiol 1999;33:471–478.
44. Porter GA, Norton T, Bennett WM. Long term follow-up of the utility of troponin T to assess cardiac risk in stable chronic hemodialysis patients. Clin Lab 2000;46:469–476.
45. Dierkes J, Domrose U, Westphal S, et al. Cardiac troponin T predicts mortality in patients with end stage renal disease. Circulation 2000;102:1964–1969.
46. Ooi DS, Zimmerman D, Graham J, Wells GA. Cardiac troponin T predicts long-term outcomes in hemodialysis patients. Clin Chem 2001;47:412–417.
47. Apple FS, Murakami MM, Pearce LA, Herzog CA. Predictive value of cardiac troponin I and T for subsequent death in end stage renal disease. Circulation 2002;106:2941–2945.
48. Apple FS, Wu AHB. Myocardial infarction redefined: role of cardiac troponin testing. Clin Chem 2001;47:377–379.

9

Cardiac-Specific Troponins
Beyond Ischemic Heart Disease

David Morrow

INTRODUCTION

Cardiac biomarkers play a pivotal role in the clinical evaluation of patients presenting with chest discomfort. Owing to their tissue specificity and high clinical sensitivity for detecting myocyte injury, the cardiac troponins have become the preferred biomarker for the diagnosis of myocardial infarction (MI) *(1)* and risk assessment of patients with suspected acute coronary syndromes (ACS) *(2,3)*. Nevertheless, clinicians often encounter increased concentrations of cardiac troponin in patients without overt coronary artery disease or low clinical probability of myocardial ischemia, leading some to concerns over biologic false-positive troponin results *(4)*. A critical distinction must be made, however, between the high specificity of cardiac troponin for myocardial injury and the lack of specificity for coronary atherothrombosis and ischemia as the mechanism of injury. As troponin assays with increasing analytic sensitivity have been developed, our ability to detect minor degrees of myocardial injury in a variety of conditions has expanded, and led to a growing list of clinical settings in which increased concentrations of cardiac troponin has been detected without evidence of overt ischemic heart disease (Table 1).

While the presence of myocyte damage and the mechanism of injury are well defined (e.g., myocarditis) in several of these conditions, the availability of assays for cardiac troponin has revealed unexpectedly prevalent myocardial injury in others, and led to important new directions for research, as well as to possibilities for novel clinical applications in nonischemic cardiac disease. This chapter describes several of these clinical settings in detail, starting with those in which some degree of myocardial damage is expected and moving toward those in the etiology of myocardial injury less well explained. Other important etiologies of troponin release are discussed individually in separate chapters (chemotherapeutic agents, cardiac surgery, angioplasty, renal failure, skeletal muscle disease, and congestive heart failure).

MYOCARDITIS

Myocarditis connotes inflammatory involvement of the myocardium that may occur in a wide range of infectious and noninfectious conditions *(5)*. Pathologic evidence from routine autopsies suggests that unrecognized myocardial involvement occurs more frequently than expected in the setting of systemic infection *(6)*. Myocarditis is an established

From: *Cardiac Markers, Second Edition*
Edited by: Alan H. B. Wu @ Humana Press Inc., Totowa, NJ

Table 1
Nonischemic^a Conditions with Elevation of Troponin

Myocarditis
Direct cardiac trauma (cardiac surgery, ablation, endomyocardial biopsy, internal defibrillator
   discharge, external cardioversion)
Blunt chest trauma
Chemotherapeutic agents (anthracyclines)
Infiltrative diseases with cardiac involvement (e.g., amyloidosis) *(116,117)*
Pericarditis *(118)*
Rhabdomyolysis with cardiac involvement *(119)*
Uncomplicated percutaneous coronary intervention
Pulmonary embolism
Hypertensive emergency (e.g., preeclampsia) *(120)*
Congestive heart failure
Uncomplicated noncardiac surgery
Acute neurologic disease, including subarachnoid hemorrhage *(121,122)*
Sepsis and related syndromes
Renal failure
Alcoholic cirrhosis *(123)*
Vital exhaustion *(124,125)*

^{a}Primary etiology is not due to coronary atherothrombosis.

cause of release of the MB isoenzyme of creatine kinase (CK-MB) in the absence of coronary artery obstruction and myocardial ischemia *(5)*. Given the difficulty in definitively establishing the presence of myocarditis in the appropriate clinical setting, sensitive and specific indicators of myocardial injury, such as the cardiac troponins, have been viewed as a potential valuable aid to diagnosis *(5)*. Viewed from an alternative perspective, abnormal concentrations of troponins resulting from unsuspected myocarditis may also be an important source of diagnostic confusion in patients with undifferentiated chest pain.

Clinical Presentation and Pathophysiology

Myocarditis is characterized by a leukocytic infiltrate and necrosis or degeneration of cardiac myocytes that may be focal or diffuse and is generally randomly distributed in the heart *(7,8)*. It is common for endomyocardial biopsies to sample relatively normal areas of myocardium when neighboring areas have significant inflammatory infiltrates *(9,10)*. Furthermore, the diverse etiologies of myocarditis may contribute to varied sensitivity of histologic findings *(11)*. In some series, histologic confirmation is made in only 10% of biopsies from patients with a clinically suspected myocarditis *(12)*. This leaves substantial room for improvement on current diagnostic techniques through the exploration of alternative markers of cellular involvement *(13)*.

Although most cases of myocarditis are viral in origin, numerous other microbiologic agents, noninfectious immunologic conditions, hypersensitivity reactions, and physical agents (e.g., radiation) may all cause clinically important myocardial inflammation. The acute phase of myocarditis may be completely asymptomatic or may result in fulminant congestive heart failure *(8)*. Long-term outcomes are similarly variable, rang-

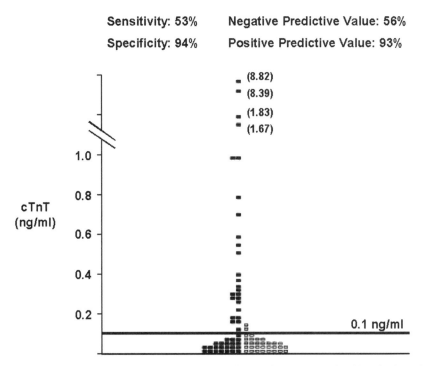

Fig. 1. Predictive performance of cTnT at a threshold of 0.1 ng/mL for histologic evidence of myocarditis. Serum levels of cTnT in 80 patients with clinically suspected myocarditis. *Solid squares* are for patients with histologic or immunohistologic criteria for myocarditis. *Open squares* indicate those with no evidence of myocarditis on biopsy. (Adapted from Lauer B, et al. J Am Coll Cardiol 1997;30:1354, with permission.)

ing from no recognizable impact, to increased risk of lethal arrhythmias, and possibly to the development of postviral dilated cardiomyopathy *(14,15)*. The symptoms are typically nonspecific, including fatigue, dyspnea, palpitations, and chest discomfort *(8),* and may be difficult to discriminate from those related to acute myocardial ischemia *(16)*.

Role of Cardiac Troponins in the Evaluation of Myocarditis

CK activities are increased in some but not all cases of myocarditis *(5,17)*, and thus the cardiac troponins have been investigated as a potential aid to the diagnosis of myocarditis *(13,18–20)*. Studies of animal models of myocarditis have shown a time-dependent rise in cardiac troponins after the onset of autoimmune myocarditis documented by histopathologic examination *(13,19)*. Human studies have extended these findings to the clinical setting and supported the use of troponins to confirm the presence of injury of cardiac myocytes and improve on the sensitivity of endomyocardial biopsy for establishing the diagnosis of myocarditis *(13,20)*.

In a population of 80 patients with clinically suspected myocarditis, increased concentrations of cardiac troponin T (cTnT) were a strong predictor of histologic or immunohistologic evidence of myocarditis on endomyocardial biopsy (Fig. 1) *(20)*. However, 44% of patients without increased concentrations of cTnT also had pathologic evidence of myocarditis, indicating that measurement of cTnT alone is not sufficient to exclude a diagnosis of myocarditis. CK-MB was increased in only one patient. Similar data are available for cardiac troponin I (cTnI) *(13)*. Among 53 patients with biopsy-proven myocarditis, 34% had increased concentrations of cTnI (≥3.1 ng/mL, Dade Stratus) compared with only 6% who had increased concentrations of CK-MB. Although it is a plausible hypothesis that patients with detectable concentrations of cardiac troponins had more active inflammation in the myocardium, no correlation between troponin elevation and the histologic severity of myocarditis was observed *(13,20)*.

The reasons for the absence of detectable troponin elevation in a large proportion of patients with histologic evidence of myocyte necrosis are likely multifactorial *(13)*. In several studies, the timing of sample acquisition relative to symptom onset was seen to be important. Specifically, patients with samples drawn earlier after the clinical onset of the syndrome were substantially more likely to have increased concentrations of cTnI, consistent with the theory that the majority of inflammatory injury occurs early in the course of myocarditis *(13)*. Depending on the specific etiology of myocardial inflammation, the timing and duration of active myocyte injury and thus increases in troponin may vary. As such, serial sampling over various stages of the illness may prove to improve sensitivity of detection of active myocarditis. It is also possible that in some cases the degree of myocardial injury was not sufficient to result in detection with the assays tested in these studies. The availability of more sensitive current generation assays for cTnI and cTnT may therefore increase the proportion of patients with suspected myocarditis who have detectable myocyte damage.

Current Use and Future Directions

Cardiac troponins frequently provide evidence of ongoing myocyte damage in patients with suspected myocarditis when CK-MB concentrations are within the normal range. However, cardiac troponins are not increased in all cases, and cannot be used to reliably exclude the disease. Nevertheless, owing to the similarly poor sensitivity of endomyocardial biopsy, some experts have recommended measurement of cardiac troponins and correlation with the results of histologic assessment in all patients with suspected myocarditis *(5)*. When increased concentrations of troponins are detected in the absence of histologic and/or immunohistologic evidence of myocarditis, sampling error is a strong possibility; however, other nonischemic and ischemic causes of myocyte necrosis should be considered. Conversely, myocarditis should be among the diagnoses considered for patients presenting with chest symptoms and increased troponins who subsequently are shown to be free of significant epicardial coronary disease *(21)*. Additional research will likely clarify the impact of timing of sampling and the cause of myocarditis as determinants of troponin elevation during the clinical course of the disease, and it is hoped will guide strategies for testing that will assist in the challenge of discerning an inflammatory vs ischemic cause of myocardial injury in patient with chest pain.

BLUNT CARDIAC TRAUMA

Blunt cardiac trauma is a syndrome that includes a broad spectrum of nonpenetrating traumatic cardiac injuries, ranging from mild pericardial inflammation to rupture of the cardiac wall *(22)*. Although the most severe cases generally demand immediate thoracotomy for diagnosis and treatment, cardiac biomarkers have traditionally been used to facilitate the detection of myocardial injury or "cardiac contusion" among patients who are hemodynamically stable. However, measurement of CK and CK-MB for this purpose has significant limitations due to the extensive skeletal muscle injury that usually occurs in association with this syndrome. Because of superior tissue specificity, the cardiac troponins have offered potential to distinguish cardiac from skeletal muscle damage in the setting of blunt chest trauma *(23,24)*.

Clinical Presentation and Pathophysiology

Blunt cardiac injury typically results from direct compression of the heart or decelerating forces delivered to the chest *(25)*. Cardiac injury may occur even after relatively low-energy chest trauma without other obvious injuries *(26,27)*. The pathologic correlates of such injury vary considerably and range from small areas of subepicardial or subendocardial hemorrhage to full thickness myocardial necrosis with or without cardiac rupture *(28)*. The relationships between the less severe pathologic findings and the risk of significant clinical manifestations of blunt cardiac trauma (e.g., severe arrhythmias) are not well characterized. Rarely, epicardial coronary thrombosis may be induced by chest trauma and result in MI due to coronary ischemia *(29,30)*. Clinical manifestations of nonpenetrating cardiac trauma include chest discomfort, dyspnea, hypotension, electrocardiographic (ECG) changes (primarily nonspecific ST and T-wave abnormalities), as well as arrhythmias including sinus tachycardia, atrial arrhythmias, ventricular conduction abnormalities, and ventricular tachycardia or fibrillation *(25)*. Cardiogenic shock is infrequent and usually indicates cardiac rupture, cardiac tamponade, or severe structural damage to a cardiac valve and/or its supporting structures. Estimates of the risk of significant clinical morbidity in the absence of such obvious catastrophic consequences vary widely *(31–35)*.

Primarily owing to difficulty in defining clear and consistent diagnostic criteria for "myocardial contusion," this term has been largely replaced by the broader designation of "nonpenetrating cardiac trauma," with some investigators and clinicians advocating categorization based on the clinical sequelae *(25,36,37)*. The traditional noninvasive tools, such as serial ECGs, are limited by poor specificity. Furthermore, there is no consensus agreement as to whether abnormalities of cardiac wall motion must be present for the diagnosis of "cardiac contusion." Thus, current strategies for evaluation are turning away from establishing strict diagnostic criteria toward an emphasis on assessing the risk of adverse clinical consequences (e.g., severe arrhythmias, or impaired ventricular or valvular function), and the need for changes in management, such as special monitoring *(37)*.

Role of Cardiac Biomarkers in Evaluating Blunt Chest Trauma

Measurement of CK and CK-MB has been used as an adjunct to the ECG and clinical evaluation in the diagnosis of blunt cardiac injury *(38)*. However, the poor tissue specificity of these markers in the setting of substantial skeletal muscle trauma has limited their clinical utility *(39,40)*. For example, in a study of 44 patients with blunt chest trauma, 70% of patients with normal echocardiograms had increased concentrations of CK-MB *(24)*. While use of a CK-MB/total CK ratio of >5% as the diagnostic criterion reduced the number of "false-positive" positive results, the sensitivity was substantially reduced. Consistent findings across multiple studies have shown similar levels of CK-MB and the CK-MB/total CK ratio in patients with and without a diagnosis of blunt cardiac injury

(35,41). These data have supported the consensus opinion that measurements of CK-MB do not have sufficient specificity to be useful in the diagnosis of blunt cardiac injury *(25)*.

Cardiac Troponins for the Diagnosis of Blunt Cardiac Injury

Multiple studies have now assessed cardiac troponins for the diagnosis of cardiac injury in the setting of nonpenetrating chest trauma *(24,35–37,41–43)*. In contrast to CK-MB, concentrations of cardiac troponins are significantly increased in patients with blunt cardiac trauma compared to those with chest trauma and no "myocardial contusion" *(24,35, 41)*. Nevertheless, the overall diagnostic performance of the cardiac troponins in studies of blunt cardiac injury has been inconsistent *(35,37,41)*. Variation in the results of these studies must be considered in the light of differing "gold standards" employed for the diagnosis and criteria for patient selection.

cTnI and cTnT have shown some promise for improving on prior methods for diagnosing blunt cardiac injury *(23,24,44)*. When compared with echocardiographic evaluation of ventricular wall motion, concentrations of cTnI above the diagnostic limit for acute MI (AMI) (≥ 3.1 ng/mL, Dade Stratus) were detected in all patients with echocardiographic evidence of cardiac injury (6/44 subjects) *(24)*. None of the patients with normal echocardiograms had increased concentrations of cTnI (Fig. 2). In this study, cTnI offered superior specificity to both CK-MB measurement and electrocardiography, which were abnormal in 70% and 95% of those with no wall motion abnormalities on cardiac echo *(24)*. Subsequent larger studies have confirmed the higher specificity of cardiac troponins for the diagnosis of blunt cardiac injury, but have found substantially lower sensitivity (12–31%) than initial reports *(35,37,41)*.

Specifically, in a prospective evaluation of 128 patients with severe chest trauma admitted to an intensive care unit, cTnT concentrations were increased (>0.5 ng/mL, ES 300, Roche Diagnostics) in 9/29 patients who developed either significant cardiac complications ($n = 9$) or echocardiographic wall motion abnormalities alone ($n = 20$) *(41)*. Nine of the remaining 99 patients who were free from these cardiac consequences of trauma had cTnT concentrations >0.5 ng/mL. Such data demonstrate adequate specificity (91%) but poor sensitivity (31%) relative to the diagnostic criteria used in this study. Receiver operating characteristics analysis suggested that the diagnostic performance could have been improved slightly by use of a lower cut point, as had been established for the diagnosis of MI. Bertinchant and colleagues had similar findings among hemodynamically stable patients with suspected blunt cardiac injury ($n = 94$) *(35)*. Based on ECG and echocardiographic findings, 28% of patients were given a diagnosis of "myocardial contusion." Increased concentrations of cTnI (≥ 0.1 ng/mL, Beckman Access) and cTnT (>0.1 ng/mL, Elecsys cTnT STAT) concentrations were highly specific (97% and 100% respectively) for the diagnosis of "myocardial contusion" but offered low sensitivity (23% and 12%, respectively).

Such data indicate the high probability of ECG and echocardiographic abnormalities among patients with chest trauma and increased troponins. However, from these results alone, it is not clear whether management of patients with suspected blunt cardiac trauma should be altered on the basis of troponin results. Is the risk of significant arrhythmias or heart failure among patients with ECG or echocardiographic abnormalities but no troponin elevation sufficiently low for them to be discharged without further observation? Conversely, does the risk of adverse clinical outcomes among patients

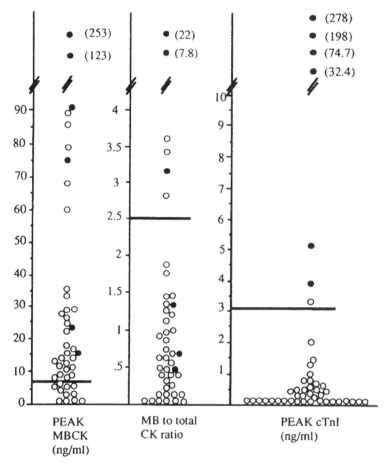

Fig. 2. Association of cTnI vs CK-MB and MB to total CK ratio with cardiac contusion. *Solid circles* indicate patients with a final diagnosis of cardiac contusion. *Open circles* indicate those without cardiac contusion. *Heavy horizontal lines* indicate the upper reference limits for each parameter. (From Adams JE, et al. Am Heart J 1996;131:310, with permission.)

with increased troponin concentrations and no appreciable abnormality of wall motion warrant prolonged monitoring for arrhythmias? From the perspective of patient management, the ability to identify those at risk for cardiac complications requiring urgent treatment takes precedence over the correlation of poorly defined diagnostic criteria *(37)*.

Cardiac Troponins and Clinical Outcomes in Blunt Chest Trauma

Few studies have evaluated cardiac troponin for predicting which patients will develop important clinical manifestations of blunt cardiac injury. In one study of 115 patients requiring intensive care for blunt chest trauma, 19 patients (16.5%) developed significant clinical manifestations (arrhythmia or pericardial effusion requiring treatment, cardiogenic shock, or hypotension unexplained by other conditions) *(36)*. cTnI (>1.5 ng/mL, Dade Dimension RxL cTnI) had a superior positive predictive value (48%) compared to the ECG (28%), while both had high negative predictive values (93% and 95%, respectively). When used together, "negative" findings on the ECG and serial measurements of

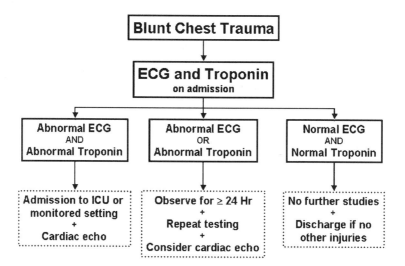

Fig. 3. A proposed algorithm for use of cardiac troponin in the triage of patients with blunt chest trauma. (Adapted with permission from Salim A, et al. J Trauma 2001;50:237.)

cTnI identified a population of patients (40%) who suffered no significant clinical manifestations of blunt cardiac trauma *(36)*. It is notable that all patients with cardiac complications in this study were already admitted to intensive care for management of noncardiac injuries. The high negative predictive capacity of the combined evaluation of the ECG and cTnI in this study supports the possibility of using such noninvasive information to identify low-risk candidates for early discharge (Fig. 3).

Other investigators have found contrasting results. In a previous study of patients with visible chest wall injuries who did not require intensive care (*n* = 74), Fulda and colleagues observed significant cardiac complications (primarily atrial or ventricular arrhythmias) in 37% *(37)*. Of patients with an increased cTnT (>0.2 ng/mL), 64% developed a cardiac complication (relative risk 2.0, $p = 0.04$). However, 73% of patients who developed subsequent cardiac events did not have elevated concentrations of cTnT. Examining the combination of the presenting ECG and cTnT, 12 of the 26 patients with cardiac complications would not have been identified based on the baseline studies alone *(37)*. Based on these findings, these investigators concluded that there is limited value to determination of cTnT in patients with blunt chest trauma. Others have made similar conclusions after finding low risk of significant morbidity among hemodynamically stable patients with chest trauma, even when concentrations of cardiac troponins were found to be increased *(35)*.

Current Use and Future Directions

The data available to date provide inconsistent observations regarding the utility of cardiac troponins in the evaluation of blunt cardiac trauma. Interpretation of the aggregate data is made difficult by substantial variation in enrollment and diagnostic criteria, troponin thresholds, and clinical end points used in these studies. Nevertheless, it is clear that the cardiac troponins offer superior specificity to CK-MB and are the preferred cardiac biomarkers for detection of cardiac injury in the setting of trauma. Further investigation is necessary to determine whether patients with normal ECGs and no elevation of troponins are at acceptably low risk to permit early discharge without observation. Moreover, the widespread clinical use of troponin assays with increasingly lower detection limits is likely to lead to detection of minor degrees of cardiac injury in the absence of ECG and echocardiographic abnormalities. Clinical studies will be necessary to determine whether such "minor" elevations are important for management or outcomes. Future research should also carefully examine the relationship between the degree of troponin elevation and clinical outcomes in this syndrome.

CARDIOVERSION

In the early 1960s external direct current electrical cardioversion (DCCV) was introduced as an approach to rapid reversion of cardiac tachyarrhythmias *(45)*. Cardioversion for hemodynamically stable arrhythmia is frequently performed as an elective procedure during which testing for myocardial necrosis is clinically unimportant and thus not performed. However, rapid electrical cardioversion is also a cornerstone of treatment for patients suffering cardiac arrest from ventricular tachycardia (VT) or fibrillation. In this setting, the subsequent clinical evaluation and management of the patient are influenced significantly by whether the cardiac arrest occurred in the setting of acute myocardial ischemia. Thus, the clinician's ability to establish or exclude the diagnosis of MI is important *(46)*.

Clinical Presentation and Pathophysiology

In part because of enhanced training and availability of electrical defibrillators, the number of patients presenting to hospitals as survivors of an out-of-hospital arrest has increased *(47,48)*. After arrival in the hospital, a substantial proportion of patients surviving prehospital resuscitation are found to have increased activities and concentrations of CK, CK-MB, and/or cardiac troponins *(49–58)*. In this circumstance, three potential etiologies should be considered: (1) the marker elevation reflects an AMI as the cause of the arrhythmia, (2) the arrhythmia has resulted in sufficient imbalance in myocardial oxygen supply and demand to result in AMI, and (3) electrical cardioversion or other resuscitative efforts have caused myocardial damage.

Biochemical and pathologic data obtained from elective procedures outside the setting of acute ischemic events have supported the hypothesis that there is some measurable damage to cardiac myocytes resulting from electrical cardioversion *(59,60)*. Histopathologic studies have demonstrated morphological and functional derangement of the myocardium following electrical shocks in animal models *(61–63)*. These studies include direct histologic evidence of myocardial damage as well as abnormal technetium pyrophosphate scintigrams *(49,60–62,64,65)*. In addition, concurrent injury to the skeletal muscle of the chest wall has been identified. Histopathologic examination has revealed pectoralis muscle damage among patients with prior cardioversion *(66)*. Furthermore, technetium pyrophosphate uptake in skeletal muscle has been demonstrated after direct current cardioversion in both animal and human series *(64,65)*. Whether from nonischemic damage to skeletal or cardiac muscle, the resulting elevation of cardiac markers of myocardial necrosis may confound the evaluation for preceding MI.

Increased Troponins in Electrical Cardioversion

DCCV for tachyarrhythmias under elective circumstances is associated with elevation of total CK in approx 50% of cases *(62,67–69)*. Although not universal *(62)*, most reported series have documented an association between the degree of CK elevation and the total number of shocks as well as the total energy delivered *(57,59,60,68,69)*. Similar observations have also been made with CK-MB among patients undergoing elective cardioversion *(57,60,62,65,68,69)*.

As in other conditions in which there may be simultaneous injury to cardiac and skeletal muscle, the availability of the cardiac-specific troponins has enabled researchers and clinicians to discriminate more effectively between the contribution of pectoralis muscle and cardiac damage to marker elevation after cardioversion. In a study of serial determinations of CK-MB mass and cardiac troponins in the setting of elective DCCV for atrial tachyarrhythmias, researchers found no elevation of cTnT, and only a mild rise in cTnI for two patients *(58)*. This observation has been consistent across multiple studies that in aggregate have shown no elevation of cTnT (>0.1 ng/mL) among 293 patients undergoing elective DCCV *(52–58)*. Several investigators have measured cTnI after elective DCCV and detected rare mild elevation of cTnI using the Dade Stratus assay *(68,69)*. Allan and colleagues *(69)* found cTnI elevations in 3/38 patients (peak values: 0.8, 1.2, and 1.5 ng/mL), while Bonnefoy *(68)* detected mild cTnI elevation in 4/28 patients studied (peak values: 0.6, 0.6, 0.6, and 0.9 ng/mL). Thus, on the basis of histopathologic data and the observed mild increases in cTnI, it remains plausible that small degrees of myocardial injury may occur during elective DCCV, dependent on the number and timing of external shocks delivered *(59,61)*. However, data from cardiac troponins indicate that such injury is less prevalent than suggested by measurements of CK and CK-MB. Moreover, substantial elevation of either of the cardiac troponins (e.g., >1.5 ng/mL for cTnI) in the setting of elective DCCV suggests causes unrelated to electrical cardioversion.

Although it is reasonable to postulate that the cardiac troponins may perform as effectively in the setting of emergency cardioversion for ventricular arrhythmias, one must be cautious about such an extrapolation as the clinical situation during prehospital resuscitation attempts is far more complex than the controlled circumstances of most studies of elective cardioversion *(46)*. More extensive skeletal muscle trauma, prolonged arrhythmia, hypoxemia, and chest compressions confound the interpretation of cardiac markers *(70)*. In at least one study of patients suffering out-of-hospital arrest, increases in CK-MB among patients without known coronary artery disease (CAD) occurred more frequently than in series involving elective cardioversion, and correlated with both the number of chest compressions as well as total energy applied *(70)*. Although, the myocardial specificity of the cardiac troponins is maintained in the setting of massive skeletal muscle trauma, the combined effects of prolonged cardiopulmonary resuscitation and repeated transthoracic shocks over a short period of time on the release of cardiac troponins have not been completely defined. Two published reports evaluating cardiac troponins after prehospital resuscitative efforts have shown elevation of cTnT among 80–85% patients without evidence of AMI by ECG criteria and/or thallium scintigraphy or autopsy *(50,51)*.

Current Use and Future Directions

At the present time, it seems reasonable to expect that elective DCCV for tachyarrhythmias causes either no elevation of troponin concentrations or only a slight increase, and that more substantial increases are indicative of myocardial damage unrelated to the external shock. More information is needed regarding interpretation of elevation of cardiac troponins in patients surviving cardioversion for out-of-hospital cardiac arrest. Until new data suggest otherwise, it is reasonable to maintain a high index of clinical suspicion for myocardial ischemia and undertake appropriate evaluation patients with increased cardiac troponins after resuscitation from cardiac arrest. Further research evaluating the interactions between components of prehospital resuscitation and elevation of cardiac-specific troponins may be helpful in clarifying the prognostic and treatment implications of such marker abnormalities.

PULMONARY EMBOLISM

Pulmonary embolism (PE) remains an under-recognized etiology of nontraumatic chest discomfort and/or shortness of breath *(71)*, and has recently been appreciated as a potential source of troponin elevation in patients with chest pain syndrome without acute coronary thrombosis *(72–74)*. PE is thus a critical alternative diagnosis to be considered by clinicians evaluating patients with unexplained chest pain or dyspnea who are found to have abnormal concentrations of cardiac troponins.

Clinical Presentation and Pathophysiology

The majority of pulmonary emboli result from thrombi that originate in the pelvic or deep veins of the leg and travel through the great veins to obstruct the branch pulmonary arteries. Dyspnea, chest discomfort, and presyncope constitute the classic presenting symptoms of PE with tachypnea and tachycardia, adding to the clinical hallmarks of the disease. Pathophysiologic consequences of PE include (1) an acute and chronic increase in pulmonary vascular resistance due to vascular obstruction and neurohormonal response, (2) impaired gas exchange due to increased ventilation/perfusion mismatch, and (3) reduced pulmonary compliance *(75)*. These factors contribute to a sudden rise in right ventricular (RV) afterload and consequent increase in RV wall stress that may be followed by RV dilatation and dysfunction *(76)*. RV dilatation and dysfunction may compromise filling of the left ventricle (LV) due to both shifting of the ventricular septum toward the LV within the constrained volume of the pericardium, and reduced RV cardiac output. Intracardiac pressures thus rise both on the left and right side of the heart, increasing myocardial oxygen demand and potentially reducing subendocardial blood supply. In some cases, myocardial oxygen demand outstrips supply resulting in subendocardial ischemia and potentially microinfarction *(76)*.

Prognostic Implications of Troponin Elevation in PE

RV infarction made evident by elevation of CK-MB is a recognized complication of massive pulmonary embolism due to the mechanisms outlined above, even in the absence of significant epicardial coronary disease *(74,77)*. However, up to 55% of patients with lesser degrees of PE may also develop RV dysfunction *(71)* that appears to be associated with less favorable outcomes *(78,79)*. Testing for cardiac troponin has now made possible detection of more subtle degrees of myocardial injury and RV dysfunction caused by PE. For example, in a study of 24 patients with documented PE who were hemodynamically stable without respiratory failure, 20.8% of this group had detectable elevation of cTnI (≥0.4 ng/mL, Abbott cTnI) *(73)*. Two other studies of similar size (36 and 56 patients) have also shown elevation of cTnI *(72)* and cTnT *(74)* in 39%

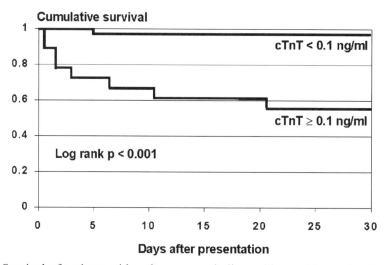

Fig. 4. Survival of patients with pulmonary embolism with or without elevation of cTnT. (Used with permission from Giannitsis E, et al. Circulation 2000;102:214.)

and 32% of patients, respectively. In the first of these studies, Giannitsis and colleagues found that patients with cTnT concentrations >0.1 ng/mL were at higher risk of death during the initial hospitalization (44% vs 3%, $p < 0.001$; Fig. 4) despite more aggressive therapy *(74)*. Notably, the prevalence of coronary disease was similar between those with and without increased troponin *(74)*. This higher mortality risk may relate to the greater number of segmental defects, the higher prevalence of RV dysfunction and the higher probability of cardiogenic shock among patients with increased troponins *(72,74)*. When framed as a test for RV dysfunction, however, sensitivity is low (42–63%) and specificity has been mixed (60–100%) *(72,74)*. As in ACS, sensitivity is maximized by serial testing *(80)*.

Lastly, data from patients with angiographically confirmed PE and serial measurements of cTnT demonstrate a lower peak than among patients with MI with a shorter duration of elevation (median 35 h), lending support to the possibility of a different mechanism of release compared with acute coronary thrombosis *(80)*.

Current Use and Future Directions

Elevation of cardiac troponins indicative of myocardial injury is evident in a substantial proportion of patients with PE and not surprisingly is related to the severity of the hemodynamic insult. It is not yet known whether measurement of cardiac troponins will improve upon other noninvasive methods such as cardiac echocardiography in assessing prognosis. Additional research is warranted to provide more comprehensive information on the prevalence and clinical implications of increased concentrations of troponins in PE, particularly among those with submassive PE for whom prognosis is not immediately evident from the clinical presentation. Moreover, there remains the exciting possibility that cardiac troponins may be useful as a rapid, widely available method for detecting patients with PE who are at high risk with probable right ventricular dysfunction and may warrant fibrinolytic therapy *(81)*.

SEPSIS

Sepsis and other syndromes of severe systemic inflammatory response, such as major trauma or pancreatitis, are characterized by considerable morbidity and high mortality risk *(82)*. The major adverse consequences of sepsis and its related syndromes are thought to be the result of an unrestrained cascade of inflammatory processes, which culminate in multiorgan dysfunction *(83)*. Up to 40% of patients with sepsis will have demonstrable myocardial dysfunction, a finding that connotes adverse prognosis *(82)*. Moreover, a high incidence of abnormal troponin concentration has been documented among patients with septic syndromes. The precise mechanisms underlying these findings as well as the prognostic and therapeutic implications of troponin elevation in this setting remain unsettled *(84)*.

Clinical Presentation and Pathophysiology

Systemic inflammatory response syndrome (SIRS) may have an infectious (sepsis) or noninfectious etiology and is defined by the presence of hyper- or hypothermia, tachypnea, tachycardia, and either leukocytosis or leukopenia. The septic syndrome involves signs of organ dysfunction such as alteration in mental status, oliguria, disseminated intravascular coagulation, or adult respiratory distress syndrome *(83)*. The cardiovascular response to sepsis is typically manifest as hypotension due to peripheral vasodilatation and consequent low systemic vascular resistance. Concurrent depression of myocardial function has been recognized for over 50 yr *(85)* but may frequently be masked by the decrease in systemic vascular resistance and increased heart rate, which usually contribute to an overall increase in cardiac output *(86)*. Parker and colleagues performed one of the first rigorous evaluations of cardiac function in sepsis and found a rapid decline in LV systolic function and increase in left end-diastolic diameter that persisted even after correction of severe acidosis and electrolyte abnormalities *(87)*. This decline in function recovered over a period of 7–10 d among survivors *(87)*.

The pathophysiologic basis for these alterations in myocardial function in the setting of sepsis remains uncertain. Although early hypotheses regarding myocardial depression in sepsis centered on the possibility of global myocardial ischemia due to disrupted coronary autoregulation and/or oxygen utilization *(86)*, subsequent studies have provided data detracting from this supposition *(88–90)* and the prevailing opinion has turned toward the potential cardiac toxicity of the broad group of inflammatory mediators released in SIRS *(91)*. In the mid-1980s researchers produced direct evidence of a circulating substance(s) in the serum of patients with sepsis that impaired contraction of isolated rat cardiac myocytes *(92)*. Further work has identified a number of candidate mediators that may act as "myocardial depressant factors" in SIRS, including lipopolysaccharide, inflammatory cytokines, prostanoids, and nitric oxide *(86)*. The inflammatory cytokines, tumor necrosis factor-α (TNF-α) and interleukin-1β, in particular have been shown to result in rapid deterioration in myocardial function in vitro *(93,94)*, in animal models *(95)* and in humans *(96)*. Although the precise mechanisms through which these factors impact myocyte function have not been elucidated, it has been proposed that the final common pathway is mediated by the pleotropic effects of nitric oxide on calcium regulation and cellular energetics *(86,97,98)*. Supportive evidence shows that up-regulation of a cytokine-inducible form of nitric oxide synthase results in the release of substantive amounts of nitric oxide *(99)*. However, others have documented direct adverse effects of TNF-α on intracellular calcium homeostasis that are independent of nitric oxide mediated pathways *(94)*. Furthermore, it is not clear whether the effects of such "myocardial depressant factors" lead only to reversible dysfunction or whether irreversible myocyte damage occurs. Determination of cardiac troponin concentrations among patients with sepsis has opened a new avenue to address this issue (84).

Elevation of Cardiac Troponins in Sepsis and Related Syndromes

A growing number of studies have demonstrated a high incidence of increased concentrations of cardiac troponins (31–85%) in patients with sepsis *(100–107)*. In a representative study among adult patients ($n = 46$) with septic shock, concentrations of cTnI (≥0.4 ng/mL, Stratus II) and cTnT (>0.1 ng/mL, Elecsys 2010) were found to be increased in 50% and 36%, respectively, with peak concentrations (median, interquartile range) of 1.4 ng/mL (0.8–6.8 ng/mL) for cTnI and 0.66 ng/mL (0.19–1.51 ng/mL) for cTnT *(106)*. Patients with increased troponins were more likely to have LV systolic dysfunction as well as an overall less favorable clinical status as captured by severity of illness indices such as the Acute Physiology and Chronic Health Evaluation (APACHE) II score (Fig. 5) *(106)*. Other studies have demonstrated consistent findings with at least modest associations between abnormal concentrations of cardiac troponins and the degree of impaired LV function *(105)* and, in some cases, evidence for increased mortality risk *(103,106)*.

A number of potential contributors to myocardial damage during sepsis should be considered. Certainly, elderly patients with sepsis are at risk for concomitant coronary atherosclerosis and may develop myocardial ischemia during the stress of major illness. However, increased concentrations of cTnI have been detected in children with meningococcal sepsis (62%) and no anticipated large or small vessel coronary atherosclerosis *(105)*. Moreover, a large proportion of adults with abnormal concentrations of cardiac troponins during sepsis have no evidence for obstructive CAD or histopathologic evidence of irreversible myocardial injury *(106,107)*. For example, in one study 58% of patients with increased cTnI had no appreciable CAD when evaluated by coronary angiography, stress echocardiography, or pathologic findings *(107)*. Although microvascular dysfunction and extreme increases in LV wall stress during aggressive vasopressor therapy may result in small territories of necrosis that may be difficult to detect on pathologic examination, evidence for a correlation between dosing of vasopressors and troponin elevation has been mixed *(103,106)*. Alternatively, disseminated microemboli are common in meningococcal sepsis and may cause microvascular occlusion in the myocardium; however, such emboli are less frequent in nonmenigococcal sepsis and other noninfectious SIRS in which troponin increases have also been observed *(108)*. In light of these and other corroborative findings *(106,107)*, it is probable that troponin elevation in sepsis often occurs due to nonischemic mechanism, in some cases through direct cytotoxic effects of myocardial depressant substances *(109,110)* or possibly through alteration of plasma membrane permeability to macromolecules *(107,111)*. In addition, in some patients the systemic infection and/or inflammatory response may also involve the myocardium resulting in myocarditis *(6)*. Given substantial heterogeneity across the clinical spectrum of sepsis and SIRS, it is also plausible that multiple mechanisms may be at play and predominate in different clinical settings. Additional research is needed

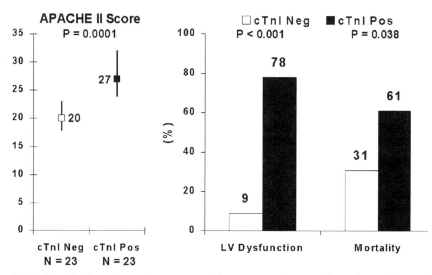

Fig. 5. Cardiac dysfunction and mortality risk among patients with sepsis and elevated troponin. (Data from Ver Elst KM, et al. Clin Chem 2000;46:650–657.)

to clarify the histological and ultrastructural changes in the myocardium, as well as the related processes that contribute to cardiac dysfunction and troponin elevation in sepsis.

Current Use and Future Directions

The release of cardiac troponins among a sizeable proportion of patients with sepsis and its related syndromes is now established and indicates the presence of at least minor degrees of myocardial injury. The debate over the mechanism(s) and whether such injury is irreversible or reversible is unresolved. In addition, it remains to be seen whether cardiac troponins will become a useful clinical tool in the care of patients with septic shock. To date, the data supporting utility for prognostic assessment are limited, and more important, no specific therapeutic strategies that might modify the risk of these patients have been identified. Application of aggressive antithrombotic, antiplatelet, and invasive therapies effective for patients presenting with ACS and increased troponin are not supported by clinical data in this setting and may expose patients with sepsis to additional, unacceptable risks. Antibodies to TNF-α used for treatment of sepsis have shown promising preliminary results in animal models *(112)* and humans with improvement in LV function *(113)*. However, subsequent larger clinical trials have not demonstrated similar efficacy *(114,115)*. Research leading to additional insight into the pathogenesis of troponin elevation in sepsis may also further elucidate the mechanisms underlying myocardial dysfunction, and guide the development of new approaches to the treatment of this highly morbid syndrome.

SUMMARY

Detectable concentrations of cardiac troponin have been discovered in the peripheral circulation of patients with a variety of nonischemic conditions affecting the myocardium, and present a challenge to clinicians who must consider alternatives to coronary

Table 2
Evidence for Clinical Use of Cardiac Troponins (Tn)

Condition	Tn aids in diagnosis	Tn associated with prognosis	Adds to other clinical tools	Aids in therapeutic decision making
Unstable angina / MI	Yes	+++	+++	+++
Myocarditis	Yes	*	+	*
Blunt chest trauma	Yes	+ / –	+	*
Chemotherapy toxicity	Yes	*	+	*
Pulmonary embolism	No	+	+	*
Congestive heart failure	No	+	*	*
Emergent cardioversion	Yes†	*	*	*
Septic shock	No	+	*	*

+++, Strong and consistent data; +, some supportive data; +/–, data remain mixed; *, insufficient/ no data; † aids in discriminating preceding MI.

thrombosis as the etiology of chest symptoms. In some instances, for example, cardiac surgery or radiofrequency ablation, the mechanism of cardiac injury is immediately apparent and is easily distinguished from an acute coronary syndrome. In other cases, where diagnosis is often more difficult, for example, myocarditis, the care providers must thoughtfully integrate biomarker and other clinical data to arrive at the correct conclusions. Frequently the peak concentration and pattern of rise and fall of troponin concentrations offer important diagnostic information.

Parallel to findings in acute coronary syndromes, troponin carries prognostic value in several nonischemic conditions (Table 2). Further research is needed to determine whether the optimal decision limits for risk assessment differ between these varied conditions, as well as to ascertain whether such information will add to current strategies for clinical care, and, in particular, whether treatment should be altered on the basis of troponin results. Such research efforts may also lead to new areas of investigation with the potential to reveal novel therapeutic targets.

ABBREVIATIONS

ACS, Acute coronary syndrome(s); AMI, acute myocardial infarction; APACHE, Acute Physiology and Chronic Health Evaluation; CAD, coronary artery disease; CK, creatine kinase; CK-MB, MB isoenzyme of CK; cTnT, cTnI, cardiac troponins T and I; DCCV, direct current electrical cardioversion; ECG, electrocardiogram; MI, myocardial infarction; PE, pulmonary embolism; RV, right ventricle; SIRS, systemic inflammatory response syndrome; TNF-α, tissue necrosis factor-α; VT, ventricular tachycardia.

REFERENCES

1. The Joint European Society of Cardiology/American College of Cardiology Committee for the redefinition of myocardial infarction. Myocardial infarction redefined—a consensus document of The Joint European Society of Cardiology/American College of Cardiology Committee for the redefinition of myocardial infarction. J Am Coll Cardiol 2000;36: 959–969.
2. Braunwald E, Antman EM, Beasley JW, et al. ACC/AHA guidelines for the management of patients with unstable angina and non-ST-segment elevation myocardial infarction. A

report of the American College of Cardiology/American Heart Association Task Force on Practice Guidelines (Committee on the Management of Patients With Unstable Angina). J Am Coll Cardiol 2000;36:970–1062.

3. Hamm CW, Braunwald E. A classification of unstable angina revisited. Circulation 2000; 102:118–122.

4. Jaffe AS. Elevations in cardiac troponin measurements: false false positives. Cardiovasc Toxicol 2001;1:87–92.

5. Feldman AM, McNamara D. Myocarditis. N Engl J Med 2000;343:1388–1398.

6. Gravanis MB, Sternby NH. Incidence of myocarditis. A 10-year autopsy study from Malmo, Sweden. Arch Pathol Lab Med 1991;115:390–392.

7. Marboe CC, Fenoglio JJ Jr. Pathology and natural history of human myocarditis. Pathol Immunopathol Res 1988;7:226–239.

8. Peters NS, Poole-Wilson PA. Myocarditis—continuing clinical and pathologic confusion. Am Heart J 1991;121:942–947.

9. Hauck AJ, Kearney DL, Edwards WD. Evaluation of postmortem endomyocardial biopsy specimens from 38 patients with lymphocytic myocarditis: implications for role of sampling error. Mayo Clin Proc 1989;64:1235–1245.

10. Dec GW, Fallon JT, Southern JF, Palacios I. "Borderline" myocarditis: an indication for repeat endomyocardial biopsy. J Am Coll Cardiol 1990;15:283–289.

11. Aretz HT. Diagnosis of myocarditis by endomyocardial biopsy. Med Clin North Am 1986; 70:1215–1226.

12. Mason JW, O'Connell JB, Herskowitz A, et al. A clinical trial of immunosuppressive therapy for myocarditis. The Myocarditis Treatment Trial Investigators. N Engl J Med 1995;333: 269–275.

13. Smith SC, Ladenson JH, Mason JW, Jaffe AS. Elevations of cardiac troponin I associated with myocarditis. Experimental and clinical correlates. Circulation 1997;95:163–168.

14. Davies MJ, Ward DE. How can myocarditis be diagnosed and should it be treated? Br Heart J 1992;68:346–347.

15. Friedman RA, Kearney DL, Moak JP, Fenrich AL, Perry JC. Persistence of ventricular arrhythmia after resolution of occult myocarditis in children and young adults. J Am Coll Cardiol 1994;24:780–783.

16. Narula J, Khaw BA, Dec GW Jr, et al. Brief report: recognition of acute myocarditis masquerading as acute myocardial infarction. N Engl J Med 1993;328:100–104.

17. Karjalainen J, Heikkila J. "Acute pericarditis": myocardial enzyme release as evidence for myocarditis. Am Heart J 1986;111:546–552.

18. Franz WM, Remppis A, Kandolf R, Kubler W, Katus HA. Serum troponin T: diagnostic marker for acute myocarditis. Clin Chem 1996;42:340–341.

19. Bachmaier K, Mair J, Offner F, Pummerer C, Neu N. Serum cardiac troponin T and creatine kinase-MB elevations in murine autoimmune myocarditis. Circulation 1995;92:1927–1932.

20. Lauer B, Niederau C, Kuhl U, et al. Cardiac troponin T in patients with clinically suspected myocarditis. J Am Coll Cardiol 1997;30:1354–1359.

21. Sarda L, Colin P, Boccara F, et al. Myocarditis in patients with clinical presentation of myocardial infarction and normal coronary angiograms. J Am Coll Cardiol 2001;37:786–792.

22. Mattox KL, Flint LM, Carrico CJ, et al. Blunt cardiac injury. J Trauma 1992;33:649–650.

23. Mair P, Mair J, Koller J, Wieser C, Artner-Dworzak E, Puschendorf B. Cardiac troponin T in the diagnosis of heart contusion. Lancet 1991;338:693.

24. Adams JE, 3rd, Davila-Roman VG, Bessey PQ, Blake DP, Ladenson JH, Jaffe AS. Improved detection of cardiac contusion with cardiac troponin I. Am Heart J 1996;131:308–312.

25. Mattox KL, Estrera AL, Wall MJ. Traumatic Heart Disease. In: Heart Disease. 6th ed. Braunwald E, Zipes DP, Libby P, eds. Philadelphia: WB Saunders, 2001, pp. 1877–1885.

26. Fein SA, Lombardo D, Daudiss K. Myocardial contusion without obvious severe chest trauma. Am J Emerg Med 1988;6:84–85.

27. Fulda G, Brathwaite CE, Rodriguez A, Turney SZ, Dunham CM, Cowley RA. Blunt traumatic rupture of the heart and pericardium: a ten-year experience (1979-1989). J Trauma 1991;31:167–172; discussion 172–173.

28. Parmley LF, Manion WC, Mattingly TW. Non-penetrating traumatic injury of the heart. Circulation 1958;18:371–396.

29. Levy H. Traumatic coronary thrombosis with myocardial infarction: postmortem study. Arch Intern Med 1949;84:261–276.

30. Stern T, Wolf RY, Reichart B, Harrington OB, Crosby VG. Coronary artery occlusion resulting from blunt trauma. JAMA 1974;215:289–291.

31. Sturaitis M, McCallum D, Sutherland G, Cheung H, Driedger AA, Sibbald WJ. Lack of significant long-term sequelae following traumatic myocardial contusion. Arch Intern Med 1986;146:1765–1769.

32. Flancbaum L, Wright J, Siegel JH. Emergency surgery in patients with post-traumatic myocardial contusion. J Trauma 1986;26:795–803.

33. Ross P Jr, Degutis L, Baker CC. Cardiac contusion. The effect on operative management of the patient with trauma injuries. Arch Surg 1989;124:506–507.

34. Silverman SH, Turner WW Jr, Gilliland MB. Delayed cardiac arrest after myocardial contusion. Crit Care Med 1990;18:677–678.

35. Bertinchant JP, Polge A, Mohty D, et al. Evaluation of incidence, clinical significance, and prognostic value of circulating cardiac troponin I and T elevation in hemodynamically stable patients with suspected myocardial contusion after blunt chest trauma. J Trauma 2000;48:924–931.

36. Salim A, Velmahos GC, Jindal A, et al. Clinically significant blunt cardiac trauma: role of serum troponin levels combined with electrocardiographic findings. J Trauma 2001;50:237–243.

37. Fulda GJ, Giberson F, Hailstone D, Law A, Stillabower M. An evaluation of serum troponin T and signal-averaged electrocardiography in predicting electrocardiographic abnormalities after blunt chest trauma. J Trauma 1997;43:304–310.

38. Michelson WB. CPK-MB isoenzyme determinations: diagnostic and prognostic value in evaluation of blunt chest trauma. Ann Emerg Med 1980;9:562–567.

39. Lindenbaum GA, Carroll SF, Block EF, Kapusnick RA. Value of creatine phosphokinase isoenzyme determinations in the diagnosis of myocardial contusion. Ann Emerg Med 1988;17:885–889.

40. Biffl WL, Moore FA, Moore EE, Sauaia A, Read RA, Burch JM. Cardiac enzymes are irrelevant in the patient with suspected myocardial contusion. Am J Surg 1994;168:523–527.

41. Ferjani M, Droc G, Dreux S, et al. Circulating cardiac troponin T in myocardial contusion. Chest 1997;111:427–433.

42. RuDusky BM. Cardiac troponins in the diagnosis of myocardial contusion: an emerging controversy. Chest 1997;112:858–860.

43. Ognibene A, Mori F, Santoni R, et al. Cardiac troponin I in myocardial contusion. Clin Chem 1998;44:889–890.

44. Mair J, Wagner I, Puschendorf B, et al. Cardiac troponin I to diagnose myocardial injury. Lancet 1993;341:838–839.

45. Lown B, Amarasingham R, Neuman J. New method for terminating cardiac arrhythmias. Use of synchronized capacitor discharge. JAMA 1962;182:548–555.

46. Morrow DA, Antman EM. Cardiac marker elevation after cardioversion: sorting out chicken and egg. Eur Heart J 2000;21:171–173.

47. Cobb LA, Eliastam M, Kerber RE, et al. Report of the American Heart Association Task Force on the Future of Cardiopulmonary Resuscitation. Circulation 1992;85:2346–2355.

48. Myerburg RJ, Conde CA, Sung RJ, et al. Clinical, electrophysiologic and hemodynamic profile of patients resuscitated from prehospital cardiac arrest. Am J Med 1980;68:568–576.

49. Krause T, Hohnloser SH, Kasper W, Schumichen C, Reinhardt M, Moser E. Assessment of acute myocardial necrosis after cardiopulmonary resuscitation and cardioversion by means of combined thallium-201/technetium-99m pyrophosphate tomography. Eur J Nucl Med 1995;22:1286–1291.
50. Grubb NR, Fox KA, Cawood P. Resuscitation from out-of-hospital cardiac arrest: implications for cardiac enzyme estimation. Resuscitation 1996;33:35–41.
51. Mullner M, Hirschl MM, Herkner H, et al. Creatine kinase-mb fraction and cardiac troponin T to diagnose acute myocardial infarction after cardiopulmonary resuscitation. J Am Coll Cardiol 1996;28:1220–1225.
52. Garre L, Alvarez A, Rubio M, et al. Use of cardiac troponin T rapid assay in the diagnosis of a myocardial injury secondary to electrical cardioversion. Clin Cardiol 1997;20:619–621.
53. Neumayr G, Hagn C, Ganzer H, et al. Plasma levels of troponin T after electrical cardioversion of atrial fibrillation and flutter. Am J Cardiol 1997;80:1367–1369.
54. Neumayr G, Schratzberger P, Friedrich G, Ganzer H, Wiedermann CJ. Effect of electrical cardioversion on myocardial cells in patients in intensive care. Br Med J 1998;316:1207–1210.
55. Rao AC, Naeem N, John C, Collinson PO, Canepa-Anson R, Joseph SP. Direct current cardioversion does not cause cardiac damage: evidence from cardiac troponin T estimation. Heart 1998;80:229–230.
56. Greaves K, Crake T. Cardiac troponin T does not increase after electrical cardioversion for atrial fibrillation or atrial flutter. Heart 1998;80:226–228.
57. Grubb NR, Cuthbert D, Cawood P, Flapan AD, Fox KA. Effect of DC shock on serum levels of total creatine kinase, MB-creatine kinase mass and troponin T. Resuscitation 1998;36:193–199.
58. Lund M, French J, Johnson R, Williams B, White H. Serum troponins T and I after elective cardioversion. Eur Heart J 1999:245–253.
59. Doherty PW, McLaughlin PR, Billingham M, Kernoff R, Goris ML, Harrison DC. Cardiac damage produced by direct current countershock applied to the heart. Am J Cardiol 1979;43:225–232.
60. Jakobsson J, Odmansson I, Nordlander R. Enzyme release after elective cardioversion. Eur Heart J 1990;11:749–752.
61. Dahl CF, Ewy GA, Warner ED, Thomas ED. Myocardial necrosis from direct current countershock. Effect of paddle electrode size and time interval between discharges. Circulation 1974;50:956–961.
62. Ehsani A, Ewy GA, Sobel BE. Effects of electrical countershock on serum creatine phosphokinase (CPK) isoenzyme activity. Am J Cardiol 1976;37:12–18.
63. DeSilva RA, Graboys TB, Podrid PJ, Lown B. Cardioversion and defibrillation. Am Heart J 1980;100:881–895.
64. Pugh BR, Buja LM, Parkey RW, et al. Cardioversion and "false positive" technetium-99m stannous pyrophosphate myocardial scintigrams. Circulation 1976;54:399–403.
65. Metcalfe MJ, Smith F, Jennings K, Paterson N. Does cardioversion of atrial fibrillation result in myocardial damage? Br Med J (Clin Res Ed) 1988;296:1364.
66. Corbitt JD Jr, Sybers J, Levin JM. Muscle changes of the anterior chest wall secondary to electrical countershock. Am J Clin Pathol 1969;51:107–112.
67. O'Neill P, Faitelson L, Taylor A, Puleo P, Roberts R, Pacifico A. Time course of creatine kinase release after termination of sustained ventricular dysrhythmias. Am Heart J 1991;122:709–714.
68. Bonnefoy E, Chevalier P, Kirkorian G, Guidolet J, Marchand A, Touboul P. Cardiac troponin I does not increase after cardioversion. Chest 1997;111:15–18.
69. Allan JJ, Feld RD, Russell AA, et al. Cardiac troponin I levels are normal or minimally elevated after transthoracic cardioversion. J Am Coll Cardiol 1997;30:1052–1056.

70. Mattana J, Singhal PC. Determinants of elevated creatine kinase activity and creatine kinase MB-fraction following cardiopulmonary resuscitation. Chest 1992;101:1386–1392.

71. Goldhaber SZ, Visani L, De Rosa M. Acute pulmonary embolism: clinical outcomes in the International Cooperative Pulmonary Embolism Registry (ICOPER). Lancet 1999;353: 1386–1389.

72. Meyer T, Binder L, Hruska N, Luthe H, Buchwald AB. Cardiac troponin I elevation in acute pulmonary embolism is associated with right ventricular dysfunction. J Am Coll Cardiol 2000;36:1632–1636.

73. Douketis JD, Crowther MA, Stanton EB, Ginsberg JS. Elevated cardiac troponin levels in patients with submassive pulmonary embolism. Arch Intern Med 2002;162:79–81.

74. Giannitsis E, Muller-Bardorff M, Kurowski V, et al. Independent prognostic value of cardiac troponin T in patients with confirmed pulmonary embolism. Circulation 2000;102:211–217.

75. Elliott CG. Pulmonary physiology during pulmonary embolism. Chest 1992;101:163S–171S.

76. Lualdi JC, Goldhaber SZ. Right ventricular dysfunction after acute pulmonary embolism: pathophysiologic factors, detection, and therapeutic implications. Am Heart J 1995;130: 1276–1282.

77. Coma-Canella I, Gamallo C, Martinez Onsurbe P, Lopez-Sendon J. Acute right ventricular infarction secondary to massive pulmonary embolism. Eur Heart J 1988;9:534–540.

78. Kasper W, Konstantinides S, Geibel A, et al. Management strategies and determinants of outcome in acute major pulmonary embolism: results of a multicenter registry. J Am Coll Cardiol 1997;30:1165–1171.

79. Ribeiro A, Lindmarker P, Juhlin-Dannfelt A, Johnsson H, Jorfeldt L. Echocardiography Doppler in pulmonary embolism: right ventricular dysfunction as a predictor of mortality rate. Am Heart J 1997;134:479–487.

80. Muller-Bardorff M, Weidtmann B, Giannitsis E, Kurowski V, Katus HA. Release kinetics of cardiac troponin T in survivors of confirmed severe pulmonary embolism. Clin Chem 2002;48:673–675.

81. Konstantinides S, Geibel A, Olschewski M, et al. Association between thrombolytic treatment and the prognosis of hemodynamically stable patients with major pulmonary embolism: results of a multicenter registry. Circulation 1997;96:882–888.

82. Parrillo JE, Parker MM, Natanson C, et al. Septic shock in humans. Advances in the understanding of pathogenesis, cardiovascular dysfunction, and therapy. Ann Intern Med 1990; 113:227–242.

83. Bone RC, Balk RA, Cerra FB, et al. Definitions for sepsis and organ failure and guidelines for the use of innovative therapies in sepsis. The ACCP/SCCM Consensus Conference Committee. American College of Chest Physicians/Society of Critical Care Medicine. Chest 1992; 101:1644–1655.

84. Wu AH. Increased troponin in patients with sepsis and septic shock: myocardial necrosis or reversible myocardial depression? Intensive Care Med 2001;27:959–961.

85. Wiggers CJ. Myocardial depression in shock. A survey of cardiodynamic studies. Am Heart J 1947;33:633–650.

86. Price S, Anning PB, Mitchell JA, Evans TW. Myocardial dysfunction in sepsis: mechanisms and therapeutic implications. Eur Heart J 1999;20:715–724.

87. Parker MM, Shelhamer JH, Bacharach SL, et al. Profound but reversible myocardial depression in patients with septic shock. Ann Intern Med 1984;100:483–490.

88. Cunnion RE, Schaer GL, Parker MM, Natanson C, Parrillo JE. The coronary circulation in human septic shock. Circulation 1986;73:637–644.

89. Dhainaut JF, Huyghebaert MF, Monsallier JF, et al. Coronary hemodynamics and myocardial metabolism of lactate, free fatty acids, glucose, and ketones in patients with septic shock. Circulation 1987;75:533–541.

90. Solomon MA, Correa R, Alexander HR, et al. Myocardial energy metabolism and morphology in a canine model of sepsis. Am J Physiol 1994;266:H757–H768.

91. Giroir BP, Stromberg D. Myocardial depression versus myocardial destruction: integrating the multiple mechanisms of myocardial dysfunction during sepsis. Crit Care Med 2000;28: 3111–3112.

92. Parrillo JE, Burch C, Shelhamer JH, Parker MM, Natanson C, Schuette W. A circulating myocardial depressant substance in humans with septic shock. Septic shock patients with a reduced ejection fraction have a circulating factor that depresses in vitro myocardial cell performance. J Clin Invest 1985;76:1539–1553.

93. Kumar A, Thota V, Dee L, Olson J, Uretz E, Parrillo JE. Tumor necrosis factor alpha and interleukin 1beta are responsible for in vitro myocardial cell depression induced by human septic shock serum. J Exp Med 1996;183:949–958.

94. Yokoyama T, Vaca L, Rossen RD, Durante W, Hazarika P, Mann DL. Cellular basis for the negative inotropic effects of tumor necrosis factor-alpha in the adult mammalian heart. J Clin Invest 1993;92:2303–2312.

95. Franco F, Thomas GD, Giroir B, et al. Magnetic resonance imaging and invasive evaluation of development of heart failure in transgenic mice with myocardial expression of tumor necrosis factor-alpha. Circulation 1999;99:448–454.

96. Cain BS, Meldrum DR, Dinarello CA, et al. Tumor necrosis factor-alpha and interleukin-1beta synergistically depress human myocardial function. Crit Care Med 1999;27: 1309–1318.

97. Balligand JL, Ungureanu D, Kelly RA, et al. Abnormal contractile function due to induction of nitric oxide synthesis in rat cardiac myocytes follows exposure to activated macrophage-conditioned medium. J Clin Invest 1993;91:2314–2319.

98. Kumar A, Brar R, Wang P, et al. Role of nitric oxide and cGMP in human septic serum-induced depression of cardiac myocyte contractility. Am J Physiol 1999;276:R265–R276.

99. Balligand JL, Ungureanu-Longrois D, Simmons WW, et al. Cytokine-inducible nitric oxide synthase (iNOS) expression in cardiac myocytes. Characterization and regulation of iNOS expression and detection of iNOS activity in single cardiac myocytes in vitro. J Biol Chem 1994;269:27580–27588.

100. Guest TM, Ramanathan AV, Tuteur PG, Schechtman KB, Ladenson JH, Jaffe AS. Myocardial injury in critically ill patients. A frequently unrecognized complication. JAMA 1995; 273:1945–1949.

101. Spies C, Haude V, Fitzner R, et al. Serum cardiac troponin T as a prognostic marker in early sepsis. Chest 1998;113:1055–1063.

102. Fernandes CJ Jr, Akamine N, Knobel E. Cardiac troponin: a new serum marker of myocardial injury in sepsis. Intens Care Med 1999;25:1165–1168.

103. Turner A, Tsamitros M, Bellomo R. Myocardial cell injury in septic shock. Crit Care Med 1999;27:1775–1780.

104. Arlati S, Brenna S, Prencipe L, et al. Myocardial necrosis in ICU patients with acute non-cardiac disease: a prospective study. Intens Care Med 2000;26:31–37.

105. Thiru Y, Pathan N, Bignall S, Habibi P, Levin M. A myocardial cytotoxic process is involved in the cardiac dysfunction of meningococcal septic shock. Crit Care Med 2000; 28:2979–2983.

106. ver Elst KM, Spapen HD, Nguyen DN, Garbar C, Huyghens LP, Gorus FK. Cardiac troponins I and T are biological markers of left ventricular dysfunction in septic shock. Clin Chem 2000;46:650–657.

107. Ammann P, Fehr T, Minder EI, Gunter C, Bertel O. Elevation of troponin I in sepsis and septic shock. Intens Care Med 2001;27:965–969.

108. Murphy JT, Horton JW, Purdue GF, Hunt JL. Evaluation of troponin-I as an indicator of cardiac dysfunction after thermal injury. J Trauma 1998;45:700–704.

109. Krown KA, Page MT, Nguyen C, et al. Tumor necrosis factor alpha-induced apoptosis in cardiac myocytes. Involvement of the sphingolipid signaling cascade in cardiac cell death. J Clin Invest 1996;98:2854–2865.

110. Bryant D, Becker L, Richardson J, et al. Cardiac failure in transgenic mice with myocardial expression of tumor necrosis factor-alpha. Circulation 1998;97:1375–1381.
111. Brett J, Gerlach H, Nawroth P, Steinberg S, Godman G, Stern D. Tumor necrosis factor/cachectin increases permeability of endothelial cell monolayers by a mechanism involving regulatory G proteins. J Exp Med 1989;169:1977–1991.
112. Van Zee KJ, Moldawer LL, Oldenburg HS, et al. Protection against lethal *Escherichia coli* bacteremia in baboons (Papio anubis) by pretreatment with a 55-kDa TNF receptor (CD120a)-Ig fusion protein, Ro 45-2081. J Immunol 1996;156:2221–2230.
113. Vincent JL, Bakker J, Marecaux G, Schandene L, Kahn RJ, Dupont E. Administration of anti-TNF antibody improves left ventricular function in septic shock patients. Results of a pilot study. Chest 1992;101:810–815.
114. Cohen J, Carlet J. INTERSEPT: an international, multicenter, placebo-controlled trial of monoclonal antibody to human tumor necrosis factor-alpha in patients with sepsis. International Sepsis Trial Study Group. Crit Care Med 1996;24:1431–1440.
115. Abraham E, Anzueto A, Gutierrez G, et al. Double-blind randomised controlled trial of monoclonal antibody to human tumour necrosis factor in treatment of septic shock. NORASEPT II Study Group. Lancet 1998;351:929–933.
116. Miller WL, Wright RS, McGregor CG, et al. Troponin levels in patients with amyloid cardiomyopathy undergoing cardiac transplantation. Am J Cardiol 2001;88:813–815.
117. Cantwell RV, Aviles RJ, Bjornsson J, et al. Cardiac amyloidosis presenting with elevations of cardiac troponin I and angina pectoris. Clin Cardiol 2002;25:33–37.
118. Bonnefoy E, Godon P, Kirkorian G, Fatemi M, Chevalier P, Touboul P. Serum cardiac troponin I and ST-segment elevation in patients with acute pericarditis. Eur Heart J 2000; 21:832–836.
119. Stelow EB, Johari VP, Smith SA, Crosson JT, Apple FS. Propofol-associated rhabdomyolysis with cardiac involvement in adults: chemical and anatomic findings. Clin Chem 2000;46:577–581.
120. Fleming SM, O'Gorman T, Finn J, Grimes H, Daly K, Morrison JJ. Cardiac troponin I in pre-eclampsia and gestational hypertension. Br J Obstet Gynaecol 2000;107:1417–1420.
121. Dixit S, Castle M, Velu RP, Swisher L, Hodge C, Jaffe AS. Cardiac involvement in patients with acute neurologic disease: confirmation with cardiac troponin I. Arch Intern Med 2000; 160:3153–3158.
122. Parekh N, Venkatesh B, Cross D, et al. Cardiac troponin I predicts myocardial dysfunction in aneurysmal subarachnoid hemorrhage. J Am Coll Cardiol 2000;36:1328–1335.
123. Pateron D, Beyne P, Laperche T, et al. Elevated circulating cardiac troponin I in patients with cirrhosis. Hepatology 1999;29:640–643.
124. Rifai N, Douglas PS, O'Toole M, Rimm E, Ginsburg GS. Cardiac troponin T and I, electrocardiographic wall motion analyses, and ejection fractions in athletes participating in the Hawaii Ironman Triathlon. Am J Cardiol 1999;83:1085–1089.
125. Chen Y, Serfass RC, Mackey-Bojack SM, Kelly KL, Titus JL, Apple FS. Cardiac troponin T alterations in myocardium and serum of rats after stressful, prolonged intense exercise. J Appl Physiol 2000;88:1749–1755.

Part III
Analytical Issues for Cardiac Markers

10

Antibody Selection Strategies
in Cardiac Troponin Assays

Alexei Katrukha

INTRODUCTION

The history of troponin assays starts from the late 1980s. In 1987, B. Cummins reported a new analyte that could be used for diagnosis of acute myocardial infarction (MI) *(1)*. The new method was based on the immunodetection of cardiac isoform of troponin I (cTnI). Two years later Katus and colleagues *(2)* suggested utilization of cardiac troponin T (cTnT) as a cardiac marker. Today dozens of commercial cTnI assays are available. Troponins are the most "popular" cardiac markers. According to Apple et al. *(3)*, in 1999 about 85% of clinical laboratories in the United States were using this analyte in their practice. But our knowledge about the nature of cTnI circulating in the blood is still only the tip of an iceberg. Limited knowledge of the antigen limits the possibilities of developing a theory of cTnI assays, and as a consequence results in huge between-method variations for existing cTnI assays *(4,5)*. Obviously the lack of an international standard *(6)* complicates assay standardization, but in the case of cTnI, the antibody standardization can be even more important *(4)*.

Immunoassays are used in clinical practice for qualitative or quantitative detection of different antigens in body fluids. Because the sought parameter is the antigen, the strategy of antibody selection should be based on our knowledge of the antigen's structure. In this chapter, we critically examine data available from the literature, which can be useful for a rational search of the antibodies suitable for the development of reliable cTnI and cTnT immunoassays.

Because of an existing patent, only one company (Roche Diagnostics) is producing cTnT assays, whereas a wide diversity of commercial cTnI assays are available. As a consequence, most studies are devoted to the peculiar properties of cTnI assays, and only a few publications discuss cTnT, as an antigen, and anti-cTnT antibodies.

CARDIOSPECIFIC ISOFORM OF TnI

The value of cTnI detection lies in its ability to differentiate cardiac from skeletal muscle injury. cTnI is able to replace the MB isoenzyme of creatine kinase (CK-MB) and other markers in diagnosis of myocardial cell necrosis because of its extraordinary

From: *Cardiac Markers, Second Edition*
Edited by: Alan H. B. Wu @ Humana Press Inc., Totowa, NJ

tissue specificity *(7,8)*. Today this protein is regarded as the most specific among known markers of myocardial cell damage *(9,10)*.

Three isoforms of TnI are expressed in human muscle tissues—one is specific to myocardial tissue, cTnI, and two others, slow skeletal (sskTnI) and fast skeletal (fskTnI) troponin I isoforms, common for skeletal muscles. The cardiac isoform is structurally different from the corresponding skeletal isoforms *(11–13)*. It contains 32 additional amino acid residues in the N-terminal part of the molecule, which are absent in the skeletal TnIs. These additional sequences, as well as 42% and 45% of sequence dissimilarity with sskTnI and fskTnI, respectively, make possible the generation of monoclonal antibodies (MAbs) that are specific to cTnI, and have no cross-reactivity with skeletal forms.

The absence of antibody cross-reactivity with skeletal forms is very important. Serum concentrations of skTnIs are increased in patients with chronic degenerative muscle disease and in marathon runners *(14)*. In the case, the assay is not sufficiently cardio-specific, and cTnI measurements can be falsely positive. As such, the monoclonal antibodies used in the immunoassays should be checked to ensure they have no cross-reactivity with the skeletal isoforms. Polyclonal antibodies, generated after animal immunization with whole cTnI molecules or any peptide different from the cardio-specific 32-amino-acid N-terminal sequence, should be affinity purified on the resins, containing corresponding skeletal TnI molecules or peptides, to remove the antibody fractions cross-reacting with the skeletal muscle motifs.

BIOCHEMICAL FORMS OF cTnI IN HUMAN BLOOD

Human cTnI is a middle-size protein with mol wt 24,007, and is highly basic (pI = 9.87) *(11)*. In muscle tissue, cTnI forms a complex with two proteins, components of the troponin complex—troponins T and troponin C (TnC) *(15,16)*. cTnI can be phosphorylated by cAMP-dependent protein kinase (kinase A) *(17)* and Ca^{2+}-phospholipid-dependent protein kinase (kinase C) *(18,19)*. The molecule is very unstable and is easily degraded by a number of different proteases.

All of these biochemical characteristics are very important for the understanding of those modifications that occur with cTnI in viable and ischemic myocytes, and that could be critical for the development of accurate diagnostic procedures for cTnI measurement.

cTnI as a Part of Troponin Complex

cTnI is a subunit of a heterotrimeric troponin complex, consisting of three different subunits—cTnI, cTnT, and TnC *(15,20)*. The troponin complex is an essential part of the cardiac and skeletal muscle contractile apparatus. Each troponin subunit performs specific functions and the letters "I," "T," and "C" in the name of the protein come from the protein's main function. TnC is a Ca^{2+}-binding protein containing four metal-binding sites. TnI *inhibits* actomyosin ATPase activity and this inhibition is reversed by the addition of Ca^{2+}-saturated TnC. TnT is a *tropomyosin*-binding subunit *(21–26)*.

The TnC molecule contains four metal-binding sites—two sites are located in the carboxy- (C)-terminal globular domain of TnC and two in the N-terminal domain. Among the components of the troponin complex, cTnI and TnC interact with each other with the highest affinity. This interaction is strongly Ca^{2+} dependent, and it is much higher when metal binding sites are saturated with Ca^{2+} ions *(24)*. The interaction between cTnI and TnC is multisite and, according to existing knowledge, cTnI wraps around the central helix of TnC in the presence of Ca^{2+}, forming contacts with both N- and C-terminal globular domains of the TnC molecule *(26)*. Complexation with TnC results in serious changes of cTnI conformation.

cTnT provides proper interaction between troponin and the actin–tropomyosin filament. Although cTnT interacts with both cTnI and TnC, this type of interaction is not as strong as the cTnI–TnC binary complex *(24)*.

In the ternary troponin complex, part of cTnI molecule is covered by two other troponin components. As a result, epitopes of some antibodies, recognizing free cTnI molecule, would be changed or inaccessible. Changes in the epitope structure could result in weakening, or vice versa, strengthening, of the antigen–antibody interaction. In 1992, Bodor et al. described anti-cTnI MAbs, produced by hybridoma cell lines, generated after animal immunization with purified cTnI. Through free, uncomplexed cTnI used as an immunogen, two out of eight tested antibodies recognized the cTnI–TnC complex with a higher response than the free cTnI molecule, whereas one MAb did not interact with cTnI in the absence of TnC *(27)*. In 1997 Katrukha et al. reported development of MAbs that, on the contrary, recognized the free form of cTnI better than the cTnI–TnC binary complex *(28,29)*. One of these antibodies MAb 414 was not able to detect complexed cTnI . Sandwich immunoassay utilizing this antibody was able to detect only free cTnI and did not recognize either binary cTnI–TnC or the ternary complexes. Later several authors confirmed that cTnI assays could be different in recognizing free and complexed forms of cTnI *(5,30,31)*. For instance, the Stratus (Dade Behring) cTnI assay responded to the cTnI–TnC complex four- to fivefold more than to free cTnI, whereas the first generation of Access (Beckman) assay revealed better sensitivity to the free form of the antigen. At the same time, several commercial immunoassays are described, which equally recognized free and complexed cTnIs *(30–32)*.

Being washed away from the necrotic tissue, cTnI retains its interaction with TnC. More than 90% of cTnI in human blood after AMI is complexed with TnC and only a small amount can be detected as a free molecule. The existence of a binary cTnI–cTnT complex or ternary cTnI–cTnT–TnC complex in AMI blood is under discussion. Some authors reported that the cTnI–cTnT binary or ternary complexes are seldom present in AMI blood *(33,34)*, whereas others detected considerable amounts of ternary complex, but not in all tested AMI serum samples *(5)*.

The fact that complexed and free cTnI forms may have different recognition patterns among different immunoassays may be the main reason for differences between commercial immunoassays. Thus, one way to eliminate such discordances is to introduce in new assays the antibodies that are insensitive to complex formation. Figure 1 illustrates the biochemical factors influencing recognition of cTnI by antibodies.

Proteolytic Degradation of cTnI

cTnI is known as a very unstable molecule. Purified antigen rapidly loses immunological activity in blood even in the presence of protease inhibitors. Stability of cTnI in the ternary troponin complex is much higher because of the protection by other troponin components, especially by TnC *(35,36)*. According to McDonough and Van Eyk *(37, 38)*, proteolytic degradation of cTnI in animal tissue starts even within the ischemic

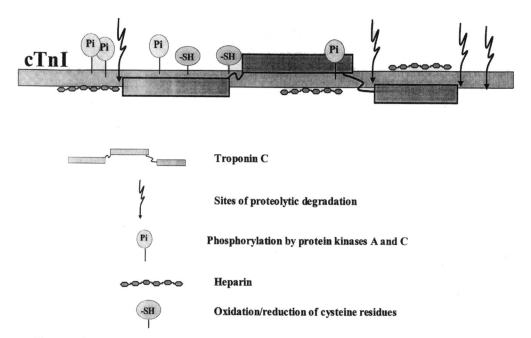

Fig. 1. Biochemical factors influencing recognition of cTnI, circulating in AMI blood, by antibodies.

myocardium, without any apparent signs of tissue necrosis and results in the appearance of different-size products. In the in vivo experiments with rat cardiac ischemia, cTnI lost the 17 amino acid residues from the C-terminal part of the molecule and the 62–72 amino acid residues from the N-terminus. In the necrotic tissue the degradation of cTnI is even more severe and variable. In the *in situ* experiments with human cardiac tissue incubated for different periods of time at 37°C, the rate of proteolytic degradation was so high that <2% of undegraded protein could be detected after 20 h of incubation *(36)*. These experiments revealed that the most stable part of cTnI is located between 28 and 110 amino acid residues *(36)*.

The rate of tissue cTnI degradation is dependent on many factors. It was demonstrated that in tissue samples obtained from different donors, the rate of cTnI degradation could differ fourfold and even more *(36)*. This discrepancy can be explained by several factors. First, different proteases are present in tissue samples collected from different donors in different concentrations. At the same time it was shown *(39)* that the rate of cTnI degradation is strongly dependent on the phosphorylation level of the protein. Phosphorylation by protein kinase A (PKA) decreases the degradation by μ-calpain *in situ,* whereas phosphorylation by protein kinase C (PKC) has a positive effect on the protease-dependent degradation. As a result, after infarction, ischemic tissue of two different patients most probably would contain different sets of cTnI fragments. The more time that passes after infarction, the less is the tissue concentration of native (uncleaved) protein, and the higher the concentration of different-size proteolytic fragments that could be detected in the patient's blood. The fragment diversity of cTnI in human blood is not studied well. Morjana *(40)* reported the existence 14- and 18-kDa cTnI fragments in patients' blood after AMI. These peptides were generated as a result of proteolytic processing from the C- and N-terminal regions of the TnI molecule. At the same time, very little unprocessed intact cTnI could be detected. Wu et al. *(5)* also observed cTnI fragments of unknown structure in the studied samples.

Specificity of antibodies to different parts of the molecule—stable or unstable—can be responsible (at least partially) for the discrepancy in the testing of blood samples from one assay to another. Assays that utilize the antibodies specific to the stable part of the antigen will be able to detect both intact and degraded cTnI molecules. On the contrary, the assay with antibodies specific to the unstable part(s) of cTnI will recognize only native (undegraded) cTnI and will fail to detect the many proteolytic fragments. As a result, assays with antibodies recognizing the intact and degraded protein should give a higher response to the patient's sample than assays with antibodies to the unstable part of the protein. The difference will be even higher with "late" samples, that is, collected several days after infarction, as the main portion of cTnI in necrotic tissue is proteolytic fragments *(36)*. Moreover, the susceptibility of cTnI to proteolytic degradation seriously complicates the preparation of stable calibrators and standards, and the procedure of blood samples collection and storage. The apparent stability of the antigen in blood samples or stability of controls (calibrators), determined by the assay to stable epitopes, will be much higher than with an assay to the unstable epitope. Venge et al. *(32)* studied the stability of cTnI by the new generation Access cTnI assay (Beckman Coulter Inc). The MAbs, utilized in this new generation assay are specific to the stable part of the cTnI molecule and their epitopes are located very close to each other. The authors stressed that in in vitro experiments, the cTnI probed by the new assay showed high stability at both room temperature and at 4°C, and could be stored up to 48 h under these conditions without any major effect on recovery. These results are in contrast to Beckman's first generation of Access cTnI assay, where storage of samples at room temperature for 1–2 h produced a decrease of 20–30% of the measured cTnI concentration. The antibodies utilized in the old generation of Access cTnI assay recognized the unstable part of the molecule *(32)*. Thus, the proper choice of antibodies helps to resolve one of the most complicated problems of cTnI assay design, that is, cTnI calibrator (standard) stability. To avoid the effect of cTnI proteolytic degradation on assay sensitivity and reproducibility and to increase the apparent stability of calibrators (standards) for the antibodies utilized in the assay, epitopes should be located in the stable part of the protein as close to each other as possible.

Phosphorylation of cTnI

Two serine residues, located at the 22nd and 23rd positions of the cTnI sequence, could be phosphorylated in vivo by PKA, as a result of epinephrine stimulation *(17)*. Recent in vitro experiments revealed that there are at least two more sites of phosphorylation on the cTnI molecule—serine residues in 38 and 165 positions, which also can be phosphorylated by PKA, although it is not clear yet whether this phosphorylation can occur only in vitro or in the living cell *(41)*. In addition to phosphorylation by PKA, cTnI can be phosphorylated by PKC *(18,19)*. Labugger et al. *(42)* reported that during ischemia, threonine amino acid residues in positions 119, 123, and/or 129 also could be phosphorylated. Thus, dephospho- and multiple monophospho-, bis-, or polyphospho-cTnI forms can coexist in the living cardiomyocyte, and after infarction all these forms could be detected in patients' blood. It was demonstrated that about the half of cTnI circulating in patients' blood is phosphorylated by PKA *(4,43)*, but it is unknown yet what part of circulating cTnI is phosphorylated by PKC.

Phosphorylation changes the structure and conformation of the cTnI molecule, and the affinity of interaction between the components of the troponin complex. Thus, phosphorylation can change the interaction of some antibodies with their epitopes. Several MAbs, recognizing only phosphorylated cTnI, or vice versa, only dephosphorylated protein, were described in literature during the last few years *(4,43,44)*. If such antibodies were to be used in cTnI immunoassay, a considerable part of the antigen in a patient's blood would remain undetected. Hence, it is preferable that the antibodies selected for the immunoassay development should be specific to the epitopes different from the sites of phosphorylation, so that interaction of such antibodies with the antigen will be unaffected by any type of phosphorylation.

Oxidation of cTnI

cTnI has two cysteines at 79 and 96 positions *(11)* that can be oxidized or reduced in vitro. Oxidation/reduction changes the structure and the conformation of the protein and thus changes the interaction of some antibodies with the number of epitopes. Wu et al. *(5)* demonstrated that three out of nine tested commercially available assays were sensitive (higher response) to the oxidation of the antigen, whereas for others there was no difference for the form of the protein tested. Although it is still unclear in what form —oxidized or reduced—cTnI releases from damaged cardiac tissue after AMI and circulates in human blood, it is preferable that antibodies used in the assay recognize both forms with the same efficiency.

Complexes of cTnI with Polyanions

As mentioned previously, cTnI is a highly basic protein with pI = 9.87 and more or less equal distribution of basic amino acid residues along the molecule. At physiological pH, cTnI carries a high positive charge. Electrostatic interaction is a main type of interaction of cTnI with other molecules. Electrostatic interaction is very important for the formation of binary complex between cTnI and highly acidic TnC (pI = 4.05 for slow skeletal isoform of TnC, expressed in cardiac tissue). Electrostatic interaction can also be responsible for the formation of different types of complexes between cTnI and other than TnC acidic molecules circulating in blood. One such known complex is that between cTnI and heparin—a drug widely used in clinical practice to prevent blood clotting. Heparin is also widely used as an anticoagulant for the collection of plasma. Recent studies demonstrated that the effect of heparin on the interaction of cTnI with antibodies is very similar to that of cTnI—TnC complex formation. In addition, similar to the sensitivity of some immunoassays to cTnI–TnC complex formation, some commercial and in-house assays are very sensitive to the presence of heparin in the sample, whereas others show no differences for samples collected with or without heparin *(4,32,45,46)*.

Studying the negative influence of heparin on the signal level in three commercial assays, Wagner et al. *(47)* demonstrated that the effect of heparin can be significantly diminished by adding to the samples heparin antagonists, such as protamine sulfate or hexadimethrine bromide. But it is absolutely clear that while developing new assays, it is preferable to check the antibodies to their sensitivity to heparin and select those that give the same response to the antigen independent of the presence or absence of heparin in the sample.

Autoantibodies to cTnI

Autoantibodies to different components of skeletal and cardiac contractile systems are described in the literature *(48–50)*. The presence of autoantibodies in the sample can complicate protein quantitative and qualitative measurements by immunological methods because of the possible competition of the autoantibodies and the antibodies utilized in the assay. To date, there has been only one case described of autoantibodies to cTnI in a patient's blood. Bohner et al. *(51)* reported on a 69-yr-old coronary artery bypass graft patient with diffuse three-vessel disease that was falsely negative when measured by Dade's cTnI assay, but positive with troponin T and CK-MB assays. It was demonstrated that the patient's blood contained anti-cTnI autoantibodies, which competed for binding sites with the antibodies utilized in the assay. The authors did not clarify the epitope specificity of autoantibodies, so we can only speculate on what part of the cTnI molecule served as an antigen for autoantibody production by the patients. Were there only one or two motifs recognized by the antibodies from Dade's assay, or were there other regions that could have been the target for host antibody production?

ANTIBODY SELECTION

Affinity of Antibodies

Affinity of the antibodies is one of the crucial factors that should be considered when antibodies are selected. The assay sensitivity strongly depends on the affinity of the antibodies used. For cTnI assays, the sensitivity is very important. cTnI concentration in the blood of AMI patients is low—usually between 0.1 and 10 ng/mL and rarely reaching a level of 50–100 ng/mL. Recent studies have shown that the detection of small changes (0.01–1 ng/mL) in the cTnI concentration in the blood of patients with unstable angina could be very important for the detection of minor myocardial damage, and have a significant prognostic value *(52–57)*. Minor myocardial cell injury as detected by cTnI is found in about 30–40% of patients with unstable angina. These patients have a poor short-term outcome *(56)*.

At the same time, the high sensitivity of cTnI assays is very important for the early diagnosis of MI during the first 2–3 h after onset of the chest pain, when cTnI concentration in the patient's blood just exceeds a normal level. Utilization of high-affinity antibodies also decreases the assay turnaround time. The original research on cTnI required 24–36 h *(1)*, whereas only 10–20 min are needed to obtain results by contemporary assays that utilize high-affinity antibodies *(58,59)*. Thus, the cTnI assay should be able to detect low and very low concentrations of the analyte in the sample within a short period of time. This is possible only in the case when both (capture and detection) antibodies recognize the antigen with high affinity.

Mono- or Polyclonal Antibodies?

As was discussed above, a wide diversity of cTnI forms is released from damaged cardiac tissue after MI. There are two approaches to extract the main part of cTnI modifications from blood samples. The first is to use as capture antibodies generated from animals immunized with either a whole cTnI molecule or, preferably, with synthetic peptides corresponding to the different parts of the molecule. Multipoint binding of the antigen by polyclonal antibodies should increase the avidity of antibody–antigen interaction, and as a result increase the sensitivity of the assay. But the utilization of polyclonal antibodies in the cTnI assay has two main shortcomings. Antibodies should be highly cardiospecific. But after animal immunization with the whole molecule or by peptides, the total pool of antibodies recognizing cTnI contains fraction that may cross-react with the skeletal isoform of the protein. Extraction of this fraction is expensive and time consuming. Another problem is the inability of duplicating the production of good polyclonal antibodies, a feature that is essential for all clinical applications. The solution here is to use several (two or three) MAbs specific to different parts of the molecule as antibodies for capture and detection. Preferably, all antibodies should not be affected by any of known cTnI modifications and biochemical factors. Such an approach—dual or triple monoclonal solid phase—helps to improve the sensitivity and reproducibility (*unpublished observations* and ref. *60*). The other option is to utilize two MAbs specific to the sites that are not affected by any known modification, with the epitopes located in the stable part of the molecule as close to each other as it is possible. Such approach works well in the new generation of Access® AccuTnI™ method *(32,60,62)*.

Epitope Mapping

The epitope location of the majority of antibodies described in literature is well documented. Some mono- or polyclonal antibodies were generated after animal immunization with synthetic peptides (e.g., polyclonal antibodies to peptides 1–4 coming from Fortron Bio Science) and in this case the epitope location is restricted by peptide sequence. Others (monoclonal) antibodies were obtained after mice were immunized with purified cTnI *(27,63,64)* or whole cardiac troponin complex *(65)*. In this case the epitope location was determined by peptide mapping *(66)* or, more precisely, by the SPOT technique *(65,67–69)*. The SPOT method utilizes the library of short (10–15 amino acid residues) overlapping peptides corresponding to the whole cTnI sequence, synthesized with steps of one to five amino acid residues. The SPOT method makes possible precise epitope mapping with the uncertainty in one or two amino acid residues.

Interestingly, among MAbs generated after animals were immunized with isolated cTnI or by whole cardiac troponin complex, 90% recognized short peptides *(65)*. Thus, the majority of produced anti-cTnI antibodies are specific to linear motives, and not to the conformational epitopes. This observation is in agreement with the present conception of the cTnI spatial pattern, that is, the cTnI molecule does not have a complex ternary structure. This feature facilitates the production of antibodies by animal immunization with predetermined specificity using short peptides. When the conformational epitopes are absent, the short synthetic peptides (10 to 12 amino acid residues), which have no ternary structure, can be used as an appropriate immunogen for antibody production.

Polyclonal and especially monoclonal antibodies, with precisely determined epitopes, are important tools in the biochemical studies of cTnI in blood, and could be very helpful in the deliberate search of the appropriate epitopes to be used as a targets for antibody production.

Antibodies Recognizing cTnI from Different Animal Species

Animal models are widely used in the trials of new drugs, in the development of new methods of surgery, and in organ transplantation. In all these cases, the effect of any new drug or technology on cardiac function and on cardiomyocyte viability should be estimated *(70–72)*. Choosing between equal possibilities, it is preferable to have in the assay the antibodies that are cross-reacting with cTnI from different animal species. Such assays could be used not only in clinical practice but also in experimental scientific work and in the preclinical studies.

TROPONIN T ANTIBODIES AND ASSAY

cTnT is very similar to cTnI as a biochemical marker of myocardial cell death. Because in the living cell they exist only as components of a heterotetrameric complex with each other and TnC, with trace amounts of free proteins, the molar concentrations of cTnI and cTnT in cardiac tissue are equal. As a consequence, after infarction, cTnT appears in a patient's blood simultaneously with cTnI and in the comparable concentrations. It reaches peak levels at the same time, and has the same time frame within which it can be detected in a patient's blood.

As the molar concentration of cTnT in human blood is the same as the concentration of cTnI, the cTnT assay should utilize high-affinity mono- or polyclonal antibodies, to be able to detect very low antigen concentrations in the sample. Specificity of antibodies to the cardiac forms of the protein is also very important. The first generation cTnT assay (cTnT enzyme-linked immunosorbent assay [ELISA]) utilized detection antibody with some cross-reactivity with the skeletal isoforms of the protein *(69)*. As a consequence, this version of the assay produced falsely positive results from blood obtained from patients with acute or chronicle muscle disease and chronic renal failure. The false-positive results were explained by cross-reaction of antibodies with the skeletal isoform of the protein. The antibodies of the current generation of cTnT assay have corrected this problem.

The interaction between cTnT and other components of the troponin complex is significantly lower, as compared to the interactions of the cTnI–TnC binary complex. In contrast with cTnI, in AMI patients' blood, cTnT is present mainly as a free molecule and its proteolytic fragments *(5)*.

cTnT undergoes rapid proteolytic degradation in ischemic and necrotic cardiac tissue. McDonough et al. *(37)* reported that in the ischemic myocytes proteolytic degradation of cTnT results in the accumulation of fragments corresponding to the 191–298 residues of cTnT sequence. In necrotic tissue (*in situ* experiments) cTnT was rapidly cleaved by proteases, forming two main peptides with apparent molecular mass 31–33 and 14–16 kDa, respectively, the products of sequential proteolysis from the N-terminal part of the molecule (*unpublished data* and ref. *72*). The epitopes of the antibodies utilized in the new version of cTnT assay are only six amino acid residues apart *(73)*, and this feature makes this assay insensitive to the proteolytic degradation of the antigen. Stability studies of cTnT in AMI serum samples described by Baum et al. *(75)* showed that as measured by the new version of the cTnT assay, cTnT had no loss of immunological activity after 5 d of storage at room temperature.

cTnT can be phosphorylated by PKC *(76,77)*, but we were unable to find studies demonstrating the effect of phosphorylation on the interaction between antigen and antibodies. Resembling some cTnI assays, the current version of the cTnT assay is sensitive to the presence of heparin in the tested sample, demonstrating a lower response to the heparin-containing blood (serum) *(45,46)*.

As the best among known markers of myocardial cell death, cTnI and cTnT have much in common as biochemical and immunochemical targets. Knowledge obtained by scientists studying the forms of cTnI in blood can be helpful for those who are developing new antibodies for the next generation cTnT assay.

ABBREVIATIONS

AMI, Acute myocardial infarction; CK, creatine kinase; CK-MB, MB isoenzyme of CK; cTnT, cTnI, and cTnC, cardiac troponin T, I, and C; MAbs, monoclonal antibodies; PKA, protein kinase A; PKC, protein kinase C.

REFERENCES

1. Cummins B, Auckland ML, Cummins P. Cardiac-specific troponin-I radioimmunoassay in the diagnosis of acute myocardial infarction. Am Heart J 1987;113:1333–1344.
2. Katus HA, Remppis A, Looser S, Hallermeier K, Scheffold T, Kubler W. Enzyme linked immuno assay of cardiac troponin T for the detection of acute myocardial infarction in patients. J Mol Cell Cardiol 1989;21:1349–1353.
3. Apple FS, Murakami M, Panteghini M, et al. International survey on the use of cardiac markers. Clin Chem 2001;47:587–588.
4. Katrukha A, Bereznikova A, Filatov V, Esakova T. Biochemical factors influencing measurement of cardiac troponin I in serum. Clin Chem Lab Med 1999;37:1091–1095.
5. Wu AH, Feng YJ, Moore R, et al. Characterization of cardiac troponin subunit release into serum after acute myocardial infarction and comparison of assays for troponin T and I. Clin Chem 1998;44:1198–1208.
6. Christenson RH, Duh SH, Apple FS, et al. Standardization of cardiac troponin I assays: round Robin of ten candidate reference materials. Clin Chem 2001;47:431–437.
7. Bodor GS, Porterfield D, Voss EM, Smith S, Apple FS. Cardiac troponin-I is not expressed in fetal and healthy or diseased adult human skeletal muscle tissue. Clin Chem 1995;41: 1710–1715.
8. Hammerer-Lercher A, Erlacher P, Bittner R, et al. Clinical and experimental results on cardiac troponin expression in Duchenne muscular dystrophy. Clin Chem 2001;47:451–458.
9. Adams JE 3rd, Sicard GA, Allen BT, et al. Diagnosis of perioperative myocardial infarction with measurement of cardiac troponin I. N Engl J Med 1994,10;330:670–674.
10. Mair J. Progress in myocardial damage detection: new biochemical markers for clinicians. Crit Rev Clin Lab Sci 1997;34:1–66.
11. Vallins WJ, Brand NJ, Dabhade N, Butler-Browne G, Yacoub MH, Barton PJR. Molecular cloning of human cardiac troponin I using polymerase chain reaction. FEBS Lett 1990;270: 57–61.
12. Wade R, Eddy R, Shows TB, Kedes L. cDNA sequence, tissue-specific expression, and chromosomal mapping of the human slow-twitch skeletal muscle isoform of troponin I. Genomics 1990;7:346–357.
13. Zhu L, Perez-Alvarado G, Wade R. Sequencing of a cDNA encoding the human fast-twitch skeletal muscle isoform of troponin I. Biochim Biophys Acta 1994;1217:338–340.

14. Takahashi M, Lee L, Shi Q, Gawad Y, Jackowski G. Use of enzyme immunoassay for measurement of skeletal troponin-I utilizing isoform-specific monoclonal antibodies. Clin Biochem 1996;29:301–308.

15. Leavis P, Gergely J. Thin filament proteins and thin filament-linked regulation of vertebrate muscle contraction. CRC Crit Rev Biochem 1984;16:235–305.

16. Filatov VL, Katrukha AG, Bulargina TV, Gusev NB. Troponin: structure, properties, and mechanism of functioning. Biochemistry (Mosc) 1999;64:969–985.

17. Wattanapermpool J, Guo X, Solaro RJ. The unique amino-terminal peptide of cardiac troponin I regulates myofibrillar activity only when it is phosphorylated. J Mol Cell Cardiol 1995;27(7):1383–1391.

18. Venema RC, Kuo JF. Protein kinase C-mediated phosphorylation of troponin I and C-protein in isolated myocardial cells is assosiated with inhibition of myofibrillar actomysoin MgATPase. J Biol Chem 1993;268:2705–2711.

19. Noland TA, Kuo JF. Protein kinase C phosphorylation of cardiac troponin I and troponin T inhibits Ca^{2+} stimulated MgATPase activity in reconstituted actomyosin and isolated myofibrils and decreases actin-myosin interaction. J Mol Cell Cardiol 1993;25:53–65.

20. Ebashi S, Wakabayashi T, Ebashi F. Troponin and its components. J Biochem (Tokyo) 1971; 69:441–445.

21. Leavis P, Gergely J. Thin filament proteins and thin filament-linked regulation of vertebrate muscle contraction. CRC Crit Rev Biochem 1984;16:235–305.

22. Zot AS, Potter JD. Structural aspects of troponin-tropomyosin regulation of skeletal muscle contraction. Annu Rev Biophys Biophys Chem 1987;16:535–559.

23. Robertson SP, Johnson JD, Potter JD. The time-course of the Ca^{2+} exchange with calmodulin, troponin, parvalbumin and myosin in response to transient increase in Ca^{2+}. Biophys J 1981;34:559–568.

24. Ingraham RH, Swenson CA. Binary interactions of troponin subunits. J Biol Chem 1984; 259:9544–9548.

25. Farah CS, Miyamoto CA, Ramos CHI, et al. Structural and regulatory functions of the NH_2- and COOH-terminal regions of skeletal muscle troponin I. J Biol Chem 1994;269:5230–5240.

26. Olah GA, Trewhella J. A model structure of the muscle protein complex $4Ca^{2+}$-troponin C-troponin I derived from small-angle scattering data: implication for regulation. Biochemistry 1994;33:12800–12806.

27. Bodor GS, Porter S, Landt Y, Ladenson JH. Development of monoclonal antibodies for an assay of cardiac troponin-I and preliminary results in suspected cases of myocardial infarction. Clin Chem 1992;38:2203–2214.

28. Katrukha AG, Bereznikova AV, Pulkki K, et al. Kinetics of liberation of free and total troponin I in sera of patients with acute myocardial infarction. Clin Chem 1997;43(S6):S106.

29. Katrukha AG, Bereznikova AV, Esakova TV, et al. Troponin I is released in the blood stream of patients with acute myocardial infarction not in the free form, but as a complex. Clin Chem 1997;43:1379–1385.

30. Katrukha A, Bereznikova A, Pettersson K. New approach to standardisation of human cardiac troponin I (cTnI). Scand J Clin Lab Invest 1999;230(Suppl):124–127.

31. Datta P, Foster K, Dasgupta A. Comparison of immunoreactivity of five human cardiac troponin I assays toward free and complexed forms of the antigen: implications for assay discordance. Clin Chem 1999;45:2266–2269.

32. Venge P, Lindahl B, Wallentin L. New generation cardiac troponin I assay for the ACCESS immunoassay system. Clin Chem 2001;47:959–961.

33. Katrukha A, Bereznikova A, Filatov V, et al. Binary cTnI –cTnT complex in AMI serum. Clin Chem Lab Med 1999;S449, H 092.

34. Giuliani I, Bertinchant JP, Granier C, et al. Determination of cardiac troponin I forms in the blood of patients with acute myocardial infarction and patients receiving crystalloid or cold blood cardioplegia. Clin Chem 1999;45:213–222.

35. Katrukha AG, Bereznikova AV, Esakova TV, Severina ME, Petterson K, Lovgren T. Troponin complex for the preparation of troponin I calibrators and standards. Clin Chem 1997;43(S6):S106.

36. Katrukha AG, Bereznikova AV, Filatov VL, et al. Cardiac troponin I degradation: application for reliable immunodetection. Clin Chem 1998;44:2433–2440.

37. McDonough JL, Arrell DK, Van Eyk JE. Troponin I degradation and covalent complex formation accompanies myocardial ischemia/reperfusion injury. Circ Res 1999;84:122–124.

38. Van Eyk JE, Powers F, Law W, Larue C, Hodges RS, Solaro RJ. Breakdown and release of myofilament proteins during ischemia and ischemia/reperfusion in rat hearts: identification of degradation products and effects on the pCa-force relation. Circ Res 1998;82: 261–271.

39. Di Lisa F, De Tullio R, Salamino F, et al. Specific degradation of troponin T and I by mucalpain and its modulation by substrate phosphorylation. Biochem J 1995;308:57–61.

40. Morjana NA. Degradation of human cardiac troponin I after myocardial infarction. Biotechnol Appl Biochem 1998;28:105–111.

41. Ward DG, Ashton PR, Trayer HR, Trayer IP. Additional PKA phosphorylation sites in human cardiac troponin I. Eur J Biochem 2001;268:179–185.

42. Labugger R, Organ L, Neverova I, Van Eyk J. Ischemia–reperfusion induced novel phosphorylation of TnI: implications for serum diagnostics. Clin Chem 2001;47(S6):A213.

43. Katrukha A, Bereznikova A, Filatov V, Kolosova O, Pettersson K, Bulargina T. Monoclonal antibodies affected by cTnI phosphorylation. Part of cTnI in the blood of AMI patients is phosphorylated? Clin Chem Lab Med 1999;S 448, H 091.

44. Cummins B, Russell GJ, Cummins P. A monoclonal antibody that distinguishes phospho- and dephosphorylated forms of cardiac troponin-I. Biochem Soc Trans 1991;19:161S.

45. Gerhardt W, Nordin G, Herbert AK, et al. Troponin T and I assays show decreased concentrations in heparin plasma compared with serum: lower recoveries in early than in late phases of myocardial injury. Clin Chem 2000;46:817–821.

46. Stiegler H, Fischer Y, Vazquez-Jimenez JF, et al. Lower cardiac troponin T and I results in heparin-plasma than in serum. Clin Chem 2000;46:1338–1344.

47. Wagner TL, Schessler HM, Liotta LA, Day AR. On the interaction of cardiac troponin I (cTNI) and heparin. A possible solution. Clin Chem 2001;47(S6):A213.

48. Dangas G, Konstadoulakis MM, Epstein SE, et al. Prevalence of autoantibodies against contractile proteins in coronary artery disease and their clinical implications. Am J Cardiol 2000;85:870-872, A6, A9.

49. Sakamaki S, Takayanagi N, Yoshizaki N, et al. Autoantibodies against the specific epitope of human tropomyosin(s) detected by a peptide based enzyme immunoassay in sera of patients with ulcerative colitis show antibody dependent cell mediated cytotoxicity against HLA-DPw9 transfected L cells. Gut 2000;47:236–241.

50. Leon JS, Godsel LM, Wang K, Engman DM. Cardiac myosin autoimmunity in acute Chagas' heart disease. Infect Immun 2001;69:5643–5649.

51. Bohner J, von Pape KW, Hannes W, Stegmann T. False-negative immunoassay results for cardiac troponin I probably due to circulating troponin I autoantibodies. Clin Chem 1996; 42:2046.

52. Tanasijevic MJ, Cannon CP, Antman EM. The role of cardiac troponin-I (cTnI) in risk stratification of patients with unstable coronary artery disease. Clin Cardiol 1999;22:13–16.

53. Morrow DA, Antman EM, Tanasijevic M, et al. Cardiac troponin I for stratification of early outcomes and the efficacy of enoxaparin in unstable angina: a TIMI-11B substudy. J Am Coll Cardiol 2000;36:1812–1817.

54. Teles R, Ferreira J, Aguiar C, et al. Prognostic value of cardiac troponin I release kinetics in unstable angina. Rev Port Cardiol 2000;19:407–422.

55. Ottani F, Galvani M, Ferrini D, et al. Direct comparison of early elevations of cardiac troponin T and I in patients with clinical unstable angina. Am Heart J 1999;137:284–291.

56. Hamm CW. Progress in the diagnosis of unstable angina and perspectives for treatment. Eur Heart J 1998;19(Suppl N):N48–N50.
57. Ottani F, Galvani M, Nicolini FA, et al. Elevated cardiac troponin levels predict the risk of adverse outcome in patients with acute coronary syndromes. Am Heart J 2000;140:917–927.
58. Heeschen C, Goldmann BU, Moeller RH, Hamm CW. Analytical performance and clinical application of a new rapid bedside assay for the detection of serum cardiac troponin I. Clin Chem 1998;44:1925–1930.
59. Apple FS, Anderson FP, Collinson P, et al. Clinical evaluation of the first medical whole blood, point-of-care testing device for detection of myocardial infarction. Clin Chem 2000; 46:1604–1609.
60. Ash J, Baxevanakis G, Bilandzic L, Shin H, Kadijevic L. Development of an automated quantitative latex immunoassay for cardiac troponin I in serum. Clin Chem 2000;46:1521–1522.
61. Uettwiller-Geiger D, Wu AHB, Apple FS, et al. Analytical performance of Beckman Coulter's Access® AccuTnI™ (Troponin I) in a multicenter evaluation. Clin Chem 2002;48:869–876.
62. Jevans AV, Apple FS, Wu AH, et al. Clinical performance of Beckmam Coulter's Access® AccuTnI™ (troponin I) in a multicenter clinical trial. Clin Chem 2000;47(S6):A205.
63. Larue C, Calzolari C, Bertinchant JP, Leclercq F, Grolleau R, Pau B. Cardiac-specific immunoenzymometric assay of troponin I in the early phase of acute myocardial infarction. Clin Chem 1993;39:972–979.
64. Suetomi K, Takahama K. A sandwich enzyme immunoassay for cardiac troponin I. Nippon Hoigaku Zasshi 1995;49:26–32.
65. Filatov VL, Katrukha AG, Bereznikova AV, et al. Epitope mapping of anti-TnI monoclonal antibodies. Biochem Mol Biol Intern 1998;45:1179–1187.
66. Larue C, Defacque-Lacquement H, Calzolari C, Le Nguyen D, Pau B. New monoclonal antibodies as probes for human cardiac troponin I: epitopic analysis with synthetic peptides. Mol Immunol 1992;29:271–278.
67. Rama D, Calzolari C, Granier C, Pau B. Epitope localization of monoclonal antibodies used in human troponin I immunoenzymometric assay. Hybridoma 1997;16:153–157.
68. Larue C, Ferrieres G, Laprade M, Calzolari C, Granier C. Antigenic definition of cardiac troponin I. Clin Chem Lab Med 1998;36:361–365.
69. Ferrieres G, Calzolari C, Mani JC, et al. Human cardiac troponin I: precise identification of antigenic epitopes and prediction of secondary structure. Clin Chem 1998;44:487–493.
70. Hansen A, Kemp K, Kemp E, et al. High-dose stabilized chlorite matrix WF10 prolongs cardiac xenograft survival in the hamster-to-rat model without inducing ultrastructural or biochemical signs of cardiotoxicity. Pharmacol Toxicol 2001;89:92–95.
71. Ricchiuti V, Sharkey SW, Murakami MM, Voss EM, Apple FS. Cardiac troponin I and T alterations in dog hearts with myocardial infarction: correlation with infarct size. Am J Clin Pathol 1998;110:241–247.
72. Ricchiuti V, Zhang J, Apple FS. Cardiac troponin I and T alterations in hearts with severe left ventricular remodeling. Clin Chem 1997;43:990–995.
73. Muller-Bardorff M, Hallermayer K, Schroder A, et al. Improved troponin T ELISA specific for cardiac troponin T isoform: assay development and analytical and clinical validation. Clin Chem 43:458–466.
74. Katrukha A, Bereznikova A, Filatov V, Kolosova O, Pettersson K, Bulargina T. Troponin T degradation in necrotic human cardiac tissue. Clin Chem Lab Med 1999;S 449, H 093.
75. Baum H, Braun S, Gerhardt W, et al. Multicenter evaluation of a second-generation assay for cardiac troponin T. Clin Chem 1997;43:1877–1884.
76. Noland TA Jr, Raynor RL, Kuo JF. Identification of sites phosphorylated in bovine cardiac troponin I and troponin T by protein kinase C and comparative substrate activity of synthetic peptides containing the phosphorylation sites. J Biol Chem 1989;264:20778–20785.
77. Jideama NM, Noland TA Jr, Raynor RL, et al. Phosphorylation specificities of protein kinase C isozymes for bovine cardiac troponin I and troponin T and sites within these proteins and regulation of myofilament properties. J Biol Chem 1996;271:23277–23283.

11

Interferences in Immunoassays for Cardiac Troponin

Kiang-Teck J. Yeo and Daniel M. Hoefner

INTRODUCTION

Cardiac troponin has largely replaced the MB isoenzyme of creatine kinase (CK-MB) as a key biochemical marker in the assessment of myocardial damage because of its high sensitivity *(1)* and cardiac specificity *(2)*. The recent joint proposal by the American College of Cardiology (ACC)/European Society for Cardiology (ESC) for the redefinition of myocardial infarction (MI) places cardiac troponin in a central role in the diagnostic workup of MI. A cardiac troponin value above the 99th percentile cut point of a reference population is considered abnormal and MI is diagnosed when serial troponins are increased in the clinical setting of acute ischemia *(3)*. Because cardiac troponin has a cornerstone role in the diagnosis of MI, has prognostic implications in patients with acute coronary syndromes (ACS) *(4–6)*, and a role in guiding antithrombotic therapy *(7–9)*, it is crucial that troponin assays have robust analytical performance to allow for reliable measurements, especially at low abnormal ranges.

Cardiac troponin assays are two-site "sandwich" immunoassays, with a primary capture antibody and a secondary detector antibody (Fig. 1A). As such, various analytical issues may affect immunoassays, in general, giving rise to occasional false-positive or false-negative results in a particular patient. In addition, assay imprecision in the upper reference cutoff region can dramatically affect the incidence of false-positive readings by that method. This chapter reviews the effects of the presence of human anti-animal antibodies and autoantibodies, low-end imprecision, and sample matrix differences (serum vs plasma) on cardiac troponin assays. Recognizing these effects will help minimize incorrect interpretations of this important marker in the assessment of ACS.

HUMAN ANTI-ANIMAL ANTIBODIES

Exposure to animal antigens can give rise to human anti-animal antibodies (HA) that can cause analytical interferences with various immunoassays *(10–13)*. The HA elicited can be of the immunoglobulin (Ig) classes IgG, IgM, IgA, and occasionally IgE. Heterophilic antibodies are human antibodies that arise from challenges by poorly defined animal immunogens; historically the term was associated with IgM antibodies observed with mononucleosis *(12)*. If exposure to a specific animal immunogen is known, the correct term should refer to the specific animal that is implicated, rather than classifying the antibodies as heterophilic *(14)*. Thus, an HA elicited by exposure to mouse antigens

From: *Cardiac Markers, Second Edition*
Edited by: Alan H. B. Wu @ Humana Press Inc., Totowa, NJ

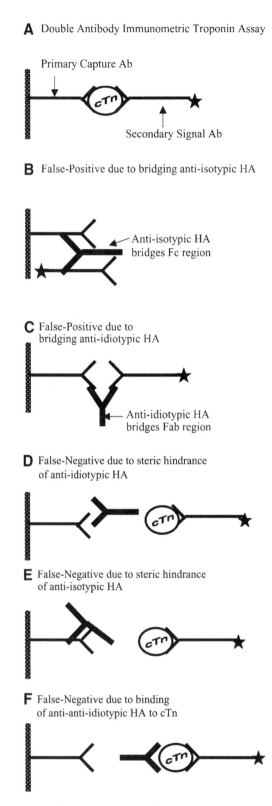

Fig. 1. Types of HA and possible mechanisms of interferences. (Adapted from Klee GG *[29]*.)

should be termed "human anti-mouse antibody" (HAMA). The prevalence of HA has previously been reported to vary from as low as 0.19% *(15)* to as high as 80% *(12)*.

Various causes that could elicit HA include iatrogenic exposure to animal-derived pharmaceuticals, such as murine monoclonal antibody-targeted imaging reagents, anti-cancer drugs, and vaccines. HA could also arise due to noniatrogenic exposure to animal proteins that occurs during veterinary and farm work, during food preparation, or by the presence of domestic animals in the home *(12)*. Owing to the increasing use of murine monoclonal antibodies for imaging and therapeutic drug targeting, the most common type of HA reported is typically a HAMA. It has been reported that even single low-dose injections of radiolabeled murine monoclonal antibodies can elicit HAMA in 41% of patients within a period of 2 wk *(16)*.

The first description of a falsely elevated cardiac troponin I (cTnI) was the case of a 69-yr-old man with an admission cTnI of 106 ng/mL (measured on the Abbott AxSYM method), but with no clinical evidence of acute MI (AMI) *(17)*. In the presence of a blocking agent containing animal immunoglobulins, the value decreased to <2.0% of the original. This indicates the presence of multispecific heterophilic antibodies that link the murine monoclonal capture and secondary labeled goat polyclonal antibodies, giving rise to a false-positive result. In addition, the original AxSYM cTnI assay appeared to be more susceptible to generating a heterophilic antibody-derived false-positive result when compared with other commercial immunoassays, which showed essentially normal values for this specimen *(17)*.

This differential susceptibility to HA with different troponin methods may be related to the effectiveness of the type of blocking agents incorporated into the formulation, the format of the immunoassay, and the type (e.g., IgG vs IgM) and concentration of the circulating HA. In addition, we and others also reported false-positive cTnI results due to presence of rheumatoid factors (RF) with the AxSYM assay *(18–20)* and other HA with the AxSYM and Beckman Access methods *(21)*. RF are usually IgM isotypic antibodies that can bind not only human IgG but also a wide variety of animal immunoglobulins *(22–24)*. Enhancement of the troponin assay by Abbott due to the inclusion of effective blocking agents has significantly reduced much of this HA interference *(15,20)*, although, in an occasional patient, a false-positive result may still occur *(20)*.

In contrast, the incidence of HA-related false-negative cTnI is less frequently encountered. Bohner et al. reported a false-negative cTnI in a patient undergoing coronary artery bypass graft surgery who had serial evolving CK-MB and cardiac troponin T (cTnT) indicative of perioperative MI *(25)*. Although they surmised that this interference on the original Stratus cTnI assay was unlikely due to HA, and attributed it to circulating cTnI autoantibodies, the presence of a type of blocking HA cannot be conclusively ruled out.

HA, once developed, are known to persist for months and can be detectable even up to 30 mo after the initial exposure *(26,27)*. Kazmierczak et al. recently reported a case study describing the sudden appearance of heterophilic antibodies in a patient that caused transient false-positive CK-MB, cTnI, and cTnT measurements with various commercial cardiac marker immunoassays *(28)*. Interestingly, over the course of several weeks, transient spikes of false-positive cTnI were observed interspersed with periods of normal values, indicating the highly variable appearance and disappearance of these heterophilic antibodies.

Table 1
Blocking Reagents and Composition

Company	Blocking reagents	Composition
Scantibodies Laboratory, Inc.	Heterophilic blocking reagent (HBR)	Specific murine immunoglobulins with high affinity for heterophilic antibodies
	Non Specific Antibody Blocking Reagent (NABR)	Nonspecific immunoglobulins that passively blocks heterophilic antibodies
Bioreclamation Inc.	Immunoglobulin Inhibiting Reagent (IIR)	Proprietary immunoglobulins formulation with high affinity for HA
Omega Biochemicals	Heteroblock reagent	Active and passive blocking mixture
Roche Diagnostics	MAB 33	Monoclonal IgG_1
	Poly MAB 33	Polymeric monoclonal IgG_1/Fab

Mechanisms of HA Interferences and Elimination

HA that bind to the Fc region of immunoglobulin are termed *antiisotypic antibodies*, while those that bind to the variable Fab region are termed *antiidiotypic antibodies*. In general, antiisotypic HA are more commonly encountered than antiidiotypic HA *(29)*. As shown in Fig. 1B,C, either type of HA can bridge the capture and secondary labeled antibodies, causing a false-positive cTn result. For example, the AxSYM cTnI immunoassay has a capture mouse monoclonal antibody/goat polyclonal-labeled second antibody format; multispecific heterophilic antibodies can bridge the two antibodies giving rise to a false-positive result in the absence of cTnI. Alternatively, it is possible that antiidiotypic or antiisotypic HA can bind the capture antibody in a way that causes steric hindrance to the binding of the ligand, resulting in a false-negative result (Fig. 1D,E). False-negative results may also arise from the presence of anti-antiidiotypic HA, which can bind to cTn directly and block access of the capture antibody to the ligand (Fig. 1F).

Various strategies have been used to reduce or eliminate interferences due to HA. Most modern commercial immunoassays have HA blockers (Table 1) incorporated in the formulation; these may include polyclonal IgG, polymeric mouse IgG, a mixture of animal serum proteins, nonimmune serum, or IgG fragments (Fab/Fc) from the species employed to develop the reagent antibodies *(12)*. The efficacy of these blocking agents is dependent on the concentration, class/subclass, specificity, and valence of the HA present *(30)*. Thus, it is impossible to eradicate completely HA interferences due to the occasional presence of a unique subclass of HA that is not blocked by these agents. Utilization of capture and detector reagent antibodies developed in different species (e.g., murine monoclonal/goat polyclonal) has been proposed to minimize the effects of HAMA *(31)*. However, the effectiveness of this method is questionable, especially in the presence of multispecific heterophilic antibodies that can cross-react with antibodies derived from different animal species *(17)*.

The format of the immunoassay, that is, one-step simultaneous vs a two-step sequential incubation, may make the former more susceptible as HA could be washed away after the first incubation in a two-step assay *(32)*. Another important consideration is that even cardiac assays with the same format (e.g., AxSYM CK-MB and original AxSYM cTnI) can show differential susceptibility to heterophilic antibodies (normal CK-MB, falsely elevated cTnI) if a blocking agent is incorporated into the first reagent step but not the second *(17)*. Another strategy is to employ Fab or F(ab')$_2$ fragments instead of intact immunoglobulin in the design of two-site immunoassays in an attempt to eliminate the interference of antiidiotypic HA with specificity to the Fc region. The other approach is to use chimeric murine/human antibodies as the capture or second labeled antibody (e.g., Roche Elecsys TSH and CEA assays) where the variable region is a murine/human construct; this should minimize the binding of HAMA and other HA *(12)*.

LOW-END PRECISION ISSUES

Owing to the recommendation to use the 99th percentile value (3 SD value above the mean) as the upper reference cutoff limit for cardiac troponin assays under the new ESC/ACC guidelines *(3)*, it is important to assess how robust these values are under realistic day-to-day operation of the clinical laboratory. Large imprecision of the assay around the 99th percentile cut point will lead to increased frequency of falsely abnormal values. It is conventional to determine reference ranges using an apparently healthy population where samples are measured in either a single analytical run or several runs spanning a short period of time, and frequently with one reagent lot. Thus, the 99th percentile cut point determined this way, although statistically valid, might be unrealistically low when between-run assay imprecision is taken into account across several lots of reagents with different analytical calibrations.

Recently, we performed a study *(33)* of six common commercial cardiac troponin assays to determine the lowest value corresponding to a coefficient of variation (CV) of 20%, which is defined as functional sensitivity. The main objective of this project was to investigate if the published upper reference values can be realistically attained under routine clinical laboratory working conditions. Precision profiles were determined with four patient pools that were assayed over a period of 8–10 wk that spanned the low normal to AMI cutoff ranges. We found that out of these six cTn assays, only one had an upper reference limit (URL) that was twice as high as the functional sensitivity. The implication was that most of the other cTn assays had URLs that were unrealistically low, and if used without modification, would result in an increased incidence of false-positive cTn values. This could cause inappropriate diagnosis or management decisions in the clinical evaluation of ACS.

The National Academy of Clinical Biochemistry *(34)* and ESC/ACC *(3)* have both recommended that cardiac troponin assays should show imprecision (CV) of ≤10% at the medical decision limits. In an attempt to translate the above guidelines to clinical trials, Apple et al. *(35)* suggested that the lowest achievable concentration with a CV of 10% be used as the cut point for cardiac injury. They also showed, however, that (based on the information derived from package inserts) at present, no manufacturer of cardiac troponin assays can meet the standard of ≤10% CV at the 99th percentile cut point, and challenged the industry to define this important cut point systematically. In addition, development of future generations of cTn assays with improved low-end precision should result in the convergence of the 10% CV and 99th percentile cut points. Such improvements in the precision at the low end are especially crucial for the ability to translate the recent research finding that minor elevations of cTn are prognostic for selection of patients with unstable angina and non-ST elevation MI for invasive therapies *(36)* to the routine clinical practice.

To this end, the Committee of Standardization of Markers of Cardiac Damage, a subcommittee of the International Federation of Clinical Chemistry, has commissioned an international collaborative study to determine the 10% CV of various commercially available cTnI and cTnT assays. Our laboratory is participating in this joint effort and has prepared eight serum pools spanning the upper reference to AMI cutoff values. Aliquots were mailed to participating vendors who will assay these specimens over 20 working days with two separate reagent lots and three separate calibrations. Precision profiles of each troponin assay will be constructed and the corresponding 10% CV value will be defined. This study is currently underway and, when completed, will provide information that will help determine whether the current 99th percentile reference and 10% CV values cited in various cTn assay product inserts can meet the 10% CV requirements as mandated by the ESC/ACC.

IMPACT OF SERUM VS PLASMA SPECIMEN ON cTn ASSAYS

The presence of fibrin strands in plasma or in serum that is processed for analysis prior to complete clot formation is well known to cause errors in many immunoassay systems. Although this is relatively common knowledge in the field of clinical chemistry, little has been detailed in the scientific literature in this regard. Nosanchuk reported on falsely increased levels of cTnI that were attributed to incomplete serum separation *(37)*. During the analysis of paired serum and plasma samples, several discordant (elevated serum) results were observed, which were reproducible on reanalysis. However, when the serum samples were recentrifuged, subsequent analysis was in agreement with the results obtained with plasma. In addition, when serum samples that deliberately contained microfibrin strands were tested, falsely elevated results were observed *(37)*. Thus, if serum is used, it is important to ensure that the clotting process is complete prior to centrifugation so as to eliminate the presence of microfibrin strands. For heparinized samples that have been in storage for extended periods, it is essential to check that fibrin strands, following heparin degradation, are not present prior to analysis.

Plasma is becoming the specimen of choice for most automated immunoassays; one of the primary reasons for this is that it allows for a decreased turn around time, which is especially important for potentially emergent assays such as those used to assess cardiac damage. Furthermore, fresh plasma may eliminate the problems associated with fibrin, mentioned above. However, most product literature for cTn assays shows a potential negative bias in plasma compared to serum. Recent reports also indicate that cTnI and cTnT may be falsely decreased in plasma from heparinized blood *(38–40)*. Gerhardt et al. *(39)* showed that mean levels of cTnT were about 15% lower in heparinized plasma samples when compared to serum samples. In addition, when heparin was added to the sera of patients with AMI, decreased cTnT results were obtained.

Troponin exists as a complex of three proteins (cTnC, cTnI, cTnT) that interact with tropomyosin, actin, and the myosin complex to form the functional unit of contraction in cardiac and skeletal muscle. Following myocardial damage, the troponins that are released circulate predominantly in one of three forms: the ternary complex containing all three molecular forms; the binary complex consisting of the cTnC–cTnI heterodimer; or they may exist in free form, of which the cTnT predominates *(41,42)*. It has been observed that the most discrepant values for plasma vs serum cTn occurred in samples that were taken during the early phase of myocardial damage, when cytosolic (free) cTnT may be proportionally most elevated in respect to the cTn complexes *(39)*. Stiegler and others noted similar but less dramatic plasma/serum changes for cTnT, which may be a result of different blood collection systems and heparin concentrations as well as different cTn complex ratios attributable to the timing of sample collection from the time of the coronary event *(40)*. Although the National Academy of Clinical Biochemistry recommends the use of plasma samples for cTn measurements *(34)*, the consensus of the Gerhardt and Stiegler studies *(39,40)* is that, until the plasma–serum bias issues can be resolved, the sample choice for cTn measurements should be serum.

The mechanism by which plasma gives falsely lower results is not fully understood. Katrukha et al. *(43)* have suggested that troponin immunoreactivity may be modified either via protein conformational changes or steric hindrance of epitopes upon heparin–cTnI complex formation. In addition, the various types of troponin complexes may create or conceal various epitopes *(42,44)*. These complexes are influenced by the availability of calcium *(45)* and, thus, anticoagulants that bind calcium (e.g., ethylene diaminetetraacetic acid [EDTA]) may have a marked impact on the assay. Whereas heparin does not appear to have a complex-dissociating effect, addition of EDTA can dissociate the troponin complexes into individual subunits *(41)*.

DEGRADATION OF cTn AND EPITOPE STABILITY

Bodor et al. *(46)* showed that the degree of cTnI phosphorylation in the failing hearts of transplant patients is reduced from the level measured in normal hearts. It is plausible that these heart failure associated changes could affect both epitope stability as well as antibody recognition. Regarding the latter, it has been shown that certain antibodies will react only with the phosphorylated form of cTnI *(47)*. In addition, oxidation of cTn may also occur, which can induce conformational changes to the protein *(45)*. Wu et al. *(41)* assessed the influence of the state of protein oxidation/reduction as measured by nine different cTnI immunoassays and found that in some assay systems the apparent concentration varied by more than fourfold, depending on the type of cTn subunit and the oxidation/reduction status of the measured complex. Because cTnI slowly oxidizes to form disulfide linkages after blood collection, they warn that unless stabilizing agents are added, some assays may yield a differential response to the reduced vs the oxidized forms *(41)*. Other studies have shown that oxidative modification allows myocardial proteins to become more vulnerable to proteolysis during ischemic episodes *(48)*. Besides the differences observed in the immunoreactivity of subunit complexes, immunoreactive fragments may also be generated as proteins undergo proteolytic cleavage.

Degradation of cTnI may have a significant effect on its stability and immunological activity, and it has been observed that cTnI fragments vary significantly in their reactivity. This has important analytical and clinical implications in that very little intact cTnI exists in serum samples that are typically collected 1–5 d following MI *(49)*. While the degradation of cTnI is associated with a loss of immunoreactivity *(49)*, cTnC may enhance the immunological activity of some, but not all, fragments *(50)*. If the cTnI fragment contains the inhibitory region of the molecule, it is relatively resistant to proteolytic degradation when complexed with cTnC *(50)*. Differential degradation of cTnI is also an important factor in assay-to-assay variability that may account for up to a 20-fold variation in results obtained with different methods *(41,51)*. Because of the many caveats that may influence immunoreactivity, it has been suggested that antibodies developed

Table 2
Cardiac Troponin Assays

Manufacturer	Immunoassay format	99th Percentile (ng/mL)[a]	AMI (ROC) cutoff (ng/mL)[a]
Abbott AxSYM cTnI	Monoclonal/goat polyclonal	0.50	2.00
Bayer ACS 180 cTnI	Monoclonal/goat polyclonal	0.10	1.00–1.50
Bayer ADVIA Centaur cTnI	Monoclonal/goat polyclonal	0.10	1.00–1.50
Bayer Immuno I cTnI	Monoclonal/goat polyclonal	0.10	0.90
Beckman Access cTnI	Monoclonal/monoclonal	0.04	0.50
BioMerieux Vidas cTnI	Monoclonal/monoclonal	0.10	0.80
Biosite Triage cTnI	Monoclonal/goat polyclonal	0.19	1.0
Byk-Santec Liason cTnI	Monoclonal/goat polyclonal	0.03	NA
Dade Dimension RxL cTnI	Monoclonal/goat polyclonal	0.07	1.50
Dade Opus cTnI	Monoclonal/goat polyclonal	0.10	1.50
Dade Stratus CS cTnI	Monoclonal/monoclonal	0.07	1.50
DPC Immulite cTnI	Monoclonal/bovine polyclonal	<1.00[d]	1.00
First Medical *Alpha Dx* cTnI	Monoclonal/goat polyclonal	0.09[b]	0.40
Innotrac cTnI	Monoclonal/monoclonal	0.10[b] (Serum) 0.08[b] (Plasma)	0.20–0.40
Tosoh cTnI	Monoclonal/monoclonal	0.45	1.35
Ortho Vitros ECi cTnI	Monoclonal/goat polyclonal	0.10[c] (Serum) 0.08[c] (Plasma)	1.00 (Serum) 0.80 (Plasma)
Roche Elecsys cTnT	Monoclonal/monoclonal	0.01	0.10

[a]Package insert information or correspondence with manufacturer.
[b]95th percentile cut point.
[c]97.5th percentile cut point.
[d]98.0th percentile cut point.
NA, Not available.

for use in troponin assays have the epitope characteristics that are not affected by complex formation, degree of phosphorylation, pI effects, and oxidation/reduction status, and have domains that are resistant to proteolysis *(42,50,52)*. The proteolysis-resistant region of cTnI lies in the central part of the molecule *(43,50);* however, one dilemma of developing antibodies to that region is that it is the amino- (N)-terminal sequence of the molecule that is suggested to generate the high cardiac specificity of the anti-cTnI antibodies *(49)*.

SUMMARY

Current cTnI assays have variable upper reference limits as well as AMI cutoff values, with differences up to 25-fold (Table 2), owing to a lack of standardization between different commercial assays. This is attributed to several factors including the use of different calibrators, use of antibodies with different epitope specificities, and the presence of various molecular forms of troponin in circulation. Occasionally, falsely elevated results may arise due to the presence of HA; this situation should be suspected in view of a nonevolving elevated cTn that either does not fit the clinical picture or the serial kinetics of an evolving AMI. False-negative cTn results may be more difficult to detect, unless a gross discrepancy exists between the clinical assessment and cTn results. If interference due to HA is suspected, this could be verified by checking the suspicious result with an alternative cTn assay made by a different manufacturer, or by reassay of the specimen in the presence of HA blocking agents. It is important for each laboratory to validate the low end of the troponin assay, that is, the value corresponding to a 10% CV, so that the incidence of false abnormal results due to analytical imprecision of the method are minimized. This is currently a very important issue to address, as recent reports have shown that minor elevations of cTn can predict benefits for patients with unstable angina and non-ST elevation MI when they are given invasive treatments *(36)*.

Recognition of the various analytical factors that can cause variable immunorecognition of cTn forms/fragments in circulation should help manufacturers develop a better generation of troponin assays that are less affected by these factors, resulting in more consistent troponin measurements across all methods.

ABBREVIATIONS

ACC, American College of Cardiology; ACS, acute coronary syndrome(s); AMI, acute myocardial infarction; CK, creatine kinase; CK-MB, MB isoenzyme of CK; cTnT, cTnI, and cTnC, cardiac troponins T, I and C; CV, coefficient of variance; EDTA, ethylenediaminetetraacetic acid; ESC, European Society for Cardiology; HA, human anti-animal antibodies; HAMA, human anti-mouse antibody; Ig, immunoglobulin; MI, myocardial infarction; RF, rheumatoid factors; URL, upper reference limit.

REFERENCES

1. Dean KJ. Biochemistry and molecular biology of troponins I and T. In: Cardiac Markers. Wu AHB, ed. Totowa, NJ: Humana Press, 1998, pp. 193–194.
2. Katus HA, Scheffold T, Remppis A, Zehlein J. Proteins of the troponin complex. Lab Med 1992;23:311–317.
3. Myocardial infarction redefined—a consensus document of The Joint European Society of Cardiology/American College of Cardiology Committee for the redefinition of myocardial infarction. J Am Coll Cardiol 2000;36:959–969.
4. Lindahl B, Venge P, Wallentin L. Relation between troponin T and the risk of subsequent cardiac events in unstable coronary artery disease. The FRISC study group. Circulation 1996; 93:1651–1657.
5. Ohman EM, Armstrong PW, Christenson RH, et al. Cardiac troponin T levels for risk stratification in acute myocardial ischemia. GUSTO IIA Investigators. N Engl J Med 1996;335: 1333–1341.
6. Antman EM, Tanasijevic MJ, Thompson B, et al. Cardiac-specific troponin I levels to predict the risk of mortality in patients with acute coronary syndromes. N Engl J Med 1996; 335:1342–1349.
7. Lindahl B, Venge P, Wallentin L. Troponin T identifies patients with unstable coronary artery disease who benefit from long-term antithrombotic protection. Fragmin in Unstable Coronary Artery Disease (FRISC) Study Group. J Am Coll Cardiol 1997;29:43–48.
8. Hamm CW, Heeschen C, Goldmann B, et al. Benefit of abciximab in patients with refractory unstable angina in relation to serum troponin T levels. c7E3 Fab Antiplatelet Therapy in Unstable Refractory Angina (CAPTURE) Study Investigators. N Engl J Med 1999;340: 1623–1629.
9. Heeschen C, Hamm CW, Goldmann B, Deu A, Langenbrink L, White HD. Troponin concentrations for stratification of patients with acute coronary syndromes in relation to therapeutic efficacy of tirofiban. PRISM Study Investigators. Platelet Receptor Inhibition in Ischemic Syndrome Management. Lancet 1999;354:1757–1762.

10. Boscato LM, Stuart MC. Heterophilic antibodies: a problem for all immunoassays. Clin Chem 1988;34:27–33.
11. Levinson SS. Antibody multispecificity in immunoassay interference. Clin Biochem 1992; 25:77–87.
12. Kricka LJ. Human anti-animal antibody interferences in immunological assays. Clin Chem 1999;45:942–956.
13. Ward G, McKinnon L, Badrick T, Hickman PE. Heterophilic antibodies remain a problem for the immunoassay laboratory. Am J Clin Pathol 1997;108:417–421.
14. Kaplan IV, Levinson SS. When is a heterophile antibody not a heterophile antibody? When it is an antibody against a specific immunogen. Clin Chem 1999;45:616–618.
15. Yeo KT, Storm CA, Li Y, et al. Performance of the enhanced Abbott AxSYM cardiac troponin I reagent in patients with heterophilic antibodies. Clin Chim Acta 2000;292:13–23.
16. Dillman RO, Shawler DL, McCallister TJ, Halpern SE. Human anti-mouse antibody response in cancer patients following single low-dose injections of radiolabeled murine monoclonal antibodies. Cancer Biother 1994;9:17–28.
17. Fitzmaurice TF, Brown C, Rifai N, Wu AH, Yeo KT. False increase of cardiac troponin I with heterophilic antibodies. Clin Chem 1998;44:2212–2214.
18. Yeo KJT, Quinn-Hall KS, Jayne JE. False increase of cardiac troponin I in a patient with rheumatoid arthritis. Diagn Endocrinol Immunol Metab 1999;17:259–261.
19. Dasgupta A, Banerjee SK, Datta P. False-positive troponin I in the MEIA due to the presence of rheumatoid factors in serum. Elimination of this interference by using a polyclonal antisera against rheumatoid factors. Am J Clin Pathol 1999;112:753–756.
20. Onuska KD, Hill SA. Effect of rheumatoid factor on cardiac troponin I measurement using two commercial measurement systems. Clin Chem 2000;46:307–308.
21. Volk AL, Hardy R, Robinson CA. False-positive cardiac troponin I results. Lab Med 1999; 30:610–612.
22. Hamako J, Ozeki Y, Matsui T, et al. Binding of human IgM from a rheumatoid factor to IgG of 12 animal species. Comp Biochem Physiol B Biochem Mol Biol 1995;112:683–688.
23. Hamilton RG, Whittington K, Warner NB, Arnett FC. Human IgM rheumatoid factor reactivity with rabbit, sheep, goat and mouse immunoglobulin (abstract). Clin Chem 1988; 34:1165.
24. Hamilton RG. Rheumatoid factor interference in immunological methods. Monogr Allergy 1989;26:27–44.
25. Bohner J, von Pape KW, Hannes W, Stegmann T. False-negative immunoassay results for cardiac troponin I probably due to circulating troponin I autoantibodies. Clin Chem 1996; 42:2046.
26. Baum RP, Niesen A, Hertel A, et al. Activating anti-idiotypic human anti-mouse antibodies for immunotherapy of ovarian carcinoma. Cancer 1994;73:1121–1125.
27. Sharma SK, Bagshawe KD, Melton RG, Sherwood RF. Human immune response to monoclonal antibody–enzyme conjugates in ADEPT pilot clinical trial. Cell Biophys 1992;21: 109–120.
28. Kazmierczak SC, Catrou PG, Briley KP. Transient nature of interference effects from heterophile antibodies: examples of interference with cardiac marker measurements. Clin Chem Lab Med 2000;38:33–39.
29. Klee GG. Human anti-mouse antibodies. Arch Pathol Lab Med 2000;124:921–923.
30. Csako G, Weintraub BD, Zweig MH. The potency of immunoglobulin G fragments for inhibition of interference caused by anti-immunoglobulin antibodies in a monoclonal immunoradiometric assay for thyrotropin. Clin Chem 1988;34:1481–1483.
31. Bartlett WA, Browning MC, Jung RT. Artefactual increase in serum thyrotropin concentration caused by heterophilic antibodies with specificity for IgG of the family Bovidea. Clin Chem 1986;32:2214–2219.
32. Madry N, Auerbach B, Schelp C. Measures to overcome HAMA interferences in immunoassays. Anticancer Res 1997;17:2883–2886.

33. Yeo KT, Quinn-Hall KS, Bateman SW, Fischer GA, Wieczorek S, Wu AHB. Functional sensitivity of cardiac troponin assays and its implications for risk stratification for patients with acute coronary syndromes. In: Markers in Cardiology: Current and Future Clinical Applications. Adams JE, III, Apple FS, Jaffe AS, Wu AHB, eds. Armonk, NY: Futura, 2001, pp. 23–30.

34. Wu AH, Apple FS, Gibler WB, Jesse RL, Warshaw MM, Valdes R Jr. National Academy of Clinical Biochemistry Standards of Laboratory Practice: recommendations for the use of cardiac markers in coronary artery diseases. Clin Chem 1999;45:1104–1121.

35. Apple FS, Wu AHB, Jaffe AS. European Society of Cardiology and American College of Cardiology guidelines for redefinition of myocardial infarction: how to use existing assays clinically and for clinical trials. Am Heart J 2001;144:981–986.

36. Morrow DA, Cannon CP, Rifai N, et al. Ability of minor elevations of troponins I and T to predict benefit from an early invasive strategy in patients with unstable angina and non-ST elevation myocardial infarction: results from a randomized trial. JAMA 2001;286: 2405–2412.

37. Nosanchuk JS, Combs B, Abbott G. False increases of troponin I attributable to incomplete separation of serum. Clin Chem 1999;45:714.

38. Dorizzi RM, Ferrari A, Giannuzzi M, Cocco C. Lower cardiac troponin I and troponin T results in heparin plasma than in serum. Clin Chem 2001;47:A200.

39. Gerhardt W, Nordin G, Herbert AK, et al. Troponin T and I assays show decreased concentrations in heparin plasma compared with serum: lower recoveries in early than in late phases of myocardial injury. Clin Chem 2000;46:817–821.

40. Stiegler H, Fischer Y, Vazquez-Jimenez JF, et al. Lower cardiac troponin T and I results in heparin-plasma than in serum. Clin Chem 2000;46:1338–1344.

41. Wu AH, Feng YJ, Moore R, et al. Characterization of cardiac troponin subunit release into serum after acute myocardial infarction and comparison of assays for troponin T and I. American Association for Clinical Chemistry Subcommittee on cTnI Standardization. Clin Chem 1998;44:1198–1208.

42. Katrukha AG, Bereznikova AV, Esakova TV, et al. Troponin I is released in bloodstream of patients with acute myocardial infarction not in free form but as complex. Clin Chem 1997;43:1379–1385.

43. Katrukha A, Bereznikova A, Filatov V, Esakova T. Biochemical factors influencing measurement of cardiac troponin I in serum. Clin Chem Lab Med 1999;37:1091–1095.

44. Bodor GS, Porter S, Landt Y, Ladenson JH. Development of monoclonal antibodies for an assay of cardiac troponin-I and preliminary results in suspected cases of myocardial infarction. Clin Chem 1992;38:2203–2214.

45. Ingraham RH, Hodges RS. Effects of Ca^{2+} and subunit interactions on surface accessibility of cysteine residues in cardiac troponin. Biochemistry 1988;27:5891–5898.

46. Bodor GS, Oakeley AE, Allen PD, Crimmins DL, Ladenson JH, Anderson PA. Troponin I phosphorylation in the normal and failing adult human heart. Circulation 1997;96:1495–1500.

47. Al-Hillawi E, Chilton D, Trayer IP, Cummins P. Phosphorylation-specific antibodies for human cardiac troponin-I. Eur J Biochem 1998;256:535–540.

48. Powell SR, Gurzenda EM, Wahezi SE. Actin is oxidized during myocardial ischemia. Free Radic Biol Med 2001;30:1171–1176.

49. Morjana NA. Degradation of human cardiac troponin I after myocardial infarction. Biotechnol Appl Biochem 1998;28:105–111.

50. Morjana N, Clark D, Tal R. Biochemical and immunological properties of human cardiac troponin I fragments. Biotechnol Appl Biochem 2001;33:107–115.

51. Shi Q, Ling M, Zhang X, et al. Degradation of cardiac troponin I in serum complicates comparisons of cardiac troponin I assays. Clin Chem 1999;45:1018–1025.

52. Katrukha AG, Bereznikova AV, Filatov VL, Esakova TV, Kolosova OV, Pettersson K, et al. Degradation of cardiac troponin I: implication for reliable immunodetection. Clin Chem 1998;44:2433–2440.

12

Cardiac Marker Measurement
by Point-of-Care Testing

Paul O. Collinson

INTRODUCTION

Point-of-care testing (POCT) for cardiac disease is not a recent innovation. Testing at the patient's bedside was described in the 7th century by the Byzantine Theophilus Protospatharios. Detailed technical manuals were published in the 16th century for POCT as a routine part of the clinical workup for a range of medical conditions including chest pain *(1)*. It is unlikely that the technique then most in vogue, examination and tasting the patient's urine, would satisfy current regulatory processes (or find favor with the modern clinical chemist).

ROLE OF BIOCHEMICAL TESTING
IN SUSPECTED ACUTE CORONARY SYNDROMES

The rationale for biochemical testing of patients with suspected acute coronary syndromes (?ACS) is to provide an accurate diagnosis and to guide patient management. The electrocardiogram (ECG) is a poor diagnostic tool, with sensitivity as low as 41% *(2)*. Conversely, ST-segment elevation on the ECG is at least 95% predictive of an occluded artery *(3,4)*. The role of the admission ECG is to identify such patients; management is aimed at opening the occluded artery by primary angioplasty or thrombolysis *(5)*. Only a minority of patients present with ST elevation acute myocardial infarction (STEMI). An audit of hospital admissions with ?ACS revealed biochemical confirmation or exclusion of myocyte necrosis is required in 90% of cases whereas 5% of patients with significant cardiac damage are discharged from the emergency department *(6)*. Measurement of the cardiac troponins (cTn), cardiac troponin T (cTnT), and cardiac troponin I (cTnI) provides a cardiospecific tool for diagnosis. Initial reports demonstrated that cTn measurement was prognostic in patients admitted with *(7)* and without ST-segment elevation *(8)*. This was followed by evidence that cTn values could be used to predict the response to a range of therapies from low-molecular-weight heparin (9) to revascularization *(10, 11)*. The paradigm shift seen in the recent proposed guidelines for diagnosis of acute MI (AMI) and management of non-ST ACS recognizes the importance of the role of cardiac marker measurements *(12,13)*. More recently, other biomarkers such as C-reactive

From: *Cardiac Markers, Second Edition*
Edited by: Alan H. B. Wu @ Humana Press Inc., Totowa, NJ

protein (CRP) *(14)* and B-type natriuretic peptide (BNP) *(15)* have been shown to provide additional prognostic data in patients admitted with ACS.

Recommendations have been made for the type and speed of service provision for cardiac marker measurement. The suggested target for turnaround time (TAT) for cardiac markers is 60 min, with the proviso that POCT should be considered as an option *(16)*. This requires that three conditions are fulfilled: that the technology for POCT is adequate, that there is evidence to support the assertion that short TAT will have clinical benefit, and that such a strategy is cost effective.

POCT SYSTEMS FOR CARDIAC MARKERS

The cardiac markers available for routine clinical measurement by POCT comprise myoglobin, creatine kinase (CK) and its MB isoenzyme (CK-MB), cTnT, cTnI, BNP, and CRP. Prototype systems have been described for other markers including fatty acid binding protein *(17)*. Although these measurement systems are designed primarily for use in the POCT environment, this distinction is artificial. POCT systems are equally usable in the emergency laboratory, in a satellite laboratory where low throughput precludes the use of a large assay platform, in the main laboratory when the main assay platform does not support the tests required, or when a stat capability is required. They can be divided into four categories.

Dry Strip Enzyme Activity Measurements

These systems have evolved from the technology used for blood glucose test strips. The basic technology is a multilayer system containing stabilized dried reagents that are solubilized by the addition of serum or plasma and undergo a series of reactions to produce an optically read end point. They were the first examples of POCT instruments for cardiac markers. The first system in clinical use was the Ames seralyzer. This system was capable of measuring CK as part of a range of analytes. The system used serum as sample and hence required serum separation by centrifugation and a sample preparation step prior to analysis. The analytical range is 0–1000 U/L with % coefficient of variation (CV) 2.9–5.5 (555–3518 U/L), and the system could be used on the coronary care unit (CCU) *(18)*. A similar approach was used with extension of multilayer dry film technology by Kodak to the measurement CK and CK-MB with the Ektachem DT-60. This was a desktop version of a larger series of analyzers using the same chemistry for CK-MB activity measurement. Again, this instrument required prior separation of serum but no other prior preparation. Experience with these systems showed good precision (% CV: 2.2–8), but agreement with other laboratory methods for CK were variable *(19,20)*. The first true whole blood system was the Reflotron (Roche Diagnostics). This used lithium heparin whole blood as the sample. Using a fixed volume pipet, 32 µL (range 28.5–31.5 µL) is applied to the reagent strip. The assay CV was 3% with a linear measuring range of 24 to 1400 U/L. Samples values may be reported up to about 1800 U/L but are flagged. Samples exceeding 1800 U/L are reported as >1400 U/L. A multicenter evaluation of the instrument found the median % CV was 3.1. Agreement with conventional laboratory methods is good ($r = 0.99$), but values are not identical *(21)*. In routine clinical use with nonlaboratory operators, greater variability is found than in the hands of trained laboratory personnel *(22)*.

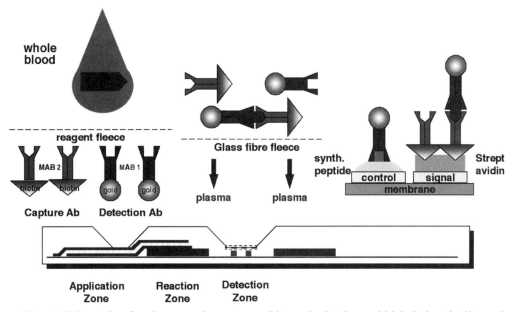

Fig. 1. Schematic of an immunochromatographic method using gold labeled optically read immunoassay (GLORIA) format.

These systems have two problems. They require a reasonable degree of operator skill, especially in pipetting blood, and the use of an independent quality control (QC) sample (a concept alien to clinicians). This has been partially or completely addressed by the subsequent categories of devices.

Dedicated Qualitative Devices ("Stick Tests") Primarily Oriented Toward POCT

These systems represent the first application of immunochromatographic technology to cardiac marker testing. The core technology is common to all the systems and utilizes three processes: an initial separation of cells from plasma, an immunoreactive phase, and a detection phase. This is illustrated for the Cardiac T system in Fig. 1. The antibodies dissolve in the plasma and react with any cTnT present to form a double-antibody–cTnT complex. The plasma containing the complex diffuses along the internal strip by capillary action and reaches the immobilized streptavidin and synthetic troponin peptides at the detection zone. Any double-antibody–cTnT complex binds by streptavidin biotin binding to the detection line and the gold complex is visualized as an optical signal. The systems include a built-in QC step. Excess gold-labeled antibody binds to the synthetic peptide to act as an internal control. The result is read as positive (two signal lines), negative (one signal line), or assay fail (no signal lines or the test line only). Precise pipetting is not required and an applicator device is used. A number of systems have been developed but clinical validation studies are available for only two.

Cardiac T (Roche Diagnostics)

The initial version of this test (first-generation, TROPT®) utilized the same antibodies as in first-generation enzyme-linked immunosorbent assay (ELISA) Troponin T but switched (M7-gold and 1B10-biotin). The assay was sold during 1994–1995, but not distributed internationally. The initial version had a reliable detection limit of 0.2–0.3 ng/mL, and hence required enhancement for use in risk stratification *(23,24)*. This was achieved with a second-generation assay using the same antibodies with enhanced sensitivity with a cutoff of 0.2 ng/mL sold from 1995 worldwide as TROPT® *(25,26)*. The improvement in the standard immunoassay with development of the enhanced Enzymun-Test Troponin T system has been reflected in the Cardiac T assay. The new M11.7 antibody has been incorporated in the third-generation assay but again switched with M11.7-gold (detection) and M7-biotin (capture). This has been sold since 1996 worldwide as TROPT sensitive® and is the only system now available *(27,28)*. However, when interpreting clinical studies, it is important to be aware of which system is being described, and to remember that diagnosis has been on the basis of the original World Health Organization (WHO) criteria for AMI. The current version has been recalibrated using recombinant human cTnT as a standard *(29)*. The detection limit of the assay is 0.05 ng/mL with 100% sensitivity to detect a value of 0.1 ng/mL.

A number of clinical studies have been performed using the second-generation device. A retrospective comparison of POCT cTnT measurement with central laboratory testing (CLT) showed 96% concordance in 191 tests with diagnostic sensitivity ranging from 17% to 71% according to time from presentation and diagnostic equivalence to CK-MB *(30)*. In a prospective observational trial, serial blood samples were obtained on presentation to the Emergency Department (ED) and 3 and 6 h later in 721 patients. CLT and POCT cTnT measurement had equivalent sensitivity for AMI detection *(31)*. Risk stratification was examined in a Thrombolysis in Myocardial Infarction (TIMI) 11A substudy in which 597 enrolled patients had POCT and simultaneous CLT of cTnT on study entry. Death, nonfatal MI, or recurrent ischemia at d 14 occurred in 33.6% of patients with a positive assay compared with only 22.5% of patients with a negative assay ($p = 0.01$) *(32)*. A Global Use of Strategies to Open Occluded Coronary Arteries in Acute Coronary Syndromes (GUSTO) III substudy of 12,666 patients presenting with ST-segment elevation found patients with a positive POCT cTnT on admission had a 15.7% mortality at 30 d compared with 6.2% in those who had a negative POCT cTnT on admission *(33)*. A retrospective comparison of POCT with CLT was performed in 773 consecutive ED patients with acute chest pain for <12 h without ST-segment elevation. cTnT and cTnI status (positive or negative) was determined at least twice by POCT on arrival and 4 or more hours later (so that one sample was taken at least 6 h after the onset of pain). Event rates at 30-d follow-up in patients with negative tests were 1.1% compared to 22.0% in patients with positive tests *(34)*.

Cardiac STATus (Spectral Diagnostics)

This system uses a dye conjugated to the detection antibody. Three systems are available: a CK-MB–myoglobin combined test, a single test strip for cTnI, and a combined CK-MB–myoglobin–cTnI test. Studies have examined analytical and clinical performance of the CK-MB–myoglobin assay. The manufacturers quoted detection sensitivity of the method is 50 ng/mL for myoglobin and 5 ng/mL for CK-MB. Comparison of 58 samples from 25 patients evaluated in the ED found diagnostically similar results to quantitative assays for CK-MB and myoglobin *(35)*. A second study of 182 consecutive ED patients found that results were not as good as for quantitative assays *(36)*. Clinical validation has been performed in a number of studies in the ED and CCU populations. In the ED, a study of 277 patients found sensitivity on serial testing over 3 h to have 95% sensitivity for diagnosis of AMI *(37)*. In the CCU, three studies of, respectively, 101 *(38)*, 99 *(39)*, and 151 *(40)* patients demonstrated sensitivity in the range 95–100%, with superior diagnostic efficiency to troponin testing in the first 6 h. The cTnI assay has been compared by enzyme immunoassay using the antibodies from Spectral cardiac STATus with an analytical cutoff for cTnI of 0.14 ng/mL with 98.9% concordance (positive test results vs cTnI values exceeding 0.14 ng/mL) *(41)*. A prospective clinical study in the 142 CCU patients gave sensitivity for diagnosis of AMI (confidence intervals in parentheses) of 100% (95.8–100) with a specificity of 82.5% (70.1–91.3) *(42)*. In 773 consecutive patients ED patients with symptoms <12 h and no ST-segment elevation, a negative cTnI at least 6 h from symptom onset had a 30-d event rate of 0.3% *(34)*.

Qualitative Immunochromatographic Devices

These use the same basic technology described above but incorporate a quantitative measuring system. Two systems are currently available.

Roche Cardiac Reader

This is a quantitative reader that uses a charge-coupled device (CCD) camera to optically read both Cardiac T strips and similar myoglobin strips (Cardiac M). There is good agreement with the quantitative methods and % CV is 10–15 for cTnT and 5–10 for myoglobin *(43)*. The assay has been recalibrated to the use of human recombinant cTnT as standard. The assay can be read quantitatively with the cardiac reader to give an effective range of 0–2 ng/mL. Values in the range 0.05–0.1 ng/mL are reported as <0.1 ng/mL. Values >2 ng/mL are above the linearity range and are recorded as >2 ng/mL. Values are equivalent to the results obtained by electrochemiluminescence immunoassay (ECLIA) *(29)*.

Triage (Biosite/Axis-Shield)

The Triage meter is slightly different. Whole blood or plasma is added to a disposable test strip and loaded into the meter. Plasma is separated is using a filter. Plasma enters the reaction and reading zone of the strip by capillary action and is controlled by a defined surface architecture. The reaction area contains fluorescent antibody conjugates and can be used to measure a cardiac panel (myoglobin, CK-MB, and cTnI) or BNP. The reaction mixture flows along the detection lane. Analyte–conjugate complexes are captured by immobilized antibodies on discrete analyte-specific zones and detected by fluorescence. The device includes a calibration check test strip. The cardiac panel has been evaluated analytically and clinically. Assay CV is reported as 12% at 0.4 ng/mL with the decision threshold for AMI 0.4 ng/mL by receiving operator characteristic (ROC) curve analysis, equivalent to conventional laboratory testing for diagnosis of AMI *(44)*. In 1024 consecutive ED admissions, a sensitivity of 96.9% with negative predictive value of 99.6% was obtained at 90 min from presentation *(45)*. POCT BNP measurement has been used to assess patients with congestive heart failure *(46)* and as a screening test for diagnosis of left ventricular dysfunction *(47)*.

Rapid Whole Blood Analytical System
Suitable for POCT or the Emergency Laboratory

These are fully quantitative dedicated analyzers that use heparinized whole blood as sample matrix. Three systems are currently available with slightly different emphases in methodology.

Stratus CS (Dade-Behring)

The Stratus CS takes heparinized whole blood but performs measurements on plasma. A compatible primary sample tube is loaded into a sample handling assembly, which is inserted into the machine. Whole blood is automatically transferred to a disposable centrifugal rotor containing an inert barrier material with density intermediate between that of plasma and blood cells. The rotor spins and this material rises to the plasma–cell interface to forms a barrier that separates plasma from cells. Samples are stable up to 2 h at room temperature in whole blood. Reagent packs for each analyte are loaded onto the machine after the sample has been loaded; hence, multiple types of test may be performed per sample, but only one sample may be loaded at a time. The reported % CV is 14.0–6.5 but in use the imprecision ranges from 6.3% (0.45 ng/mL) to 1.75% (18 ng/mL). The detection limit of the assay is 0.01–0.02 ng/mL with a functional sensitivity of 0.03 ng/mL and an upper reference limit of 0.08 ng/mL *(48,49)*. QC is conventional by analysis of QC materials as sample. In 412 ED patients diagnostic sensitivity was 98% and for patients with unstable angina and a cTnI ≥0.08 ng/mL, the 30-d event rate was 25.9% compared to 1.5% for those <0.08 ng/mL *(48)*. In a multicenter evaluation of biochemical diagnostic pathways in 1005 ED patients, a combined strategy using myoglobin plus cTnI was considered optimal for risk stratification *(50)*.

Innotrac Aio

This is available as a small CLT instrument (Aio central) or a stat analyzer (Aio Satellite). The instrument and measuring system is the same, but sample handling is different with Aio central including an 88-tube sample conveyor. The system uses whole blood or plasma as the sample matrix and can take primary sample tubes. As for the Stratus CS, QC is by analysis of QC materials as samples. The system utilizes biotinylated capture antibodies preimmobilized by streptavidin binding to the solid phase and europium-labeled detection antibodies. Reagents are preloaded onto the machine as prepackaged sample "pens" with all the reagents required for each single immunoassay in a dry stable form in a single use sample cup. The system can analyze cTnI (analytical sensitivity 0.05 ng/mL, % CV 6.4–7.6), myoglobin (analytical sensitivity 0.5 µg/L, % CV 8.7–9.4), and CK-MB mass (analytical sensitivity 0.5 ng/mL, % CV 7.3–8.2).

Alpha Dx (Sigma Diagnostics)

This is the most innovative system as it is a robust true POCT device. It uses K-EDTA anticoagulated whole blood as the sample matrix for measurement of a cardiac panel of CK-MM, CK-MB, myoglobin, and cTnI, and incorporates QC into the analytical process. The instrument is a desktop, portable, integrated immunoassay analyzer. The consumable components are a fluid cassette, containing a stabilized, buffered detergent solution used for all reaction and wash steps and reagents, supplied in the form of test-disks. Each test disk is a complete immunoassay system that contains all the required test-specific reagents together with bilevel quality controls for each test in stabilized form. A diskette contains lot-specific calibration information, limits for system quality control, and expiration date for each lot. The test disk is a rotor comprised of three geometrically equivalent segments in a radial design. The three segments comprise one for the test sample and one each for the high- and low-quality control. Assay % CV is reported as 7.4–8.8% with diagnostic sensitivity and specificity for AMI of 93% and 94%, respectively *(51)*. In patients admitted with non-ST elevation ACS, measurement of cTnI by this system can be used for outcome prediction.

In considering selection of a POCT it is important that the results produced have similar (ideally identical) clinical cutoffs to values produced by CLT. This is less of a problem for myoglobin and CK-MB but is a potential source of confusion for cTnI. Either methods should be chosen that produce comparable cTnI values or the same method used in both CLT and POCT.

IMPACT OF POCT ON PATIENT MANAGEMENT

Although it is self-evident that POCT will improve TAT, there is a need for objective evidence. Studies on POCT have suffered from a range of definitions of TAT and have largely been observational. Comparison of stat lab testing blood gas and glucose with central laboratory testing using analytical TAT (sample number accession by the analyzer to result posting) showed median TAT reduced to 4 min from 10 min *(52)*. The same group, in a prospective observational study utilizing a more robust definition of time from order initiation to time that the result was acted upon (designated therapeutic turnaround time, TTAT), found median TTAT was 13 min for POCT vs 25 min for CLT. The consistent finding in this and other studies of POCT is that improvement in TAT alone is not the significant factor. The principal delay is the time from result availability to clinical action being taken. This has been neatly summarized as the concept of "vein to brain" time.

There are limited but similar data for cardiac POCT. Improvement in TAT has been shown for the Triage system with reduction in median TAT from 71 min (CLT) to 24 min (POCT) *(45)*. In a prospective randomized controlled trial of POCT we found a significant decrease in TAT for measurements of CK (median TAT Reflotron 5 min POCT vs 69 min CLT; median TAT AlphaDx 20 min POCT vs 72 min CLT) and for cTnT and cTnI (median TAT Cardiac T and Spectral Cardiac STATUS 20 min vs 79 min CLT).

Assessment of TAT or TTAT by POCT suffers from one common flaw. TAT for such instruments is based on time to process an individual sample rather than sample throughput. Hence it may take 60 min for the laboratory to produce the first result but they can be produced at 10-s intervals thereafter. Conversely, for a single POCT instrument, once the sample is loaded, it is committed until analysis is complete in 15–20 min. This means that for the busy ED or CCU assessment of multiple patients simultaneously may prove difficult. This factor is overlooked in both evaluation and choice of POCT instrumentation. If it is necessary to process multiple patients simultaneously, multiple POCT instrumentation will be required.

The actual target for TAT is not evidence based but makes the assumption that faster is better and that most laboratories can achieve a TAT of 60 min. What evidence is there that this reduction in TAT (or TTAT) can be converted into improved clinical outcomes, either length of stay (LOS) or more direct measures such as time to treatment, morbidity, or mortality? Such evidence can be divided into that which addresses the impact of TAT alone and that which addresses the impact of POCT directly.

There are data that support the concept that improved TAT alters objective measures such as LOS. In a prospective observational study of a rapid diagnostic cardiac enzyme policy compared with a conventional strategy, there was a significant reduction in mean LOS on CCU from 3 to 2 d *(53)*. Provision of a more frequent assay service showed a similar reduction *(54)*. Conversely, a survey of hospitals found that a more rapid and frequent assay service was associated with reduced LOS in patients with a diagnosis of AMI, not, as might be expected, the low risk "rule-out" patient *(55)*. There is a tendency to focus on TAT rather than process but it is the combination of both that is important. The development of chest pain evaluation units (CPEUs) illustrates this. A randomized clinical trial (RCT) of rapid rule-out in a CPEU compared to conventional management by hospital admission showed significant reduction in LOS and cost *(56)*. This was achieved by change in process and without use of POCT. The exponential growth of CPEUs in the United States and their growing popularity in other countries reflects a desire to improve process and reduce costs. The strategy in these units utilizes rapid sequential cardiac marker measurement. This would be expected to be a rate-limiting step in the decision making and POCT would be expected to be of value. However, objective evidence for this is lacking.

The direct impact of POCT on patient care will depend on the data produced and the impact on clinical decision making. Studies in the ED have shown no impact of POCT electrolyte and blood gas measurement on LOS or patient outcomes *(57,58)*. ED studies of cardiac marker measurement have shown that POCT is diagnostically accurate and can be used to support rapid (90-min) rule-out protocols but have not looked at the impact on the outcome *(45,59)*. In a prospective RCT of POCT vs CLT on the CCU the improvement in TAT improved time to reach a definitive diagnosis for CK (16.2 h CLT vs 12.2 h POCT) and cTn (16.2 h CLT vs 14.7 h POCT). This affected LOS only in a subset of low-risk patients in a protocol-driven decision-making process. The impact was large, with reduction of total hospital LOS from 209.3 h (CLT) to 149.9 h *(42)* in 24.8% of all CCU admissions.

There is evidence to support the role of rapid cardiac marker measurement and POCT on the process. As cardiac markers are integral to therapy it would be expected that POCT should have a place in therapeutic decision making. A direct impact of POCT cardiac marker measurement has been demonstrated. A study of CK measurements by POCT on 117 patients with nondiagnostic ECG showed that management was altered and treatment instituted (in this case thrombolysis) in 15/29 (52%) solely on the basis of POCT measurements *(60)*. This finding has not been confirmed for the ED *(61)*. A role could be envisaged for POCT measurements in stopping low molecular weight heparin in cTn-negative patients or commencing glycoprotein IIb/IIIa (GP IIb/IIIa) antagonists prior to angioplasty and stent placement. Such pathways are ideal for POCT but depend on the configuration of the service. Institutions with on-site catheterization and an early aggressive invasive strategy may proceed straight to immediate catheterization in all cases. The merits of such a strategy in the troponin era deserve a critical review. In the majority of cases (even in the United States only 37% of hospitals have catheter labs and only 25% can perform angioplasty) immediate catheterization is not available and the use of rapid cardiac marker measurement prior to decision to treat and transfer would be logical.

COST-EFFECTIVENESS OF POCT CARDIAC MARKER TESTING

Assessment of POCT costs is difficult owing to a failure to compare like with like *(62)*. Often CLT price (including overheads) is compared with marginal cost for POCT and purports to show that POCT will be more cost effective than purchasing laboratory tests. The true cost of POCT needs to be assessed realistically, including equipment cost, staff cost for operation of the equipment, as well as consumables. There are other implementation costs including training costs (both initial training and subsequent training of new staff) and ongoing quality assurance. An accurate assessment of costs is best achieved by using semifixed (including staff time for analysis, costs for training and quality management) and variable costs. When this type of analysis is rigorously performed, POCT is more expensive. Semifixed costs are lower because staff costs are lower for CLT. Salary scales are lower for laboratory staff than for critical care nurses. The only time this may not be the case is when nursing assistants are employed whose duties include POCT. However, time taken per sample analyzed is less for CLT than POCT so that net labor cost always remains lower. Consumable costs are significantly lower for CLT as laboratory testing can achieve economies of scale, producing lower variable costs.

The justification of POCT is difficult when analytical costs alone are considered. A more pragmatic approach is to consider the costs of the process of health care. The largest cost components in each patient episode cost are hospital stay and treatment. As discussed previously, the major driver for CPEUs is reduction in LOS and number of hospitalizations, hence costs. This can be illustrated for a strategy for rule-out of low risk in patients utilizing reduction of LOS from an average of 4 d to 2 d. Average cost per CCU day is $3000 and average cost per day for a medical bed is $1000. Typical figures for LOS would be 1.5 d CCU plus 2.5 d medical (total cost $7000). For an accelerated rule-out protocol this would decrease to 1 d on CCU and 1 d medical (total cost $4000). Hence the net saving per patient is $3000. Typical POCT costs would be $80 per patient for a combination of myoglobin plus cTn, performed twice compared with $20 for comparable tests by CLT. The typical profile of ?ACS admissions would be 12% STEMI, 18% non-STEMI (4% non-Q WHO AMI plus 14% cTn-positive unstable angina by the old criteria). The relative impact of POCT vs CLT costs compared with process costs is illustrated in Table 1 for 100 admissions. The estimate of a halving in hospital stay is supported by the RCT data shown previously which demonstrated a halving of LOS in the low-risk group and a net overall cost reduction over the duration of the study.

The use of POCT to guide interventions can be shown to be cost efficient. The cost of 24 h of therapy with low molecular weight heparin is $30, but it has been shown that treatment in cTn-negative patients confers no benefit *(9)*. Hence, a strategy of stopping low molecular weight heparin at 12 h in cTn-negative patients can be compared with the conventional clinical strategy of 24 h of therapy. Similarly, the benefits of GP IIb/IIIa antagonists and revascularization are confined to cTn-positive patients *(10,11,63,64)*.

Table 1
Relative Impact of Laboratory Testing
Strategies and Length of Stay on Patient Episode Costs

Cost components	4-d stay	2-d stay	Difference
CCU bed cost for STEMI + NSTEMI patients	135,000	135,000	0
Medical bed cost for STEMI + NSTEMI patients	75,000	75,000	0
CCU bed cost for low risk patients	315,000	210,000	105,000
Medical bed cost for low risk patients	175,000	70,000	105,000
Test costs	2000	8000	−6000
Total cost	702,000	498,000	204,000

Costs are based on a typical case mix for 100 patients and are given in dollars.

Table 2
Relative Impact of Treatment Costs on Patient Episode Costs

Treatment strategy	All cases on clinical grounds	cTn-positive patients only after 12 h	Cost difference for treatment	Additional test cost difference	Net cost benefit
Low molecular weight heparin	2640	1590	1050	1000	50
Glycoprotein IIb/IIIa antagonist	44,000	9000	35,000	1000	34,000
Cardiac catheter	440,000	90,000	350,000	1000	349,000

Costs are based on a typical case mix for 100 patients and are given in dollars.

Hence administration of GP IIb/IIIa antagonists with angiography on all patients can be compared with treatment of only cTn-positive patients followed by angiography ("upstream" therapy). This is illustrated in Table 2. The same case mix as in the preceding is used for 100 admissions and the following costs assumed: POCT cTn $20, CLT cTn $10, 24-h low molecular weight heparin $30, $500 for GP IIb/IIIa antagonist therapy, and $5000 for angiography and percutaneous intervention coronary (excluding the cost of stents). It can be seen that the savings from unnecessary treatment and interventions, all of which have a level of risk, recoup the additional costs of POCT.

In conclusion, the technology for POCT is reliable and robust. There is evidence that POCT does improve TAT and that this can improve objective measures such as LOS and interventions. There is the potential for this to be converted in improvement in cost efficiency. However, improvement in TAT alone is not sufficient. Unless the biochemical testing is incorporated within a decision-making protocol the benefits of the improved TAT will not be realized either in an improvement of patient care or improved cost efficiency.

ABBREVIATIONS

ACS, Acute coronary syndrome(s); AMI, acute myocardial infarction; BNP, B-type natriuretic peptide; CCU, coronary care unit; CK, creatine kinase; CK-MB, MB isoenzyme of CK; CLT, central laboratory test; CPEU, chest pain evaluation unit; CRP, C-reactive protein; ctnT and cTnI, cardiac troponins T and I; CV, coefficient of variation; ECG, electrocardiogram; ED, emergency department; GP IIb/IIIa, glycoprotein IIb/IIIa; LOS, length of stay; PEC, patient episode cost; POCT, point-of-care testing; QC, quality control; RCT, randomized clinical trial; STEMI, ST elevation myocardial infarction; TAT, turnaround time; TTAT, therapeutic TAT; WHO, World Health Organization.

REFERENCES

1. Anon. Seynge of Urynes. London: R. Kele, 1552.
2. Zarling EJ, Sexton H, Milnor P Jr. Failure to diagnose acute myocardial infarction. The clinicopathologic experience at a large community hospital. JAMA 1983;250:1177–1181.
3. Topol EJ, Bates ER, Walton JA Jr, et al. Community hospital administration of intravenous tissue plasminogen activator in acute myocardial infarction: improved timing, thrombolytic efficacy and ventricular function. J Am Coll Cardiol 1987;10:1173–1177.
4. Yusuf S, Pearson M, Sterry H, et al. The entry ECG in the early diagnosis and prognostic stratification of patients with suspected acute myocardial infarction. Eur Heart J 1984;5:690–696.
5. Indications for fibrinolytic therapy in suspected acute myocardial infarction: collaborative overview of early mortality and major morbidity results from all randomised trials of more than 1000 patients. Fibrinolytic Therapy Trialists' (FTT) Collaborative Group (published erratum appears in Lancet 1994 Mar 19;343[8899]:742) (see comments). Lancet 1994;343:311–322.
6. Collinson PO, Premachandram S, Hashemi K. Prospective audit of incidence of prognostically important myocardial damage in patients discharged from emergency department. Br Med J 2000;320:1702–1705.
7. Stubbs P, Collinson P, Moseley D, Greenwood T, Noble M. Prognostic significance of admission troponin T concentrations in patients with myocardial infarction. Circulation 1996;94:1291–1297.
8. Hamm CW, Ravkilde J, Gerhardt W, et al. The prognostic value of serum troponin T in unstable angina (see comments). N Engl J Med 1992;327:146–150.
9. Lindahl B, Venge P, Wallentin L. Troponin T identifies patients with unstable coronary artery disease who benefit from long-term antithrombotic protection. Fragmin in Unstable Coronary Artery Disease (FRISC) Study Group. J Am Coll Cardiol 1997;29:43–48.
10. Stubbs P, Collinson P, Moseley D, Greenwood T, Noble M. Prospective study of the role of cardiac troponin T in patients admitted with unstable angina (see comments). Br Med J 1996;313:262–264.
11. Diderholm E, Andren B, Frostfeldt G, Genberg M, Jernberg T, Lagerqvist B, et al. The prognostic and therapeutic implications of increased troponin T levels and ST depression in unstable coronary artery disease: the FRISC II invasive troponin T electrocardiogram substudy. Am Heart J 2002;143:760–767.
12. Myocardial infarction redefined—a consensus document of The Joint European Society of Cardiology/American College of Cardiology Committee for the redefinition of myocardial infarction. Eur Heart J 2000;21:1502–1513.
13. Bertrand ME, Simoons ML, Fox KA, et al. Management of acute coronary syndromes: acute coronary syndromes without persistent ST segment elevation. Recommendations of the task force of the European Society of Cardiology (in process citation). Eur Heart J 2000;21:1406–1432.
14. de Winter RJ, Bholasingh R, Lijmer JG, et al. Independent prognostic value of C-reactive protein and troponin I in patients with unstable angina or non-Q-wave myocardial infarction. Cardiovasc Res 1999;42:240–245.

15. de Lemos JA, Morrow DA, Bentley JH, et al. The prognostic value of B-type natriuretic peptide in patients with acute coronary syndromes. N Engl J Med 2001;345:1014–1021.

16. Wu AH, Apple FS, Gibler WB, Jesse RL, Warshaw MM, Valdes R Jr. National Academy of Clinical Biochemistry Standards of Laboratory Practice: recommendations for the use of cardiac markers in coronary artery diseases. Clin Chem 1999;45:1104–1121.

17. Watanabe T, Ohkubo Y, Matsuoka H, et al. Development of a simple whole blood panel test for detection of human heart-type fatty acid-binding protein. Clin Biochem 2001;34: 257–263.

18. Ramhamadany EM, Collinson PO, Evans DH, Fink RS, Baird IM. Reliability of the Ames Seralyser for creatine kinase measurement in the coronary care unit. Clin Chem 1988;34: 1914.

19. Ng RH, Altaffer M, O'Neill M, Mukadam H, Statland BE. Measurement of six enzymes with the Kodak DTSC Module, a physician's office analyzer. Clin Chem 1987;33:1911–1913.

20. Hafkenscheid JC, van d V. Two dry-reagent systems evaluated for determinations of enzyme activities. Clin Chem 1988;34:155–157.

21. Horder M, Jorgensen PJ, Hafkenscheid JC, et al. Creatine kinase determination: a European evaluation of the creatine kinase determination in serum, plasma and whole blood with the Reflotron system. Eur J Clin Chem Clin Biochem 1991;29:691–696.

22. Romer M, Haeckel R, Henco A, et al. A multicentre evaluation of the Ektachem DT60-, Reflotron- and Seralyzer III systems. Eur J Clin Chem Clin Biochem 1992;30:547–583.

23. Collinson PO, Thomas S, Siu L, Vasudeva P, Stubbs PJ, Canepa-Anson R. Rapid troponin T measurement in whole blood for detection of myocardial damage. Ann Clin Biochem 1995;32(Pt 5):454–558.

24. Collinson PO, Gerhardt W, Katus HA, Muller-Bardorff M, Braun S, Schricke U, et al. Multicentre evaluation of an immunological rapid test for the detection of troponin T in whole blood samples. Eur J Clin Chem Clin Biochem 1996;34:591–598.

25. Christenson RH, Fitzgerald RL, Ochs L, et al. Characteristics of a 20-minute whole blood rapid assay for cardiac troponin T. Clin Biochem 1997;30:27–33.

26. Gerhardt W, Ljungdahl L, Collinson PO, et al. An improved rapid troponin T test with a decreased detection limit: a multicentre study of the analytical and clinical performance in suspected myocardial damage. Scand J Clin Lab Invest 1997;57:549–557.

27. Herkner H, Waldenhofer U, Laggner AN, et al. Clinical application of rapid quantitative determination of cardiac troponin-T in an emergency department setting. Resuscitation 2001; 49:259–264.

28. Hirschl MM, Herkner H, Laggner AN, et al. Analytical and clinical performance of an improved qualitative troponin T rapid test in laboratories and critical care units. Arch Pathol Lab Med 2000;124:583–587.

29. Collinson PO, Jorgensen B, Sylven C, et al. Recalibration of the point-of-care test for CARDIAC T Quantitative with Elecsys Troponin T 3rd generation. Clin Chim Acta 2001; 307:197–203.

30. Hirschl MM, Lechleitner P, Friedrich G, et al. Usefulness of a new rapid bedside troponin T assay in patients with chest pain. Resuscitation 1996;32:193–198.

31. Evaluation of a bedside whole-blood rapid troponin T assay in the emergency department. Rapid Evaluation by Assay of Cardiac Troponin T (REACTT) Investigators Study Group. Acad Emerg Med 1997;4:1018–1024.

32. Antman EM, Sacks DB, Rifai N, McCabe CH, Cannon CP, Braunwald E. Time to positivity of a rapid bedside assay for cardiac-specific troponin T predicts prognosis in acute coronary syndromes: a Thrombolysis in Myocardial Infarction (TIMI) 11A substudy. J Am Coll Cardiol 1998;31:326–330.

33. Ohman EM, Armstrong PW, White HD, et al. Risk stratification with a point-of-care cardiac troponin T test in acute myocardial infarction. GUSTO III Investigators. Global Use of Strategies to Open Occluded Coronary Arteries. Am J Cardiol 1999;84:1281–1286.

34. Hamm CW, Goldmann BU, Heeschen C, Kreymann G, Berger J, Meinertz T. Emergency room triage of patients with acute chest pain by means of rapid testing for cardiac troponin T or troponin I (see comments). N Engl J Med 1997;337:1648–1653.
35. Schwartz JG, Gage CL, Farley NJ, Prihoda TJ. Evaluation of the cardiac STATus CK-MB/myoglobin card test to diagnose acute myocardial infarctions in the ED. Am J Emerg Med 1997;15:303–307.
36. Schouten Y, de Winter RJ, Gorgels JP, Koster RW, Adams R, Sanders GT. Clinical evaluation of the CARDIAC STATus, a rapid immunochromatographic assay for simultaneous detection of elevated concentrations of CK-MB and myoglobin in whole blood. Clin Chem Lab Med 1998;36:469–473.
37. Brogan GX, Jr., Bock JL, McCuskey CF, et al. Evaluation of cardiac STATus CK-MB/myoglobin device for rapidly ruling out acute myocardial infarction. Clin Lab Med 1997; 17:655–668.
38. Panteghini M, Cuccia C, Pagani F, Turla C. Comparison of the diagnostic performance of two rapid bedside biochemical assays in the early detection of acute myocardial infarction. Clin Cardiol 1998;21:394–398.
39. Luscher MS, Ravkilde J, Thygesen K. Clinical application of two novel rapid bedside tests for the detection of cardiac troponin T and creatine kinase-MB mass/myoglobin in whole blood in acute myocardial infarction. Cardiology 1998;89:222–228.
40. Sylven C, Lindahl S, Hellkvist K, Nyquist O, Rasmanis G. Excellent reliability of nurse-based bedside diagnosis of acute myocardial infarction by rapid dry-strip creatine kinase MB, myoglobin, and troponin T. Am Heart J 1998;135:677–683.
41. Heeschen C, Goldmann BU, Moeller RH, Hamm CW. Analytical performance and clinical application of a new rapid bedside assay for the detection of serum cardiac troponin I. Clin Chem 1998;44:1925–1930.
42. Collinson PO, John CM, Cramp DRG, Carson ER, Morgan SH. Point of care testing or central laboratory testing: an evaluation. Health Technology Assessment 2003; in press.
43. Muller-Bardorff M, Sylven C, Rasmanis G, et al. Evaluation of a point-of-care system for quantitative determination of troponin T and myoglobin (in process citation). Clin Chem Lab Med 2000;38:567–574.
44. Apple FS, Christenson RH, Valdes R Jr, et al. Simultaneous rapid measurement of whole blood myoglobin, creatine kinase MB, and cardiac troponin I by the triage cardiac panel for detection of myocardial infarction. Clin Chem 1999;45:199–205.
45. McCord J, Nowak RM, McCullough PA, et al. Ninety-minute exclusion of acute myocardial infarction by use of quantitative point-of-care testing of myoglobin and troponin I. Circulation 2001;104:1483–1488.
46. Maisel A. B-type natriuretic peptide in the diagnosis and management of congestive heart failure. Cardiol Clin 2001;19:557–571.
47. Maisel AS, Koon J, Krishnaswamy P, et al. Utility of B-natriuretic peptide as a rapid, point-of-care test for screening patients undergoing echocardiography to determine left ventricular dysfunction. Am Heart J 2001;141:367–374.
48. Heeschen C, Goldmann BU, Langenbrink L, Matschuck G, Hamm CW. Evaluation of a rapid whole blood ELISA for quantification of troponin I in patients with acute chest pain. Clin Chem 1999;45:1789–1796.
49. Altinier S, Mion M, Cappelletti A, Zaninotto M, Plebani M. Rapid measurement of cardiac markers on Stratus CS. Clin Chem 2000;46:991–993.
50. Newby LK, Storrow AB, Gibler WB, et al. Bedside multimarker testing for risk stratification in chest pain units: the chest pain evaluation by creatine kinase-MB, myoglobin, and troponin I (CHECKMATE) study. Circulation 2001;103:1832–1837.
51. Apple FS, Anderson FP, Collinson P, et al. Clinical evaluation of the first medical whole blood, point-of-care testing device for detection of myocardial infarction (In process citation). Clin Chem 2000;46:1604–1609.

52. Kilgore ML, Steindel SJ, Smith JA. Evaluating stat testing options in an academic health center: therapeutic turnaround time and staff satisfaction. Clin Chem 1998;44:1597–1603.

53. Collinson PO, Ramhamadamy EM, Stubbs PJ, et al. Rapid enzyme diagnosis of patients with acute chest pain reduces patient stay in the coronary care unit. Ann Clin Biochem 1993; 30(Pt 1):17–22.

54. Apple FS, Preese LM, Riley L, Gerken KL, Van Lente F. Financial impact of a rapid CK-MB-specific immunoassay on the diagnosis of myocardial infarction. Arch Pathol Lab Med 1990;114:1017–1020.

55. Wu AH, Clive JM. Impact of CK-MB testing policies on hospital length of stay and laboratory costs for patients with myocardial infarction or chest pain (see comments). Clin Chem 1997;43:326–332.

56. Gomez MA, Anderson JL, Karagounis LA, Muhlestein JB, Mooers FB. An emergency department-based protocol for rapidly ruling out myocardial ischemia reduces hospital time and expense: results of a randomized study (ROMIO). J Am Coll Cardiol 1996;28:25–33.

57. Kendall J, Reeves B, Clancy M. Point of care testing: randomised controlled trial of clinical outcome. Br Med J 1998;316:1052–1057.

58. Parvin CA, Lo SF, Deuser SM, Weaver LG, Lewis LM, Scott MG. Impact of point-of-care testing on patients' length of stay in a large emergency department. Clin Chem 1996;42: 711–717.

59. Hamm CW. Cardiac biomarkers for rapid evaluation of chest pain. Circulation 2001;104: 1454–1456.

60. Downie AC, Frost PG, Fielden P, Joshi D, Dancy CM. Bedside measurement of creatine kinase to guide thrombolysis on the coronary care unit. Lancet 1993;341:452–454.

61. Gibler WB, Hoekstra JW, Weaver WD, et al. A randomized trial of the effects of early cardiac serum marker availability on reperfusion therapy in patients with acute myocardial infarction: the serial markers, acute myocardial infarction and rapid treatment trial (SMARTT). J Am Coll Cardiol 2000;36:1500–1506.

62. Foster K, Despotis G, Scott MG. Point-of-care testing. Cost issues and impact on hospital operations. Clin Lab Med 2001;21:269–284.

63. Hamm CW, Heeschen C, Goldmann B, et al. Benefit of abciximab in patients with refractory unstable angina in relation to serum troponin T levels. c7E3 Fab Antiplatelet Therapy in Unstable Refractory Angina (CAPTURE) Study Investigators (published erratum appears in N Engl J Med 1999 Aug 12;341(7):548) (see comments). N Engl J Med 1999; 340:1623–1629.

64. Heeschen C, Hamm CW, Goldmann B, Deu A, Langenbrink L, White HD. Troponin concentrations for stratification of patients with acute coronary syndromes in relation to therapeutic efficacy of tirofiban. PRISM Study Investigators. Platelet Receptor Inhibition in Ischemic Syndrome Management (see comments). Lancet 1999;354:1757–1562.

13

Standardization of Cardiac Markers

Mauro Panteghini

INTRODUCTION

The development of commercially available assays for the determination of cardiac proteins has been one of the most important innovations in the field of cardiovascular diagnostics in the last decade. The availability of innovative procedures to detect myoglobin, creatine kinase isoenzyme MB (CK-MB) mass concentration, and, above all, cardiac troponins now represents a major opportunity to improve significantly clinical assessment of the acute coronary syndrome (ACS) (1). The routine clinical use of the measurement of the catalytic activity of "cardiac" enzymes, that is, lactate dehydrogenase, aspartate aminotransferase, CK and CK-MB, has gradually been replaced—although at different speeds in various countries—by automated quantitative immunoassays for mass determination of myoglobin, CK-MB, cardiac troponin I (cTnI), and cardiac troponin T (cTnT) (2).

In the 1970s, the first cardiac marker to be measured by immunochemical methods (at that time radioimmunoassays) was myoglobin. However, this marker did not initially gain popularity because of the lack of a rapid emergency methodology. More recently, assay techniques with an analytical turnaround time of <15 min have been developed, so that myoglobin has been revisited as a potentially useful early biochemical marker (3). In the 1980s, the introduction of automated immunoassays based on monoclonal anti-CK-MB antibodies allowed the measurement of the protein concentration (= mass) instead of the catalytic activity of the CK-MB isoenzyme. This significantly improved the analytical sensitivity and specificity of the assays (4). With these CK-MB immunoassays, analytical interferences—often leading to false-positive results using traditional immunoinhibition assays—were eliminated. Finally, in the 1990s, the introduction of immunoassays for the measurement of the cardiac troponins resulted in a revolution in the use of cardiac markers. Cardiac troponins are at present regarded as the most specific of the currently commercially available biochemical markers for myocardial damage and the redefined criterion used to classify ACS patients presenting with ischemic symptoms as myocardial infarction (MI) patients is heavily predicated on an increased concentration of these markers in blood (5).

It is of course important that these clinically relevant biomarkers, on which critical decisions will rest, are measured with highly reliable and standardized methods to achieve

From: *Cardiac Markers, Second Edition*
Edited by: Alan H. B. Wu @ Humana Press Inc., Totowa, NJ

comparability of results among different assays. Interchangeability of results over time and space would significantly contribute to improvements in health care, as results of clinical studies undertaken in different locations or times could be applied universally.

Myoglobin, CK-MB mass, and troponins are in fact measured by a number of different immunoassays using specific antibodies directed to the respective antigens. These immunoassays can therefore be influenced by the nature of both the antibody and the antigen. For instance, different monoclonal antibodies may recognize different epitopes of the same antigen present in the blood. Multiple forms of troponins (I or T) may also exist in blood, free or bound to other troponins. The numerical results of a measurement procedure may also be dependent on the matrix (e.g., buffer or artificial serum, instead of true human serum) in which the calibration material is dissolved. The nature and behavior of the calibrator become paramount in immunoassays in which the measurement is entirely a matter of comparison of a test with a calibrator. As a final consequence, analytical systems may give results that are typical for a certain method or instrument, so that different results from different assays and platforms may be obtained and this problem may cloud interpretations of reported data, creating a substantive problem for the clinical and laboratory communities.

For a solution of this problem, it is important to reflect on the concept of a metrologically correct measurement system and to discuss how this concept can be applied to immunoassays measuring cardiac markers *(6)*.

REFERENCE MEASUREMENT SYSTEM

It has been realized for some time that durable standardization of quantitative measurements in laboratory medicine requires the consistent application of a generally accepted reference system for calibration and validation of routine methods *(7)*. Such a structure is based on the concepts of metrological traceability and of hierarchy of analytical measurement procedures. Key elements of the system are the reference measurement procedure and different kinds of reference materials. The traceability model for quantities that are not fully physicochemically characterized and for which results of measurements are not traceable to International System of Units (SI), such as cardiac markers, emphasizes in particular the importance of the definition of the analyte and its interrelationship with the primary reference material (Fig. 1). Some standardization problems of cardiac markers are associated with an insufficient definition of the entity involved, an example of which is cTnI. In biological samples, cTnI is present as a heterogeneous mixture of different molecular species. Intact cTnI and a spectrum of up to 11 modified products have been detected in sera from patients with MI *(8)*. In turn, for the definition of the analyte cTnI, it will have to be decided whether it refers to:

- A mixture of different forms, that is, free and complexed with troponin C and T, or to only one prevalent form.
- Composition classes (in terms of oxidation, phosphorylation, etc.).
- Content classes (in terms of percent of phosphorylation, etc.).

This microheterogeneity may be circumvented by definition of a unique, invariant part of the molecule that is common to all components of the mixture, for example, the epitopes that are located in the stable part of the molecule and are not affected by IC or ITC complex formation and other in vivo modifications. In consequence, antibodies

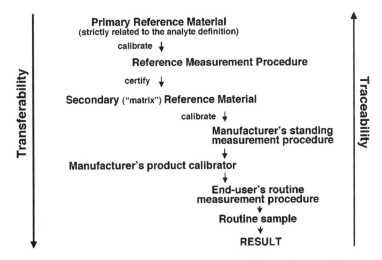

Fig. 1. The reference measurement system for cardiac markers.

used for the development of reliable cTnI assays should preferably recognize these epitopes *(9)*.

Once the secondary reference material is certified, this material and the manufacturer's standing procedure can be used in industry to assign values to commercial calibrators. Clinical laboratories use routine procedures with validated calibrators, both from commercial sources, to measure human specimens. In this way, the obtained value will be traceable to the primary reference material and the standardization of measurement, that is, the process of realizing traceability, will be reached (Fig. 1). The scheme shown in Fig. 1 is, however, valid only as long as the following two conditions are fulfilled: (1) The materials involved in the transfer of values from the reference procedure to the routine laboratory procedures must be commutable with the human specimens, and (2) reference procedure and routine methods must have identical specificities for the analyte.

REFERENCE MATERIALS

A prerequisite for guaranteeing comparability of results among different methods is the availability of suitable reference materials. By definition, a reference material is a material or substance one or more of whose property values are sufficiently homogeneous and well established to be used for the calibration of an apparatus, the assessment of a measurement method, or assigning values to other materials *(10)*.

A reliable reference material for application in clinical laboratory measurements should be appropriately and thoroughly defined by a set of characteristics *(11,12)*. General characteristics comprise the origin, the mode of production, the physical state and phase, homogeneity, additives, storage conditions, and stability. Specific characteristics describe the molecular composition, purity, matrix, assigned value, and uncertainty of measurement. Additional characteristics concern the procedures for assessing homogeneity and stability, the protocol followed for assigning the value and the uncertainty, as well as instructions for use and the intended function *(11)*.

Primary Reference Materials

The primary materials should be homogeneous, pure, and identical to the corresponding substance in the blood. They should be characterized as far as possible by advanced spectroscopic, chromatographic, and other methods.

The primary structures of all clinically important cardiac markers are known, and they can either be purified from natural sources or expressed by recombinant techniques *(13–20)*. A pure protein for use as a primary calibrant should, however, reflect the heterogeneity to be encountered in the test sample *(21)*. For some cardiac markers, for example, for cTnI, pure protein that shows the same microheterogeneity as the protein present in plasma cannot be prepared. Because of this heterogeneity, Ekins has argued that standardization of immunoassays for heterogeneous antigens such as cTnI is impossible, the only long-term solution being the measurement of individual components *(22)*. However, an acceptable practical solution to make cTnI standardization possible can be the definition of preferable antibody-binding epitopes on the cTnI molecule and then the use as reference material of a compound representing the natural and major form of the antigen in blood after tissue release, that is, the complexed form *(9)*. The subcommittee for cTnI standardization of the American Association for Clinical Chemistry (AACC) targeted three candidate reference materials that are complexes of troponins C, I, and T *(23)*. It is hoped that one of these can be proposed in the near future as cTnI primary reference material.

The situation for myoglobin and CK-MB seems simpler. For a single polypeptide chain protein with molecular mass of about 17 kDa such as myoglobin, the purification from human sources, for example, cardiac tissue, can be easily used to produce primary immunogens and calibrators. Conversely, for a heterodimeric protein such as CK-MB, the alternative use of recombinant DNA technology may provide more homogeneous and pure protein *(17)*.

Theoretically, primary reference materials can be used for calibration of reference procedures and routine methods. However, when primary materials are intended for direct value assignment to manufacturers' calibrators, they should be tested extensively for commutability *(6)*. In fact, purification procedures can lead to a partial degradation resulting in noncommutability of reference materials with native samples *(24,25)*, but also pure compounds prepared by recombinant techniques may have altered structures with the consequence that the probability of matrix effects is high *(26)*.

A still unsolved aspect is the way to assign values to primary reference materials. Stenman proposed that concentrations of these materials should be determined by amino acid analysis and the results expressed as substance concentrations in moles per liter, on the grounds that substance concentrations of pure protein solutions can be accurately determined by amino acid analysis *(27)*. For Whicher, the most practical way to express concentration is in mass per volume rather than in moles per volume, as molecular weight may vary according to the biological state of the protein *(21)*. For these reasons, dry mass should be used as the basis for assigning value to a primary calibrant *(21)*. Other authors have described an alternative approach for assigning a mass concentration value to primary materials, based on the existence of a protein (albumin) certified reference material (SRM 927, National Institute of Standards and Technology [NIST]) and a procedure, such as the Doetsch method, able to measure protein mass, free of interference and independent of the particular amino acid composition of the protein *(25)*.

Table 1
General Requirements for a Secondary Matrixed Reference Material

- Properly documented characteristics and properties of the antigen contained in the material
- Possibly serum-based matrix
- Same immunochemical behavior in all methods of measurement
- No matrix effects different from clinical samples
- Documented stability and storage characteristics
- Documented overlap between new and old lot production
- Documentation of all certification steps
- Approved by international institutions, e.g., IFCC

Adapted from ref. *12*.

Secondary ("Matrix") Reference Materials

The use of serum-based reference materials has the advantage that the matrix is similar to that in clinical samples. If useful, pure protein may be added to them to increase the marker concentration *(28,29)*. Detailed requirements for a secondary "matrix" reference material for immunoassays are reported in Table 1. For clinical applications, human serum (or defibrinated, delipidized plasma) is the preferred base matrix. The effects of the natural variation between donors can be minimized by using pooled collections from a number of individuals.

Although matrix-based materials are desirable as they are more likely to behave in a similar fashion to test samples, this does not eliminate *a priori* the matrix problem because different immunoassays may have different matrix problems *(24)*. Thus, also "patient-like" reference materials should be used for calibration of commercial methods only if their commutability has been proven.

Standardization of the majority of plasma protein determinations has been accomplished by preparation of a serum-based material *(30)*. A similar way was selected by the Committee on Standardization of Markers of Cardiac Damage (C-SMCD) of the International Federation of Clinical Chemistry and Laboratory Medicine (IFCC) for myoglobin standardization *(12)*. An international collaborative study was organized with the involvement of seven companies using 12 different platforms. Five candidate secondary reference materials were assayed in relation to linearity, recovery rate, and commutability to demonstrate a possible identity between the materials and the usual routine samples. The study produced data of major scientific importance, and also provided the basis for the selection of human heart myoglobin material, prepared in a lyophilized form, as the most suitable candidate secondary reference material. As an example, Fig. 2 shows the "recovery rates" (experimental values divided by the nominal values provided by the companies submitting each material) for the candidate materials, demonstrating that materials 1 and 3 cannot be correctly measured by the assays currently on the market. Using the selected material (2 in Fig. 2) as an *a posteriori* common calibrator, a significant harmonization effect was immediately demonstrated, by reducing the interassay bias from 32% to 13%.

Table 2 summarizes the hierarchy and the main characteristics of reference materials useful for cardiac marker standardization:

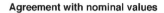

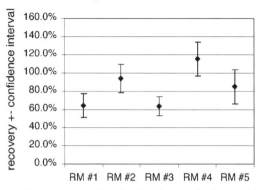

Fig. 2. Recovery (experimental value divided by the nominal value) in percentage for the five candidate secondary reference materials for myoglobin, evaluated in the Project for Standardization of Immunoassays for Myoglobin Determination organized by the Committee on Standardization of Markers of Cardiac Damage (C-SMCD) of the International Federation of Clinical Chemistry and Laboratory Medicine (IFCC).

Table 2
Hierarchy of Reference Materials for Cardiac Markers

1. Primary reference material: recombinant or human purified protein
2. Secondary reference material:
   a. Pool of human sera spiked with the corresponding purified antigen
   b. Pool of human sera containing the corresponding antigen ("native") in elevated concentrations

1. Primary reference material, that is, pure analyte, with values possibly assigned by mass determination/calculation.
2. Secondary reference material, that is, matrixed, with values assigned by a reference method against the primary material.

Commutability of Reference Materials

As discussed previously, reference materials for cardiac markers should be extensively investigated for commutability before use for directly assigning values to manufacturers' calibrators. The physical–chemical properties of calibrators and control materials used in immunoassays for cardiac markers may differ significantly from the analyte in clinical specimens. Cattozzo et al. *(31)* clearly showed the perverse effect of recalibrating with noncommutable materials for myoglobin and CK-MB and the consequent misinterpretation of patient results.

Commutability has been defined as the ability of a reference/control material for a given analyte to show interassay properties comparable to those of the same analyte in human serum *(32)*. This characteristic of reference materials and calibrators can be affected by many factors (Table 3).

Commutability of cardiac marker–containing materials and samples between procedures is so fundamental for the use of these materials to calibrate immunoassays directly that it should not be accepted uncritically or without the most rigorous experimental verification *(24)*. In fact, any significant difference in the behavior of the materials and

Table 3
Factors Involved in Commutability of Reference and Calibration Materials

- Nonhuman origin of the protein (e.g., pure compounds prepared by recombinant techniques may have altered structure by lacking carbohydrate side chains)
- Procedures that result in physical changes, e.g., purification or lyophilization
- Matrix of the solution (e.g., use of bovine serum albumin can be inadequate in reflecting any nonanalyte constituents of patient samples)
- Addition of preservatives, antimicrobial agents, stabilizers, or other additives

the clinical specimens in measurement systems will result in measurement errors. Commutability, or the convertibility of results between methods, thus requires the experimental demonstration of the same constant ratio between results given by the procedures for the reference material and for all unknown samples *(24)*. When available, one method should be the recognized reference method, used to certify the concentration of the reference material. The reference material and the samples should also show proportional dilution curves in the methods to be used *(33)*.

REFERENCE MEASUREMENT PROCEDURE

The development of reference procedures is indispensable for the success of standardization. These methods should be used for certification of secondary reference materials (Fig. 1). Unfortunately, for cardiac proteins the search and the assessment of candidate reference materials has not been so far supported by the contemporaneous development of reference procedures. This may have been due to technical difficulties, but another reason might be that it was thought that a common reference material would be sufficient for reaching method comparability *(17)*.

Recent developments in mass spectrometry have made it possible to analyze proteins in detail that is not possible by other methods *(34)*. However, this technique is still not useful for proteins occurring at low concentrations, such as cardiac troponins. As an alternative, some authors have proposed the development of immunological reference methods, based on the availability of monoclonal antibodies with well-defined epitope specificity *(27)*. They may have the advantage of a level of analytical sensitivity that is unmatched by technologies that would otherwise be preferred for standardization. The main argument against this proposal is that an immunological procedure may be too dependent on a certain assay technology as this technique is an indirect measurement approach *(27)*. For all these reasons, reference procedures for cardiac markers will most probably not be available in the near future. As a practical interim solution, an European working group suggested the selection of a "consensus method," understood in the sense of "the most effective method for solving clinical questions that is available at a given time" *(6)*.

In addition to the need of commutability with the human specimens of the different reference and calibrator materials, the concept of a reference system is valid only if the reference procedure and corresponding routine procedures have similar specificities for the measured cardiac protein *(35)*. Where the routine method shows insufficient or different specificity, recalibration is indeed impossible and the method in question should be reengineered *(6)*.

The specificity of an immunoassay is dependent mainly on the epitope specificity of the antibodies used. Problems of differing antibody specificities are often more evident when the target analyte is cTnI. In a study, serial blood samples from a patient with MI were tested by two assays, both nominally intended to measure cTnI, one with antibodies recognizing the stable part of the molecule and another with antibodies specific to the amino- (N)- and carboxy- (C)-terminal parts of the molecule, which are very susceptible to proteolysis *(36)*. Within 24 h after onset of the chest pain, the ratio of cTnI concentrations measured by the first and second assay was close to 1, but 2–3 d later it was close to 3 or even higher. Four days after MI, there was no detectable cTnI with the second assay, but significant amounts of the antigen were still measured by the assay with antibodies recognizing the stable part of the molecule *(36)*. The differences could be explained by the different specificities of the assays (the tests measured in fact "different analytes," that is, the intact cTnI and nicked forms the former, only the intact molecule the latter): in this case no standardization between the assays is possible. Therefore, acceptable cTnI standardization could not be possible for all assays on all comercially available platforms if differences in assay specificity are not minimized *(9)*.

FEASIBILITY OF CARDIAC MARKER STANDARDIZATION

The final objective of the standardization projects of cardiac marker measurements must be the promotion of result traceability by means of a reference measurement system by providing reference measurement procedures and reference materials. At present, there are, however, no reference methods; certified reference materials, preferably in the matrix to be measured routinely, should still be established, and, at least for cardiac troponins, the analyte in patients' blood can be significantly different from newly synthesized or recombinant protein. The progress in standardization of cardiac protein immunoassays will therefore be slow. As an interim solution, some authors have proposed assay harmonization by recalibrating various assays to give the same results *(37)*. Although methods can produce more or less similar results, these may, however, be far from the traceability *(38)*. Furthermore, maintenance of calibration may be very problematic in the absence of reference procedures *(27)*. Therefore, standardization should be the goal whenever possible.

In recent years, a number of meaningful efforts toward standardization of cardiac markers have been initiated by several organizations *(39,40)*. For a general account of the organizations and agencies involved in various aspects of immunoassay standardization and of the offices controlling their use, the reader may refer to the recent review of Stenman *(27)*. It should be remembered that the European Community has recently issued a new in vitro diagnostics (IVD) directive, which should be implemented by December, 2003, and will require that calibration of all IVD assays be traceable to the highest available reference material or method *(41)*. However, it is obvious that reference systems for cardiac markers will not be available by 2003, when this directive should be implemented. Furthermore, the authority responsible for authorization of reference systems has not yet been determined. Very recently, a Joint Committee on Traceability in Laboratory Medicine (JCTLM) has been established with the aim to support worldwide traceability, comparability, and equivalence of measurement results in laboratory medicine (Table 4). The work of JCTLM shall be based on existing international or intergovernmental agreements and it will operate by consensus (Fig. 3). In particular,

Table 4
Objectives of the Joint Committee on Traceability in Laboratory Medicine (JCTLM)

- Promoting the concept of traceability of measurement results to the SI or to other internationally agreed references where traceability to the SI is not yet feasible
- In cases where traceability to the SI is not yet feasible (e.g., measurement of cardiac proteins), coordinating and giving guidance in the establishment of a Reference Measurement System with respect to medical needs where such an international conventional system is applicable
- Identifying and prioritizing the measurands requiring international traceability and comparability and encouraging appropriate organizations to accept responsibility for the development of suitable reference measurement procedures and certified reference materials
- Disseminating relevant information to all interested parties
- Providing scientific and organizational expertise to the parties involved
- Encouraging the application of reference systems by the In Vitro Diagnostics (IVD) industry

JCTLM states that " in cases where traceability to SI is not feasible [e.g., measurement of cardiac protein] an international conventional reference measurement system will be established. Such a reference system comprises the definition of the measurand, validated measurement methods and certified reference materials. This system is expected to be implemented by internationally recognized reference measurement laboratories in Laboratory Medicine."

The actual work on cardiac marker standardization is performed by capable experts in Committees and Working Groups (Table 5). Because standardization is an international rather than a national problem, it is desirable that one international organization is responsible for the coordination of various standardization projects. For this reason, in 1998 IFCC decided to establish the C-SMCD, inviting members from the previously established American and European groups to become members of this Committee (39). The plan of action of the C-SMCD was developed taking into account work already done by the existing national and international groups. Regarding assay standardization, the C-SMCD decided to concentrate its attention on immunoassays for determination of CK-MB mass, myoglobin, and cTnI. Owing to the existence of an international patent, all commercial assays for cTnT are marketed by one manufacturer, and therefore standardization for cTnT is not so urgent.

In the case of CK-MB, two projects related to the preparation of reference materials were conducted (17,25). A project of the AACC subcommittee on CK-MB mass assay standardization led to identification and characterization of a CK-MB primary lyophilized material (in recombinant form) (17). Although this material did not have a certified mass concentration value or any uncertainty statement, it was very effective in obtaining assay harmonization, achieving a reduction of the systematic error among methods from 40% to 13% (17). A second project, supported by the European Community—Standards, Measurements, and Testing Programme, has assigned a mass concentration value to the already available CK-MB BCR 608 primary material (enzyme purified from human heart), with previously certificated catalytic activity (13,25). Unfortunately, the material is not commutable and cannot therefore be used to calibrate directly the manufacturers' measurement procedures (24).

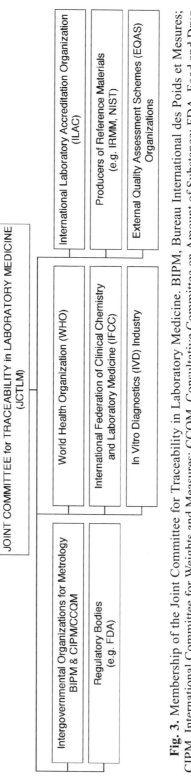

Fig. 3. Membership of the Joint Committee for Traceability in Laboratory Medicine. BIPM, Bureau International des Poids et Mesures; CIPM, International Committee for Weights and Measures; CCQM, Consultative Committee on Amount of Substance; FDA, Food and Drug Administration; IRMM, Institute for Reference Materials and Measurements; NIST, National Institute of Standards and Technology.

Table 5
State of the Art of Cardiac Marker Standardization

Marker	Reference procedure	Reference materials					
		Type	Status	Characterization study	Availability	Limitations	Commutability
CK-MB	NA	Primary: recombinant tissue isoform	Lyophilized	AACC	Seradyn	No certification of mass concentration	Not tested (the material is to be diluted in the manufacturer diluent to compensate matrix effects)
		Primary: purification from human heart	Lyophilized	European Community	IRMM	Lack of commutability	No
Myoglobin	ID-MS in development	Secondary: normal human serum spiked with human heart myoglobin	Lyophilized	IFCC C-SMCD	IRMM[a]	Complete characterization and value certification to be performed	Yes
Cardiac troponin I	NA	Primary: ITC ternary complex purified from human heart[b]	Liquid frozen/ Lyophilized	AACC	NIST[a]	No homogeneity and stability informations Validation and selection to be completed	To be performed
		Primary: recombinant IC binary complex[b]	Liquid frozen/ Lyophilized	AACC	NIST[a]	No homogeneity and stability informations Validation and selection to be completed	To be performed
		Secondary: human serum spiked with "degraded" recombinant ITC complex	Liquid frozen	AACC	?	Complete characterization to be performed No homogeneity and stability informations Validation to be completed	To be performed

[a]When the material will be available.
[b]These are alternative candidate materials. After the study completion, only one material will be selected and certified.
NA, Not available; AACC, American Association for Clinical Chemistry; IRMM, Institute for Reference Materials and Measurements; ID-MS, isotope dilution mass spectrometry; IFCC C-SMCD, Committee on Standardization of Markers of Cardiac Damage of the International Federation of Clinical Chemistry and Laboratory Medicine; NIST, National Institute of Standards and Technology.

In the case of myoglobin, a dedicated effort by the IFCC C-SMCD is in progress to prepare a secondary reference material *(42)*. The producer of the selected candidate material was requested to prepare a second larger batch of this material, providing all data necessary to characterize it for submission to the Institute for Reference Materials and Measurements (IRMM). To certify the proposed material, the establishment of a reference method based on mass spectrometry was the option selected by the C-SMCD in agreement with IRMM. When the certified reference material is available, a round robin study will be carried out involving all the interested companies to show assay standardization through the use of this material.

In the case of cTnI, AACC established in 1996 a subcommittee for standardization of cTnI immunoassays *(43)*. The subcommittee's primary mission was to develop and characterize a reference material for cTnI to minimize between-method variation. At present, the AACC subcommittee is starting a round robin study, including serum pools for comparison and a preliminary evaluation of inter-method commutability of the five selected candidate reference materials (four primary and one secondary) (Table 5). Preliminary characterization studies to verify the material composition were conducted at NIST. Of particular interest is the evaluation, as secondary material, of a preparation based on the hypothesis that incubation of a recombinant human cardiac ITC complex in human serum may generate a material that closely resembles cTnI composition from clinical samples *(44)*.

DEFINITION OF QUALITY SPECIFICATIONS FOR CARDIAC MARKER ASSAYS

Standardization is not only the process of realizing traceability by the creation of a reference system, but also the attempt to reduce the sources of variability of immunoassays (Table 6). The quality of a method and its analytical performance characteristics should be judged against objective quality specifications, for example, published state-of-the-art data or recommendations documented by expert professional groups. On this particular topic, a document on quality specifications for cardiac troponin assays was recently prepared by C-SMCD *(9)*. The main goals of this document were:

1. Manufacturers endorse or at minimum address the enclosed recommendations.
2. All package inserts and instructions for use of troponin immunoassays include adequate information on method design, as well as on preanalytical and analytical performance characteristics.
3. The scientific community selects research projects that consider with priority the definition of the issues addressed in the document.

Relevant points in the document were related to analytical factors, that is, antibody specificity, calibrator characterization, sample dilution, detection limit, analytical imprecision, and assay interferences, and preanalytical factors, that is, sample type and storage *(9)*. Many of these issues have already been discussed in this chapter and in other chapters of this book. The issue of analytical imprecision of cardiac marker assays and its importance for medical decision making is discussed briefly.

Analytical imprecision is not uniform between commercial assays for cardiac markers. The C-SMCD recommends a total imprecision (as coefficient of variation [CV]) at MI decision limit of <6% for myoglobin and of <10% for CK-MB mass and troponins *(1,9)*. It was shown, however, that some commercial assays for myoglobin determination do

Table 6
Sources of Analytical and Preanalytical
Variability in Immunoassays for Cardiac Marker Measurement

Heterogeneity of analyte
Antibody used in the assay: specificity, species/nature, stability of corresponding epitopes
Technique of measurement
Separation technique
Label and detection method
Calibration procedure
Curve-fitting algorithm
Dilution medium
Matrix effects of sample
Sample collection and processing
Laboratory environment

Adapted from ref. *12.*

not meet this target of quality, and that an improvement in precision is required if these assays are to be offered on a routine basis *(45)*. Also, for troponin determination, not all the assays perform equally well in routine clinical settings. Individual assay imprecisions are summarized in Table 7; these are based on information supplied by the peer-reviewed literature *(46–59)*.

Efforts to improve the imprecision of myoglobin and cardiac troponin assays are therefore warranted. Clinical laboratories should carefully consider the effect of imprecision on clinical decision making when they implement and evaluate new assays for cardiac marker determination. In the interest of cost-effectiveness, the implementation of an assay for cardiac markers in clinical laboratories often occurs on the analyzers already available in the laboratory. In this way, the costs for performing markers are only incremental (for the additional reagents and disposables needed) to those already invested in the acquisition of the hardware. While this author does not oppose in principle a strategy of cost-effectiveness, considerations related to the imprecision of the values obtained must be paramount in the selection of a platform for measuring cardiac marker panel *(60)*.

To highlight the issue of imprecision of troponin assays, the C-SMCD have recently prepared a protocol to evaluate objectively the analytical imprecision of commercially available troponin assays around the decision limit for MI, through the careful definition of the imprecision profile for each assay. The imprecision profile, namely, a scattergraph showing on the ordinate the CV vs increasing troponin concentrations on the abscissa, will be obtained using the NCCLS EP5-A protocol for evaluation of the imprecision by assessing pools of human sera containing troponin concentrations that cover the low-concentration range of the assay *(46)*. From this profile, the troponin concentration associated with a 10% CV, determined from the intercept of the total CV (*y*-axis) equal to 10% with the imprecision profile curve, will be determined and the performance of each assay evaluated. The C-SMCD hopes that the results of this study can help to clarify this pivotal point for the right implementation of the new diagnostic strategies in ACS patients *(61)*.

Table 7
Total Imprecision Around the Diagnostic Cutoffs for MI
of Commercial Assays for Cardiac Troponin Determination

Company/platform	Troponin concentration (ng/mL)	CV_{TOT} (%)	Reference
Abbott AxSYM	1.25	20.0	Yeo et al. *(46)*
Bayer ACS:180	1.33	4.1	Pagani et al. *(47)*
Bayer ACS:Centaur	0.52	13.0	Stiegler et al. *(48)*
Bayer Immuno 1	1.00	4.9	Wu *(49)*
Beckman Access 2nd gen.	0.09	10.0	Wu et al. *(50)*
BioMerieux Vidas	0.27	8.4	Bataillon et al. *(51)*
Biosite Triage	0.34	19.5	Wu *(49)*
Dade Dimension RxL 2nd gen.	0.14	11.4	Kaminski et al. *(52)*
Dade Opus 2nd gen.	0.22	17.7	Sanhai et al. *(53)*
Dade Stratus CS	0.08	14.0	Altinier et al. *(54)*
DPC Immulite	1.00	9.8	Kao et al. *(55)*
DPC Immulite Turbo	1.26	20.0	Yeo et al. *(46)*
First Medical Alpha Dx	0.30	7.4	Apple et al. *(56)*
Ortho-Clinical Diagn. Vitros	0.35	10.0	Apple et al. *(57)*
Roche Cardiac Reader	0.33	18.0	Muller-Bardorff et al. *(58)*
Roche Elecsys 3rd gen.	0.11	3.6	Pagani et al. *(59)*

CV_{TOT}, Total coefficient of variation; gen., generation.

The demand for very precise cardiac marker assays undoubtedly presents a difficult challenge, but comparison of different generation assays performed on the same instruments clearly shows that there has been a significant improvement in the precision offered by the newer assays and that this improvement has been considered by manufacturers as the main goal in the design of new assays *(50,52)*.

CONCLUSIONS

Owing to a very complicated situation, it is clear that the problems of cardiac marker standardization will not be solved within the next few years. Nevertheless, a number of projects are at present underway under the auspices of IFCC and other organizations. In this situation, it is above all essential that a uniform and rigorous outlook be maintained to ensure optimal utilization of all expertise available, including that in the diagnostic industry.

ABBREVIATIONS

AACC, American Association for Clinical Chemistry; ACS, acute coronary syndrome(s); CK, creatine kinase; CK-MB, MB isoenzyme of CK; C-SMCD, Committee on Standardization of Markers of Cardiac Damage; cTnI, cardiac troponin I; cTnT, cardiac troponin T; CV, coefficient of variation; IFCC, International Federation of Clinical Chemistry and Laboratory Medicine; IRMM, Institute for Reference Materials and Measurements; IVD, in vitro diagnostics; JCTLM, Joint Committee on Traceability in Laboratory Medicine; MI, myocardial infarction; NIST, National Institute for Standards and Technology; SI, International System of Units.

REFERENCES

1. Panteghini M, Apple FS, Christenson RH, Dati F, Mair J, Wu AH. Use of biochemical markers in acute coronary syndromes. IFCC Scientific Division, Committee on Standardization of Markers of Cardiac Damage. Clin Chem Lab Med 1999;37:687–693.
2. Apple FS, Murakami M, Panteghini M, et al., on behalf of the IFCC Committee on Standardization of Markers of Cardiac Damage. International survey on the use of cardiac markers. Clin Chem 2001;47:587–588.
3. Panteghini M, Pagani F, Bonetti G. The sensitivity of cardiac markers: an evidence-based approach. Clin Chem Lab Med 1999;37:1097–1106.
4. Panteghini M. Diagnostic application of CK-MB mass determination. Clin Chim Acta 1998; 72:23–31.
5. Alpert J, Thygesen K, Antman E, Bassand JP, for the Joint European Society of Cardiology/American College of Cardiology Committee. Myocardial infarction redefined—A consensus document of the Joint European Society of Cardiology/American College of Cardiology Committee for the Redefinition of Myocardial Infarction. J Am Coll Cardiol 2000;36:959–969.
6. Stöckl D, Franzini C, Kratochvila J, Middle J, Ricos C, Thienpont LM. Current stage of standardization of measurements of specific polypeptides and proteins discussed in light of steps needed towards a comprehensive measurement system. Eur J Clin Chem Clin Biochem 1997;35:719–732.
7. Müller MM. Implementation of reference systems in laboratory medicine. Clin Chem 2000; 46:1907–1909.
8. Labugger R, Organ L, Collier C, Atar D, Van Eyk JE. Extensive troponin I and T modification detected in serum from patients with acute myocardial infarction. Circulation 2000; 102:1221–1226.
9. Panteghini M, Gerhardt W, Apple FS, Dati F, Ravkilde J, Wu AH. Quality specifications for cardiac troponin assays. International Federation of Clinical Chemistry and Laboratory Medicine (IFCC). IFCC Scientific Division Committee on Standardization of Markers of Cardiac Damage. Clin Chem Lab Med 2001;39:174–178.
10. International Organization for Standardization—ISO. Terms and definitions used in connection with reference materials. ISO Guide 30:1992.
11. Dybkaer R. Reference materials—a main element in a coherent measurement system. Eur J Clin Chem Clin Biochem 1991;29:241–246.
12. Dati F, Panteghini M, Apple FS, Christenson RH, Mair J, Wu AH. Proposals from the IFCC Committee on Standardization of Markers of Cardiac Damage (C-SMCD): strategies and concepts on standardization of cardiac marker assays. Scand J Clin Lab Invest 1999; 59(Suppl 230):113–123.
13. Gella FJ, Frey E, Ceriotti F, et al. Production and certification of an enzyme reference material for creatine kinase isoenzyme 2 (CRM 608). Clin Chim Acta 1998;276:35–52.
14. Schreiber A, Specht B, Pelsers MMAL, Glatz JFZ, Börchers T, Spener F. Recombinant human heart-type fatty acid-binding protein as standard in immunochemical assays. Clin Chem Lab Med 1998;36:283–288.
15. Liu SG, Shi QW, Song QL, et al. Development and analysis of recombinant human cardiac troponin complexes for immunoassay controls and calibrators. Clin Chem 1998;44(Suppl):A21.
16. Zhang MY, Song QL, Shi QW, Kadijevic L, Liu SG. Recombinant single chain cardiac troponin I-C polypeptide: an ideal stable control material for cardiac troponin I immunoassays. Clin Chem 1999;45(Suppl):A53.
17. Christenson RH, Vaidya H, Landt Y, et al. Standardization of creatine kinase-MB (CK-MB) mass assays: the use of recombinant CK-MB as a reference material. Clin Chem 1999;45: 1414–1423.
18. Liu S, Zhang M, Ling Q, et al. The second generation of recombinant single chain cardiac troponin I-C polypeptide: a superior stable control material for cardiac troponin I immunoassays. Clin Chem 2000;46(Suppl):A179–A180.

19. Sunahara Y, Uchida K, Tanaka T, Matsukawa H, Inagaki M, Matuo Y. Production of recombinant human creatine kinase (r-hCK) isozymes by tandem repeat expression of M and B genes and characterization of r-hCK-MB. Clin Chem 2001;47:471–476.

20. Tobias R, Pekatch T, Frater Y, Styba G, McClure S, Jackowski S. Heme reconstitution and folding of recombinant myoglobin. Clin Chem 1997;43:S158.

21. Whicher JT. Calibration is the key to immunoassay but the ideal calibrator is unattainable. Scand J Clin Lab Invest 1991;51(Suppl 205):21–32.

22. Ekins R. Immunoassay standardization. Scand J Clin Lab Invest 1991;51(Suppl 205):33–46.

23. Christenson RH, Duh SH, Apple FS, et al. Standardization of cardiac troponin I assays: round robin of ten candidate reference materials. Clin Chem 2001;47:431–437.

24. Sánchez M, Canalias F, Palencia T, Gella FJ. Creatine kinase 2 mass measurement: methods comparison and study of the matrix effect. Clin Chim Acta 1999;288:111–119.

25. Sánchez M, Gella FJ, Profilis C, et al. Certification of the mass concentration of creatine kinase isoenzyme 2 (CK-MB) in the reference material BCR 608. Clin Chem Lab Med 2001; 39:858–865.

26. Kahn SE, Apple FS, Bodor GS, et al. Standardization of cardiac troponin I assays: pilot evaluation of ten candidate reference materials. Clin Chem 2000;46(Suppl):A89.

27. Stenman UH. Immunoassay standardization: is it possible, who is responsible, who is capable? Clin Chem 2001;47:815–820.

28. Bender D, Tobias R, Shaikh N. Patient-based CK-MB calibrators: a potential commutable/secondary standard for CK-MB immunoassay instrumentation. Clin Chem 2001;47(Suppl): A202.

29. Tobias RB, Bender D, Pituley A, Shi Q, Shaikh N. Development of clinical-based and recombinant calibrators for myoglobin diagnostic tests. Clin Chem 2001;47(Suppl):A203–A204.

30. Whicher JT, Ritchie RF, Johnson AM, et al. New international reference preparation for proteins in human serum (RPPHS). Clin Chem 1994;40:934–938.

31. Cattozzo G, Franzini C, Melzi d'Eril GV. Myoglobin and creatine kinase isoenzyme MB mass assays: intermethod behaviour of patient sera and commercially available control materials. Clin Chim Acta 2001;303:55–60.

32. Rej R, Drake P. The nature of calibrators in immunoassays: Are they commutable with test samples? Must they be? Scand J Clin Lab Invest 1991;51(Suppl 205):47–54.

33. Moss DW, Whicher JT. Commutability and the problem of method-dependent results. Eur J Clin Chem Clin Biochem 1995;33:1003–1007.

34. Barr JR, Maggio VL, Patterson DG, et al. Isotope dilution-mass spectrometric quantification of specific proteins: model application with apoliprotein A-I. Clin Chem 1996;42:1676–1682.

35. Panteghini M, Ceriotti F, Schumann G, Siekmann L. Establishing a reference system in clinical enzymology. Clin Chem Lab Med 2001;39:795–800.

36. Katrukha AG, Bereznikova AV, Filatov VL, et al. Degradation of cardiac troponin I: implication for reliable immunodetection. Clin Chem 1998;44:2433–2440.

37. Green S, Onoroski M, Moore R, Wu A, Lehrer M, Vaidya H and the AACC CK-MB mass assay standardization subcommittee (MB-MASS). Standardization of CK-MB mass immunoassays. Clin Chem 1994;40:1032.

38. Panteghini M. Update on cardiac troponin standardization. Biochim Clin 2001;25:275–276.

39. Panteghini M. IFCC Committee on Standardization of Markers of Cardiac Damage: premises and project presentation. Clin Chem Lab Med 1998;36:887–893.

40. Panteghini M. Standardization activities of markers of cardiac damage: the need of a comprehensive approach. Eur Heart J 1998;19(Suppl N):N8–N11.

41. International Organization for Standardization, European Committee for Standardization. In vitro diagnostic medical devices—measurement of quantities in samples of biological origin—metrological traceability of values assigned to calibrators and control materials. ISO/TC 212/WG2 N65 prEN 17511. Geneva, Switzerland: International Organization for Standardization, 2000.

42. Panteghini M, Apple FS, Christenson RH, Dati F, Mair J, Wu AH. Recent approaches in standardization of cardiac markers. Clin Chem Lab Med 1999;37(Suppl):S112.
43. Wu AHB, Feng YJ, Moore R, Apple FS, McPherson PH, Buechler KF, Bodor G, for the American Association for Clinical Chemistry subcommittee on cTnI standardization. Characterization of cardiac troponin subunit release into serum after acute myocardial infarction and comparison of assays for troponin T and I. Clin Chem 1998;44:1198–1208.
44. Shi Q, Zhang MY, Kadijevic L, Liu S. Creation of a commutable cardiac troponin I calibration material. Clin Chem 2001;47(Suppl):A27.
45. Zaninotto M, Pagani F, Altinier S, et al. Multicenter evaluation of five assays for myoglobin determination. Clin Chem 2000;46:1631–1637.
46. Yeo KTJ, Quinn-Hall KS, Bateman SW, Fischer GA, Wieczorek S, Wu AHB. Functional sensitivity of cardiac troponin assays and its implications for risk stratification of patients with acute coronary syndromes. In: Markers in Cardiology: Current and Future Clinical Applications. Adams JE III, Apple FS, Jaffe AS, Wu AHB, eds. Armonk, NY: Futura, 2001, pp. 23–29.
47. Pagani F, Bonetti G, Stefini F, Cuccia C, Panteghini M. Determination of decision limits for ACS: systems cardiac troponin I. Clin Chem Lab Med 2000;38:1155–1157.
48. Stiegler H, Fisher Y, Vazquez-Jimenez JF, et al. Lower cardiac troponin T and I results in heparin-plasma than in serum. Clin Chem 2000;46:1338–1344.
49. Wu AHB. Laboratory and near patient testing for cardiac markers. J Clin Ligand Assay 1999; 22:32–37.
50. Wu A, Apple F, Venge P, et al. Analytical performance of Beckman Coulter's Access AccuTnI (troponin I) in a multicenter evaluation. Clin Chem Lab Med 2001;39(Suppl):S191.
51. Bataillon S, Incaurgarat B, Varret F, et al. Preliminary evaluation of the Vidas cardiac troponin I assay. Clin Chem Lab Med 2001;39(Suppl):S195.
52. Kaminski D, Sivakoff S, McCormack B, Pierson-Perry J. Development and analytical performance of an improved method for cardiac troponin-I on the Dade Behring Dimension clinical chemistry system. Clin Chem 2001;47(Suppl):A211.
53. Sanhai WR, Romero LF, Hickey G, Ruttle D, Christenson RH. Performance characteristics of a revised cardiac troponin I assay for the Opus plus immunoassay system. Clin Biochem 2001;34:579–582.
54. Altinier S, Mion M, Cappelletti C, Zaninotto M, Plebani M. Rapid measurement of cardiac markers on Stratus CS. Clin Chem 2000;46:991–993.
55. Kao JT, Wong IL, Lee JY, Chen RC. Comparison of Abbott AxSYM, Behring Opus Plus, DPC Immulite and Ortho-Clinical Diagnostics Vitros ECi for measurement of cardiac troponin I. Ann Clin Biochem 2001;38:140–146.
56. Apple FS, Anderson FP, Collinson P, et al. Clinical evaluation of the First Medical whole blood, point-of-care testing device for detection of myocardial infarction. Clin Chem 2000; 46:1604–1609.
57. Apple FS, Koplen B, Murakami MM. Preliminary evaluation of the Vitros ECi cardiac troponin I assay. Clin Chem 2000;46:572–574.
58. Muller-Bardorff M, Rauscher T, Kampmann M, et al. Quantitative bedside assay for cardiac troponin T: a complementary method to centralized laboratory testing. Clin Chem 1999; 45:1002–1008.
59. Pagani F, Bonetti G, Panteghini M. Evaluation of the Elecsys electrochemiluminescent immunoassay for cardiac troponin T determination. Clin Chem. 1999;45(Suppl):A144.
60. Jaffe AS, Ravkilde J, Roberts R, et al. It's time for a change to a troponin standard. Circulation 2000;102:1216–1220.
61. Panteghini M. Recent approaches in standardization of cardiac markers. Clin Chim Acta 2001;311:19–25.

14

Analytical Issues and the Evolution of Cutoff Concentrations for Cardiac Markers

Alan H. B. Wu

INTRODUCTION

Cardiac troponin has been shown to be very useful for the determination of minor myocardial damage (MMD) for patients who present with chest pain. Subsequent outcome studies have shown that patients with an increase in troponin are at high short-term risk (4 wk) for death and myocardial infarction (MI). These clinical trials together with a better understanding of the pathophysiology of acute coronary syndromes (ACS) have led the European Society of Cardiology (ESC) and the American College of Cardiology (ACC) to formulate a joint committee to redefine the criteria for acute myocardial infarction (AMI) (1). Their recommendation was that, in the context of cardiac ischemia, any increase in the concentration of cardiac troponin or creatine kinase (CK) in blood is indicative of AMI. A working subgroup of the ESC/ACC Committee have recommended that the cutoff concentration for cardiac markers be set at the 99% of the reference range (2). However, as summarized in Table 1, the acceptance and implementation of these new standards have been slowed by the continued lack of sensitivity for commercial troponin assays. Another of the major issues is the proper determination of the appropriate cutoff concentrations. These issues are discussed in this chapter.

TROPONIN VS CK-MB IN MMD

When cardiac troponins T and I (cTnT and cTnI) were first introduced into clinical practice, there were questions concerning the interpretation of an increased cTnT or cTnI with a normal CK and MB isoenzyme of CK (CK-MB), in the clinical context of ACS. Because of the discrepancies with troponin test results vs CK-MB, then considered the gold standard marker for cardiac damage, cardiologists, emergency department physicians, and clinical laboratory practitioners were confused about how to interpret results. The early concern was that troponin was possibly not specific for cardiac damage. However, numerous analytical studies (3,4) and clinical outcomes studies (5,6) have shown that troponin is a highly specific and sensitive marker of cardiac damage. The specificity is derived from the fact that skeletal muscle troponin T and I are structurally distinct from cardiac isotypes and monoclonal antibodies toward the cardiac form do not cross-react with the skeletal muscle forms. Moreover, studies have shown that cardiac troponin is not released from regenerating skeletal muscle or renal tissue (7,8).

From: *Cardiac Markers, Second Edition*
Edited by: Alan H. B. Wu @ Humana Press Inc., Totowa, NJ

Table 1
Factors Leading to Ambiguities in the Use of Cardiac Troponin Assays

1. Changing criteria for diagnosis of AMI
2. Disagreement of troponin results vs CK-MB (previously considered the "gold standard" cardiac marker)
3. Lack of assay standardization and differences in the performance of commercial troponin assays
4. Lack of assay standardization between central laboratory based and point-of-care testing platforms for cardiac troponin assays
5. Confusion in the assignment of cutoff concentrations

The sensitivity is the result of the higher myocardial tissue content of troponin vs CK (6–10 mg/g wet wt for troponin vs 1 mg/g wet wt for CK).

LACK OF STANDARDIZATION

There is a uniform lack of standardization for the three most widely used cardiac markers, myoglobin, CK-MB, and cTnI. These problems are being addressed by Standardization Subcommittees of the International Federation of Clinical Chemistry (IFCC) for myoglobin and the American Association for Clinical Chemistry (AACC) for CK-MB and cTnI. The objectives and activities of these committees are summarized in Chapter 13. The initial standardization effort was for CK-MB *(9)*. Although a commercial standard for CK-MB has been characterized and is now available for use, manufacturers of CK-MB have been slow to adopt it. Differences in results between myoglobin and CK-MB from different manufacturers can vary by one- to twofold from each other. Of the three cardiac markers, the greatest discrepancies among commercial assays is seen for cTnI. Results from one assay to another can differ by as much as 40-fold. There are two major reasons for these discrepancies: the lack of an accepted troponin I standard and the use of different antibody pairs in commercial kits. The problem of standardization was caused by use of different materials as the standard (peptides, free and complexed troponin forms). Much of this was caused by uncertainties as to how troponin is released after myocardial injury. The nature of differences in antibody specificity and strategies for optimum antibody selection are discussed in Chapter 10.

Until standardization for cardiac markers can be achieved, results from one assay are not directly comparable to results from another. If a patient is transferred from one facility to another, repeat testing of previous samples will be necessary to interpret data from more recent blood collections.

ESTABLISHMENT OF THE PROPER CUTOFF CONCENTRATIONS FOR CARDIAC MARKERS

Basic Concepts for Assignment of the Reference Range

Normal ranges and cutoff concentrations for disease detection are essential elements for clinical use and interpretation of clinical laboratory tests. Once a laboratory test has been developed, it is necessary to determine the normal range of the analyte, that is, the

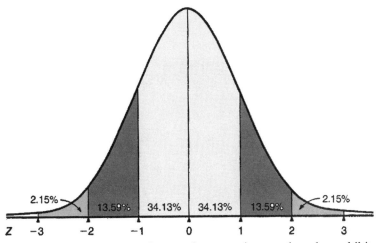

Fig. 1. Determination of the normal range for normal range data that exhibits a Gaussian distribution.

distribution of test results from a presumably healthy population. If the distribution of results falls under a Gaussian distribution ("bell-shaped curve," *see* Fig. 1), the normal range is calculated as the mean plus or minus two times the standard deviation (SD). This analysis will include 95% of the test population. If the distribution is non-Gaussian, the data are listed in ascending or descending order, and the normal range is calculated as the central 95% of test results. When the normal range is used for clinical diagnosis, it is termed the "reference range." It should be noted that when the normal range is established in this manner, 5% of a healthy population will have an abnormal test result. Use of the 99th percentile raises the upper limit of normal (and the lower limit if applicable) and reduces the number of false-positives to 1% total.

These statistical treatments are applicable for tests that have clinical significance at both high and low concentrations, for example, thyroid-stimulating hormone (TSH) for detection of hypo- and hyperthyroidism, respectively. For cardiac markers, only high results are significant, and therefore only an upper reference range limit is necessary. This is calculated as the mean plus 2 SD (Gaussian distribution) or the lower 97.5% of the test results (non-Gaussian). Use of the 99th percentile results in the mean plus 3 SD or the lower 99.5% of test results.

The population of healthy individuals tested for the normal range determination should be age, race, and gender matched to the population for which the test is intended. For example, in the case of cardiac markers, the reference range determination in pediatric patients is largely unnecessary. If there are significant differences between the normal range of subpopulations, separate determinations and assignments should be made.

The use of the normal range as the reference range for interpretation of laboratory tests is appropriate when the analyte is used to determine multiple disease processes, abnormalities, or etiologies. Glucose is used to determine stress, diabetes mellitus, hypoglycemia, and other clinical conditions. Serum creatinine is generically used to indicate glomerular disease, irrespective to the underlying etiology (e.g., nephrotic syndrome or glomerular nephritis).

Some laboratory tests are used not to detect the presence of disease, but for determining the likelihood of future disease risk. Thus, it is not appropriate to use the normal range as the reference range. In a Western population, the normal range for total, high-density lipoprotein (HDL), and low-density lipoprotein (LDL) cholesterol is higher than the target concentrations established by the National Cholesterol Education Program cutoffs for low risk. This simply indicates that the average individual on a Western diet is at higher risk than ideal. In a similar manner, tests on amniotic fluid for Down's syndrome (so-called "triple markers") are expressed as relative risk ratios and not on the basis on whether or not the test is normal or abnormal. This approach is used because these tests are not diagnostic for Down's syndrome.

CUTOFF CONCENTRATIONS FOR CARDIAC MARKERS

CK is a test for which a separate normal range for gender is necessary. The total CK enzyme activity and myoglobin concentrations from normal individuals originate from the turnover and remodeling of skeletal muscles. Owing to higher skeletal muscle contents, men have higher reference ranges than women for both tests, although separate reference ranges are not always used. The cutoff for total CK is determined from the upper 97.5% of a Gaussian distribution, and myoglobin from the upper 97.5% of a non-Gaussian distribution of results from a healthy population.

Cutoff concentrations for cardiac markers, particularly CK-MB, have also not been traditionally established from the normal range. This is partly because CK-MB was used only for diagnosis of a single disease, that is, AMI. Therefore cutoff concentrations were established by the value that discriminated between patients with AMI, as defined by criteria established by the World Health Organization (WHO), from other patients presenting with chest pain, but for whom the diagnosis of AMI was ruled out. As such, patients with unstable angina were ruled out under the original WHO definition of AMI *(10)*. Using this designation, the AMI cutoff concentration for CK-MB is substantially higher than the upper limit of normal, as determined from a healthy population.

THE WHO ROC CUTOFF CONCEPT

Optimum AMI cutoff concentrations were determined by the use of receiver operating characteristic (ROC) curve analysis *(11)*. ROC curves are graphical plots of clinical sensitivity vs 1–clinical specificity at different marker concentrations (Fig. 2)[1]. The cutoff concentration that produces a point closest to the 100% values for both axes ("ideal test," *see upper left hand corner* of Fig. 2) defines the optimum cutoff. The area-under-the-curve (AUC) can be calculated when comparing the results of one ROC curve to another. The curve that produces an area closest to 1.00 is the more valuable test. Prior to the redefinition of AMI by the ESC/ACC, The National Academy of Clinical Biochemistry (NACB) recommended that the AMI cutoff be established from ROC curve analysis *(12)*. This cutoff was based on the definition of AMI established by the

---

[1]The sensitivity of a test is the number of true positives (positive test result in the presence of a disease) divided by the sum of the true positives and false negatives (negative test result in the presence of a disease). The specificity of a test is the number of true negatives (negative test result in the absence of a disease) divided by the sum of the true negatives and false positives (positive test result in the absence of a disease).

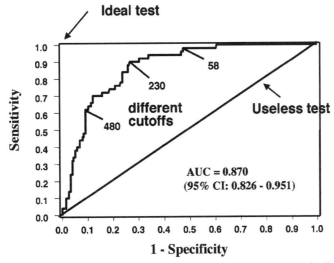

Fig. 2. ROC curve. The AUC and 95% confidence interval for the AUC is shown. Individual cutoff concentrations are plotted on the curve. An ideal test is one that has 100% sensitivity and specificity (plots as a single point at the *upper right hand corner*). A useless test is a line that runs from the *lower left corner* to the *upper right corner*.

WHO. Because of the importance of MMD for risk stratification of patients with unstable angina, the NACB recommended a second lower cutoff at the 95th percentile of the normal range.

The 99th Percentile and 10% Coefficient of Variation Cut Point Concepts

ROC curve analysis is appropriate for diseases or conditions that are either present or absent (e.g., either a woman is pregnant or not pregnant). ACS, however, present as a continuum of events that begins with plaque rupture, clot formation, reversible injury and MMD and non-ST elevation MI, and ST-elevation MI (Fig. 3). Therefore two cutoffs as suggested by the NACB was not consistent with the pathophysiology of a disease continuum. The high sensitivity and specificity of cardiac troponin makes it possible to tract the progression of this disease from the first onset of irreversible injury. Because irreversible cardiac damage can occur by a number of mechanisms besides ischemic disease, for example, congestive heart failure, myocarditis, and other disorders, cardiac troponin should be considered as a marker of myocardial damage, and not just a marker of AMI. The Joint ESC/ACC Committee have recommended that any statistically significant increase in cardiac troponin should be considered as a positive indication of cardiac disease. The finding of any significant increase in a cardiac marker, notably cardiac troponin, in the context of ischemia, has become the predicate for the new definition of AMI *(1)*.

What remains to be established is what constitutes an analytically and clinically significant increase. A cardiac markers subcommittee of the ESC/ACC have recommended that the 99th percentile of the normal range be used as the cutoff for cardiac markers *(2)*. This group has also suggested that the precision of the assay be at least 10%. While the 99% cutoff designation is sufficient for CK-MB, this presents a problem for the current

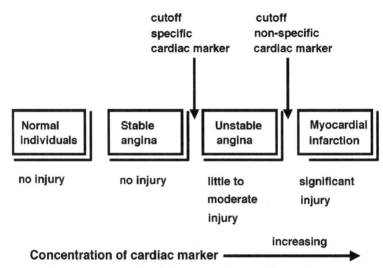

Fig. 3. The continuum of myocardial injury in ACS. Cutoffs for CK-MB are set to differentiate between unstable angina and MI. Troponin is more sensitive and detects release during the early stages of ACS.

generation of cardiac troponin assays, as these tests do not have the predicate sensitivity to detect troponin in health individuals. Therefore the 99% of the normal range cannot be calculated with statistical reliability. As a compromise, Apple and Wu suggested that for any given troponin assay, the cutoff be determined as the troponin concentration that produces a 10% coefficient of variation (CV), as determined by between-run precision studies *(13)*. This value was selected because it is an estimate of the biological variation for cardiac markers (*see* next section).

Figure 4A illustrates the concentration vs precision profile for the Beckman Access (second-generation) troponin assay. The 95th and 99th percentiles were determined to be 0.03 and 0.04 ng/mL, respectively. However, the precision at these are >10%. Therefore the more appropriate cutoff concentration is higher, that is, 0.06 ng/mL. For cTnT, the 95% and 99% are 0.01 ng/mL, with a 10% CV cut point of 0.03 (Fig. 4B). Precision studies are normally conducted over several weeks using a single instrument and lot number of reagents.

Assessment of the Biological Variability

The selection of the 10% CV value as the cutoff for cardiac markers has not been documented with clinical trials. It was derived from the "functional sensitivity" concept used for defining the specific generation and applicable cutoff concentrations for assays for TSH. The functional sensitivity for TSH assays is defined as the concentration that produces a 20% CV *(14)*. Use of this limit for cardiac markers will produce a limit that is very low relative to the current ROC-based cutoff. Rather than go to this extreme, the ESC/ACC opted to use a slightly higher cutoff, the value that produces a 10% CV.

For cardiac markers, the concentration at 10% CV is based on the biological variation of these markers. The biological variation (BV) is calculated from:

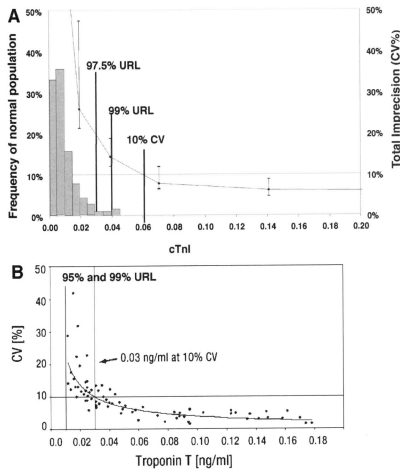

Fig. 4. The precision vs concentration profile for the (**A**) Beckman Access cTnI assay and (**B**) Roche Elecsys cTnT assay. The 95%, 99%, and 10% CV cutoffs are identified.

$$\text{Intraindividual biological variance, } \delta_I^2 = \delta_{total-W}^2 - \delta_A^2$$

$$\text{Interindividual biological variance, } \delta_G = \delta_{total-B}^2 - \delta_A^2 - \delta_I^2$$

where $\delta_{total-W}$ = total within-subject variation, $\delta_{total-B}$ = total between-subject variation, and δ_A = analytical variation. The corresponding CVs are determined by the (variance/ mean) × 100.

The analytical goal for precision will be determined as: $CV_I^{1/2}/2$. The critical difference required for a serial change is 2.77 $(CV_I^2 + CV_G^2)^{1/2}$. The biological variability for myoglobin and CK have been experimentally determined to be 9.3% *(15)* and 5.6% *(16)*, respectively. The biological variability for troponin cannot be determined by current commercial assays because of the lack of assay sensitivity. The 10% CV is an estimate based on the data from myoglobin and CK-MB.

The Limit of Detection Concept as a Cutoff for Cardiac Markers

There are at least two alternative procedures for determining the sensitivity of an assay and are candidates to be used as the cut point for cardiac markers (Table 2). The

Table 2
Methods for Determining Assay Sensitivity

Method	Description
10% CV	In precision studies, the concentration that produces a 10% between-run precision
Dilution	A high sample is diluted and the concentration calculated from a calibration curve. The last dilution that remains within 10% of the target value is the limit of sensitivity.
Statistical	Repeated measurement of a sample devoid of the sample. The limit of sensitivity is determined as the mean of results plus three times the standard deviation.

statistical method is to determine the analyte concentration that produces a signal-to-noise ratio that exceeds 3.0 *(17)*. This can be accomplished experimentally by repeatedly measuring a sample devoid of the analyte into an appropriate matrix, and taking the mean of results and adding three times the standard deviation. In the dilution method, one serially dilutes a sample containing the analyte and determines the concentration of the dilutions from a standard curve *(18)*. When the concentration at which the dilution deviates by some fixed amount, for example, 10% of the expected value based on the undiluted result divided by the dilution factor, the limit of detection has been exceeded.

The limit of detection concept has been proposed as a cutoff for cardiac markers and has produced cutoff concentrations that are below the 10% CV cutoff concept *(19)*. Clinical trials studies such as Treat Angina with Aggrastat and determine Cost of Therapy with an Invasive or Conservative Strategy (TACTICS) *(20)* and Fragmin in Unstable Coronary Artery Disease (FRISC) II *(21)* have shown that use of very low cutoff concentrations for cTnT and cTnI have resulted in the identification of additional patients with non-ST elevation AMI deemed to be at future risk. In this author's opinion, use of this very low cutoff may be appropriate for patients identified as having non-ST elevation AMI such as those enrolled in these trials. However, use of this cutoff in a general group of patients who present with chest pain to an emergency department, who have a low prevalence of ACS, will degrade the positive predictive value of the test due to larger numbers of false-positive results *(22)*.

Cutoffs for the Natriuretic Peptides

Problems regarding cutoff concentrations and the lack of standardization for B-type natriuretic peptides (BNPs) are also anticipated to occur. In a manner similar to cTnT and cTnI, there is only one manufacturer of assays for amino- (N)-terminal proBNP (Roche Diagnostics) and several manufacturers for the intact BNP hormone (Shionogi, Biosite, Bayer, and Abbott). The use of different antibodies and different calibrating materials among the BNP assays will lead to standardization issues and confusion over diagnostic cutoffs. One advantage BNP has over cTnI is that assay sensitivity issues will not be a problem, as BNP concentrations are measurable in healthy individuals.

SUMMARY

Figure 5 summarizes the various definitions of cutoff concentrations for AMI, beginning with the lowest (limit of detection concept) to the highest concentration (WHO

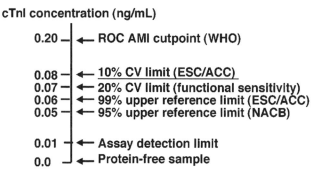

cTnI concentration (ng/mL)

0.20 — ← ROC AMI cutpoint (WHO)

0.08 — ← 10% CV limit (ESC/ACC)
0.07 — ← 20% CV limit (functional sensitivity)
0.06 — ← 99% upper reference limit (ESC/ACC)
0.05 — ← 95% upper reference limit (NACB)

0.01 — ← Assay detection limit
0.0 — ← Protein-free sample

Fig. 5. Cutoff concentrations for a hypothetical cTnI assay based on various criteria. The assay's detection limit should not be used as the diagnostic cut point.

ROC cut point concept) *(23)*. The concentration of a hypothetical cTnI assay is used for comparative purposes. The ESC/ACC have suggested that the concentration of the marker that produces a 10% CV is the best cut point (shown underlined) until there are improvements in analytical assays to enable the use of the 99% cut point value. Consistent with the IFCC Committee for Standardization of Markers of Cardiac Damage, use of error limits to this 10% CV cut point are also shown.

The selection of the appropriate cutoff concentration, especially for cardiac troponin, is far from settled. A major part of the problem is the lack of universal acceptance of the redefinition of the ESC/ACC guidelines. The criticisms to the redefinition began immediately after its publication in 2000. Most of the criticisms to this document have centered around the impact the redefinition will have on past and future epidemiology studies, therapeutic selection, and societal and other issues *(24–27)*. What is underappreciated by most clinicians is the inability of existing cardiac troponin assays to meet the performance goals set by the joint committees. This has led to continued confusion among laboratory and clinical practitioners alike as to the proper cutoff and interpretation of results. This debate will likely continue well into the next decade.

ABBREVIATIONS

AACC, American Association for Clinical Chemistry; ACC, American College of Cardiology; ACS, acute coronary syndrome(s); AMI, acute myocardial infarction; AUC, area-under-the curve; BNP, B-type natriuretic peptide; CK, creatine kinase; CK-MB, MB isoenzyme of CK; cTnT, cTnI, cardiac troponins T and I; CV, coefficient of variation; ESC, European Society of Cardiology; IFCC, International Federation of Clinical Chemistry; MI, myocardial infarction; MMD, minor myocardial damage; NACB, National Academy of Clinical Biochemistry; ROC, receiver operating characteristic; SD, standard deviation; TSH, thyroid-stimulating hormone; WHO, World Health Organization.

REFERENCES

1. Joint ESC/ACC Committee. Myocardial infarction redefined—a consensus document of The Joint European Society of Cardiology/American College of Cardiology Committee for the redefinition of myocardial infarction. J Am Coll Cardiol 2000;36:959–969.

2. Jaffe AS, Ravkilde J, Roberts R, et al. It's time to change to a troponin standard. Circulation 2000;102:1216–1220.

3. Adams J, Bodor G, Davila-Roman V, et al. Cardiac troponin I: a marker with high specificity for cardiac injury. Circulation 1993;88:101–106.

4. Ishii J, Ishikawa T, Yukitake J. Clinical specificity of a second generation cardiac troponin T assay in patients with chronic renal failure. Clin Chim Acta 1998;270:183–188.

5. Lindahl B, Venge P, Wallentin L. Troponin T identifies patients with unstable coronary artery disease who benefit from long-term antithrombotic protection. Fragmin in Unstable Coronary Artery Disease (FRISC) Study Group. J Am Coll Cardiol 1997;29:43–48.

6. Morrow DA, Antman EM, Tanasijevic M, et al. Cardiac troponin I for stratification of early outcomes and the efficacy of enoxaparin in unstable angina: a TIMI-11B substudy. J Am Coll Cardiol 2000;36:1812–1817.

7. Ricchiuti V, Voss EM, Ney A, Odland M, Anderson PAW, Apple FS. Cardiac troponin T isoforms expressed in renal diseased skeletal muscle will not cause false-positive results by the second generation cardiac troponin T assay by Boehringer Mannheim. Clin Chem 1998;44:1919–1924.

8. Haller C, Zehelein J, Remppis A, Muller-Bardorff M, Katus HA. Cardiac troponin T in patients with end-stage renal disease: absence of expression in truncal skeletal muscle. Clin Chem 1998;44:930–938.

9. Christenson RH, Vaidya H, Landt Y, et al. Standardization of creatine kinase-MB (CK-MB) mass assays: the use of recombinant CK-MB as a reference material. Clin Chem 1999;45:1414–1423.

10. World Health Organization. Report of the Joint International Society and Federation of Cardiology/World Health Organization Task Force on Standardization of Clinical Nomenclature. Nomenclature and criteria for diagnosis of ischemic heart disease. Circulation 1979;59:607–609.

11. Zweig MH, Campbell G. Receiver-operating characteristic (ROC) plots: a fundamental evaluation tool in clinical medicine. Clin Chem 1993;39:561–577.

12. Wu AHB, Apple FS, Gibler WB, Jesse RL, Warshaw MM, Valdes R Jr. National Academy of Clinical Biochemistry Standards of Laboratory Practice: recommendations for use of cardiac markers in coronary artery diseases. Clin Chem 1999;45:1104–1121.

13. Apple FS, Wu AHB. Myocardial infarction redefined: role of cardiac troponin testing (editorial). Clin Chem 2001;47:377–379.

14. Spencer CA, Takeuchi M, Kazarosyan M, MacKenzie F, Beckett GJ, Wilkinson E. Interlaboratory/intermethod differences in functional sensitivity of immunometric assays of thyrotropin (TSH) and impact on reliability of measurement of subnormal concentrations of TSH. Clin Chem 1995;41:367–374.

15. Panteghini M, Pagani F. Biological variation of myoglobin in serum (letter). Clin Chem 1997;42:2435.

16. Ross SM, Fraser CG. Biological variation of cardiac markers: analytical and clinical considerations. Ann Clin Biochem 1998;35:80–84.

17. Long GL, Winefordner JD. Limits of detection. A closer look at the IUPAC definition. Analyt Chem 1983;55:712A–719A.

18. Needleman SB, Romberg RW. Limits of linearity and detection for some drugs of abuse. J Analyt Toxicol 1990;14:34–38.

19. Tate J, Badrick T, Koumantakis G, Potter JM, Hickman PE. Reporting of cardiac troponin concentration. Clin Chem 2002;48:2077–2080.

20. Morrow DA, Cannon CP, Rifai N, et al. Ability of minor elevations of troponins I and T to predict benefit from an early invasive strategy in patients with unstable angina and non-ST elevation myocardial infarction. JAMA 2001;286:2405–2412.

21. Lindahl B, Diderhohn E, Lagerqvist B, Venge P, Wallentin L. Troponin T 0.1 mg/L is an inappropriate cutoff value for risk stratification in unstable coronary artery disease using the new third generation troponin T assay. J Am Coll Cardiol 2000;102(Suppl II):522.

22. Wu AHB, Apple FS. Reporting of cardiac troponin concentration [letter]. Clin Chem 2002; 48:2077–2082.

23. Apple FS, Wu AHB, Jaffe AS. European Society of Cardiology and American College of Cardiology guidelines for redefinition of myocardial infarction: how to use existing assays clinically and for clinical trials. Am Heart J 2002;144:981–986.

24. Tunstall-Pedoe H. Redefinition of myocardial infarction by a consensus dissenter. J Am Coll Cardiol 2001;37:1472–1473.

25. Richards AM, Lainchbury JG, Nicholls MG. Unsatisfactory redefinition of myocardial infarction. Lancet 2001;357:1635–1636.

26. Norris RM. Dissent from the consensus on the redefinition of myocardial infarction. Eur Heart J 2001;22:1626–1627.

27. Tormey W, Birkhead JS, Norris RM, Jolobe OMP. Redefinition of myocardial infarction. Lancet 2001;358:764.

Part IV
Early Cardiac Markers of Myocardial Ischemia and Risk Stratification

15

Rationale for the Early Clinical Application of Markers of Ischemia in Patients with Suspected Acute Coronary Syndromes

Robert L. Jesse

INTRODUCTION

Coronary artery disease accounted for well over half a million deaths in 1999, or about one out of every five deaths *(1)*. It had been projected that in 2002 were approx 1,250,000 acute coronary syndromes (ACS) of which about 60% were new and 40% recurrent events. More than 45% of the people who experience an ACS in a given year will die from it; 250,000 will die without being hospitalized. It is estimated that there are 12.5 million people alive today with a history of acute myocardial infarction (AMI), angina, or both. The incidence is equal between men and women.

In the setting of coronary atherosclerosis, a relatively benign plaque can precipitously become unstable, resulting in a myriad of clinical consequences. Risk stratification is a fundamental first step in the assessment of patients presenting with ACS; the success of a specific intervention is often directly linked to risk in a given patient. It is intuitive, then, that the ability to detect the higher-risk patients early would permit more expedient treatments aimed at minimization of the more severe outcomes. Failure to intervene in a timely fashion could result in myocardial cell death as detected by the presence of specific markers of necrosis in the peripheral blood.

A recent European Society of Cardiology/American College of Cardiology (ESC/ACC) consensus conference endorsed cardiac troponins T and I (cTnT and cTnI) as the necrosis markers of choice due to their superior sensitivity and specificity *(2)*. This document specifically proposed that, "*any amount of troponin caused by ischemia should be labeled as an infarct.*" In the presence of ischemia, troponin clearly defines a higher-risk cohort, but more important, also identifies the subset of patients in whom several interventions have proven most successful. However, the majority of studies showing benefit in troponin-positive patients predate the ESC/ACC report, and in many of these, the single most preventable outcome was AMI *(3-7)*. Thus, where even low levels of troponin were the best predictors of success for the interventions *(8)*, under the new definition, the presence of troponin now assigns the diagnosis of AMI, the very outcome we are trying to prevent. Confusion will certainly result from the change in nomenclature, but the lessons learned provide a very strong argument for the need to detect ischemia in

From: *Cardiac Markers, Second Edition*
Edited by: Alan H. B. Wu @ Humana Press Inc., Totowa, NJ

suspected ACS patients before necrosis occurs, or in conjunction with necrosis to assign correctly the diagnosis of AMI.

This chapter explores the rationale for diagnosing myocardial ischemia in advance of the occurrence of necrosis, the current capability to do so, and the therapeutic implications for such findings.

PATHOPHYSIOLOGY

ACS is a pathophysiological sequence that can ultimately lead to the death of myocytes. A precipitating event appears to be disruption of a "vulnerable" atherosclerotic plaque resulting in the exposure of highly thrombogenic subendothelial structures. Platelet adhesion, activation, and aggregation occur, and along with initiation of the plasma coagulation cascade, lead to formation of an intracoronary thrombus *(9,10)*. Obstruction of the vessel lumen due to thrombus may be minimal, with little or no impairment to blood flow, and in such cases is entirely asymptomatic. On the other extreme it could result in total occlusion of the artery with classic AMI symptoms. More often, however, it is a combination of reduced blood flow and increased oxygen demand that contributes to the critical oxygen insufficiency leading to ischemic myocardium. Symptomatic ischemia defines unstable angina. If ischemia persists, then myocytes will eventually die. In some circumstances, myocytes can also die due to injury sustained as a result of reperfusion. The detection of products of myocardial necrosis in the peripheral blood, in the setting of ischemia, defines AMI *(2)*.

CLINICAL CORRELATION

In addition to direct myocardial injury, there is significant risk associated with ischemia due to arrhythmias, including both those that occur around the time of reperfusion and those that occur late. Any focus of necrosis within the myocardium can potentially lead to arrhythmias, and thus any damage, no matter how small, can ultimately be fatal. Therefore, for patients presenting with ACS, it is imperative that we define our fundamental goal as the prevention of myocardial necrosis. To do so, the pivotal concern must be with the presence of ischemia. The ability to detect ischemia and intervene on this basis is needed to protect against early ischemic complications, to prevent progression to irreversible cell injury, and ultimately to prevent necrosis and the related complications.

The distribution of risk is relatively broad among the large population of patients who seek medical attention for chest pain, including at the lower end those who have benign noncardiac symptoms. But for those who do have ACS, the detection of events comprising this continuum will in turn aid in risk stratification. For instance, ST-segment elevation representing myocardial injury traditionally indicates one of the highest risk conditions and defines the population of patients whose outcomes can be markedly improved through early use of specific interventions including fibrinolytics and percutaneous intervention (PCI). Other electrocardiographic (ECG) indicators, for example, ST-segment depression, identify higher-risk individuals, as does increased troponin concentrations in the absence of ischemic ECG changes. These relatively limited objective descriptors are the basis for categorization of the ACS patient: ST-segment or non-ST-segment elevation AMI, and unstable angina. Some patients who lack any of these findings may also be at high risk, as seen in those patients having nonischemic ECGs, normal cardiac markers, and large perfusion/wall motion defects noted with myocardial perfusion imaging (MPI) *(11)*.

The ability to accurately detect ever smaller amounts of myocardial necrosis has led to confusion regarding clinical diagnoses. Early work comparing troponin with creatine kinase (CK)/MB isoenzyme of CK (CK-MB), suggested that approximately one third of patients with a clinical diagnosis of unstable angina had small elevations in either cTnT or cTnI *(12)*. In contrast to the two-level troponin cutoff proposed by in the National Academy of Clinical Biochemistry Standards of Laboratory Practice *(13)*, the ESC/ACC consensus statement took the definitive stance that any troponin elevation resulting from ischemia be diagnostic for an AMI *(12)*. However, it must be remembered that, regardless of the nomenclature, the occurrence of myocardial necrosis is in fact a terminal event and includes inherent delays in time to detection due to the release kinetics specific to a given marker. Thus, relying on these markers as the sole diagnostic criterion will be relatively late in the course of ACS, could fail to identify patients that present early, and could falsely label patients as having an AMI who have troponin elevations not secondary to ischemia. The coupling of necrosis to ischemia in the diagnostic criteria places increased importance on the need to detect ischemia accurately. The ability to detect ACS must consider both severity and duration of ischemia. While the duration of myocardial ischemia will ultimately determine whether necrosis will occur, it is the severity and extent of an occlusion (i.e., a large proximal left anterior descending vs a small marginal branch of a left circumflex) that will affect our ability to detect it.

WHY DO WE NEED TO DETECT ISCHEMIA?

Ischemia is the link between coronary disease and myocardial dysfunction (Fig. 1). It exists when oxygen supply is inadequate to meet myocardial oxygen demands, and can occur through both supply-side and demand-side etiologies. Events that occur at the level of the artery mirror those of the ventricle: injury, dysfunction, activation of autocrine/endocrine pathways, and remodeling. When plaque rupture occurs in an ACS, intracoronary thrombus and superimposed vasoconstriction can limit oxygen supply. There can also be increased oxygen demand due to enhanced sympathetic activity from pain or in response to reduced cardiac output. Ischemia can result in myocardial injury from both reperfusion and from failing to reperfuse. In the latter case myocytes die following prolonged hypoxia. In the former, direct myocardial injury results from oxygen free radicals generated during reperfusion. In either case there will be systolic dysfunction in proportion to the extent of ischemia initially, and later in proportion to the extent of myocardial damage. Ischemia can cause arrhythmias through several mechanisms including reperfusion injury, electrolyte shifts, altered automaticity, and altered conduction. Ischemia can cause both systolic and diastolic dysfunction, with short-, intermediate-, and long-term consequences, for example, acute regional wall motion deficits, stunning, hibernation, and so forth. Ischemia can be rapidly reversible and have little prolonged effect, or can have catastrophic consequences including infarction and death due to fatal arrhythmias or pump failure.

HOW CAN WE DETECT ISCHEMIA?

Opportunities to detect an ACS prior to the onset of necrosis are suggested by the specific components of the pathophysiological processes involved. At the present time we do not have adequate assays to detect either acute plaque rupture or intracoronary thrombosis. Biochemical testing may detect inflammation (C-reactive protein) *(14)* or

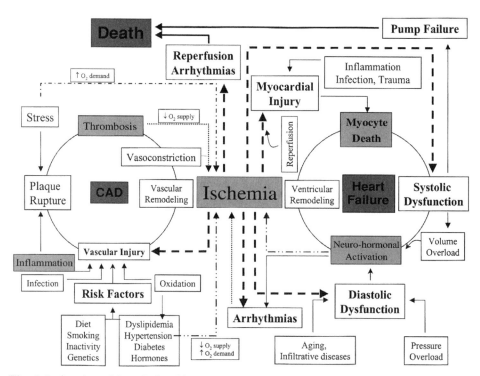

Fig. 1. Ischemia and its relationship to coronary events and ventricular function. Ischemia is at the center of pathologic coronary events and their impact on left ventricular function. Vascular injury leads to the formation of coronary plaques that can rupture and promote intracoronary thrombosis. This can result in obstruction to blood flow and thus reduced oxygen supply (••••). Ischemia can also result in increased oxygen demand (•-•-•), from stress, neurohormonal responses, and arrhythmias. In some cases, such as hypertension, both supply and demand are affected (-••-••-). The effects of ischemia are widespread and varied (----). Prolonged ischemia can cause damage to both the artery and to the ventricular myocardium; in the case of the latter, this includes both systolic and diastolic dysfunction, as well arrhythmias. Damage can occur via mechanisms related to anoxia/hypoxia, or through reperfusion injury.

oxidation (malondialdehyde-modified low-density lipoprotein [MDA-LDL]) *(15)* associated with vulnerable plaques, but it has not been established that these provide a clear indication of an acute or impending event. For this reason these assays should be considered disease state markers rather than acute event markers. Plaques with active inflammation can be identified by heat, a cardinal sign of inflammation. Thermography catheters have been used to localize "vulnerable" plaques *(16)*, although the relationship between the "hot" plaque and an acute event has not been established. Although we have a good understanding of the processes involved in thrombosis, despite early hopes with assays such as p-selectin, there is at present no reliable indicator for an acute intracoronary thrombus.

We do, however, have reliable methods for the detection of ischemia. Historically, electrical changes seen on the ECG have been the primary diagnostic criteria for ischemia. More recently, <u>acute</u> perfusion abnormalities with single-photon emission computed tomography (SPECT) MPI and mechanical dysfunction demonstrated by either echocardiogram (ECHO) or gated MPI have been used as surrogate markers *(17,18)*. Ischemia precedes necrosis, and therefore early identification, stabilization, and intervention can prevent significant myocardial injury. This occurs primarily through protection of myocardium at risk by restoration of blood flow/oxygenation, although perhaps in the near future it may be through induction of cytoprotective measures aimed at protecting against cell death. A reliable biochemical marker for ischemia could rapidly become the gold standard for the diagnosis and treatment of the ACS, much in the way the necrosis markers are for AMI.

Despite technological advancements, the mainstay of our diagnostic approach to the evaluation of chest pain remains the detection of myocardial ischemia by the ECG. Simply stated, the ECG is the easiest, fastest, and least expensive test for myocardial ischemia. The ECG represents the summed electrical vectors generated by depolarization and repolarization of the myocardium. Repolarization in ischemic myocardium differs from that of normal myocardium and generates the ST-segment and T-wave changes that are the hallmarks of ischemia and injury. Unfortunately, the major failure of the ECG is in sensitivity. This is especially true for a single tracing at the time of initial evaluation, at which the diagnostic sensitivity for AMI is approx 50%, and for unstable angina only approx 35% *(19-22)*. Furthermore, approx 10% of the patients who ultimately are diagnosed with AMI have an entirely normal presenting ECG *(23)*. This occurs in part due to anatomic location, where certain areas of the heart may be electrically silent on the surface ECG, and in part to the temporal considerations. Ischemic ECG changes occur in real-time; thus signs may not be present if there is not ongoing ischemia at the exact moment the tracing is being performed. In addition, the ECG can be affected by concurrent treatments; for example, prior use of nitrates may resolve ischemic ECG changes and may actually interfere with the diagnosis.

Ischemia impairs myocardial contractility, and therefore analysis of regional wall motion can also be used to document ACS. Gated SPECT MPI can provide information on both regional and global left ventricular function *(11,24)*. It should be noted that SPECT perfusion imaging is an ischemia-driven test: uptake of the isotope requires active membrane transport and a functioning mitochondrial electron transport system. Thus, both perfusion and function contribute to the diagnosis of ischemia when used acutely. Similar information is obtained with ECHO where regional wall motion abnormalities have both diagnostic and prognostic information *(25,26)*, and as a result there is increasing interest in the ability to demonstrate myocardial ischemia in the acute setting through ECHO. Both techniques have high sensitivity and specificity, and especially high negative predictive value when the study is entirely normal. However, both are limited to some degree by the logistics of performing and interpreting the tests in a timely manner, and the cost of providing these studies in the emergency department with a 7 d/wk, 24 h/d availability. Another significant limitation is that without previous studies with which to compare, it is often impossible to determine if an abnormal area is new due to ischemia, or is old representing an area of scar (i.e., prior MI). However, any abnormality, whether old or new, contributes significantly to the risk assessment.

Ideally, we should be able to detect ischemic events through simple biochemical tests. Such markers must be held to the same sensitivity, specificity, and kinetic criteria/standards as are the necrosis markers. Fortunately, there does appear to be some progress toward the development of an ischemia marker. Holvoet recently demonstrated that

MDA-LDL was a sensitive marker for ACS and equally present in unstable angina as in AMI *(15).* This would be expected for an ischemia marker, as the initial pathophysiologic events leading to ischemia and AMI are indistinguishable. Only later does progression to necrosis, the outcome differentiating the two, occur. Although MDA-LDL may distinguish stable from unstable coronary disease, a direct relationship to the occurrence of an acute event has not been established. Thus, MDA-LDL appears to be a marker of unstable coronary disease, although it may still not be useful for identification of patients having acute events.

The distinction between an event marker and a disease state marker is very important for the management of ACS patients. Although disease state markers add to an overall risk analysis, they are less useful for directing or monitoring acute therapy. A new assay to detect the acute occurrence of ischemia has been reported, and is currently in clinical trials. The "IMA" test (*I*schemia-*M*odified *A*lbumin, Ischemia Technologies, Denver, CO) is based on alterations to the amino- (N)-terminus of serum albumin as it passes through an ischemic tissue bed *(27).* Human albumin that has been damaged by oxygen free radicals is both functionally and immunologically distinct from native albumin and can be readily differentiated. The assay appears to correlate well to clinical diagnoses across the spectrum of ACS, and appears to have favorable kinetics for use as a true event marker for ACS. Other biochemical assays reported to diagnose myocardial ischemia that are in clinical development include those for unbound free fatty acids (ADIFAB™, FFA Sciences, San Diego, CA) and sphingosine-1-phosphate (Medlyte, San Diego, CA).

CLINICAL IMPLICATIONS
FOR THE DIAGNOSIS AND TREATMENT OF ISCHEMIA

It is somewhat simplistic to say that the sole consequence of unrelieved ischemia is myocardial necrosis secondary to hypoxia/anoxia, as this is only partially responsible for the damage observed. Reperfusion following ischemia can itself result in significant injury to viable myocardium through the generation of reactive oxygen species, including superoxide anion, hydroxyl radical, hydrogen peroxide, and singlet oxygen. These compounds can in turn lead to lipid peroxidation and destruction of proteins resulting in membrane destabilization, cell dysfunction, and cell death (Fig. 2). Clinically these also become manifest as electrical instability, and thus arrhythmias are common.

Brief ischemia followed by reperfusion can also be beneficial. A biological form of myocardial protection, called ischemic preconditioning, occurs via both rapid and delayed onset mechanisms. The rapid form develops almost immediately but is short in duration. The delayed phase becomes manifest well after 12 h, requires activation of specific genes and synthesis of proteins, and persists for a significantly longer time. Although this phenomenon has been best characterized in animal models, ischemic preconditioning does appear to be clinically important in humans *(28,29).* The stuttering angina seen in some patients is thought to represent the physiological equivalent of ischemic preconditioning. If true, patients who have intermittent ischemia should have smaller infarcts than those who abruptly occlude arteries. A substudy from Global Use of Strategies to Open Occluded Coronary Arteries in Acute Coronary Syndromes (GUSTO)-I suggests that this may indeed be the case. Bahr et al. (Fig. 3) reported that among patients present-

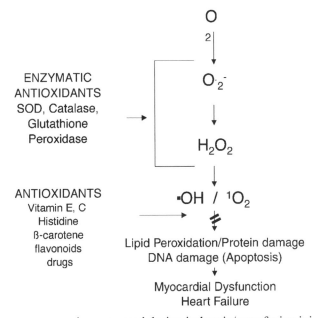

Fig. 2. Reactive oxygen species generated during ischemia/reperfusion injury and the action of antioxidants. When ischemia is followed by reperfusion reactive-oxygen species are generated. These include superoxide anion ($^\bullet O_2^-$), which rapidly dismutates to hydrogen peroxide (H_2O_2), and in the presence of iron, $^\bullet OH$ radical or possibly $^1O_2$ may be formed via the iron-catalyzed Haber–Weiss reaction. These compounds are highly destructive. They initiate lipid peroxidation in the cell membranes, damage proteins, and cause DNA fragmentation, resulting in the apoptotic (programmed) cell death of myocyte. Traditional enzymatic antioxidants scavenge oxyradicals or prevent their formation. These are not always effective because of their limited accessibility to the site of free radical generation. However, a large number of natural or synthetic compounds have the ability to inhibit the oxidative damage.

ing with ST-segment elevation AMI, prodromal symptoms were present in a higher proportion of those with aborted AMI or low levels of myocardial damage than among patients with extensive cardiac injury. As expected, this was also associated with improved 1-yr and 5-yr mortality rates *(30)*. Similar findings were seen among the subset of patients enrolled in the Thrombolysis in Myocardial Infarction (TIMI)-4 study who had angina within the 48 h before the AMI compared to those who did not. There was a lower incidence of congestive heart failure (CHF) or shock (1% vs 6%, $p = 0.008$), smaller infarct size by CK (115 IU vs 151 IU, $p = 0.03$), and a lower combined end point of death, CHF, or shock (3% vs 10%, $p = 0.006$) *(31)*.

Controlled ischemic preconditioning prior to planned interventional procedures such as coronary artery bypass graft (CABG) and PCI could be employed to prevent focal necrosis. The ability to promote cytoprotective mechanisms for patients presenting with an ACS could potentially reduce the progression to AMI. This would obviously require the capability to detect ischemia early to identify the patients who should receive treatment. If successful, the difference between risk zones in unstable angina and infarct zones in AMI could be considerable. The Na^+/K^+ exchange pump inhibitor cariporide

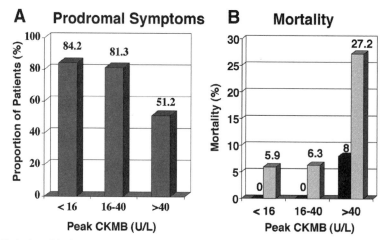

Fig. 3. Relationship between prodromal symptoms and outcomes in AMI. Among the 207 patients enrolled at a single site in the GUSTO-I study, 196 survived the first 24 h following presentation. The extent of prodromal anginal symptoms preceding the AMI was analyzed along with the peak CK-MB level as a predictor of survival (*black bar*: 1 yr, *grey bar*: 5 yr). CK-MB < 16 was considered "aborted AMI" (*n* = 19); between 16 and 40, "minor myocardial damage" (*n* = 32); and >40 was "extensive cardiac injury" (*n* = 163) *(30)*.

in ACS patients preserved left ventricular volumes and ejection fraction among the treated group compared to controls, suggesting an attenuation of reperfusion injury *(32)*. Selective activation of the adenosine A-1 receptor also appeared to protect from myocardial injury through both acute and delayed pathways in mouse and rabbit hearts *(33,34)*. Clinical trials of adenosine agonists to limit infarct size are underway in humans *(35)*.

Early initiation of antithrombotic regimens may also serve to reduce ischemic injury. This has been shown repeatedly for patients presenting with ST-segment elevation AMI *(36,37)*. However, this benefit is not simply via dissolution of clots in the larger epicardial arteries, and it has been hypothesized that the low-level troponin elevations seen in many ACS patients are actually from microembolization *(38)*. In general, when there is normal epicardial flow (TIMI flow grade 3), mortality is low (3.5%). However, there is still a significant differentiation in mortality based on microvascular flow. Normal microvascular flow (TIMI perfusion grade 3) has the lowest mortality, 0.73%, vs abnormal microvascular flow (TIMI myocardial perfusion grade 0–2), where it is 4.7% *(39)*. The white blood cells may also be a major participant in embolic downstream ischemic damage, including reperfusion injury and the "no-reflow phenomenon, as platelet–white blood cell aggregates are known to occur in ACS *(40)*.

A consistent finding from major ACS trials, including Platelet Receptor Inhibition in Ischemic Syndrome Management (PRISM) *(41,42)*, Treat Angina with Aggrastat and determine Cost of Therapy with an Invasive or Conservative Strategy (TACTICS) *(8)*, (tirofiban), Chimeric c7E3 AntiPlatelet Therapy in Unstable Angina Refractory to Standard Treatment Trial (CAPTURE) *(43)*, (abciximab), Fragmin in Unstable Coronary Artery Disease (FRISC) *(44,45)*, FRISC-II *(46)*, (dalteparin), and Efficacy and Safety of Subcutaneous Enoxaparin in Non-Q-wave Coronary Events (ESSENCE) *(47)* (enoxaparin), was the reduction in progression to AMI among the higher risk, non-ST elevation, unstable coronary syndrome patients who underwent medical stabilization prior to intervention. Retrospective analyses in each case showed that most of the treatment benefit occurred in the patients who were troponin positive.

Indeed, a glaring paradox in the treatment of ACS is that the majority of the benefit appears to lie in the patients who are troponin positive. If the advantage to treatment is to prevent MI and death, then why would those who have already sustained an MI stand to benefit most? One possibility is that the troponin analyses were retrospective, and the reference sample was not drawn immediately on presentation. In many studies, troponin was drawn at the time of enrollment into the study, which often was several hours after presentation. The observed benefit is based on an attenuation of further damage. Had the analysis been prospective based on the presenting sample, the troponin might not yet have been elevated, and would have added little to the analysis. In the recently published Chest Pain Evaluation by Creatine Kinase-MB, Myoglobin, and Troponin I (CHECK-MATE) trial, the time of chest pain onset to first marker was 6.4 h for the troponin-positive group and 5.3 h for the troponin-negative group *(48)*. Using multimarker strategies including troponin and CK-MB, only 14.3% of patients were positive at presentation. Another possibility is that the presenting troponin elevation was not from the acute event, but rather from an event hours or even days before representing post-infarct angina, a high-risk clinical condition that was attenuated with more aggressive treatment strategies. The CHECKMATE suggests that this could be the case; only 5.2% of the patients were positive at baseline when CK-MB was the only marker used vs the 14.9% when troponin is added. Because troponin generally rises later than CK-MB, the additional 9.1% positive with troponin might well be "old" elevations representing post-MI angina. It is clear that a trial using a rapid troponin assay to determine therapy prospectively is needed to understand this relationship fully.

There is evidence that it is the prevention of myocardial necrosis that provides the most substantive short- and long-term benefit for patients presenting with non-ST-segment ACS. Fintel reported that the 6-mo mortality for patients hospitalized with non-ST elevation ACS who experienced an AMI prior to undergoing a PCI was 15.2%, vs 3.5% for those who didn't experience a prior AMI, an 11.7% absolute reduction in mortality ($p = 0.001\%$). For patients having an AMI within the first 72 h of hospitalization mortality was 18.3% vs 5.5% for those who did not have an AMI, a 12.8% absolute reduction in mortality ($p = 0.0001$) *(49)*. Progression to AMI among patients presenting with non-ST elevation ACS carries adverse risk that is presumably preventable with rapid intervention. Compared to standard treatment, including aspirin and heparin, additions of abciximab, eptifibatide, and tirofiban have all shown reduction in progression to AMI, which also demonstrates late mortality benefit *(50)*. TACTICS compared an early invasive to conservative strategy in high-risk ACS patients treated with the glycoprotein IIb/IIIa receptor blocker tirofiban. There was a definite advantage to the invasive arm, which was most prominent in the troponin-positive patients *(51)*. Combining data from GUSTO IIb and PURSUIT, Roe noted that the incidence of AMI was only 2.2% in patients having PCI within the first 24 h vs 8.9% among those having PCI in d 2–3 *(52)*. Thus, rapid identification of high-risk patients and early intervention including medical stabilization and PCI appears to provide the greatest outcomes benefit through the prevention of myocardial necrosis.

We believe that early detection of ischemia is the key to defining and intervening in the higher risk ACS patients, not troponin. In many cases troponin will rise too late to direct the early initiation of therapy. It has been well established that ischemic changes on the ECG portend a bad prognosis *(53)*; however, the poor sensitivity for the ECG is a strong argument for the need to develop better biochemical markers for ischemia. In all such cases, the explicit goal is maintain microcirculatory flow to prevent even minor infarctions *(54)*. Only a marker that precedes necrosis can do this.

SUMMARY

1. Plaque rupture and the associated thrombosis are seminal events in an ACS. However, it appears likely that these occur frequently, are often silent, and are thus of little immediate clinical consequence. If myocardial oxygen supply is inadequate, and **if ischemia is present, significant immediate problems may result**: the most pressing of these are myocardial necrosis and the related complications.
2. **Myocardial necrosis resulting from ischemia defines AMI**. This is an important distinction as myocardial necrosis can occur from many etiologies. Strictly speaking, one must therefore demonstrate evidence of both ischemia and necrosis to diagnose AMI. Cardiac troponin is now the preferred marker for detecting necrosis. For most studies, and in clinical practice, ischemia is defined by the ECG findings, and to a lesser extent, clinical findings. The ECG is currently the standard method for diagnosing ischemia, being rapid, easy to perform, and only slightly difficult to interpret. However, it lacks both sensitivity and specificity, especially for non-ST elevation ACS.
3. Many clinical trials have documented that troponin-positive ACS patients are both a higher risk cohort, as well as one in whom more aggressive treatments will provide the greatest benefit. Paradoxically, the primary benefit from these treatments has been prevention of progression to AMI. Under new definitions, in this clinical context the very presence of these markers now defines AMI and thus would make demonstration of that clinical benefit more difficult. In addition, **the greatest benefit actually lies in the prevention of necrosis** prior to intervention. This demands the ability to detect ischemia and prevent its consequences.
4. **Methods to document ischemia are imperative for diagnostic, treatment, and prognostic reasons**. The high sensitivity, specificity, and negative predictive values for imaging confirm that this is possible, albeit at great logistical difficulty.
5. **A simple, rapid, near-patient biochemical assay for ischemia is needed** to identify higher risk ACS patients who might benefit from treatments designed to prevent progression to AMI and other consequences of ischemia.

ABBREVIATIONS

ACC, American College of Cardiology; ACS, acute coronary syndromes; AMI, acute myocardial infarction; CABG, coronary artery bypass graft; CAPTURE, Chimeric c7E3 AntiPlatelet Therapy in Unstable Angina Refractory to Standard Treatment Trial; CHECKMATE, Chest Pain Evaluation by Creatine in Kinase-MB, Myoglobin, and Troponin I Study; CHF, congestive heart failure; CK, creatine kinase; ECG, electrocardiogram; ECHO, echocardiogram; ESC, European Scoiety of Cardiology; ESSENCE, Efficacy and Safety of Subcutaneous Enoxaparin in Non-Q-wave Coronary Events; FRISC, Fragmin in Unstable Coronary Artery Disease; GUSTO, Global Use of Strategies to Open Occluded Coronary Arteries in Acute Coronary Syndromes; IMA, Ischemia-Modified Albumin; IU, international units; LDL, low-density lipoprotein; MDA, malondialdehyde mondified; MPI, myocardial perfusion imaging; PCI, percutaneous intervention;

PRISM, Platelet Receptor Inhibition in Ischemic Syndrome Management; PURSUIT, Platelet IIa/IIIb in Unstable Angina Receptor Suppression Using Integrilin Therapy; SPECT, single photon emission computed tomography; TACTICS, Treat Angina with Aggrastat and determine Cost of Therapy with an Invasive or Conservative Strategy.

REFERENCES

1. 2002 Heart and Stroke Statistical Update. 2001. Dallas, TX, American Heart Association.
2. Myocardial Infarction Redefined—A Consensus Document of The Joint European Society of Cardiology/American College of Cardiology Committee for the Redefinition of Myocardial Infarction. J Am Coll Cardiol 2002;36:959–969.
3. Randomized placebo-controlled trial of abciximab before and during coronary intervention in refractory unstable angina: the CAPTURE Study. Lancet 1997;349:1429–1435.
4. Platelet Receptor Inhibition in Ischemic Syndrome Management in Patients Limited by Unstable Signs and Symptoms (PRISM-PLUS) study investigators. Inhibition of the platelet glycoprotein IIb/IIIa receptor with tirofiban in unstable angina and non-Q-wave myocardial infarction. N Engl J Med 1998;338:1488–1497.
5. Lindahl B, Diderholm E, Kontny F, et al. Long term treatment with low molecular weight heparin (dalteparin) reduces cardiac events in unstable coronary artery disease with troponin T elevation: a FRISC II substudy. Circulation 1999;100:I–498.
6. Morrow DA, Antman EM, Tanasijevic M, et al. Cardiac troponin I for stratification of early outcomes and the efficacy of enoxaparin in unstable angina: a TIMI-11B substudy. J Am Cardiol 2001;36:1812–1817.
7. Inhibition of platelet glycoprotein IIb/IIIa with eptifibatide in patients with acute coronary syndromes. N Engl J Med 1998;339:436–443.
8. Morrow DA, Cannon CP, Rifai N, et al. Ability of minor elevations of troponins I and T to predict benefit from an early invasive strategy in patients with unstable angina and Non-ST elevation myocardial infarction. JAMA 2001;286:2405–2412.
9. Fuster V, Badimon L, Badimon JJ, Chesebro JH. The pathogenesis of coronary artery disease and the acute coronary syndromes (Part 1). N Engl J Med 1992;326:242–250.
10. Fuster V, Badimon L, Badimon JJ, Chesebro JH. The pathogenesis of coronary artery disease and the acute coronary syndromes (Part 2). N Engl J Med 1992;326:310–318.
11. Kontos MC, Jesse RL, Schmidt KL, Ornato JP, Tatum JL. Value of acute rest sestamibi perfusion imaging for evaluation of patients admitted to the emergency department with chest pain. J Am Coll Cardiol 1997;30:976–982.
12. Katus HA, Remppis A, Neumann FJ, et al. Diagnostic efficiency of troponin T measurements in acute myocardial infarction. Circulation 1991;83:902–912.
13. Wu AHB, Apple FS, Warshaw MM, Valdes R Jr, Jesse RL, Gibler WB. National Academy of Clinical Biochemistry Standards of Laboratory Practice reccomendations for use of cardiac markers in coronary artery disease. Clin Chem 1999;45:1104–1121.
14. Ridker PM, Hennekens CH, Buring JE, Rifai N. C-reactive protein and other markers of inflammation in the prediction of cardiovascular disease in women. N Engl J Med 2000; 342:836–843.
15. Holvoet P, Collen D, Van de Werf F. Malondialdehyde-modified LDL as a marker of acute coronary syndromes. JAMA 1999;281:1718–1721.
16. Stefanadis C, Diamantopoulos L, Vlachopoulos C, et al. Thermal heterogeneity within human atherosclerotic coronary arteries detected in vivo: a new method of detection by application of a special thermography catheter. Circulation 1999;99:1965–1971.
17. Kontos MC, Jesse RL, Anderson FP, Schmidt KL, Ornato JP, Tatum JL. Comparison of myocardial perfusion imaging and cardiac troponin I in patients admitted to the emergency department with chest pain. Circulation 1999;99:2073–2078.

18. Kontos MC. Role of echocardiography in the emergency department for identifying patients with myocardial infarction and ischemia. Echocardiography 1999;16:193–205.

19. Rouan GW, Lee TH, Cook EF, Brand DA, Weisberg MC, Goldman L. Clinical characteristics and outcome of acute myocardial infarction in patients with initially normal or nonspecific electrocardiograms (a report from the multicenter chest pain study). Am J Cardiol 1989;64:1087–1092.

20. Lee TH, Rouan GW, Weisberg MC, et al. Clinical characteristics and natural history of patients with acute myocardial infarction sent home from the emergency room. Am J Cardiol 1987;60:219–224.

21. Slater DK, Hlatky MA, Mark DB, Harrell FE Jr, Pryor DB, Califf RM. Outcome in suspected acute myocardial infarction with normal or minimally abnormal admission electrocardiographic findings. Am J Cardiol 1987;60:766–770.

22. Brush JE Jr, Brand DA, Acampora D, Chalmer B, Wackers FJ. Use of the initial electrocardiogram to predict in-hospital complications of acute myocardial infarction. N Engl J Med 1985;312:1137–1141.

23. Karlson BW, Herlitz J, Wiklund O, Richter A, Hjalmarson A. Early prediction of acute myocardial infarction from clinical history, examination and electrocardiogram in the emergency room. Am J Cardiol 1991;68:171–175.

24. Kontos MC, Arrowood JA, Jesse RL, et al. Comparison of echocardiography and myocardial perfusion imaging for diagnosing emergency department patients with chest pain. Am Heart J 1998;136:724–733.

25. Sabia P, Abbott RD, Afrookteh A, Keller MW, Touchstone DA, Kaul S. Importance of two-dimensional echocardiographic assessment of left ventricular systolic function in patients presenting to the emergency room with cardiac-related symptoms. Circulation 1991;84:1615–1624.

26. Sabia P, Afrookteh A, Touchstone DA, Keller MW, Esquivel L, Kaul S. Value of regional wall motion abnormality in the emergency room diagnosis of acute myocardial infarction. A prospective study using two-dimensional echocardiography. Circulation 1991;84:I85–I92.

27. Bar-Or D, Lau E, Rao N, Bampos N, Winkler JV, Curtis CG. Reduction in the cobalt binding capacity of human albumin with myocardial ischemia. Ann Emerg Med 1999;34:4.

28. Kloner RA, Jennings RB. Consequences of brief ischemia: stunning, preconditioning, and their clinical implications. Part 1. Circulation 2001;104:2981–2989.

29. Kloner RA, Jennings RB. Consequences of brief ischemia: stunning, preconditioning, and their clinical implications. Part 2. Circulation 2001;104:3158–3159.

30. Bahr RD, Leino EV, Christenson RH. Prodromal unstable angina in acute myocardial infarction: prognostic value of short- and long-term outcome and predictor of infarct size. Am Heart J 2000;140:126–133.

31. Kloner RA, Shook T, Przyklenk K, et al. Previous angina alters in-hospital outcome in TIMI 4: a clinical correlate to preconditioning? Circulation 1995;91:37–45.

32. Rupprecht HJ, vom Dahl J, Terres W, et al. Cardioprotective effects of the Na^+/H^+ exchange inhibitor cariporide in patients with acute anterior myocardial infarction undergoing direct PTCA. Circulation 2001;101:2902–2908.

33. Bernardo NL, Okubo S, Maaieh M, Wood M, Kukreja RC. Delayed preconditioning with adenosine is mediated by opening of ATP-sensitive K^+ channels in rabbit heart. Am J Physiol 1999;277:H128–H135.

34. Zhao T, Xi L, Chelliah J, Levasseur JE, Kukreja RC. Inducible nitric oxide synthase mediates delayed protection induced by activation of adenosine A1 receptors: evidence from gene knockout mice. Circulation 2000;108:902–907.

35. Mahaffey KW, Puma JA, Barbagelata NA, et al. Adenosine as an adjunct to thrombolytic therapy for acute myocardial infarction: results of a multicenter, randomized, placebo-controlled trial. The Acute Myocardial Infarction STudy of ADenosine (AMISTAD) trial. J Am Coll Cardiol 1999;34:1711–1720.

36. Weaver WD, Cerqueira M, Hallstrom AP, et al. Prehospital-initiated vs. hospital-initiated thrombolytic therapy. The Myocardial Infarction Triage and Intervention Trial. JAMA 1993; 270:1211–1216.

37. The GUSTO investigators. An international randomized trial comparing four thrombolytic strategies for acute myocardial infarction. N Engl J Med 1993;329:673–682.

38. Topol EJ, Yadav JS. Recognition of the importance of embolization in atherosclerotic vascular disease. Circulation 2000;101:570–580.

39. Gibson CM, Cannon CP, Murphy SA, et al. Relationship of TIMI myocardial perfusion grade to mortality after administration of thrombolytic drugs. Circulation 2000;101:125–130.

40. Ott I, Neumann FJ, Gawaz M, Schmitt M, Schomig A. Increased neutrophil-platelet adhesion in patients with unstable angina. Circulation 1996;94:1239–1246.

41. Hamm CW, Heeschen C, Goldmann BU, White HD. Benefit of tirofiban in high-risk patients with unstable angina identified by troponins in the PRISM study. Circulation 1999;100: I-775–I-775.

42. Heeschen C, Hamm C, Goldmann B, Deu A, Langenbrink L, White HD. Troponin concentrations for stratification of patients with acute cornary syndromes in relation to therapeutic efficacy of tirofiban. Lancet 1999;354:1757–1762.

43. Hamm CW, Heeschen C, Goldmann B, et al. Benefit of abciximab in patients with refractory unstable angina in relation to serum troponin T levels. c7E3 ab Antiplatelet Therapy in Unstable Refractory Angina. N Engl J Med 1999;340:1623–1629.

44. Lindahl B, Venge P, Wallentin L. Relation between troponin T and the risk of subsequent cardiac events in unstable coronary artery disease. Circulation 1996;93:1651–1657.

45. Lindahl B, Venge P, Wallentin L. Troponin T identifies patients with unstable coronary artery disease who benefit from long-term antithrombotic protection. Fragmin in Unstable Coronary Artery Disease (FRISC) Study Group. J Am Coll Cardiol 1997;29:43–48.

46. Lindahl B, Diderholm E, Lagerqvist B, Venge P, Wallentin L, and the FRISC II Investigators. Mechanisms behind the prognostic value of troponin T in unstable coronary artery disease: a FRISC II substudy. J Am Coll Cardiol 2001;38:979–986.

47. Lange RA, Hillis D. Cardiovascular complications of cocaine use. N Engl J Med 2001;345: 351–358.

48. Newby LK, Storrow AB, Gibler WB, et al. Bedside multimarker testing for risk stratification in chest pain units. The Chest Pain Evaluation by Creatine Kinase-MB, Myoglobin, and Troponin I (CHECKMATE) study. Circulation 2001;103:1832–1837.

49. Fintel DJ, Ledley GS. Management of patients with non-ST-segment elevation acute coronary syndromes: insights from the PURSUIT Trial. Clin Cardiol 2000;23:V1–V12.

50. Boersma E, Akkerhuis M, Theroux P, Califf RM, Topol EJ, Simoons ML. Platelet glycoprotein IIb/IIIa receptor inhibition in non-ST-elevation acute coronary syndromes. Early benefit during medical treatment only, with additional protection during percutaneous coronary intervention. Circulation 1999;100:2045–2048.

51. Cannon CP, Weintraub WS, Demopoulos L, et al. Troponin T and I to predict 6 month mortality and relative benefit of invasive vs conservative strategy in patients with unstable angina: primary results of the TACTICS-TIMI 18 troponin substudy. J Am Coll Cardiol 2001; 37:325A.

52. Roe MT, Alexander JH, Pacchiana CM, et al. Elevated CK-MB following coronary intervention in patients with acute coronary syndromes is associated with a four-fold increase in mortality: results from the GUSTO-IIb and PURSUIT Trials. J Am Coll Cardiol 2000; 35:40A.

53. Savonitto S, Ardissino D, Granger CB, et al. Prognostic value of the admission electrocardiogram in acute coronary syndromes JAMA 1999;281:707–713.

54. Roe MT, Ohman EM, Maas AC, et al. Shifting the open-artery hypothesis downstream: the quest for optimal reperfusion. J Am Coll Cardiol 2001;37:9–18.

16

Ischemia-Modified Albumin, Free Fatty Acids, Whole Blood Choline, B-Type Natriuretic Peptide, Glycogen Phosphorylase BB, and Cardiac Troponin

Alan H. B. Wu, Peter Crosby, Gary Fagan, Oliver Danne, Ulrich Frei, Martin Möckel, and Joseph Keffer

INTRODUCTION

There is increasing need to make accurate early diagnosis and rule out acute coronary syndromes (ACS) in patients who present to the emergency department (ED) with chest pain. Accurate diagnosis will reduce the number of inappropriate management decisions, and the number of malpractice lawsuits relating to these decisions. Early diagnosis will facilitate faster entry to treatment protocols such as anticoagulant and antiplatelet therapies resulting in reduced morbidity, mortality, and hospital length of stay. Rapid rule-out of ischemia will facilitate discharge of patients at no or low risk for cardiovascular complications and alleviate the diminishing resources available to EDs. Although the presence of ST-segment depressions on the electrocardiogram (ECG) is evidence of ischemia, the ECG is nondiagnostic in the majority of unstable angina patients. Radionuclide imaging is a sensitive marker for ischemia, but is expensive and requires a high degree of technical expertise.

Cardiac markers are not reliably increased at the time of patient presentation to be useful for ED triaging purposes. The prevailing view is that cardiac troponin, creatine kinase (CK), and myoglobin are released only following myocardial necrosis (1,2), although there are data that suggest that troponin may be released during reversible ischemia (3). Given the need for early detection of myocardial ischemia, there is active ongoing research to find such a serologic marker. This chapter supplements the other chapters in this section regarding markers of ischemia.

ISCHEMIA-MODIFIED ALBUMIN

The discovery that albumin in serum of patients with myocardial ischemia exhibited lower metal binding capacity for Co(II) than the albumin in serum of normal subjects was originally made by Bar-Or (4). A manual chemistry assay for the detection of cobalt was configured and used in clinical investigations to determine if the test had value for

The section on Ischemia-Modified Albumin was authored by Peter Crosby and Gary Fagan.
The section on Whole Blood Choline was authored by Oliver Danne, Ulrich Frei, and Martin Möckel.
The section on glycogen phosphorylase BB was authored by Joseph Keffer.

From: *Cardiac Markers, Second Edition*
Edited by: Alan H. B. Wu @ Humana Press Inc., Totowa, NJ

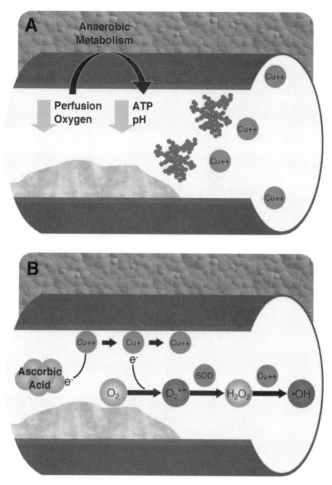

Fig. 1. Pathophysiologic mechanism for the IMA test. (**A**) Ischemia leads to the release of redox active metals like copper and iron. (**B**) Free Cu (II) reacts with reducing agents like ascorbic acid to form Cu (I). Cu (I) plus oxygen produces superoxide anion ($O_2^{\bullet-}$). Superoxide anion is converted to hydrogen peroxide (H_2O_2) and O_2 by superoxide dismutase (SOD). H_2O_2 produces hydroxyl free radical ($OH^\bullet$) in the presence of copper (Fenton reaction). (**C**) Albumin scavenges free copper. (**D**) Site specific Fenton reactions damage the metal binding site, releasing copper to begin the process again.

detecting ischemia. Preliminary results from evaluation of patients presenting with signs and symptoms of acute myocardial infarction (AMI) *(5)* and angioplasty patients made transiently ischemic with balloon inflation *(6)* proved encouraging. The following mechanism was proposed.

Ischemia occurs when there is an imbalance between oxygen supply and demand. Inadequate tissue oxygen induces anaerobic metabolism, which increases lactic acid and reduces pH *(7,8)*. Reduced pH concentrations lead to the release of metals such as copper and iron from proteins and intracellular stores. Copper and iron are physiologically abundant ions, which may produce tissue damaging reactive oxygen species under certain conditions *(9)*.

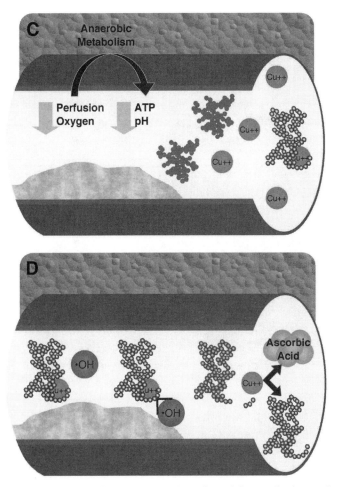

Fig. 1. (C) Albumin scavenges free copper. **(D)** Hydroxyl free radicals attack the N-terminus of albumin, releasing Cu^{2+} to begin the process again.

Metal-catalyzed oxidative damage requires a cation capable of redox cycling (copper or iron), a substance such as ascorbic acid to reduce the oxidized cation, a supply of oxygen to generate hydrogen peroxide or other potential reactive oxygen species, and a cation binding site on a target molecule (lipid, protein, or nucleic acid). In the presence of ascorbic acid, Cu (II) is reduced to Cu (I), which can react with oxygen to produce superoxide anion ($O_2^{\bullet-}$) and regenerate Cu (II). This allows one Cu (II) to recycle and produce large quantities of $O_2^{\bullet-}$ as long as there is an abundant supply of ascorbic acid present. Superoxide anion is converted to hydrogen peroxide (H_2O_2) and oxygen in the presence of superoxide dismutase (SOD), an enzyme abundantly distributed in tissue. When H_2O_2 is generated in the presence of redox reactive metals, a Fenton reaction (superoxide–metal–H_2O_2 system) *(9)* can occur producing highly reactive OH$^{\bullet}$ free radicals that can damage proteins, lipids, and DNA in a site-specific manner *(10–12)*. Figure 1 summarizes this mechanism.

In the presence of redox reactive metals, a Fenton reaction (superoxide–metal–H_2O_2 system) *(9)* can occur producing highly reactive OH$^{\bullet}$ free radicals that can damage proteins, lipids, and DNA in a site-specific manner *(10–12)*. Trace amounts of metal ions can be highly effective in inducing damage in molecular targets because the oxidized form of the metal, generated in the Fenton reaction, is continually reduced or redox cycled in a chain reaction by reducing agents. In an example by Halliwell et al. *(13)*, a 1 µmol/L of Fe(II) and an equal concentration of H_2O_2 are able to produce 4.58×10^{13} hydroxyl radicals per dm^3/s. Because the rate constant for Cu(I) is larger $(4.7 \times 10^3 \ M^{-1}s^{-1})$ than Fe(II) $(76 \ M^{-1}s^{-1})$, substituting Cu(I) for Fe(II) in this same example would produce 2.83×10^{17} hydroxyl radicals per dm^3/s, enabling a significant amount of damage to targeted proteins.

Numerous studies have demonstrated that the primary high-affinity binding site for the transition metals copper(II), nickel(II), and cobalt(II) in human albumin is located at the amino- (N)-terminus, and involves coordination of the metal to the first three amino acids: aspartic acid, alanine, and histidine *(14–17)*. Other binding sites for transition metals on albumin have been described including a second strong binding site and numerous weak (monodentate) binding sites (thiols, histidines, tryptophans, and tyrosines) *(15)*. Titration experiments with molar equivalents of copper have shown that the difference in affinity between site 1 (N-terminus) and site 2 is so high that the second site becomes populated only after saturation of the first site *(15)*.

It was postulated that ischemia-induced modifications to binding site 1 were responsible for the decreased metal binding phenomenon seen in patients with myocardial ischemia. Using synthetic peptides representing the amino acids present at the N-terminus of albumin, Bar-Or was able to demonstrate that acetylation or removal of the N-terminal aspartate or both the aspartate and alanine residues eliminated the cobalt metal binding capacity of the N-terminal tetrapeptide. Substitution of the position 2 alanine with proline also eliminated metal binding *(18)*. Copper bound to the N-terminus site will also prevent cobalt binding, because the binding constant for copper $(K_a = 1.5 \times 10^{16}$ L/mol) *(19)* is much higher than for cobalt $(K_a = 6.5 \times 10^3$ L/mol) *(20)* and no significant exchange between copper and cobalt will occur with the concentration of cobalt present during the incubation time of the assay.

Albumin in which the N-terminus is either damaged or occupied by copper is termed Ischemia-Modified Albumin (IMA™) and is characterized by the inability to bind transition metals such as cobalt at the N-terminus.

The Albumin Cobalt Binding Test (ACB™ Test, Ischemia Technologies, Denver, CO) was originally developed by Bar-Or in prototype form *(5)*. A cobalt solution is added to serum. Cobalt not sequestered (bound) at the N-terminus of albumin is detected using dithiothreitol (DTT) as a colorimetric indicator. In sera of normal patients, more cobalt is sequestered at the N-terminus of albumin, leaving less cobalt to react with DTT and form a colored product. Conversely, in sera of patients with ischemia, cobalt is not sequestered at the N-terminus of IMA, leaving more free cobalt to react with DTT and form a darker color. This prototype assay was subsequently developed for use on an automated clinical chemistry platform, the Roche Cobas Mira® Plus Analyzer *(21)*, and called the ACB™ Test. Second-generation versions of the ACB Test have improved analytical performance, and are able to run on other chemistry platforms such as the Hitachi 911 and KoneLab 20 analyzers.

IMA is produced as a result of cardiac ischemia. Anecdotal evidence suggests that IMA may be increased in patients with brain ischemia (stroke) and perhaps gastrointestinal ischemia, but does not appear to be increased in patients with skeletal muscle ischemia. Therefore, although IMA is not cardiac specific, it is specific enough to offer promise as a diagnostic test for patients presenting with suspected ACS.

Extensive clinical studies have been conducted on IMA as measured by the ACB Test. The clinical data show that IMA rises rapidly (within minutes) in response to transient ischemia induced by balloon angioplasty *(6,22)*, and appears to return to baseline within 6–12 h. IMA is not increased (i.e., ACB Test result within normal range) as a result of anaerobic metabolism in skeletal muscle, at least as measured in a group of marathon runners *(23)*. A negative IMA at acute presentation in chest pain patients (i.e., ACB Test result within normal range) can be used to predict subsequent negative troponin, indicating that IMA has value as an early rule out of AMI *(24)*. IMA from acute presentation blood draw from patients presenting to a hospital emergency room with suspected ACS has twice the sensitivity of cardiac troponin for detecting patients with AMI, and when used in conjunction with troponin, almost three times as many patients with AMI can be detected from a presentation blood test than with troponin alone *(25,26)*. IMA is also an effective diagnostic tool for cardiac ischemia. In a group of 69 patients, IMA showed a sensitivity of 93.3% and a specificity of 72.2% for detection of cardiac ischemia as determined by myocardial perfusion imaging (sestamibi) and 12-lead ECG *(27)*. The test has value in diagnosing cardiac ischemia in non-ST-segment elevation ACS patients in the ED *(28)*. The sensitivity of IMA taken at acute presentation to predict positive angiography was 75%, which was double that of ECG. The combined test of IMA with ECG was 90% sensitive to predict positive angiography or final diagnosis of ACS *(29)*.

The ACB Test is a quantitative in vitro diagnostic test that detects IMA by measuring the cobalt binding capacity of albumin in human serum. In the product distributed outside the United States, IMA is indicated for use as an adjunct to cardiac troponin to aid in the diagnosis of AMI in patients presenting with symptoms of ACS. It is likely that IMA may prove to be useful as a biochemical marker of ischemia, and several clinical studies are underway now to test this hypothesis, and to apply for Food and Drug Administration (FDA) approval for this use.

Work is under way to develop a point of care device for IMA testing, including immunoassay and other analytical techniques, which may allow a test to be performed on a small amount of whole blood (venipuncture or finger prick) within minutes. This will accelerate the adoption of IMA as a useful test for managing possible ACS patients in the ED.

FREE FATTY ACIDS

Fatty acids are straight-chain carboxylic acids containing none or variable numbers of unsaturated double bonds. High concentrations of these lipids are found in adipose tissue and serve as a reservoir for energy production. Fatty acids are oxidized in the mitochondria during starvation or if the cell is devoid of a glucose source. Because of the lipid and nonaqueous solubility of fatty acids, the majority of fatty acids in serum are bound to albumin. The free fatty acid concentration (FFA) ranges from 5 to 10 nmol/L. Previous studies have shown that the presence of unbound FFAs can have a deleterious effect on myocardial function by inducing a proarrhythmic effect *(30)*. In a study of 5250 men, FFAs were measured and the outcomes of subjects were followed for 22 yr. FFAs were found to be an independent risk factor for sudden death (odds ratio 1.70, 95% CI:

1.21–2.13) *(31)*. It was hypothesized that FFAs have an arrhythmogenic role and contributed to the death by contributing to a higher frequency of premature ventricular complexes.

Abnormal concentrations of FFAs may be a sensitive marker for cardiac ischemia and have been evaluated in preliminary studies. In the work of Kleinfeld et al., FFAs were measured before and 30 min after coronary angioplasty in 22 patients *(32)*. The mean FFA concentration increased 14-fold over baseline concentrations, with the highest concentrations seen in patients with ischemic ST-segment changes on the ECG. In a follow-up study, these investigators measured FFAs on 458 patients enrolled in the Thrombolysis in Myocardial Infarction (TIMI) II trial *(33)*. Blood was collected at presentation and 50 min, 5 h, and 8 h after administration of TPA. Using a cutoff of 5 nmol/L, the sensitivity of FFAs was 91% at admission and 98% when the 50-min sample was included. The specificity was 93% for normal individuals and patients with noncardiovascular diseases. FFA values also correlated with mortality, with a fourfold higher rate of death from low to high concentrations.

FFAs can be measured by fluorometry using acrylodated intestinal fatty acid binding protein as a fluorescent probe *(34)*. Using this procedure, the FFA concentration in normal individuals is normally distributed and is not influenced by age or gender. However, higher concentrations of FFAs are observed after fasting.

WHOLE BLOOD CHOLINE

Choline and phosphatidic acid are the major products generated by phosphodiesteric cleavage of membrane phospholipids (i.e., phosphatidylcholine) catalyzed by phospholipase D (PLD) enzymes *(35)*. Several experimental studies have demonstrated that PLD activation is involved in the major processes of coronary plaque destabilization: platelet activation by collagen and thrombin *(36–38)*, macrophage activation by oxidized low-density lipoproteins *(39)*, matrix metalloproteinase secretion *(40)*, and endothelial cell dysfunction *(41–43)* (Fig. 2). Isomers of PLD are emerging as important components in the cellular signal transduction pathways involved in coronary plaque destabilization *(44,45)*. While second messengers such as phosphatidate, lysophosphatidate, and diacylglycerol are enzymatically generated, choline is used as a marker of PLD activation. Furthermore, phospholipases are activated early after onset of myocardial ischemia and represent a major mechanism of early sarcolemmal damage *(46,47)*. Based on these processes, increased concentrations of choline have to be anticipated after plaque destabilization and myocardial ischemia, and were first demonstrated in patients with ACS using high-resolution 600-MHz nuclear magnetic resonance (NMR) spectroscopy of whole blood ultrafiltrate. Plasma or serum was found to contain much lower concentrations of choline, as blood cells possess a specific choline transporter leading to the concentrative intracellular accumulation of choline *(48)*.

Analytical Considerations

For clinical studies whole blood choline is currently measured by high-performance liquid chromatography–electrospray ionization mass spectrometry (HPLC-ESI-MS) using external calibration samples. This method allows highly specific and sensitive determination of free unbound choline in whole blood ultrafiltrate (WBCHO). Other methods like high-resolution 600-MHz NMR spectroscopy show an excellent correla-

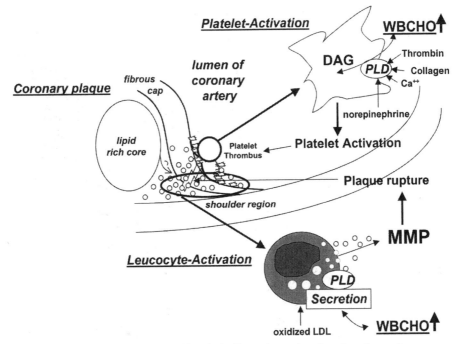

Fig. 2. PLD activation and whole blood choline release is related to the major processes of coronary plaque destabilization: platelet activation by collagen, thrombin, calcium, and norepinephrine; macrophage activation by oxidized low density lipoproteins (LDL), matrixmetalloproteinase (MMP) secretion, and endothelial cell dysfunction. These processes represent major causative events in the pathophysiology of acute coronary syndromes. DAG, Diacylglycerol; other abbreviations as in text.

tion to the HPLC-ESI-MS method ($r^2 = 0.998$). Commercial assays of WBCHO are under development.

Clinical Studies

One clinical study has been completed examining the clinical utility of whole blood choline in 327 patients with suspected ACS *(49)*. Patients were classified according to new American College of Cardiology/European Society of Cardiology (ACC/ECS) criteria of MI and Agency for Health Care Policy and Research (AHCPR) guidelines of unstable angina. WBCHO was measured by HPLC-ESI-MS and patients were followed for 30 d. This study indicates that whole blood choline was an independent predictor of cardiac death and nonfatal cardiac arrest and adds prognostic information to cardiac troponins (Figs. 3 and 4). Whole blood choline is also significantly predictive for life-threatening arrhythmias, MI, heart failure, and percutaneous coronary revascularization. Interestingly WBCHO still preserves its predictive value for major cardiac events, when looking only at patients with a negative troponin test on admission, which implicates an important clinical utility (Fig. 5). Furthermore, whole blood choline has the highest sensitivity (86%) for early diagnosis of high-risk unstable angina in troponin-negative patients without AMI. In this troponin-negative population other myocardial markers such as myoglobin or

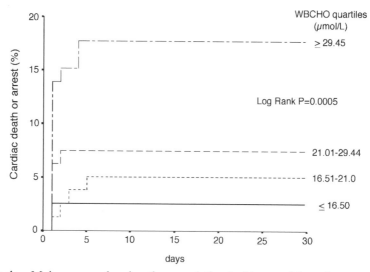

Fig. 3. Kaplan–Meier curves showing the cumulative incidence of the primary end point cardiac death or nonfatal cardiac arrest within 30 d according to WBCHO concentration on admission in 317 patients with suspected ACS. Data were analyzed in relation to WBCHO quartiles. Increasing concentrations of WBCHO on admission implicate a significant increase of risk for cardiac death and arrest within 30 d. The rate of cardiac death or arrest increased with rising quartiles of WBCHO on admission (log rank test $p = 0.0005$). Reproduced with permission from Danne O, et al. Am J Cardiol 2003, in press.

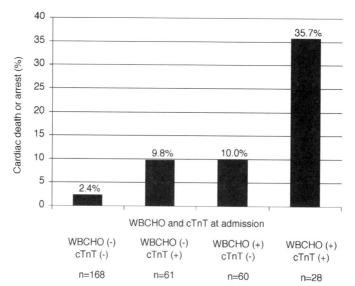

Fig. 4. Early risk stratification by WBCHO and cardiac troponin T (cTnT) expressed as the 30-d rate of cardiac death and nonfatal cardiac arrest. Results of the first blood sample were analyzed and positive tests (+) were defined according to the following cutoff values: WBCHO > 28.2 μmol/L, cTnT ≥ 0.03 ng/mL. The combination of whole blood choline and cTnT provides additional prognostic information for rapid biochemical risk stratification based on the results of a single blood sample on admission. WBCHO and troponins are strong and additive predictors of cardiac death and arrest. Reproduced with permission from Danne O, et al. Am J Cardiol 2003, in press.

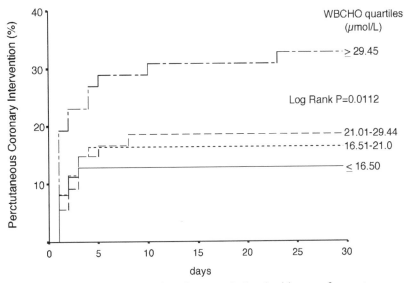

Fig. 5. Kaplan–Meier curves showing the cumulative incidence of percutaneous coronary intervention within 30 d according to WBCHO concentration on admission in patients with a negative cardiac troponin T (<0.03 ng/mL) on admission. Data were analyzed in relation to WBCHO quartiles. Increasing concentrations of WBCHO on admission implicate a significant increase of need for percutaneous coronary intervention in troponin-negative patients (log rank test $p = 0.0112$). As a marker of coronary plaque destabilization WBCHO is independent of myocardial necrosis and also serves as a risk predictor in troponin-negative patients.

CK-MB mass failed to detect high-risk patients; thus markers of coronary plaque destabilization, such as WBCHO, may have an important clinical utility (Fig. 6).

In contrast to other cardiac markers, the optimal time of testing of whole blood choline is the admitting blood sample. Many patients show a decline of WBCHO after antiplatelet, antithrombotic, and antiischemic therapies.

WBCHO was positive in 86% of patients with unstable angina, 45% with non-ST elevation MI (NSTEMI), and 32% with ST elevation MI (STEMI) in this first study. These differences have caused some controversies and have been explained by differences in the pathophysiology of plaque destabilization, which is speculative at this point.

In contrast to conventional cardiac markers, whole blood choline does not reflect myocardial necrosis but the initiating events of plaque fissure and cell activation, explaining a high sensitivity of whole blood choline in high-risk unstable angina at presentation. The findings of 83% of patients with high-risk unstable angina and increased whole blood choline concentrations may be related to the rate of 70–80% of unstable angina patients with platelet-rich white thrombi on coronary angioscopy *(50,51)* and 73% of patients with eccentric or complex coronary lesions *(52)*. Patients with acute STEMI have a red thrombus on angioscopy, corresponding to a lower rate of whole blood choline-positive patients in this group and a different pathophysiology of coronary thrombus formation *(53)*. In many of these STEMI patients with sudden onset of chest pain without prior symptoms, the interval from plaque rupture to formation of a covering red thrombus is short and leaves no time for activation of circulating blood cells by collagen and

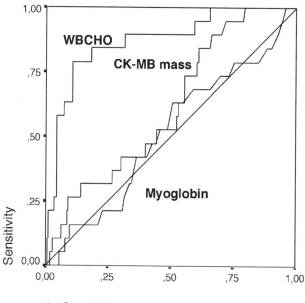

1 - Specificity

Fig. 6. Receiver operating characteristic curves for diagnosis of high-risk unstable angina in troponin T-negative patients without AMI defined according to new ACC/ESC criteria. WBCHO showed the largest area under the curve (AUC: 0.869; 95% CI: 0.781–0.956) when compared to CK-MB mass (AUC: 0.611; 95% CI: 0.490–0.732) and myoglobin (AUC: 0.510; 95% CI: 0.374–0.645), indicating a superior diagnostic power of WBCHO for detection of high-risk unstable angina with a single blood test on admission. After the ACC/ESC redefinition of MI myocardial markers such as myoglobin or CK-MB mass fail to detect patients with high-risk unstable angina. Markers of coronary plaque destabilization, such as WBCHO, may have an important clinical utility for early diagnosis of unstable angina.

other plaque-related tissue factors. These patients remain WBCHO silent unless other factors contribute to increased WBCHO concentrations. This is essentially different in many patients with non-ST elevation ACS in whom plaque destabilization is often a fluctuating process with intermittent formation of non-occluding white thrombi causing intermittent symptoms of variable degree. The process of plaque-related intermittent stimulation of cell surface receptors on blood cells presumably leads to PLD activation and measurable increases of whole blood choline. Other factors that are involved in amplification of PLD activity are norepinephrine concentrations *(54)* and the formation of leukocyte/platelet aggregates, both representing important causative factors for arrhythmias and sudden cardiac death *(55,56)*. These major cardiac events were also associated with increased WBCHO concentrations.

Furthermore, it should be noted that the concentrations of WBCHO in control patients are not normally distributed, and we have indications of families with persistent high WBCHO concentrations. It will be an interesting field of research to investigate whether these individuals have acquired or inborn forms of increased PLD expression, and whether this disposition also represents a risk factor for long-term vascular events.

Additional studies are needed to investigate the process, time course of PLD activation, and WBCHO release in ACS as well as the clinical significance of this marker. Current data suggest a possible clinical utility for early risk stratification of patients with a negative troponin test on admission and for diagnosis of high-risk unstable angina.

B-TYPE NATRIURETIC PEPTIDE

The biochemistry of the natriuretic peptides and the pathophysiology of congestive heart failure (CHF) are described in Chapters 23 and 22, respectively. With regard to CHF, this marker is important in the diagnosis, staging severity, risk stratification for future adverse events such as death or CHF complications, and for monitoring the success of drug therapy. There have been a few clinical studies that suggest that B-type natriuretic peptide (BNP) might also have a role in cardiac ischemia in patients with ACS. Tateishi et al. measured BNP in 30 patients who underwent percutaneous transluminal coronary angioplasty (PTCA) and compared results to 49 control patients who underwent coronary angiography *(57)*. Blood was collected immediately before and at regular intervals up to 96 h thereafter. These investigators showed that after 24 h, the BNP doubled in the angioplasty group, while no change was observed in the angiography group. Their presumption was that the balloon induced a transient ischemia, which caused release of BNP in the absence of significant myocardial necrosis. In another study, Sabatine et al. measured BNP before, immediately after, and 4 h after stress testing with myocardial perfusion imaging (MPI)*(58)*. In patients with severe ischemia as assessed by MPI, median BNP concentration increased from baseline to 15 pg/mL, while an increase of 12.7 pg/mL was observed in those with mild to moderate ischemia. Only a 5.7 pg/mL change was observed in patients without ischemia. Given the fact that BNP release from myocytes is due to up-regulation at the genome concentration and not from cytoplasmic storage granules (such as for atrial natriuretic peptide), it is difficult to hypothesize that BNP will prove to be useful as an early marker for myocardial ischemia caused by ACS. The origin of BNP release immediately after stress testing is currently unclear. It is likely that a small cytoplasmic pool of peptides exists.

GLYCOGEN PHOSPHORYLASE BB

Human glycogen phosphorylase (GP) b (EC 2.4.1.1) (GP-BB) exists in the form of three isoezymes, which have been exhaustively studied. There are three isoenzyme forms: BB (brain), MM (muscle), and LL (liver). The heart contains principally the BB form although MM is also present *(59)*. Tissue concentrations in the heart and brain are comparable. In the absence of GP-BB arising from breach of the blood–brain barrier, the assay of serum or plasma for this isoenzyme reveals principally this isoenzyme from cardiac sources. There is also evidence of this enzyme in leukocytes, platelets, spleen, kidney, bladder, testis, digestive tract, and aorta although in low concentrations compared to the predominant LL form. As such, GP-BB is not totally cardiospecific. However, the underlying pathophysiology is particularly intriguing because it is known that the enzyme release from the myocardial cell is primed by preexistent ischemia. The high concentration of the enzyme in the myocardial cell preexisting in a macromolecular complex in the sarcoplasmic reticulum is released into the cytosol by phosphorylase kinase activating the enzyme. A gradient is created that favors rapid release and entry into the peripheral circulation on further ischemic insult *(59)*. This well studied patho-physiology correlates with the clinical timing of early appearance of the marker in the peripheral blood following infarction.

Analytical Considerations

An immunoassay for GP-BB was initially announced in a published letter *(60)*. A detailed description of the method was reported subsequently *(61)*. Given the unique structure of the three isoenzyme forms of GP-BB, epitopes could be identified that conveyed analytical specificity to the immunoenzymometricassay. The monoclonal antibodies showed no cross-reactivity to the other isoenzymes. Approximately 20% of the amino acid sequence is unique to the BB form. Peroxidase was employed as the label for signal generation.

Clinical Applications

In the initial clinical data, the impressive earlier appearance of GP-BB was noted, significantly improved as contrasted not only with CK-MB but also superior to myoglobin. In addition, the elevation remained detectable longer than that of myoglobin. In ROC analysis, the performance was described as superior to all markers including cardiac troponin T. Patient classification was by clinical and ECG criteria. As such, the relevance to the current classification of these patients may be questionable. In this report and in another *(62)*, considerable discussion centered on the elevation of GP-BB in the absence of other cardiac markers and is more elaborately discussed referencing the basic science studies in another publication *(63)*. While there is much speculation with regard to whether the enzyme is released during ischemia in the absence of necrosis, the authors acknowledge that the answer to that question is not known. With regard to the cardiospecificity, the most telling remark is as follows: "As long as the diagnostic specificity of GP-BB for myocardial damage is not fully delineated, a positive GP-BB result should be later confirmed by cardiac troponin I measurement" *(63)*.

An intriguing exploration of the sensitivity of GP-BB in detecting "minimal myocardial damage" was reported by Lang et al. by serially testing individuals subjected to endomyocardial biopsy. These patients were studied predominantly for cardiomyopathy or myocarditis and were not ischemic. Troponin T (enzyme-linked immunosorbent assay [ELISA], apparently second-generation assay) was increased following the biopsy promptly within 10 min and to a significant degree in approximately half of the group. GP-BB did not significantly increase in any patients. This puzzling difference from the initial studies in patients with ACS is explained by the authors on the basis of the pathophysiology of GP-BB. Clearly, ischemic insult primes the myocardial cell and induces increased glyocogenolysis. These patients were not exposed to ischemic insult. In addition, the earlier comparison employed the less sensitive first-generation cTnT assay, while this study used a cutoff of 0.1 ng/mL—apparently the second-generation cTnT assay. Of interest, although there is no currently available commercial source of these GP-BB assay reagents in North America, Lang et al. reference the assay to have been provided by a commercial source (Laboserv GmbH, Staufenberg, Germany) *(64)*. To date, studies of renal failure, trauma, and other complex patients with coexistent ACS are not available.

Summary for GP-BB

Glycogen phosphorylase BB isoenzyme appears comparable to CK-MB in diagnostic specificity while appearing significantly earlier. It has been proposed as a potential partner with cardiac troponin for a combination of an early marker, clearly earlier than myoglobin, along with the later cardiospecific confirming marker. To date, most of the published work has been produced based on one assay but that is not widely available. Reviews of the field continue to reference the potential of this diagnostic test. However, original data investigating the complex spectrum of patients encountered in acute chest pain triage are limited.

In view of the known lack of absolute cardiospecificity, one may expect that enthusiasm for basing early therapy on the finding of a positive GP-BB assay will be tempered. As with myoglobin, the known high cardiospecificity of the troponins, I and T, has minimized the value of alternative markers. If therapy cannot be reliably based on the test data, the impetus for use of the assay is minimized.

CARDIAC TROPONINS

As documented in a recent editorial *(65)*, the prevailing view among most laboratory scientists and cardiologists is that protein-based cardiac markers such as myoglobin (17 kDa), CK (84 kDa), lactate dehydrogenase (140 kDa), and cardiac troponins T (37 kDa) and I (24 kDa) are most likely released only after the onset of irreversible injury. Animal studies for CK have confirmed this notion *(66)*. The release kinetics for cardiac troponin from the heart to the blood is more complicated than for cytoplasmic markers such as CK. Figure 7A illustrates the release of cardiac troponin following irreversible injury. The initial release is thought to be due to the cytoplasmic component while the prolonged appearance is due to the gradual breakdown of the myofibrils. Once into blood, cardiac troponin has a relative short half-life of about 120 min *(67)*. Patients with minor myocardial damage can have an increased concentration of troponin in the absence of increased CK-MB. The logical explanation for this apparent discrepancy is the higher myocardial tissue content of cardiac troponin, at 10.8 mg/g wet wt for cardiac troponin T and 6.0 mg/g for cardiac troponin I, relative to CK-MB at 1.4 mg/g *(68)*. Increased analytical specificity can also improve the clinical sensitivity. As cardiac troponin is not expressed in skeletal muscle tissue, and there is little day-to-day turnover of cardiac myocytes, very low concentrations of cardiac troponin are found in blood of healthy individuals. Thus, any increase due to minor myocardial damage can be readily discernible. In contrast, CK is released from all contractile tissue and there can be a substantial amount of CK in normal blood. As such, the release of enzymes following minor myocardial damage must exceed the existing the ambient background concentration observed in healthy individuals. An analogy would be the differences in a lit candle in daylight (high background) vs the same candle at night (low background).

Controlled animal studies, clinical observations, and research studies have challenged the notion that cardiac troponin is released only during irreversible injury *(69–72)*. In a porcine model of ischemia, troponin was released into blood in the absence of histologic evidence of irreversible myocyte damage at significantly higher concentrations than in sham controls *(70)*. When myoglobin and CK-MB were also measured, there was

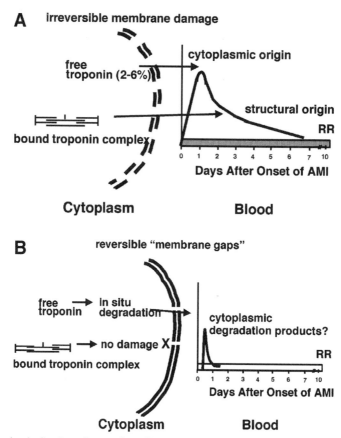

Fig. 7. Hypothesis for the release of cardiac markers from cytoplasms and myofibrils to blood following (**A**) irreversible and (**B**) reversible injury.

no difference between controls and ischemic animals. In humans, it has been known for many years that some patients with unstable angina exhibit a transient release of cardiac troponin in blood, that is, abnormal concentrations for only 1 or 2 d (71). The absence of a delayed release from the myofibrillar pool and appearance in blood suggest that in these cases, the myocytes might be reversibly damaged. This implies that ischemic injury can result in a transient release of cytosolic proteins due to leaky membranes but without permanent injury. Other evidence of the reversibility concept is suggested in patients with septic shock. Troponin concentrations are increased in a large fraction of these patients (72), putatively due to the release of myocardial depressive factors. On recovery, however, these patients do not exhibit permanent cardiac damage as assessed by nuclear perfusion imaging (73,74). Moreover, histologic evidence of irreversible myocardial damage is not consistently observed in autopsies of patients with high troponin who died of sepsis (75,76).

The mechanism for the release of troponin in reversible injury may be related to the presence of myocardial depressive factors (e.g., tumor necrosis factor-α) that are released during inflammation. These factors have been shown to increase the permeability of endothelial cell monolayers in cell culture to the point of releasing albumin (67 kDa) *(77)*. An alternate explanation is the degradation of troponin *in situ* during periods of ischemia. The release of lower-molecular-weight fragments, as described in Chapter 7, may enable release of troponin during ischemia and detection in blood with the initial hours after the onset of chest pain. By Western blot analysis, cardiac troponin can be detected from blood samples collected from patients with chest pain at the time of their ED presentation *(78)*. Suleiman et al. showed that short periods (3 min) of regional ischemia followed by reperfusion produced of significant amounts of troponin in peripheral blood *(79)*. Figure 7B illustrates how troponin might be released during reversible ischemia to produce a transient and minor increase of this protein in blood.

It may not be possible to definitely prove with definitive experimentation that troponin is release during reversible ischemia. Some question the significance of the pathophysiologic mechanism of cardiac marker release to the clinical practice of cardiology *(65)*. However, the utility of cardiac troponin for detecting minor myocardial damage and the identification of more patients at risk for future cardiovascular events may be improved with the development of next-generation assays with substantially improved analytical sensitivity, and possibly specificity toward important epitopes found early in blood.

ABBREVIATIONS

ACB, Albumin Cobalt Binding; ACC/ESC, American College of Cardiology/European Society of Cardiology; ACS, acute coronary syndromes; AHCPR, Agency for Health Care Policy and Research; AMI, acute myocardial infarction; BNP, B-type natriuretic peptide; CHF, congestive heart failure; CI, confidence interval; CK, creatine kinase; CK-MB, MB isoenzyme of CK; DTT, dithiothreitol; ECG, electrocardiogram; ED, emergency department; ELISA, enzyme-linked immunosorbent assay; FDA, Food and Drug Administration; FFA, free fatty acid; GP-BB, glycogen phosphorylase BB; HPLC-ESI-MS, high-performance liquid chromatography electrospray ionization mass spectrometry; IMA, Ischemia-Modified Albumin; MPI, myocardial perfusion imaging; NMR, nuclear magnetic resonance; NSTEMI, non-ST elevation myocardial infarction; PLD, phospholipase D; PTCA, percutaneous transluminal coronary angioplasty; TIMI, Thrombolysis in Myocardial Infarction; WBCHO, whole blood choline.

REFERENCES

1. Jaffe AS, Ravkilde J, Roberts R, et al. It's time for a change to a troponin standard. Circulation 2000;102:1216–1220.
2. Ishikawa Y, Saffitz JE, Mealman TL, Grace AM, Roberts R. Reversible myocardial ischemic injury is not associated with increased creatine kinase activity in plasma. Clin Chem 1997;43:467–475.
3. Wu AHB, Ford L. Release of biochemical markers in acute coronary syndromes: ischemia or only necrosis? Clin Chim Acta 1999;284:161–171.
4. Bar-Or D, Lau E, Rao N, Bampos N, Winkler J, Curtis CG. Reduction in cobalt binding capacity of human albumin with myocardial ischemia. Annual Meeting of the American College of Emergency Physicians, 1999.
5. BarOr D, Lau E, Winkler J. A novel assay for the cobalt-albumin binding and its potential as a marker for myocardial ischemia: a preliminary report. J Emerg Med 2000;19:311–315.

6. BarOr D, Winkler J, VanBenthuysen K, Harris L, Lau E, Hetzel F. Reduced cobalt binding of human albumin with transient myocardial ischemia following elective percutaneous transluminal coronary angioplasty compared to CK-MB, myoglobin and troponin I. Am Heart J 2001;141:985–991.

7. Cobbe SM, Poole-Wilson PA. The time of onset and severity of acidosis in myocardial ischaemia. J Mol Cell Cardiol 1980;12:745–760.

8. Levine RL. Ischemia: from acidosis to oxidation. FASEB J 1993;7:1242–1246.

9. Wardman P, Candeias LP. Fenton Centennial Symposium. Fenton chemistry: an introduction. Radiat Res 1996;145:523–531.

10. Samuni A, Aronovitch J, Godinger D, Chevion M, Czapski G. On the cytotoxicity of vitamin C and metal ions. A site-specific Fenton mechanism. Eur J Biochem 1983;137:119–124.

11. Marx G, Chevion M. Site-specific modification of albumin by free radicals. Biochem J 1985;236:397–400.

12. McCord JM. Oxygen-derived free radicals in post-ischemic tissue injury. N Engl J Med 1985;312:159–163.

13. Halliwell B, Gutteridge JMG. Free Radicals in Biology and Medicine. New York: Oxford University Press, 1999, p. 45.

14. Laussac JP, Sarkar B. Characterization of the copper (II)- and nickel (II)- transport site of human serum albumin. Studies of copper (II) and nickel (II) binding to peptide 1–24 of human serum albumin by 13C and 1H NMR spectroscopy. Biochemistry 1984;23:2832–2838.

15. Bal W, Christodoulou J, Sadler P, Tucker A. Multi-metal binding site of serum albumin. J Inorgan Biochem 1998;70:33–39.

16. Glennon JD, Sarkar B. Nickel (II) transport in human blood serum. Studies of nickel (II) binding to human albumin and to native-sequence peptide, and ternary-complex formation with L-histidine. Biochem J 1982;203:15–23.

17. Mohanakrishnan P, Chignell CF, Cox RH. Chloride ion nuclear magnetic resonance spectroscopy probe studies of copper and nickel binding to serum albumins. J Pharmaceut Sci 1985;74:61–62.

18. BarOr D, Curtis G, Rao N, Bampos N, Lau E. Characterization of the Co^{2+} and Ni^{2+} binding amino-acid residues of the N-terminus of human albumin. Eur J Biochem 2001;268:42–47.

19. Masuoka J, Hegenauer J, Van Dyke BR, Saltman P. Intrinsic stoichiometric equilibrium constants for the binding of zinc (II) and copper (II) to the high affinity site of serum albumin. J Biol Chem 1993;268:21533–21537.

20. Nandedkar AK, Hong MS, Friedberg F. Co^{2+} binding by plasma albumin. Biochem Med 1974; 9:177–183.

21. Painter PC, Branham E, Morris D, et al. Analytical studies of an assay to detect myocardial ischemia. Clin Chem 2000;47:A75.

22. Sinha MK, Gaze DC, Collinson PO, Kaski JC. A novel assay for the detection of ischaemia in percutaneous coronary artery intervention by assessment of the albumin cobalt binding (ACB) test. AHA Meeting on Cardiac Ischemia, Seattle, WA:2001.

23. Apple FS, Quist HE, Otto AP, Mathews WE, Murakami MM. Release characteristics of cardiac biomarkers and ischemia-modified albumin as measured by the albumin cobalt-binding test after a marathon race. Clin Chem 2002;48:1097–1100.

24. Christenson RL, Duh SH, Sanhai WR, et al. Characteristics of an albumin cobalt binding test for assessment of acute coronary syndrome patients: a multicenter study. Clin Chem 2001; 47:464–470.

25. Wu AHB, Morris DL, Fletcher DR, Apple FS, Christenson RH, Painter PC. Analysis of the Albumin Cobalt Binding (ACB™) test as an adjunct to cardiac troponin I for the early detection of acute myocardial infarction. Cardiovasc Toxicol 2001;1:147–152.

26. Morris DL, Fletcher DR, Apple FS, et al. The Albumin Cobalt Binding test (ACB Test) as an adjunct to troponin for early diagnosis of acute myocardial infarction. Eur Heart J 2001; 22(Suppl);P608.

27. Heller GV, Cyr G, Storrow AB, et al. The Albumin Cobalt Binding test (ACB™ Test) to diagnose ischemia in patients with symptoms of coronary artery disease. Clin Chem 2001; 47(S6):A205.

28. Sinha MK, Gaze DC, Collinson PO, Kaski JC. The Albumin Cobalt Binding (ACB) test diagnoses cardiac ischaemia in patients with non-ST-elevation chest pain in the emergency department. Presented at the AHA Meeting on Cardiac Ischemia, Seattle, WA, 2001.

29. Sinha MK, Gaze DC, Collinson PO, Kaski JC. Ischemia Modified Albumin (IMA™): a marker of ischaemia in patients presenting to the emergency department with chest pain. Presented at the Ninth International Conference on Emergency Medicine, Edinburgh, UK, 2002.

30. Kurien VA, Oliver MF. A metabolic cause of arrhythmias. Lancet 1970;1:813–815.

31. Jouven X, Charles MA, Desnos M, Ducimetiere P. Circulating nonesterified fatty acid concentration as a positive risk factor for sudden death in the population. Circulation 2001; 104:756–761.

32. Kleinfeld AM, Prothro D, Brown DL, Dais RC, Richieri GV, DeMaria A. Increases in serum unbound free fatty acid concentrations following coronary angioplasty. Am J Cardiol 1996;78:1350–1354.

33. Kleinfeld AM, Kleinfeld KJ, Adams JE. Serum concentrations of unbound free fatty acids reveal high sensitivity for early detection of AMI in patient samples from the TIMI II Trial (abstract). J Am Coll Cardiol 2002;39(Suppl):312A.

34. Richieri GV, Kleinfeld AM. Unbound free fatty acid concentrations in human serum. J Lipid Res 1995;36:229–240.

35. Morris AJ, Frohman MA, Engebrecht J. Measurement of phospholipase D activity. Analyt Biochem 1997;252:1–9.

36. Chiang TM. Activation of phospholipase D in human platelets by collagen and thrombin and its relationship to platelet aggregation. Biochim Biophys Acta 1994;1224:147–155.

37. Martinson EA, Scheible S, Greinacher A, Presek P. Platelet phospholipase D is activated by protein kinase C via an integrin alpha IIb beta 3-independent mechanism. Biochem J 1995;310(Pt 2):623–628.

38. Martinson EA, Scheible S, Marx-Grunwitz A, Presek P. Secreted ADP plays a central role in thrombin-induced phospholipase D activation in human platelets. Thromb Haemost 1998; 80:976–981.

39. Gomez-Munoz A, Martens JS, Steinbrecher UP. Stimulation of phospholipase D activity by oxidized LDL in mouse peritoneal macrophages. Arterioscler Thromb Vasc Biol 2000; 20:135–143.

40. Williger BT, Ho WT, Exton JH. Phospholipase D mediates matrix metalloproteinase-9 secretion in phorbol ester-stimulated human fibrosarcoma cells. J Biol Chem 1999;274: 735–738.

41. Cox DA, Cohen ML. Lysophosphatidylcholine stimulates phospholipase D in human coronary endothelial cells: role of PKC. Am J Physiol 1996;271(4 Pt 2):H1706–H1710.

42. Cox DA, Cohen ML. Relationship between phospholipase D activation and endothelial vasomotor dysfunction in rabbit aorta. J Pharmacol Exp Ther 1997;283:305–311.

43. Garcia JG, Fenton JW, Natarajan V. Thrombin stimulation of human endothelial cell phospholipase D activity. Regulation by phospholipase C, protein kinase C, and cyclic adenosine 3'5'-monophosphate. Blood 1992;79:2056–2067.

44. O'Brien KD, Pineda C, Chiu WS, Bowen R, Deeg MA. Glycosylphosphatidylinositol-specific phospholipase D is expressed by macrophages in human atherosclerosis and colocalizes with oxidation epitopes. Circulation 1999;99:2876–2882.

45. Houle MG, Bourgoin S. Regulation of phospholipase D by phosphorylation-dependent mechanisms. Biochim Biophys Acta 1999;1439:135–149.

46. Kurz T, Schneider I, Tolg R, Richardt G. Alpha 1-adrenergic receptor-mediated increase in the mass of phosphatidic acid and 1,2-diacylglycerol in ischemic rat heart. Cardiovasc Res 1999;42:48–56.

47. Barry WH. Mechanisms of myocardial cell injury during ischemia and reperfusion. J Card Surg 1987;2:375–383.

48. Deves R, Krupka RM. The comparative specificity of the inner and outer substrate transfer sites in the choline carrier of human erythrocytes. J Membr Biol 1984;80:71–80.

49. Danne O, Möckel M, Lueders C, Muegge C, Zschunke GA, Lufft H, Mueller CH, Frei U. Prognostic implications of whole blood choline levels in acute coronary syndromes. Am J Cardiol 2003; in press.

50. Mizuno K, Satomura K, Miyamoto A, et al. Angioscopic evaluation of coronary-artery thrombi in acute coronary syndromes. N Engl J Med 1992;326:287–291.

51. Mizuno K, Arakawa K, Isojima K, et al. Angioscopy, coronary thrombi and acute coronary syndromes. Biomed Pharmacother 1993;47:187–191.

52. Haft JI, Goldstein JE, Niemiera ML. Coronary arteriographic lesion of unstable angina. Chest 1987;92:609–612.

53. Ambrose JA. Plaque disruption and the acute coronary syndromes of unstable angina and myocardial infarction: if the substrate is similar, why is the clinical presentation different? J Am Coll Cardiol 1992;19:1653–1658.

54. Jones AW, Shukla SD, Geisbuhler BB. Stimulation of phospholipase D activity and phosphatidic acid production by norepinephrine in rat aorta. Am J Physiol 1993;264(3 Pt 1): C609–C616.

55. Davies MJ, Thomas AC, Knapman PA, Hangartner JR. Intramyocardial platelet aggregation in patients with unstable angina suffering sudden ischemic cardiac death. Circulation 1986;73:418–427.

56. Falk E. Unstable angina with fatal outcome: dynamic coronary thrombosis leading to infarction and/or sudden death. Autopsy evidence of recurrent mural thrombosis with peripheral embolization culminating in total vascular occlusion. Circulation 1985;71:699–708.

57. Tateishi J, Masutani M, Ohyanagi M, Iwasaki T. Transient increase in plasma brain (B-type) natriuretic peptide after percutanoues transluminal coronary angioplasty. Clin Cardiol 2000; 23:776–780.

58. Sabatine MS, Morrow DA, De Lemos JA, et al. Elevation of B-type natriuretic peptide in the setting of myocardial ischemia. Circulation 2001;104:II–485.

59. Mair J. Glycogen phosphorylase isoenzyme BB to diagnose ischaemic myocardial damage. Clin Chim Acta 1998;272:79–86.

60. Rabitzsch G, Mair J, Lechleitner P, et al. Isoenzyme BB of glycogen phosphorylase b and myocardial infarction. Lancet 1993 Apr 17;341:1032–1033.

61. Rabitzsch G, Mair J, Lechleitner P, et al. Immunoenzymometric assay of human glycogen phosphorylase isoenzyme BB in diagnosis of ischemic myocardial injury. Clin Chem 1995; 41:966–978.

62. Mair P, Mair J, Krause EG, Balogh D, Puschendorf B, Rabitzsch G. Glycogen phosphorylase isoenzyme BB mass release after coronary artery bypass grafting. Eur J Clin Chem Clin Biochem 1994;32:543–547.

63. Krause EG, Rabitzsch G, Noll F, Mair J, Puschendorf B. Glycogen phosphorylase isoenzyme BB in diagnosis of myocardial ischaemic injury and infarction. Mol Cell Biochem 1996;160–161:289–295.

64. Lang K, Borner A, Figulla HR. Comparison of biochemical markers for the detection of minimal myocardial injury: superior sensitivity of cardiac troponin—T ELISA. J Intern Med 2000;247:119–123.

65. Jaffe AS, Ravkilde J, Roberts R, et al. It's time for a change to a troponin standard. Circulation 2000;102:1216–1220.

66. Ishikawa Y, Saffitz JE, Mealman TL, Grace AM, Roberts R. Reversible myocardial ischemic injury is not associated with increased creatine kinase activity in plasma. Clin Chem 1997;43:467–475.

67. Katus HG, Remppis A, Scheffold T. Intracellular compartmentation of cardiac troponin T and its release kinetics in patients with reperfused and nonreperfused myocardial infarction. Am J Cardiol 1991;67:1360–1367.

68. Dean KJ. Biochemistry and molecular biology of troponins I and T. In: Cardiac Markers. Wu AHB, ed. Totowa, NJ: Humana Press, 1998, pp. 193–204.

69. Sobel BE, LeWinter MM. Ingenuous interpretation of elevated blood levels of macromolecular markers of myocardial injury: a recipe for confusion. J Am Coll Cardiol 2000;35: 1355–1358.

70. Feng YJ, Chen C, Fallon JT, Ma L, Waters DD, Wu AHB. Comparison of cardiac troponin I, creatine kinase-MB, and myoglobin for detection of acute myocardial necrosis in a swine myocardial ischemic model. Am J Clin Pathol 1998;110:70–77.

71. Hamm CW, Ravkilde J, Gerhardt W, Jorgensen P, Peheim E, Ljungdahl L. The prognostic value of serum troponin T in unstable angina. N Engl J Med 1992;327:146–150.

72. Wu AHB. Increased troponin in patients with sepsis and septic shock: myocardial necrosis or reversible myocardial depression (editorial). Crit Care Med 2001;27:959–960.

73. Parker MM, Shelhamer JH, Bachrach SL, et al. Profound but reversible myocardial depression in aptients with septic shock. Ann Intern Med 1984;100:483–490.

74. Ellrod AG, Riedinger MS, Kimchi A, et al. Left ventricular performance in septic shock: reversible segmental and global abnormalities. Am Heart J 1985;110:402–409.

75. ver Elst KM, Spapen HD, Nguyen DN, et al. Cardiac troponins I and T are biological markers of left ventricular dysfunction in septic shock. Clin Chem 2000;46:650–657.

76. Ammann P, Fehr T, Minder EI, et al. Elevation of troponin I in sepsis and septic shock. Crit Care Med 2001;29:965–969.

77. Brett J, Gewrlach H, Nawroth P, et al. Tumor necrosis factor/cachectin increases permeability of endothelial cell monolayers by a mechanism involving regulatory G proteins. J Exp Med 1989;169:1977–1991.

78. Suleiman MS, Lucchetti V, Caputo M, Angelini GD. Short periods of regional ischaemia and reperfusion provoke release of troponin I from the human hearts. Clin Chim Acta 1999; 284:25–30.

79. Colantonio DA, Pickett W, Brison RJ, Collier CE, Van Eyk JE. Detection of cardiac troponin I early after onset of chest pain in six patients. Clin Chem 2002;48:668–671.

17

C-Reactive Protein for Primary Risk Assessment

Gavin J. Blake and Paul M. Ridker

INTRODUCTION

Accumulating evidence suggests that inflammatory processes play a key role in the pathogenesis of atherosclerosis *(1)*. Given that over half of all myocardial infarctions (MIs) occur in individuals without overt hyperlipidemia, attention has focused on whether plasma concentrations of inflammatory biomarkers can help predict cardiovascular risk *(2)*.

Of these inflammatory biomarkers, C-reactive protein (CRP) has been the most extensively studied. Produced mainly by the liver in response to interleukin-6 (IL-6), CRP was initially considered to be a sensitive but innocent bystander marker of low-grade vascular inflammation. Accumulating data, however, suggest that CRP may play a more direct role in atherogenesis. CRP opsonization of low-density lipoprotein (LDL) mediates LDL uptake by macrophages *(3)*, and CRP stimulates monocyte release of other pro-inflammatory cytokines such as IL-1b, IL-6, and tumor necrosis factor-α (TNF-α) *(4)*. Furthermore, CRP mediates monocyte chemoattractant protein-1 (MCP-1) expression by endothelial cells *(5)* and causes endothelial cells to express intercellular adhesion molecule-1 (ICAM-1) and vascular cell adhesion molecule-1 (VCAM-1) *(6)*. Recent data suggest that arterial tissue can produce CRP, with CRP and complement mRNA being substantially up-regulated in atherosclerotic plaque *(7)*. Thus CRP may serve as an endogenous activator of complement in atheroma.

As shown in Fig. 1, there is robust evidence from several large-scale prospective studies in the United States and Europe that increased concentrations of CRP are a strong predictor of future MI, stroke, and peripheral vascular disease among healthy men and women *(8–17)*. For example, in a cohort of 22,000 healthy middle-aged men, those with CRP concentrations in the highest quartile had a twofold increased risk of stroke or peripheral vascular disease and a threefold increased risk of MI *(9,10)*. These findings were independent of lipid levels and other traditional cardiovascular risk factors.

Other promising inflammatory markers include soluble intercellular adhesion molecule-1 (sICAM-1), p-selectin, soluble CD 40 ligand, and lipoprotein-associated phospholipase A_2. sICAM-1 and p-selectin are cell adhesion molecules involved in the tethering and adhesion of inflammatory cells to the diseased endothelium. Interestingly, CRP induces expression of cellular adhesion molecules in human endothelial cells *(6)*. Plasma concentrations of sICAM-1 and p-selectin have been found to be increased among apparently healthy individuals at risk for future cardiovascular events in prospective studies

From: *Cardiac Markers, Second Edition*
Edited by: Alan H. B. Wu @ Humana Press Inc., Totowa, NJ

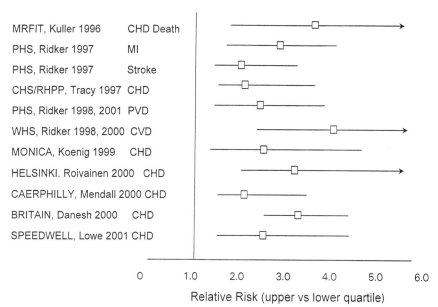

Fig. 1. Prospective studies of CRP and future cardiovascular events among healthy individuals. Risk estimates and 95% confidence intervals are calculated as comparison of top vs bottom quartile within each study group. (Adapted from Blake GJ, Ridker PM. Circ Res 2001;89:766–768 and Ridker PM. Circulation 2001;103:1814–1815.)

from both the United States and Europe, although the predictive effect of these inflammatory biomarkers may be attenuated after adjustment for traditional cardiovascular risk factors *(18–21)*.

Lipoprotein-associated phospholipase A_2 circulates in association with LDL cholesterol and may contribute directly to the progression of atherosclerosis by hydrolyzing oxidized phospholipids into proatherogenic fragments and by generating lysolecithin, which has proinflammatory properties. In a study among hyperlipidemic men, baseline levels of lipoprotein-associated phospholipase A_2 were an independent predictor of future cardiovascular events *(22)*. However, in a recent study among lower risk women, the predictive effect of lipoprotein-associated phospholipase A_2 was markedly attenuated in adjusted analyses, while CRP remained a strong independent predictor of risk (Fig. 2) *(23)*. Lipoprotein-associated phospholipase A_2 is highly correlated with LDL cholesterol, which may in part account for these different results.

CD 40 ligand is a transmembrane protein structurally related to TNF-α, which binds to CD40 leading to the activation of macrophages and T lymphocytes. Both CD40 and CD40 ligand are abundantly expressed in the shoulder regions of atherosclerotic plaque *(24)*. Recent data show that apparently healthy women with increased plasma levels of soluble CD40 ligand at baseline are at increased risk for future cardiovascular events *(25),* and that CD40 ligand concentrations are increased among patients with unstable angina *(26)*. Intriguingly, the administration of antiCD40 ligand antibody to hyperlipidemic mice leads to a dramatic reduction in lesion size and lipid content *(27)*. These data suggest that novel targeted antiinflammatory interventions may soon have a role to play in the treatment of atherosclerosis and its complications.

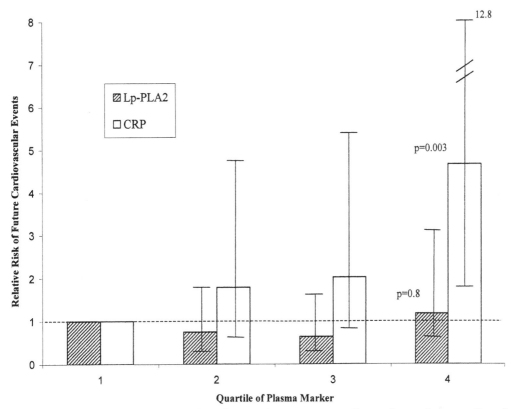

Fig. 2. Adjusted relative risks of cardiovascular events according to increasing quartiles of lipoprotein-associated phospholipase A_2 (Lp-PLA$_2$) and CRP compared to the lowest quartile. (Adapted from Blake GJ, et al. JACC 2001:38;1305.)

As shown in Fig. 3, a recent analysis seeking to compare the predictive value of several traditional and inflammatory biomarkers found that CRP and the ratio of total cholesterol to high-density lipoprotein cholesterol were the strongest predictors of future cardiovascular risk among apparently healthy middle-aged women *(8)*. Moreover, the predictive effect of CRP was additive to that of total cholesterol (TC) to high-density (HDL) lipoprotein cholesterol ratio.

Consistent data from large well-conducted prospective studies are a prerequisite for potential clinical application of any novel risk factor. However, in addition, the candidate risk marker should improve on traditional risk assessment, should direct potential therapeutic intervention, and screening for the risk factor should be relatively cost effective. Of the inflammatory markers currently investigated, CRP meets most, if not all, of these criteria. Moreover, the potential prognostic utility of CRP is increased by its relatively long half-life, lack of circadian variation *(28)*, and low coefficients of variation when measured with high-sensitivity assays *(29)*, such as those now commercially available.

CAN CRP TESTING IMPROVE ON STANDARD LIPID TESTING?

In current clinical practice, lipid screening is the only blood test routinely advocated for cardiovascular risk assessment. However, data suggest that CRP testing may have

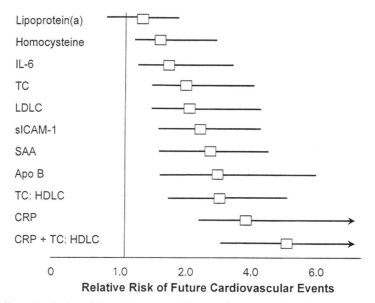

Fig. 3. Adjusted relative risks of future cardiovascular events for the highest quartile compared to the lowest quartile of plasma concentration of each risk marker among apparently healthy women. (Adapted from Ridker PM, et al. N Engl J Med 2000:342;839.)

the potential to improve cardiovascular risk prediction when used as an adjunct to lipid testing *(8,30,31)*. In this regard, in the Women's Health Study, the area under the receiver–operator curve was significantly greater (*p* < 0.001) when CRP testing was added to lipid screening, compared with lipid screening alone *(8)*. Furthermore, when the relative risks associated with combined lipid and CRP testing were estimated, it was evident that increasing concentrations of CRP had additive predictive value at all lipid levels. Figure 4 shows the interactive effects of CRP and lipid testing among healthy men and women *(32)*. Men and women with both CRP and lipid levels in the highest quintile are at markedly increased risk, but even among those with average or low lipid levels, CRP testing can identify individuals with high relative risks of future cardiovascular events. For instance, among postmenopausal women with LDL concentrations below 130 mg/dL (the current National Cholesterol Education Program target for lipid reduction in primary prevention *[33]*), women with high CRP concentrations were at markedly increased risk of future MI, coronary revascularization, and stroke, even after adjustment for other traditional cardiovascular risk factors *(8)*. Recent data also suggest that CRP may be a strong predictor of prognosis at 30 d among patients undergoing percutaneous coronary intervention, and that the risk associated with increased CRP concentrations is independent of, but additive to, the American College of Cardiology/American Heart Association (ACC/AHA) lesion score (Fig. 5) *(34)*.

CLINICAL ROLE OF CRP TESTING

The finding that combining CRP testing with routine lipid assessment may significantly improve risk prediction has important clinical implications. More than half of all MIs occur in individuals without increased lipid levels, and these individuals are at

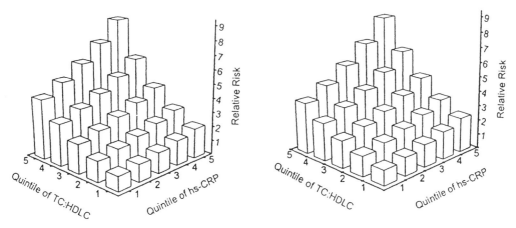

Fig. 4. Interactive effects of CRP and lipid tests in men (**left**) and women (**right**). (Adapted from Ridker PM. Circulation 2001;103:1814–1815.)

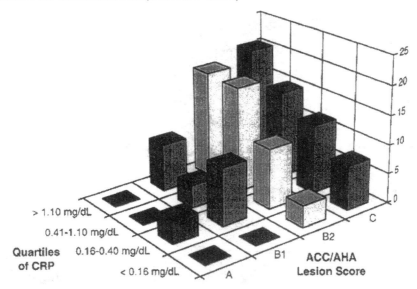

Fig. 5. Progressive increase in risk of death or MI stratified by increasing ACC/AHA lesion complexity score and CRP concentrations. Numeric values indicate number of patients. (Adapted from Chew DP, et al. Circulation 2001:104;995.)

higher risk if CRP concentrations are increased. Thus, CRP testing might indicate a group to whom aggressive risk factor modification should be targeted, including weight loss, exercise, smoking cessation, and diet. This concept also has pathophysiological appeal, given that CRP concentrations are higher in diabetics and individuals with obesity *(35, 36)*. Indeed, adipose tissue is a potent source of IL-6, which is the main stimulus for CRP production in the liver. Interestingly, recent data show that baseline concentrations of CRP and IL-6 are also strong independent predictors of the risk of incident type II diabetes among apparently healthy women *(37)*.

Although no studies have directly assessed the impact of CRP reduction on cardio-vascular risk, intriguing data suggest that antiplatelet and statin therapy may be most effective among individuals with chronic low-grade vascular inflammation, as evidenced by increased CRP concentrations. For example, in the Physicians' Health Study, randomization to aspirin was associated with a 56% risk reduction among those with baseline CRP concentrations in the highest quartile (9). The risk reduction declined with decreasing quartile concentrations of CRP. Moreover, recent data suggest that the benefits of clopidogrel pretreatment in addition to aspirin for patients undergoing percutaneous coronary intervention may be greatest among those patients with increased CRP concentrations (38).

Accumulating evidence suggests that statins may have powerful antiinflammatory effects (39,40). Indeed the risk reduction observed with these agents in large-scale clinical trials have been greater than that explained on the basis of changes in lipid parameters alone. In this regard, several studies have recently demonstrated that statins reduce CRP concentrations, and that this effect is independent of lipid lowering (41–44).

Data from the Cholesterol and Recurrent Events (CARE) trial, a secondary prevention study, indicates that statins may be most effective among patients with evidence of persistent inflammation (45). The CARE trial randomized patients with a prior history of MI to receive either pravastatin or placebo (46). Patients with evidence of persistent inflammation (as evidenced by an increase of both CRP and serum amyloid A) were at increased risk of recurrent cardiovascular events (45). The study group with the highest risk of recurrent events was that of patients with persistent evidence of inflammation who were assigned to placebo (relative risk 2.81; $p = 0.007$). The proportion of recurrent cardiovascular events prevented by pravastatin was 54% among those patients with high CRP and serum amyloid protein A (SAA) concentrations compared to 25% among those without persistent inflammation. This difference was observed despite identical baseline LDL levels in these two groups.

A recent analysis from the Air Force/Texas Atherosclerosis Prevention Study (AFCAPS/TexCAPS) population provides new data regarding the interaction between CRP concentrations and the benefits of statin therapy for primary prevention (31). In this analysis, individuals were divided into four groups according to median LDL (149 mg/dL) and CRP (0.16 mg/dL) concentrations. The group with LDL < 149 mg/dL and low CRP concentrations were at low risk and showed no benefit from therapy with lovastatin compared to placebo. Individuals with LDL >149 mg/dL were at more than twofold increased risk, regardless of CRP concentrations, and randomization to lovastatin for these individuals resulted in a large reduction in cardiovascular events compared to placebo. However, the most intriguing results pertained to the group with low LDL (<149 mg/dL) but with high CRP concentrations. This group had a high risk of future cardiovascular events, similar to those with high LDL values. Moreover, the benefit of lovastatin therapy for prevention of future cardiovascular events among these individuals with low LDL but high CRP was similar to that seen among those with overt hyperlipidemia (Fig. 6).

These findings, although hypothesis generating, have potentially important implications for clinical practice. The recently presented results of the Heart Protection Study suggest that the risk reduction with statin therapy may be similar for those with low LDL concentrations (<100 mg/dL) as for those with increased LDL concentrations (47). Thus the benefits of statin therapy may extend to many millions of individuals currently outside of National Cholesterol Education Program guidelines. If supported by randomized trials designed to test this hypothesis directly, CRP testing may identify a group of patients with LDL levels below current treatment guidelines who may derive the greatest bene-

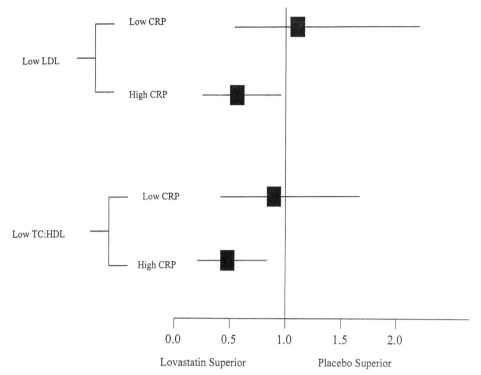

Fig. 6. Relative risks associated with lovastatin therapy, according to baseline of lipid and CRP concentrations. LDL indicates low-density lipoprotein, TC:HDL indicates total cholesterol to high-density cholesterol ratio. (Adapted from Blake GJ, Ridker PM. Circ Res 2001;89:763–771. Data derived from Ridker PM, et al. N Eng J Med 2001:344:1964.)

fit from statin therapy *(48)*. Furthermore, preliminary data suggest that a strategy of CRP screening to target statin therapy among those without overt hyperlipidemia may prove rela-tively cost-effective among selected middle-aged men and women *(49)*.

ALGORITHM FOR CARDIOVASCULAR RISK ASSESSMENT COMBINING CRP AND LIPID SCREENING

Because the population distribution of CRP is right-skewed, for practical application it may be convenient to divide CRP concentrations into an ordinal system such as quintiles. In such analyses *(8,9)*, for each quintile increase in CRP, the adjusted relative risk of a future cardiovascular event increased by 26% for healthy American men and 33% for healthy American women. These data were adjusted for traditional cardiovas-cular risk factors such as age, smoking, body mass index, diabetes, hypertension, hyper-lipidemia, family history of premature MI, and exercise. Given that risk estimates appear to be linear across CRP quintiles, these quintiles can be considered to represent individ-uals with low, mild, moderate, high, and highest relative risks of future cardiovascular events.

A proposed cardiovascular risk assessment tool is shown in Fig. 7 *(50)*. For practical purposes, risk assessment may be divided into three steps as shown in Fig. 7A. After determination of quintile of TC/HDL ratio and quintile of CRP a relative risk for future

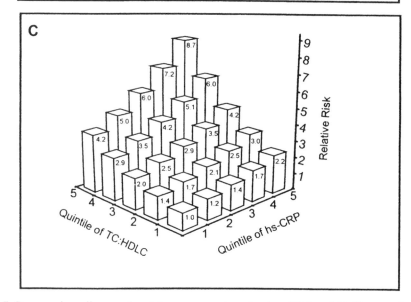

Fig. 7. Proposed cardiovascular risk assessment tool using CRP and lipid screening. (From Rifai N, Ridker PM. Clin Chem 2001:47:29.)

cardiovascular events may be estimated from Fig. 7C. The distribution of CRP shown in Fig. 7B was derived from population-based studies and the relative risks were derived from analyses from the Physicians' Health Study and the Women's Health Study. In is important to note that the clinical cut points in these algorithms may require revision as more data become available.

POTENTIAL LIMITATIONS TO CRP SCREENING

Use of hormone replacement therapy is associated with higher CRP concentrations *(51)*. Trauma or acute infection may cause a transient rise in CRP, and testing for CRP may be best deferred for 2–3 wk in these circumstances. Similarly, testing for CRP concentrations for cardiovascular risk prediction will be of limited value among patients with chronic inflammatory conditions such as rheumatoid arthritis. However, recent data suggest that fewer than 2% of all CRP assays are greater than 1.5 mg/dL, a concentration that may be associated with an alternative inflammatory condition. Moreover, data from the CARE trial suggest that the correlation coefficient for two samples of

CRP obtained 5 yr apart was 0.6, a figure similar or superior to that seen for lipid parameters *(42).* Furthermore, in contrast to other inflammatory cytokines such as IL-6, no circadian variation has been found to exist for CRP *(28).*

SUMMARY

Inflammation plays a key role in atherosclerosis, and CRP, a sensitive marker of chronic low-grade vascular inflammation, may provide a novel method for detecting individuals at high risk for plaque rupture. Data suggesting a direct role for CRP in cellular adhesion molecule expression *(6)* and describing CRP localized within atheromatous plaque *(52)* further raise the possibility that CRP may be directly involved in the atherosclerotic process.

Several large-scale prospective studies have consistently demonstrated that CRP is a strong independent predictor of cardiovascular risk. Inexpensive assays for CRP testing are now commercially available, and recent data suggest that CRP testing may add to the ability of lipid testing alone to identify individuals at high risk for plaque rupture. Moreover, preventive therapies such as aspirin and statins may be especially effective among patients with high CRP concentrations. Although further research is required, available data suggest that CRP testing may have an important role for global risk assessment for primary prevention of cardiovascular disease.

ABBREVIATION

ACC, American College of Cardiology; AFCAPS/TexCAPS, Air Force/Texas Atherosclerosis Prevention Study; AHA; American Heart Association; CARE, Cholesterol and Recurrent Events; CRP, C-reactive protein; HDL, high-density lipoprotein; ICAM, intercellular adhesion molecule; IL, interleukin; LDL, low-density lipoprotein; MCP, monocyte chemoattractment protein; MI, myocardial infarction; SAA, serum amyloid protein A; TC, total cholesterol; TNF, tumor necrosis factor; VCAM, vascular cell adhesion molecule.

REFERENCES

1. Ross R. Atherosclerosis—an inflammatory disease. N Engl J Med 1999;340:115–126.
2. Blake GJ, Ridker PM. Novel clinical markers of vascular wall inflammation. Circ Res 2001; 89:763–771.
3. Zwaka TP, Hombach V, Torzewski J. C-reactive protein-mediated low density lipoprotein uptake by macrophages: implications for atherosclerosis. Circulation 2001;103:1194–1197.
4. Ballou SP, Lozanski G. Induction of inflammatory cytokine release from cultured human monocytes by C-reactive protein. Cytokine 1992;4:361–368.
5. Pasceri V, Chang J, Willerson JT, Yeh ET. Modulation of c-reactive protein-mediated monocyte chemoattractant protein-1 induction in human endothelial cells by anti-atherosclerosis drugs. Circulation 2001;103:2531–2534.
6. Pasceri V, Willerson JT, Yeh ET. Direct proinflammatory effect of C-reactive protein on human endothelial cells. Circulation 2000;102:2165–2168.
7. Yasojima K, Schwab C, McGeer EG, McGeer PL. Generation of C-reactive protein and complement components in atherosclerotic plaques. Am J Pathol 2001;158:1039–1051.
8. Ridker PM, Hennekens CH, Buring JE, Rifai N. C-reactive protein and other markers of inflammation in the prediction of cardiovascular disease in women. N Engl J Med 2000; 342:836–843.

9. Ridker PM, Cushman M, Stampfer MJ, Tracy RP, Hennekens CH. Inflammation, aspirin, and the risk of cardiovascular disease in apparently healthy men. N Engl J Med 1997;336: 973–979.

10. Ridker PM, Buring JE, Shih J, Matias M, Hennekens CH. Prospective study of C-reactive protein and the risk of future cardiovascular events among apparently healthy women. Circulation 1998;98:731–733.

11. Danesh J, Whincup P, Walker M, et al. Low grade inflammation and coronary heart disease: prospective study and updated meta-analyses. Br Med J 2000;321:199–204.

12. Harris TB, Ferrucci L, Tracy RP, et al. Associations of elevated interleukin-6 and C-reactive protein concentrations with mortality in the elderly. Am J Med 1999;106:506–512.

13. Mendall MA, Strachan DP, Butland BK, et al. C-reactive protein: relation to total mortality, cardiovascular mortality and cardiovascular risk factors in men. Eur Heart J 2000;21: 1584–1590.

14. Koenig W, Sund M, Frohlich M, et al. C-Reactive protein, a sensitive marker of inflammation, predicts future risk of coronary heart disease in initially healthy middle-aged men: results from the MONICA (Monitoring Trends and Determinants in Cardiovascular Disease) Augsburg Cohort Study, 1984 to 1992. Circulation 1999;99:237–242.

15. Kuller LH, Tracy RP, Shaten J, Meilahn EN. Relation of C-reactive protein and coronary heart disease in the MRFIT nested case-control study. Multiple Risk Factor Intervention Trial. Am J Epidemiol 1996;144:537–547.

16. Tracy RP, Lemaitre RN, Psaty BM, et al. Relationship of C-reactive protein to risk of cardiovascular disease in the elderly. Results from the Cardiovascular Health Study and the Rural Health Promotion Project. Arterioscler Thromb Vasc Biol 1997;17:1121–1127.

17. Roivainen M, Viik-Kajander M, Palosuo T, et al. Infections, inflammation, and the risk of coronary heart disease. Circulation 2000;101:252–257.

18. Hwang SJ, Ballantyne CM, Sharrett AR, et al. Circulating adhesion molecules VCAM-1, ICAM-1, and E-selectin in carotid atherosclerosis and incident coronary heart disease cases: the Atherosclerosis Risk In Communities (ARIC) study. Circulation 1997;96:4219–4225.

19. Ridker PM, Hennekens CH, Roitman-Johnson B, Stampfer MJ, Allen J. Plasma concentration of soluble intercellular adhesion molecule 1 and risks of future myocardial infarction in apparently healthy men. Lancet 1998;351:88–92.

20. Ridker PM, Buring JE, Rifai N. Soluble P-selectin and the risk of future cardiovascular events. Circulation 2001;103:491–495.

21. Malik I, Danesh J, Whincup P, et al. Soluble adhesion molecules and prediction of coronary heart disease: a prospective study and meta-analysis. Lancet 2001;358:971–976.

22. Packard CJ, O'Reilly DS, Caslake MJ, et al. Lipoprotein-associated phospholipase A2 as an independent predictor of coronary heart disease. West of Scotland Coronary Prevention Study Group. N Engl J Med 2000;343:1148–1155.

23. Blake GJ, Dada N, Fox JC, Manson JE, Ridker PM. A prospective evaluation of lipoprotein-associated phospholipase A(2) concentrations and the risk of future cardiovascular events in women. J Am Coll Cardiol 2001;38:1302–1306.

24. Mach F, Schonbeck U, Sukhova GK, et al. Functional CD40 ligand is expressed on human vascular endothelial cells, smooth muscle cells, and macrophages: implications for CD40-CD40 ligand signaling in atherosclerosis. Proc Natl Acad Sci USA 1997;94:1931–1936.

25. Schonbeck U, Varo N, Libby P, Buring J, Ridker PM. Soluble CD40L and Cardiovascular Risk in Women. Circulation 2001;104:2266–2268.

26. Aukrust P, Muller F, Ueland T, et al. Enhanced concentrations of soluble and membrane-bound CD40 ligand in patients with unstable angina. Possible reflection of T lymphocyte and platelet involvement in the pathogenesis of acute coronary syndromes. Circulation 1999;100:614–620.

27. Mach F, Schonbeck U, Sukhova GK, Atkinson E, Libby P. Reduction of atherosclerosis in mice by inhibition of CD40 signalling. Nature 1998;394:200–203.

28. Meier-Ewert HK, Ridker PM, Rifai N, Price N, Dinges DF, Mullington JM. Absence of diurnal variation of C-reactive protein concentrations in healthy human subjects. Clin Chem 2001;47:426–430.
29. Ockene IS, Matthews CE, Rifai N, Ridker PM, Reed G, Stanek E. Variability and classification accuracy of serial high-sensitivity C-reactive protein measurements in healthy adults. Clin Chem 2001;47:444–450.
30. Ridker PM, Glynn RJ, Hennekens CH. C-reactive protein adds to the predictive value of total and HDL cholesterol in determining risk of first myocardial infarction. Circulation 1998;97:2007–2011.
31. Ridker PM, Rifai N, Clearfield M, et al. Measurement of C-reactive protein for the targeting of statin therapy in the primary prevention of acute coronary events. N Engl J Med 2001; 344:1959–1965.
32. Ridker PM. High-sensitivity C-reactive protein (hs-CRP): a potential adjunct for global risk assessment in the primary prevention of cardiovascular disease. Circulation 2001;103: 1813–1818.
33. Executive Summary of the Third Report of the National Cholesterol Education Program (NCEP) Expert Panel on Detection, Evaluation, and Treatment of High Blood Cholesterol in Adults (Adult Treatment Panel III). JAMA 2001;285:2486–2497.
34. Chew DP, Bhatt DL, Robbins MA, et al. Incremental prognostic value of elevated baseline C-reactive protein among established markers of risk in percutaneous coronary intervention. Circulation 2001;104:992–997.
35. Visser M, Bouter LM, McQuillan GM, Wener MH, Harris TB. Elevated C-reactive protein concentrations in overweight and obese adults. JAMA 1999;282:2131–2135.
36. Ford ES. Body mass index, diabetes, and C-reactive protein among U.S. adults. Diabetes Care 1999;22:1971–1977.
37. Pradhan AD, Manson JE, Rifai N, Buring JE, Ridker PM. C-reactive protein, interleukin 6, and risk of developing type 2 diabetes mellitus. JAMA 2001;286:327–334.
38. Chew DP, Bhatt DL, Robbins MA, et al. Effect of clopidogrel added to aspirin before percutaneous coronary intervention on the risk associated with C-reactive protein. Am J Cardiol 2001;88:672–674.
39. Frenette PS. Locking a leukocyte integrin with statins. N Engl J Med 2001;345:1419–1421.
40. Blake GJ, Ridker PM. Are statins anti-inflammatory? Curr Control Trials Cardiovasc Med 2000;1:161–165.
41. Ridker PM, Rifai N, Lowenthal SP. Rapid reduction in C-reactive protein with cerivastatin among 785 patients with primary hypercholesterolemia. Circulation 2001;103:1191–1193.
42. Ridker PM, Rifai N, Pfeffer MA, Sacks F, Braunwald E. Long-term effects of pravastatin on plasma concentration of C-reactive protein. The Cholesterol and Recurrent Events (CARE) Investigators. Circulation 1999;100:230–235.
43. Jialal I, Stein D, Balis D, Grundy SM, Adams-Huet B, Devaraj S. Effect of hydroxymethyl glutaryl coenzyme a reductase inhibitor therapy on high sensitive C-reactive protein concentrations. Circulation 2001;103:1933–1935.
44. Albert M, Danielson E, Rifai N, Ridker PM. Effect of statin therapy on C-reactive protein concentrations. The Pravastatin Inflammation/ CRP Evaluation (PRINCE): a Randomized Trial and Cohort Study. JAMA 2001;286:64–70.
45. Ridker PM, Rifai N, Pfeffer MA, et al. Inflammation, pravastatin, and the risk of coronary events after myocardial infarction in patients with average cholesterol concentrations. Cholesterol and Recurrent Events (CARE) Investigators. Circulation 1998;98:839–844.
46. Sacks FM, Pfeffer MA, Moye LA, et al. The effect of pravastatin on coronary events after myocardial infarction in patients with average cholesterol concentrations. Cholesterol and Recurrent Events Trial investigators. N Engl J Med 1996;335:1001–1009.
47. Collins R. Results of the Heart Protection Study. Presented at the American Heart Association meeting, Anaheim, November 2001.

48. Ridker PM. Should statin therapy be considered for patients with elevated C-reactive protein? The need for a definitive clinical trial. Eur Heart J 2001;22:2135–2137.
49. Blake GJ, Ridker PM, Kuntz KM. Cost-effectiveness of CRP screening to target statin therapy. Am J Med 2003;114 (in press).
50. Rifai N, Ridker PM. Proposed cardiovascular risk assessment algorithm using high-sensitivity C-reactive protein and lipid screening. Clin Chem 2001;47:28–30.
51. Ridker PM, Hennekens CH, Rifai N, Buring JE, Manson JE. Hormone replacement therapy and increased plasma concentration of C-reactive protein. Circulation 1999;100:713–716.
52. Torzewski M, Rist C, Mortensen RF, et al. C-reactive protein in the arterial intima: role of C-reactive protein receptor-dependent monocyte recruitment in atherogenesis. Arterioscler Thromb Vasc Biol 2000;20:2094–2099.

18

Prognostic Role of Plasma High-Sensitivity C-Reactive Protein Levels in Acute Coronary Syndromes

Luigi M. Biasucci, Antonio Abbate, and Giovanna Liuzzo

INTRODUCTION

Prediction of future adverse cardiac events in patients with known coronary artery disease (CAD) remains extremely challenging for the clinical cardiologist. Patients presenting with acute coronary syndromes (ACS) have a relatively high risk of recurrent angina, acute myocardial infarction (AMI), and death during hospitalization and follow-up. Data from multicenter trials show mortality rates >5% during the intermediate term *(1,2)*. Early assessment of left ventricular (LV) function at echocardiography and the extension of CAD (in terms of number of vessels affected at angiography) constitute the most important tools available to estimate cardiac risk. However, although age, depressed LV function, and multivessel CAD are considered high-risk features, prognosis in low-risk subjects remains difficult to establish and therefore optimal management remains an issue. Earlier in the 1970s and 1980s, experimental data were produced supporting an active role of inflammatory reaction in promoting atherosclerotic plaque formation and complications *(3,4),* but only in the past few years has evidence of a prognostic role of systemic inflammatory markers in terms of prediction of short- and long-term risk been presented. This is particularly true for C-reactive protein (CRP), a prototypic acute phase protein. Its levels rapidly rise after an inflammatory stimulus and, depending on the intensity of the stimulus, even a several-hundred-fold increase in plasma levels may occur *(5)*. CRP is not consumed to a significant extent in any process and its clearance is not influenced by any known condition; therefore, its concentration appears to be dependent only on the rates of production and excretion. The long half-life of CRP, approx 19 h, makes its detection in blood easy even several hours after the acute stimulus. Because of all these characteristics CRP can be considered an "ideal marker."

The major inducer of CRP synthesis by the liver is interleukin (IL)-6, which, in turn, is induced by tumor necrosis factor-α, IL-1, platelet-derived growth factor, antigens, and the endotoxins. Thus, CRP is the marker of a cascade of inflammatory mediators. Physiologically, CRP is a molecule involved in defense mechanism, being part of the "innate defense." It binds to monocytes, macrophages, and neutrophils and triggers the cascade that leads to complement activation favoring opsonization and phagocytosis of intruder molecules. CRP also modulates cell-mediated immune response, stimulating B- and

From: *Cardiac Markers, Second Edition*
Edited by: Alan H. B. Wu @ Humana Press Inc., Totowa, NJ

T-lymphocyte activation and enhancing tissue factor and oxygen-free species production by mononuclear cells. Accumulating data support an active role of CRP not only in lipoprotein–cell interaction and atherosclerosis promotion but also as a central mediator in tissue damage during ischemia–infarction *(6–10)*.

As a marker of inflammatory reaction, CRP is a well-established tool in acute and chronic illnesses, in which CRP levels are increased well beyond the reference range and thus use of high-sensitivity methods is not requested. Conversely, ischemic heart disease is not an overt inflammatory disease, and CRP levels within the reference range may contain important prognostic and pathophysiological information. Recent reinterpretation of this reactant, favored by the use of a high-sensitivity method, lead to extensive use in cardiovascular disease. Interestingly the large European Concerted Action on Thrombosis and Disabilities Angina Pectoris Study Group (ECAT) study including more than 2000 patients, published in 1995 *(11)*, showed, among patients with stable or unstable angina followed for 2 yr, a significant risk prediction by plasma fibrinogen levels and less important correlation with CRP levels. In 1997, however, the same group published new data showing that, when obtained by an ultrasensitive method, quintiles of CRP levels distribution were strong predictors of adverse events, with a twofold increase of coronary events for CRP levels >3.6 mg/L after adjustment for a number of confounders *(12)*. Easy-to-use, inexpensive, and precise kits allowing reproducible high-sensitivity CRP (hs-CRP) measurement are now commercially available; its stability in blood samples even after prolonged storage at room temperature and delayed analysis allows accurate determinations. Reliability and reproducibility are further guaranteed by the World Health Organization (WHO) standardization for CRP levels.

Since publication in 1994 by Liuzzo et al. *(13)* of the different risk profile in patients with unstable angina according to the inflammatory status, as shown by hs-CRP plasma levels, the number of reports on this issue has been steadily increasing, cumulating data on thousands of patients. Details of the different studies are presented and discussed.

RISK PREDICTION IN ACS

CRP as a Marker of In-Hospital Events

Several prospective studies are present in the literature in which the utility of a specific cutoff level for plasma CRP in predicting adverse events among medically treated patients with non-ST-segment elevation ACS was analyzed *(13–17)* (Fig. 1). The original osservation by Liuzzo et al. *(13)* showed that patients with Braunwald's class IIIb unstable angina (UA) with hs-CRP levels above 3 mg/L (90th percentile of normal hs-CRP determination) had an approximately fivefold increased risk of recurrent angina, AMI, or death. All patients had normal troponin T concentrations. Eighteen of the 20 patients with UA and CRP >3 mg/L suffered adverse events compared to only 1 of the 11 patients in the low-CRP-level group. Similar results were observed in patients with AMI presenting with ST-segment elevation (STEAMI): 77% of the patients with increased CRP concentrations (vs 14% among the remaining) experienced one of the composite end points. In this study, hs-CRP levels above 3 mg/L had a predictive value for in-hospital events of 90% in UA and 77% in STEAMI. Interestingly all patients with CRP >10 mg/L (99th percentile of normal distribution) had either recurrent angina, AMI, or death. Secondary analysis on incidence of hard end point (AMI or death), however, did not

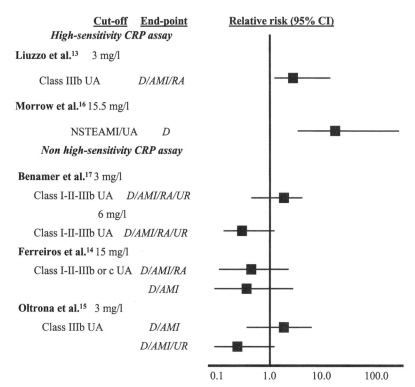

Fig. 1. Overview of the studies analyzing the in-hospital prognostic value of CRP levels. The figure reports relative risk and 95% confidence interval for the different studies in consideration of the population, end point analyzed, and cutoff used (not a meta-analysis). AMI, Acute myocardial infarction; CRP, C-reactive protein; D, death; NSTEAMI, non-ST elevation acute myocardial infarction; RA, refractory angina; UA, unstable angina; UR, urgent revascularization.

show significant predictivity, possibly due to the small number of cases. A larger series enrolling 251 patients (recently presented by the same authors at the 2000 American Heart Association annual meeting) showed independent predictive value of hs-CRP levels >19 mg/L for in-hospital death and AMI *(18)*.

Conversely, three studies *(14,15,17)* enrolling in total about 400 patients with UA failed to show a significantly increased risk of in-hospital events among patients with increased CRP. These studies have important differences compared to the original observation by Liuzzo et al. *(13)*, because in their case, non-hs-CRP assays were used. Moreover, the studies also differed substantially in the cutoff levels chosen to define the high levels of CRP and in the enrolling criteria. Notably, while Liuzzo et al. included only troponin-negative unstable patients in the original report, Ferreiros et al. *(14)* and Oltrona et al. *(15)* showed no data about troponin levels. Ferreiros et al. *(14)* considered the entire spectrum of UA, including post-infarction angina, a condition in which the prognosis is dependent mostly on the extent of myocardial necrosis. However, the largest study published to date on the short-term prognostic role of CRP (437 patients) supports the findings that increased hs-CRP concentrations are predictors for short-term mortality *(16)*. Morrow et al. *(16)* showed an 18-fold increased risk of death among patients with

UA and NSTEAMI using a hs-CRP determination and a cutoff value of 15.5 mg/L. Verheggen et al. *(19)* described a significantly higher occurrence rate of refractory angina among patients with UA with levels in the IVth quartile (>6 mg/L) (vs the lowest [<1.2 mg/L]); in this study also fibrinogen and white blood cell count were associated with the short-term prognosis. According to the data derived from the studies so far available, while 3 mg/L appears a good marker of an increased risk of the combined end point of death, AMI, and refractory angina in well-selected patients with negative troponin levels, a cutoff level of 10 mg/L appears to be more suitable for the prediction of hard events, such as death *(20)*. Interestingly, in the data presented by Oltrona et al. *(15)*, using a cutoff level of 10 mg/L, a trend toward increased risk was found for death and AMI and not for the composite end point of death, AMI, and urgent revascularization.

To date, definite conclusions on the role of hs-CRP in predicting in-hospital cardiac events cannot be drawn, as different studies had different enrolling criteria, end point definitions, CRP cutoff levels, and determination assays. When homogeneous groups of patients were selected, hs-CRP determination and different cutoff levels specific for the end point analysis were used, elevated CRP levels significantly predicted adverse events. Therefore, although use of hs-CRP determination appears advisable, confounding factors need to be cautiously avoided. Interestingly, low levels of hs-CRP in combination with low levels of troponins are associated with low risk of in-hospital events *(13,16)*, suggesting an important negative predictive value of CRP.

CRP as a Marker of Mid- to Long-Term Prognosis

All the studies *(14,21–27)* prospectively analyzing the recurrence of cardiac events in the intermediate term have shown a significant predictive value of high CRP levels in patients with ACS. In the different studies, with a follow-up ranging from 90 d to 4 yr, CRP levels predicted not only the composite end point of death, AMI, recurrent angina, and need for coronary revascularization procedures but also the incidence of the single end point of death during follow-up (Fig. 2).

Interestingly hs-CRP concentrations appeared to be persistently increased for at least 12 mo in up to 39% of cases in a series of 53 patients with class IIIb unstable angina followed for 1 yr *(21)*, suggesting a persistent inflammatory activation in many unstable patients. In this report by Biasucci et al. *(21)*, in a multivariate analysis including fibrinogen levels, age, diabetes, and hypertension, hs-CRP levels >3 mg/L at discharge were an independent predictor of new unstable ischemic events including death, AMI, and new hospitalization for unstable angina. The persistence of increased concentrations during follow-up and the strong correlation with clinical recurrence suggested hs-CRP as a marker of persistent instability in the coronary tree. The difference in the 1-yr outcome between patients with CRP levels below and above 3 mg/L remained significant also when the outcome was analyzed according to medical or interventional treatment. A limitation of this study is the relatively small number of patients and the highly selected population (indeed all had negative troponin levels); however, other studies have looked at larger unselected cohorts.

In the large ECAT study *(12)* 2121 patients (>50% with unstable angina) were enrolled from 1984 to 1987 and followed for 2 yr. A twofold increase of coronary events was observed with hs-CRP >3.6 mg/L after adjustment for a number of confounders. More recently, more than 900 patients presenting with ACS from the Fragmin in Unstable

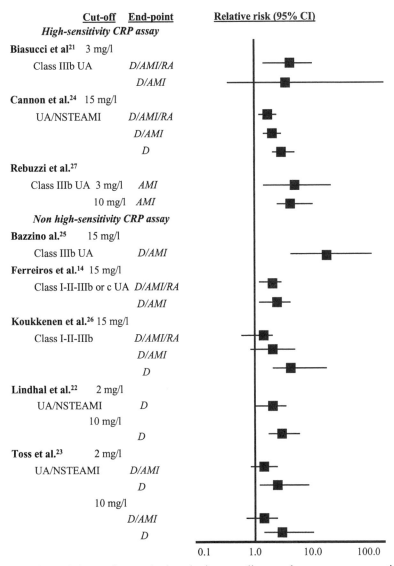

Fig. 2. Overview of the studies analyzing the intermediate- to long-term prognostic value of CRP levels. The figure reports relative risk and 95% confidence interval for the different studies in consideration of the population, end point analyzed, and cutoff used (not a meta-analysis). AMI, Acute myocardial infarction; CRP, C-reactive protein; D, death; NSTEAMI, non-ST elevation acute myocardial infarction; RA, refractory angina; UA, unstable angina; UR, urgent revascularization.

Coronary Artery Disease (FRISC) study population were followed up to 50 mo *(22)* (mean 37 mo) after the initial event for evaluation of the primary end point of cardiac death. The authors observed 70 deaths in the entire group (7.6%), 39 among the 309 patients (12.6%) with high CRP levels (above 10 mg/L) and 31 in the remaining (5.1%), with a relative risk (RR) of 2.48 (1.58–3.89). A significant difference was observed already after the first 5 mo of follow-up *(23)*. Recently, similar results have been presented by

Cannon et al. *(24)* at the 2001 American College of Cardiology annual meeting, an RR >3 for cardiac death at 6 mo follow-up among 1804 presenting with ACS in the Treat Angina with Aggrastat and Determine Cost of Therapy with an Invasive or Conservative Strategy (TACTICS)–Thrombolysis in Myocardial Infarction (TIMI) 18 Substudy was found in patients with hs-CRP >15 mg/L.

Ferreiros et al. *(14)* showed in 1999 a very strong correlation of CRP levels with 90-d mortality among unselected patients with unstable angina. Recently, Bazzino et al. *(25)* not only have shown the clinical usefulness of CRP levels at discharge in patients with UA but also have suggested superiority of CRP determination compared to a well-established noninvasive test for risk assessment as stress test in prediction of death and AMI at 90 d. CRP levels >15 mg/L compared to a positive result on cardiac stress test showed a higher sensitivity (88% vs 47%), specificity (81% vs 70%), positive predictive value (37.5% vs 18.2%), and negative predictive value (98% vs 90%). The authors thereby speculate that the two different evaluations looked at different mechanisms: plaque instability for the inflammatory marker and reduced coronary flow reserve for the positive stress test.

CRP and STEAMI

Although no large studies have prospectively assessed the value of CRP for the prognostic short- and long-term stratification of patients with STEAMI, many data suggest that CRP might be of value even in this group of patients *(13,28–31)*. As previously described, the report by Liuzzo et al. *(13)* has shown a prognostic role of hs-CRP levels not only in patients with UA but also in patients with STEAMI. Other studies have looked at this issue. CRP levels in the IVth quartile was an independent predictive factor for composite end point in the series of 64 patients presented by Tommasi et al. *(28)*. Nikfardjam et al. *(29)* have presented prospective data on 729 patients presenting with STEAMI and followed for 3 yr. Although a twofold increase risk for mortality was apparent for patients with CRP levels in the upper quintile (vs the others), this association was less evident after correction for other parameters.

As for myocardial necrosis markers (i.e., creatine kinase [CK]), peak CRP levels during in-hospital course of AMI have clinical implications, predicting cardiac rupture *(30)* and mortality *(30,31)*, however, on a different pathophysiological basis. In fact, while CK and other markers reflect the amount of myocardial damage, CRP levels are only partially related to the amount of necrosis, being associated with clinical presentation and possibly with an individual response, as patients with preinfarction angina have higher CRP levels *(32)*. In experimental AMI models, human CRP binds to damaged cells, activates complement, and enhances infarct size, playing a central role in mediating cellular damage during prolonged ischemia *(8)*. This observation may help to explain the increased risk of death and cardiac rupture in patients with high CRP peak levels *(30,31)*.

When more than 700 patients with previous AMI (>2 mo) of the Cholesterol and Recurrent Events (CARE) study were followed in a long-term follow-up recurrence of cardiac events was greatest in the highest vs the lowest quintile *(33)*.

CRP and Coronary Revascularization Procedures

Recent data suggest that CRP may be a useful marker also in patients undergoing coronary revascularization procedures. Although the data published so far are convincingly strong on the the long-term prognosis, data on the short-term prognostic role of hs-CRP are less consistent.

In a series of patients with UA undergoing balloon angioplasty presented by Buffon et al. *(34),* high hs-CRP levels were associated with an increased risk of in-hospital death, AMI, and refractory angina. Similar results were found in patients undergoing primary percutaneous revascularization in STEAMI *(35).* However, a large study on contemporary percutaneous coronary intervention (with optimal medical therapy—including glycoprotein IIb/IIIa inhibitors—and routine stent implantation) failed to show any significant influence of hs-CRP levels on in-hospital events *(36).* It is possible that the state of the art therapy in the latter study might have largely modified the clinical course and reduced the number of early events by such a large amount that the prognostic role of CRP is no longer evident.

Conversely, all studies analyzing predictive value of CRP levels for recurrence of events after coronary revascularization procedures *(36–39)* have confirmed the original observation by Buffon et al. *(34)* of a strong correlation between preprocedural levels and recurrence rate (Fig. 3). Data from the Chimeric c7E3 AntiPlatelet Therapy in Unstable Angina Refractory to Standard Treatment Trial (CAPTURE) trial are particularly useful to analyze this issue *(36).* Baseline hs-CRP values were determined in 447 patients with UA enrolled in the placebo arm of the trial. All underwent percutaneous early coronary intervention and were followed for a 6-mo period. Using a multivariate analysis (including troponin T levels) hs-CRP emerged as an independent predictor of mortality at 6 mo. Moreover, those patients with elevated levels (>10 mg/L) had an RR >2 for urgent 30-d revascularization procedures, non-urgent procedures, and incidence of AMI. Similar results were evident in data presented by Chew et al. *(37)* from a series of more than 700 patients (56% of whom had UA) with a RR of 30-d mortality of 23.11 (95% CI: 2.86–186.54; $p < 0.001$). Versaci et al. *(38)* have demonstrated a 60% recurrence of events in patients with UA and preprocedural CRP levels >5 mg/L treated by coronary stenting (vs 3% among patients with CRP levels <5 mg/L, $p < 0.001$); no AMI or death occurred among patients with low CRP levels.

Interestingly, in the different studies, the rate of major complications (death and AMI) in the low CRP levels group was very low and ranged from 0 to 1%. A higher recurrence rate were reported also for patients with high CRP levels undergoing coronary artery bypass surgery *(40).* On the other hand, in consideration of the wide use of atheroablative percutaneous coronary interventions, Zhou et al. have looked at the eventual prognostic use of CRP levels in patients undergoing directional atherectomy *(41).* No significant difference was found in this study among patients with high vs low CRP levels.

Additional Value of CRP in Combination with Troponin Levels

A major issue is the role of hs-CRP compared to troponins in the prognostic stratification of the patients. Cardiac troponins T and I (cTnT and cTnI) are excellent markers of myocardial necrosis and cardiac risk in ACS. Elevation of CRP after necrosis is expected, however, CRP levels appear not to be correlated with troponin levels, but to rise and fall in the acute-phase response in an amount that varies widely among individuals *(32).* Thus it is not surprising that growing evidence suggests an incremental value of CRP on top of the myocardial necrosis markers.

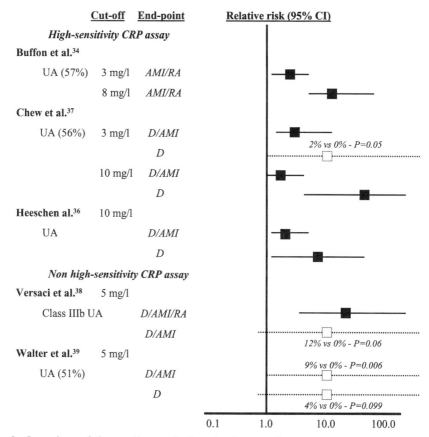

Fig. 3. Overview of the studies analyzing the intermediate-term prognostic value of CRP levels in patients undergoing percutaneous coronary interventions. The figure reports relative risk and 95% confidence interval for the different studies in consideration of the population, end point analyzed, and cutoff used (not a meta-analysis). When relative risk could not be calculated, because of 0% of event rate in the low CRP levels group, recurrence rate (in terms of percentage) and *p* values were shown for each group of patients. AMI, Acute myocardial infarction; CRP, C-reactive protein; D, death; NSTEAMI, non-ST elevation acute myocardial infarction; RA, refractory angina; UA, unstable angina; UR, urgent revascularization.

While the reports by Liuzzo et al. *(13)* and by Biasucci et al. *(21)* considered only unstable patients without elevation of cTnT levels, to obviate the confounding factor of myocardial necrosis, other authors evaluated CRP predictive value independently and in combination with cTnT *(16,17,23,26,27,36)*. The first studies to address this issue were published in 1998. In a substudy of the TIMI 11A, Morrow et al. *(16)* showed that hs-CRP and cTnT levels were additive in the prediction of death in patients with UA and NSTEAMI. Rebuzzi et al. *(27)* showed similar results on 102 patients with UA. These results were further confirmed in the FRISC trial *(23)* (on more than 900 patients) and in the interventional CAPTURE trial *(36)* (447 patients). All these studies have shown how the worse prognosis was for those patients with elevation of both troponin and CRP levels and, interestingly, the best prognosis in terms of adverse events is expected in patients with normal CRP and troponin levels. While aggressive therapy is indicated for high-risk patients, early discharge of double-negative patients appears to be a safe strategy.

In consideration of the different pathophysiologic significance that may be associated with troponin and CRP increase, attention should be paid to the results of these studies. In the CAPTURE trial, Heeschen et al. *(36)* have shown how elevated cTnT levels were the strongest predictors for in-hospital events and hs-CRP was an independent predictor at 6 mo follow-up. Indeed the elevation of the two markers reflects two different mechanisms: whereas the former reflects myocardial necrosis (and possibly the presence of complex coronary plaques) and predicts immediate complication, the latter is associated with coronary tree instability and recurrence of adverse events.

Thereby, the two markers should not be considered alternatives for each other. Troponin is the marker of choice to define AMI in the setting of the ACS and has a definite short-term prognostic role in these syndromes *(42–44)*. CRP should be considered a useful tool to define the risk in the short- and long-term follow-up, being in the combination of the two markers the stronger prognostic factor. Although measurement of CRP is classified "of not proven usefulness (Class IIb, level of evidence B)" in the American College of Cardiology/American Heart Association Guidelines *(43)*, the continuously growing body of evidence that CRP is associated with prognosis in ACS suggests that its use should be encouraged. In fact, a Task Force of the European Society of Cardiology has evaluated the usefulness of CRP levels in ACS. As indicated in the recommendations recently published *(44)*, CRP is considered a reliable marker of long-term risk.

CONCLUSIONS AND PRACTICAL CONSIDERATIONS

In conclusion, available data strongly recommend the use of hs-CRP as a prognostic marker in patients with ACS, on top of other prognostic factors including troponin levels. The data are very consistent for intermediate- to long-term follow-up and less consistent for in-hospital outcome. Evaluation of hs-CRP levels at the time of admission should be included in the assessment of the patient including clinical setting, associated diseases, markers of myocardial necrosis (especially troponin levels), LV function, and age. Cutoff levels for CRP should be judged on the basis of the clinical scenario (in particular if myocardial necrosis is present) and in consideration of the end point of interest. Patients with elevated hs-CRP levels do worse at the short- and long-term follow-up, independently of the cutoff value used. However, if is true that patients with hs-CRP levels >3 mg/L but <10 mg/L may not have an increased risk of death in the in-hospital and out-of-hospital follow-up, they experience a worse in-hospital course, in terms of refractory angina, AMI, and urgent revascularization. On the other hand, the use of a cutoff point of 10 mg/L definitively identifies patients at higher risk of death but may not distinguish, among the survivors, those who may suffer from recurrent myocardial ischemia. Moreover, a stronger association of CRP with fatal AMI than with nonfatal AMI has been suggested *(18,22,24,26,36,37)*. Colocalization in the necrotic myocardium during AMI of CRP and complement has been described leading to a greater extent of necrosis *(8,10)*. Therefore, a worse prognosis in patients with high plasma CRP levels experiencing an AMI may be partially correlated to this pathophysiological mechanism.

Most of the studies analyzed used determination of CRP levels at the time of hospital admission and thereby these values should be the reference value to estimate prognosis.

However, on the basis of the observation that some patients have persistently increased CRP concentrations beyond the acute phase reaction (48–72 h) and up to 12 mo after the acute event, some authors *(14,21)* suggested that CRP levels 7-10 d after admission may be a better predictor of the long-term prognosis. From our point of view, the two determinations probably have additive value. The first is especially useful for the in-hospital course; the other may offer additional information for the out-of-hospital events. Moreover, when possible, blood sampling 1–3 mo later may be useful because it is likely that the highest risk of future events is confined to patients with persistently elevated levels of CRP.

CRP levels should be determined by high-sensitivity methods (as very low levels may be markers of very low risk) according to WHO standards. Data should be cautiously interpreted in the presence of overt inflammatory and infectious disease.

CRP DETERMINATION BEYOND RISK PREDICTION

CRP levels predict the risk of adverse cardiac events, but it is unclear whether they can guide the management of patients in ACS. This issue has not been explored by any controlled randomized trials, but some suggestions come from retrospective analysis. As described, patients with low hs-CRP and troponin levels have a very favorable prognosis. Mortality among these patients is extremely low and therefore the assumption of a lesser need for aggressive therapy in this group appears reasonable. Targeting of drug therapy on the basis of CRP levels was shown to be effective in a primary prevention trial *(45)*. Interestingly, medical therapy known to be effective in the treatment of ACS (i.e., aspirin *[46]*, clopidogrel *[47]*, abciximab *[48,49]*, and statins *[50]*) appears to lower cardiac risk together with CRP levels. Controlled, prospective studies are needed to define better the role of hs-CRP as a guide to therapy.

ABBREVIATIONS

ACS, Acute coronary syndrome(s); AMI, acute myocardial infarction; CAD, coronary artery disease; CAPTURE, Chimeric c7E3 AntiPlatelet Therapy in Unstable Angina Refractory to Standard Treatment Trial; CARE, Cholesterol and Recurrent Events; CK, creatine kinase; CRP, C-reactive protein; cTnI and cTnT, cardiac troponins I and T; ECAT, European Concerted Action on Thrombosis and Disabilities Angina Pectoris Study Group; FRAXIS Fraxiparine in Ischemic Syndrome; FRISC, Fragmin in Unstable Coronary Artery Disease; hs-CRP, high-sensitivity C-reactive protein; IL, interleukin; LV, left ventricle; RR, relative risk; STEAMI, ST elevation acute myocardial infarction; TACTICS, Treat Angina with Aggrastat and Determine Cost of Therapy with an Invasive or Conservative Strategy; TIMI, Thrombolysis in Myocardial Infarction; UA, unstable angina; WHO, World Health Organization.

REFERENCES

1. Wallentin L, Lagerqvist B, Husted S, et al. for the FRISC II investigators. Outcome at 1 year after an invasive compared with a non-invasive strategy in unstable coronary-artery disease: the FRISC II invasive randomised trial. Lancet 2000;356:9–16.
2. Platelet Receptor Inhibition in Ischemic Syndrome Management in Patients Limited by Unstable Signs and Symptoms (PRISM- PLUS) Study Investigators. Inhibition of the plate-

let IIb/IIIa receptor with tirofiban in unstable angina and non-Q-wave myocardial infarction. N Engl J Med 1998;338:1488–1497.

3. Ross R. Atherosclerosis—an inflammatory disease. N Engl J Med 1999;340:115–126.

4. Alexander WR, Dzau VJ. Vascular biology—the past 50 years. Circulation 2000;102:112–116.

5. Pepys MB, Baltz ML. Acute phase proteins with special reference to C-reactive protein and related proteins (pentaxins) and serum amyloid A protein. Adv Immunol 1983;34:141–212.

6. Lagrand WK, Visser CA, Hermens WT, et al. C-reactive protein as a cardiovascular risk factor—more than an epiphenomenon. Circulation 1999;100:96–102.

7. Zwaka TP, Hombach V, Torzewski J. C-reactive protein-mediated low density lipoprotein uptake by macrophages—implications for atherosclerosis. Circulation 2001;103:1194–1196.

8. Griselli M, Herbert J, Hutchinson WL, et al. C-reactive protein and complement are important mediators of tissue damage in acute myocardial infarction. J Exp Med 1999;190:1733–1740.

9. Torzewski J, Torzewski M, Bowyer DE, et al. C-reactive protein frequently colocalizes with the terminal complement complex in the intima of early atherosclerotic lesions of human coronary arteries. Arterioscler Thromb Vasc Biol 1998;18:1386–1392.

10. Lagrand WK, Niessen HWM, Wolbink GJ, et al. C-reactive protein colocalizes with complement in human hearts during acute myocardial infarction. Circulation 1997;95:97–103.

11. Thompson SG, Kienast J, Pyke SD, et al. for the European Concerted Action on Thrombosis and Disabilities Angina Pectoris Study Group. Haemostatic factors and the risk of myocardial infarction or sudden death in patients with angina pectoris. N Engl J Med 1995;332:635–641.

12. Haverkate F, Thompson SG, Pyke SD, Gallimore RJ, Pepys MB for the European Concerted Action on Thrombosis and Disabilities Angina Pectoris Study Group. Production of C-reactive protein and the risk of coronary events in stable and unstable angina. Lancet 1997;3349:462–466.

13. Liuzzo G, Biasucci LM, Gallimore JR, et al. The prognostic value of C-reactive protein and serum amyloid A protein in severe unstable angina. N Engl J Med 1994;331:417–424.

14. Ferreiros ER, Boissonnet CP, Pizarro R, et al. Independent prognostic value of C-reactive protein in unstable angina. Circulation 1999;100:1958–1963.

15. Oltrona L, Ardissino D, Merlini PA, et al. C-reactive protein elevation and early outcome in patients with unstable angina pectoris. Am J Cardiol 1997;80:1002–1006.

16. Morrow DA, Rifai N, Altman EM, et al. C-reactive protein is a potent predictor of mortality independently of and in combination with troponin T in acute coronary syndromes: a TIMI 11A substudy. Thrombolysis in Myocardial Infarction 11A. J Am Coll Cardiol 1998;31:1460–1465.

17. Benamer H, Steg PG, Benessiano J, et al. Comparison of the prognostic value of C-reactive protein and troponin I in patients with unstable angina pectoris. Am J Cardiol 1998;82:845–850.

18. Biasucci LM, Meo A, Buffon A, et al. Independent prognostic value of C-reactive protein levels for in-hospital death and myocardial infarction in unstable angina. Circulation 2000;102(Suppl II):140.

19. Verheggen PWHM, de Maat MPM, Manger Cats V, et al. Inflammatory status as a main determinant of outcome in patients with unstable angina, independent of coagulation activation and endothelial cell function. Eur Heart J 1999;20:567–574.

20. Biasucci LM, Liuzzo G, Colizzi C, Rizzello V. Clinical use of C-reactive protein for the prognostic stratification of patients with ischemic heart disease. Ital Heart J 2001;2:164–171.

21. Biasucci LM, Liuzzo G, Grillo RL, et al. Elevated levels of C-reactive protein at discharge in patients with unstable angina predict recurrent instability. Circulation 1999;99:855–860.

22. Lindhal B, Toss H, Siegbahn A, et al. for the FRISC Study Group. Markers of myocardial damage and inflammation in relation to long-term mortality in unstable coronary artery disease. N Engl J Med 2000;343:1139–1147.

23. Toss H, Lindhal B, Siegbahn A, Wallentin L, for the FRISC Study Group. Prognostic influence of increased fibrinogen and C-reactive protein levels in unstable coronary artery disease. Circulation 1997;96:4204–4210.

24. Cannon CP, Weintraub WS, Demopoulos L, et al. High-sensitivity C-reactive protein (hs-CRP) to predict 6 month mortality and relative benefit of invasive vs. conservative strategy in patients with unstable angina: primary results of the TACTICS-TIMI 18 C-reactive protein substudy (abstract). J Am Coll Cardiol 2001;37(Suppl A):315A.

25. Bazzino O, Ferreiros ER, Pizarro R, Corrado G. C-reactive protein and the stress tests for risk stratification of patients recovering from unstable angina pectoris. Am J Cardiol 2001; 87:1235–1239.

26. Koukkenen H, Penttilä K, Kemppainen A, et al. C-reactive protein, fibrinogen, interleukin-6 and tumor necrosis factor-α in the prognostic classification of unstable angina pectoris. Ann Med 2001;33:37–47.

27. Rebuzzi A, Quaranta G, Liuzzo G, et al. Incremental prognostic value of serum levels of troponin T and C-reactive protein on admission in patients with unstable angina pectoris. Am J Cardiol 1998;82:715–719.

28. Tommasi S, Carluccio E, Bentivoglio M, et al. C-reactive protein as a marker for cardiac ischemic events in the year after a first uncomplicated myocardial infarction. Am J Cardiol 1999;83:1595–1599.

29. Nikfardjam M, Mullner M, Schreiber W, et al. The association between C-reactive protein on admission and mortality in patients with acute myocardial infarction. J Intern Med 2000; 247:341–345.

30. Anzai T, Yoshikawa T, Shiraki H, et al. C-reactive protein as a predictor of infarct expansion and cardiac rupture after a first Q-wave acute myocardial infarction. Circulation 1997; 96:778–784.

31. Pietila KO, Harmoinen AP, Jokiniitty J, Pasternak AI. Serum C-reactive protein concentration in acute myocardial infarction and its relationship to mortality during 24 months of follow-up in patients under thrombolytic treatment. Eur Heart J 1996;17:1345–1349.

32. Liuzzo G, Biasucci LM, Gallimore JR, et al. Enhanced inflammatory response in patients with preinfarction unstable angina. J Am Coll Cardiol 1999;34:1696–1703.

33. Ridker PM, Rifai N, Pfeffer MA, et al. Inflammation, pravastatin and the risk of coronary events after myocardial infarction in patients with average cholesterol levels. Cholesterol and Recurrent Events (CARE) Investigators. Circulation 1998;98:839–844.

34. Buffon A, Liuzzo G, Biasucci LM, et al. Preprocedural serum levels of C-reactive protein predict early complications and late restenosis after coronary angioplasty. J Am Coll Cardiol 1999;34:1512–1521.

35. Tomoda H, Aoki N. Prognostic value of C-reactive protein levels within six hours after the onset of acute myocardial infarction. Am Heart J 2000;140:324–328.

36. Heeschen C, Hamm CW, Bruemmer J, et al. for the CAPTURE Investigators. Predictive value of C-reactive protein and troponin T in patients with unstable angina: a comparative analysis. J Am Coll Cardiol 2000;35:1535–1542.

37. Chew DP, Bhatt DL, Robbins MA, et al. Incremental prognostic value of elevated baseline C-reactive protein among established markers of risk in percutaneous coronary intervention. Circulation 2001;104:992–997.

38. Versaci F, Gaspardone A, Tomai F, et al. Predictive value of C-reactive protein in patients with unstable angina pectoris undergoing coronary artery stent implantation. Am J Cardiol 2000;85:92–95.

39. Walter DH, Fichtlscherer S, Swelling M, et al. Preprocedural C-reactive protein levels and cardiovascular events after coronary stent implantation. J Am Coll Cardiol 2001;37:839–846.

40. Milazzo D, Biasucci LM, Luciani N, et al. Elevated levels of C-reactive protein before coronary artery bypass grafting predict recurrence of ischemic events. Am J Cardiol 1999; 84:459–461.

41. Zhou YF, Csako G, Grayston JT, et al. Lack of association of restenosis following coronary angioplasty with elevated C-reactive protein levels or seropositivity to *Chlamydia pneumoniae*. Am J Cardiol 1999;84:595–598.

42. Antman EM, Bassand JP, Klein W, et al. Myocardial infarction redefined—a consensus document of the Joint European Society of Cardiology/American College of Cardiology committee for the redefinition of myocardial infarction. J Am Coll Cardiol 2000;36:959–969.

43. Braunwald E, Antman EM, Beasley JW, et al. ACC/AHA Guidelines for the management of patients with unstable angina and non-ST-segment elevation myocardial infarction. A report of the American College of Cardiology/American Heart Association Task Force on practice guidelines (Committee on the management of patients with unstable angina). J Am Coll Cardiol 2000;36:970–1062.

44. Bertrand ME, Simoons ML, Fox KAA, et al. Management of acute coronary syndromes without persistent ST segment elevation. Recommendations of the Task Force of the European Society of Cardiology. Eur Heart J 2000;21:1406–1432.

45. Ridker PM, Rifai N, Clearfield M, et al. for the Air Force/Texas Coronary Atherosclerosis Prevention Study Investigators. Measurement of C-reactive protein for targeting of statin therapy in the primary prevention of acute coronary events. N Engl J Med 2001;344:1959–1965.

46. Kennon S, Price CP, Mills PG, et al. The effect of aspirin on C-reactive protein as a marker of risk in unstable angina. J Am Coll Cardiol 2001;37:1266–1270.

47. Robbins MA, Chew DP, Bhatt DL, et al. ADP-antagonist therapy added to aspirin prior to coronary intervention markedly attenuates the risk associated with baseline CRP status (abstract). J Am Coll Cardiol 2001;37(Suppl A):813A.

48. Buffon A, Liuzzo G, Angiolillo DJ, et al. Abciximab decreases cytokine production by circulating monocytes in patients with unstable angina and elevated inflammatory markers (abstract). J Am Coll Cardiol 2001;37(Suppl A):818A.

49. Lincoff AM, Kereiakes DJ, Mascelli MA, et al. Abciximab depresses the rise in levels of circulating inflammatory markers after percutaneous coronary revascularization. Circulation 2001;104:163–167.

50. Jialal I, Stein D, Balis D, et al. Effect of hydroxymethyl glutaryl coenzyme A reductase inhibitor therapy on high sensitive C-reactive protein levels. Circulation 2001;103:1933–1935.

19

Preanalytic and Analytic Sources of Variations in C-Reactive Protein Measurement

Thomas B. Ledue and Nader Rifai

INTRODUCTION

In 1930, Tillet and Francis observed a substance in the sera of individuals infected with pneumococcal pneumonia that formed a precipitate when mixed with the C-polysaccharide fraction of *Streptococcus pneumoniae (1)*. They noted that this "C-reactive" activity was absent from the sera of healthy individuals. MacLeod and Avery subsequently characterized this substance as a protein that required calcium ions for its reaction with C-polysaccharide and introduced the term "acute phase" to describe the sera of patients with various acute infections *(2)*. Despite its name, the acute phase response was subsequently identified by Lofstrom to be present in both acute and chronic inflammatory conditions; consequently, C-reactive protein (CRP) became recognized as a nonspecific acute phase protein *(3)*.

Structure

CRP is composed of five identical, noncovalently bonded subunits or "pentamers" with a total molecular mass of 118,000 daltons. This arrangement is similar to that of another acute phase protein known as serum amyloid P component. Moreover, the CRP gene has been located on the proximal long arm of chromosome 1, band q2.1, as are the inflammation-related genes for serum amyloid P component and Fc receptors. Synthesis of CRP occurs in hepatocytes whose activity is stimulated by cytokines, especially interleukin (IL)-6, IL-1β, and tumor necrosis factor *(4)*.

Function

In the presence of calcium ions, CRP can bind to polysaccharides of many bacteria, fungi, and certain parasites. In addition, CRP will also bind to phosphorylcholine, phosphatidylcholines such as lecithin, and nucleic acids, and demonstrates a non-calcium-dependent binding to cationic molecules such as protamine, heparin, and histones *(5)*. More recently, CRP has been shown to bind to various lipid structures such as liposomes and lipoproteins, which on aggregation are incorporated into low-density lipoprotein and very-low-density lipoprotein *(6)*. Once bound, CRP is a powerful activator of the classical complement system. In a fashion similar to antigen–antibody complexes, CRP promotes opsonization, phagocytosis, and lysis of foreign substances in response to the

From: *Cardiac Markers, Second Edition*
Edited by: Alan H. B. Wu @ Humana Press Inc., Totowa, NJ

inflammatory reaction. It is one of the most consistently elevated and fastest reacting acute phase proteins (biological half-life of 19 h). Levels may rise 1000-fold or more within 24–48 h of tissue injury.

Clinical Significance

Owing to the speed and magnitude of its response, CRP has been used to detect, predict outcome, and assess the efficacy of treatment for various infectious, inflammatory, and necrotic processes. As a nonspecific marker of inflammation, levels of CRP should always be interpreted in the context of the patient's clinical history, preferably with review of prior results. No known deficiency states for CRP have been described.

There is growing interest in the relationship between inflammation and the pathogenesis of atherosclerosis. Current research suggests that CRP is a good marker of plaque vulnerability. It has been shown to be present in atherosclerotic plaques, but absent from the normal vessel wall *(7,8)*. Elevated levels of CRP *(9–11)*, serum amyloid protein A (SAA) *(9,10)*, and IL-6 *(12)* appear to reflect the hyperresponsiveness of the inflammatory system to stimuli affecting the walls of the coronary artery. CRP is also predictive of poor outcome in acute coronary syndromes (ACS), for example, unstable angina and non-Q-wave myocardial infarction (MI) *(13)*. In patients undergoing coronary artery bypass grafting, increased preoperative CRP (≥ 3.0 mg/L) is a risk factor for recurring ischemic events as well as a predictor of adverse events following angioplasty *(14,15)*. For additional information, refer to Chapter 17.

In direct comparisons with traditional (total cholesterol [TC], low-density-lipoprotein cholesterol, high-density-lipoprotein cholesterol [HDL-C]) and "novel" risk factors (Lp[a], homocysteine, apolipoprotein B) of coronary heart disease, baseline levels of CRP within the normal reference range were the single strongest predictor of future coronary events in apparently healthy adult men and women *(16–20)*. In patients experiencing their first MI, the predictive value of CRP was found to be additive to that of the ratio of total cholesterol to HDL-C *(21)*.

Laboratory Methodology

Various commercial methods have been developed to measure CRP in serum and plasma. Historically, many laboratories have relied on the semiquantitative latex agglutination assay for visual end point estimation of the extent of inflammation. Unfortunately, the assay suffers from a lack of sensitivity and interpretation is subjective, making correlation with clinical disease activity difficult. Throughout the 1970s and 1980s, more reliable methods including nephelometry and turbidimetry began to appear *(22)*. The advantage of these assays is that they are automated, rapid, and accurate; however, most have a lower detection limit approx 10 mg/L, which precludes their use in risk assessment for coronary heart disease, where significant changes in the range of 0.5–3.5 mg/L have been reported *(16,17)*.

More recently, investigators have worked to improve assay performance by developing highly sensitive immunoassays for CRP (hs-CRP). Numerous approaches including the use of fluorescent, luminescent, or radioactive adducts to antibodies to enhance the immunoprecipitate have been developed with success. Although these assays have enabled measurement of CRP in apparently healthy individuals, they tend to be more laborious and expensive to perform. An alternative design has been to amplify the light-scattering

Table 1
Variables Known to Affect CRP Results

Preanalytic	Analytic
Physiologic	Sensitivity
Race	Precision
Age	Antigen excess
Sex	Calibration/curve-fitting
Season	Reference materials/standardization
Altitude	Quality assurance
Pregnancy	Matrix effects
Lifestyle (exercise, smoking, obesity, alcohol, hormone therapy)	
Specimen collection	
Fasting	
Time of collection	
Specimen type	
Time and temperature of storage	

properties of the antigen–antibody complex by covalently coupling latex particles to specific antibody. This approach has found a wide appeal among clinical laboratories owing to the flexibility of chemistry analyzers for turbidimetric applications.

With increased availability of hs-CRP immunoassays much discussion concerning their performance and clinical utility has arisen *(19,20,23)*. A recently proposed algorithm for assessment of future coronary risk employing CRP, TC, and HDL-C has spawned debate as to whether the assay should be used for routine screening *(24)*. Indeed, different studies using various assays have resulted in different cut points and emphasize the need for additional standardization. Variables associated with the preanalytic and analytic phase of CRP determination must also be factored before routine screening can be seriously considered (see Table 1).

The preanalytic phase can be divided into two categories, those that are non-modifiable or physiologic factors and those that are modifiable such as specimen collection.

PHYSIOLOGIC CONSIDERATIONS

Race

There is relatively scant information on the effects of race on CRP concentration. Chambers et al. *(25)* found the geometric mean for CRP to be 17% higher in Indian Asians compared with European whites; however, the difference dropped after adjustment for central obesity and insulin resistance. Data from the National Health and Nutrition Evaluation Survey (NHANES III) revealed higher CRP values for non-Hispanic blacks (particularly women) than for non-Hispanic whites or Mexican Americans *(26)*.

Age and Sex

As mentioned above, traditional CRP immunoassays are unable to measure CRP reliably below 10 mg/L. Historically, laboratories have reported these values as "less than"

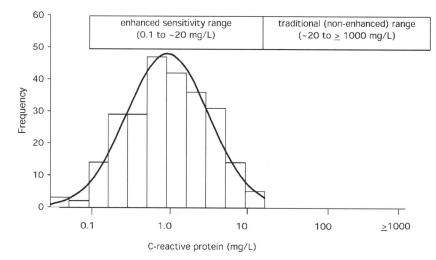

Fig. 1. Distribution of CRP results in 252 apparently healthy adults. The *horizontal bars* indicate approximate assay ranges for enhanced (hs-CRP) and traditional (nonenhanced) assay dynamic ranges.

the assays lower detection limit; however, with the introduction of hs-CRP immuno-assays there has been renewed interest in conducting reference range studies. Using a particle-enhanced nephelometric assay for hs-CRP, we have previously shown the distribution of CRP values in males, females, and both genders to be non-Gaussian when evaluated for skewness and kurtosis *(27)*. We observed no gender-related differences of serum CRP, and a common log-normal reference interval (2.5–97.5th percentile) was calculated to be <0.17–10.1 mg/L (Fig. 1). No relationship was found between age and serum CRP concentration (Fig. 2). These data are very consistent with those of Erlandsen et al. *(28)*. However, in a recent study by Hutchinson et al. that included more than 5000 subjects, CRP levels increased with age. The authors, however, could not exclude the possibility that such an increase may be attributed to the increased incidence of obesity that is associated with aging *(29)*.

Seasonal Variation

At present, there are limited data on CRP levels and seasonal cycles. In a group of 24 elderly subjects (age ≥75 yr) whose blood was collected monthly for 1 yr, Crawford and co-workers observed a winter/summer change of 3.7 mg/L, but found no evidence for infection to explain the differences *(30)*. In contrast, no consistent pattern of change in CRP values was reported from SEASON, a study specifically designed to examine seasonal changes in cardiovascular risk biomarkers *(31)*.

Within- and Between-Subject Variation

The within-subject CV for 19 healthy adults studied over 20 wk was 63% compared with 76% for between-subject CV *(32)*. In a separate study, Macy et al. reported within-subject CVs of 42% and between-subject CVs of 92% *(33)*. Such variation makes it difficult to reliably predict cardiovascular disease risk using smaller groups such as tertiles, quartiles, or quintiles. Data from Kluft and co-workers summarizing the bio-

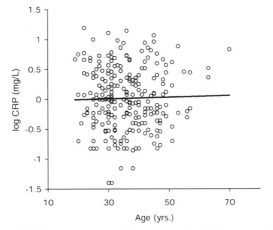

Fig. 2. Distribution of CRP results according to age in 252 apparently healthy adults. Log CRP = 0.0014*age + 0.0035, $r = 0.078$, $p = 0.71$.

logical variability for CRP indicate that although the intraindividual CV was rather large (averaging 30%), it was acceptable when the estimated composite CV for the group of individuals was 120% *(34)*. They suggested multiple blood sampling to establish an individual's baseline CRP. Macy et al. determined that three measurements at monthly intervals were sufficient to define an individual's normal range, provided there is no intercurrent infection *(33)*. In an effort to refine sampling techniques and decision limits for CRP, deMaat et al. proposed a practical working scheme for determining low levels of CRP *(35)*. Recently Ockene et al. demonstrated that two independent measurements of CRP can classify up to 90% of subjects into the exact or immediately adjacent quartile *(31)*.

Altitude

CRP levels in 15 adult males increased from 3.4 ± 0.15 mg/L to 5.6 ± 0.35 mg/L after changing from sea level to >3600 m *(36)*. In evaluating the effect of high altitude on blood chemistries, it is important to adjust for the significant increase in hemoglobin concentration as a result of height.

Pregnancy

CRP levels were slightly higher in pregnant than in nonpregnant women; however, there was no reported change associated with gestational age *(37)*.

Lifestyle (Exercise, Smoking, Obesity, Alcohol, Hormone Therapy)

Strenuous exercise has been shown to increase CRP levels. In 30 male marathon runners, median CRP concentrations rose from a prerace level of 1.1 mg/L to a postrace level of 4 mg/L, and further increased to 22.7 mg/L 24 h after the race ended *(38)*.

Numerous studies have documented a significant correlation between CRP and smoking *(39–41)*. In general, CRP concentrations increase among smokers with increased cigarette consumption *(39)*. In the elderly, CRP levels are associated with lifetime exposure to cigarette smoke. This association was independent of cessation, suggesting that some of the smoking-related damage may be irreversible *(42)*. These data support the hypothesis that CRP is primarily related to lifetime exposure (pack-years) and not to years since cessation of smoking. Lowe et al. found CRP levels doubled in current smokers compared with never-smokers, and although CRP levels decreased with time since quitting, they remained elevated more than 10 yr after quitting when compared with never-smokers *(40)*.

Visser et al. found higher CRP concentrations among individuals with increased body mass index and concluded that a state of low-grade systemic inflammation and obese persons existed *(43)*. Yudkin et al. demonstrated relationships between CRP levels and measures of obesity to be consistent with in vivo release of IL-6 from adipose tissue *(44)*. In fact, nearly one fourth of IL-6 produced in vivo originates from adipose tissue *(45),* and is thought to modify adipocyte glucose, lipid metabolism, and body weight (46,47). Among children aged 10–11 yr, adiposity was the major determinant of CRP levels with levels nearly threefold higher in the top fifth of the Ponderal index than in the bottom fifth *(48)*.

Among patients with a first MI, alcohol use was associated with CRP levels, with never-users having higher levels compared with regular users. However, no difference in levels was found among control subjects *(49)*. In 17 patients who drank for more than 3 wk, the median CRP levels decreased from 6 to 4 mg/L 1 wk after alcohol withdrawal *(50)*.

Estrogen replacement therapy has been shown to increase serum CRP concentrations, suggesting a proinflammatory effect. After 1 yr of treatment, CRP concentrations were 85% higher than at baseline (51). In the Women's Health Study, those who received hormone replacement therapy had median CRP levels twice as high as those who did not receive therapy or to those of age-matched males *(52)*.

SPECIMEN COLLECTION

Fasting

In an evaluation of paired samples collected from 10 subjects in the fasting state and 3 h postprandially, we observed no significant difference in CRP concentrations between the two groups (mean ± SD fasting 6.60 ± 13.5 mg/L, nonfasting 6.30 ± 14.0 mg/L; $p < 0.37$) *(53)*. Nevertheless, in assays that depend on optical clarity, such as turbidimetry and nephelometry, fasting before sampling is recommended.

Time of Collection

It is important to establish if CRP exhibits a circadian rhythm to determine whether the time for sample collection for the purpose of assessing future coronary risk should be standardized. Interest in the diurnal variation of CRP is stimulated by the fact that proinflammatory cytokines such as IL-6, which are responsible for CRP synthesis, have been shown to exhibit diurnal variation *(54,55)*. Meier-Ewert found no evidence of diurnal variation for CRP from hourly blood samples collected from 13 healthy adults *(56)*.

Specimen Type

Most immunoassays are designed to work with either serum or plasma; however, differences between these two fluids are a commonly unrecognized source of variability in CRP assays. Ledue et al. have previously reported that the use of EDTA or citrated plasma specimens resulted in biases of −12 and −16% in hs-CRP concentration when compared to serum *(53)*. They concluded that the differing water content of serum compared to plasma, due to the osmotic shifting effect of the anticoagulant on erythrocytes, was the likely explanation for the difference. These substantial differences must be appreciated, particularly if cut points are based on serum and cardiovascular risk assessment strategies are to be used.

Time and Temperature of Storage

CRP has been shown to be stable at 4°C for 60 d *(57)*. In a study of long-term storage, no significant changes in CRP levels were seen in normal subjects or subjects with an acute phase response when serum or plasma were stored at −70°C for more than 20 yr *(58)*. Ideally, when storing samples long term, they should be dispensed into cryotubes so there is minimal air space and placed at ≤−20°C, preferably in a noncycling freezer. On removal, samples should be thawed slowly in the refrigerator and mixed by gentle inversion before use.

ANALYTICAL CONSIDERATIONS

Sensitivity

The current algorithms for cardiovascular risk assessment require that hs-CRP results be reported in terms of quintiles of risk *(23)*. Therefore, for an assay to be clinically relevant, it must be able to measure hs-CRP reliably at least at a concentration of 0.7 mg/L. This level corresponds to the 20th percentile of the reference population and is the lowest cut point used in the risk assessment algorithm. Assays used for clinical research, however, should possess a higher level of sensitivity. Of the nine hs-CRP assays examined by Roberts et al. all had a lower limit of quantification of ≤0.3 mg/L *(59)*.

Precision

Assay imprecision expressed as the percentage of coefficient of variation (% CV) is the result of combined variables including antibody affinity, specimen dilution (i.e., degree of turbidity), instrument performance (i.e., lamp deterioration), and operator technique. For hs-CRP, the within-laboratory imprecision should be <10% at 0.2 mg/L *(60)*. In a recent evaluation of nine different hs-CRP methods, five of the methods met these criteria *(59)*.

Antigen Excess

In light-scattering immunoassays, as the antigen concentration increases beyond the equivalence point, smaller immune complexes are formed that result in diminished signal. This diminished signal may correspond to an antigen concentration in antibody excess or beyond the equivalence point in antigen excess. This problem is common with analytes such as CRP where there is a very wide pathological range of values. Indeed, among nine hs-CRP immunoassays reviewed by Roberts et al., antigen excess was detected among three of the assays *(59)*. To minimize this effect one could perform a second assay on a dilute sample, perform serum protein electrophoresis, or assay another acute phase protein to see whether the levels may be high. Although these approaches are admittedly impractical, time consuming, and costly, the laboratory must remain vigilant to avoid erroneous value assignment. The second generation hs-CRP turbidimetric methods can measure CRP over a wide range of concentrations, similarly to the nephelometric methods which can automatically dilute samples with high concentrations.

Curve-Fitting Algorithms

All quantitative methods use some sort of curve-fitting routine to determine CRP concentrations in patient sera. Before implementing hs-CRP assays, the laboratory should validate the curve-fitting algorithm for goodness of fit to ensure they do not introduce imprecision or bias into the reported value. Validation techniques including back-calculation of calibrator values is a relatively straightforward procedure and will reveal concentration-dependent bias. In general, multipoint calibration methods result in more accurate and precise results than single- or two-point calibration curves *(61)*.

Reference Materials

The vast majority of hs-CRP immunoassays are calibrated to either the World Health Organization (WHO) First International Reference Preparation for C-reactive Protein Immunoassay (85/506), introduced in 1986 *(62)*, or the Certified Reference Material 470 (CRM 470) introduced in 1993 *(63)*. The value assigned to CRM 470 was derived from WHO IRP 85/506 using a very high precision transfer protocol *(64)*.

Despite the availability of valid reference materials there have been several published reports of bias-related problems thought to be related to standardization or to poor value transfer by the manufacturer *(27,59,60)*. In addition, lack of commutability among different assays (e.g., nephelometric vs turbidimetric) from a single manufacturer can arise when the manufacturer's calibrators and controls are not compared directly to CRM 470/ RPPHS in each assay system in which they are to be used *(65)*.

Matrix Effects

Matrix effects typically result in a consistent bias between two sources of matrix, such as that between serum and the matrix used to prepare a calibrator, for example. These differences might also include variation in optical clarity, protein structure (e.g., monomeric vs the native pentameric protein), and binding to other proteins. In the presence of differences in the protein itself, variations in antibody specificity and reactivity could also contribute to divergence in assayed values. Roberts et al. observed biases ranging from −31 to +28% of the mean calculated for nine methods (calibrated to CRM 470) for a single serum specimen with a CRP concentration of 0.5 mg/L *(59)*. They concluded that matrix effects among the various calibrators were a likely factor contributing to the lack of agreement among the methods.

Standardization of hs-CRP Assays

As indicated above, several reports that examined the performance of hs-CRP methods indicated a discrepancy among reported results and suggested the need for standardizing these assays. This is a clinically important issue considering the CRP result of an individual patient will be interpreted in the context of nationally established cut points. Therefore, it is imperative that all commercially available methods give comparable results. The Centers for Disease Control and Prevention has taken the lead and initiated a

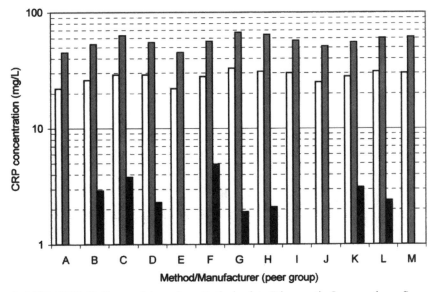

Fig. 3. 2000–2001 College of American Pathologists Diagnostic Immunology Survey Program results for three specimens. Specimen 1 (*clear column*) overall mean CRP = 56.3 mg/L, CV = 12.1%; specimen 2 (*shaded column*) overall mean CRP = 28 mg/L, CV = 12.1%; specimen 3 (*solid column*) overall mean CRP = 2.9 mg/L, CV = 34.4%.

standardization program to which manufacturers of all hs-CRP reagents worldwide have been invited to participate. Phase I of the program, which will determine whether CRM 470 is the appropriate reference material for hs-CRP methods and identify other potential secondary calibrators, is scheduled to begin in the fall of 2001. After the appropriate reference material is identified, the effect of using a single calibrator in the various methods on the harmonization of CRP results will be evaluated in Phase II.

Quality Assurance Schemes

The majority of external quality assurance programs worldwide reflect the nonenhanced CRP assays. Most published reports reflect unusually large within- and among-manufacturer CVs that are concentration dependent. Data from the 2000–2001 CAP proficiency program revealed that at CRP concentrations of 28 and 56 mg/L the average among-manufacturer CVs were 12% compared with 34% at 2.9 mg/L (Fig. 3). These data are consistent with a recent study that showed that at CRP concentrations <6 mg/L, among-manufacturer CVs range from 30% to 60%, with within-manufacturer (among-laboratory) CVs as high as 160% (65). At CRP concentrations >20 mg/L, among-manufacturer CVs were <20%, with within-manufacturer CVs 3–15%. Similar findings have been reported in earlier studies from Belgium (61) and the United Kingdom (66). These high CVs underscore the need for more sensitive immunoassays and virtually preclude the use of most traditional assays for estimating atherosclerotic cardiovascular disease risk (65). The College of American Pathologists plans to include hs-CRP in upcoming surveys as a separate reportable analyte.

SUMMARY

Although CRP was discovered more than 70 yr ago, its clinical utility has been hampered by lack of understanding of its function and by the difficulties associated with accurate quantitation. With growing awareness of the role of CRP in health and disease we will undoubtedly see a continued expansion in the use of this test. The utility of CRP to predict future coronary events in apparently healthy subjects and assess prognosis in patients with ACS have renewed interest in its measurement. A better control of pre-analytical and analytical sources of variations will undoubtedly lead to improvement in CRP measurement. hs-CRP methods are currently available and appear to be reliable. A standardization of these methods will further improve their accuracy and assure harmonization among reported CRP results.

ABBREVIATIONS

ACS, Acute coronary syndrome(s); CRM, Certified Reference Material; CRP, C-reactive protein; CV, coefficient of variance; HDL-C, high-density-lipoprotein cholesterol; Hs-CRP, high-sensitivity C-reactive protein; IL, interleukin; MI, myocardial infarction; NHANES III, National Health and Nutrition Evaluation Survey III; SAA, serum amyloid protein A; TC, total cholesterol; WHO, World Health Organization.

REFERENCES

1. Tillet WS, Francis T. Serological reaction in pneumonia with a non-protein somatic fraction of pneumococcus. J Exp Med 1930;52:561–571.
2. MacLeod CM, Avery OT. The occurrence during acute infections of a protein not normally present in the blood. II. Isolation and properties of the reactive protein. J Exp Med 1943;73:183–190.
3. Lofstrom G. Comparison between the reaction of acute phase serum with pneumococcus C-polysaccharide and with pneumococcus type 27. Br J Exp Pathol 1944;25:21–26.
4. Castell JV, Gomez-Lechon MJ, Fabra R, Trullenque R, Heinrich PC. Acute phase response of human hepatocytes: regulation of acute phase protein synthesis by interleukin-6. Hepatology 1990;12:1179–1186.
5. Johnson AM, Rohlfs E, Silverman LM. Proteins. In: Tietz Textbook of Clinical Chemistry, 3rd edit., Burtis CA, Ashwood ER, eds. WB Saunders, Philadelphia, 1999, pp. 477–540.
6. Bienvenu J, Whicher JT, Aguzzi F. C-reactive protein. In: Serum Proteins in Clinical Medicine, Vol. II. Ritchie RF, Navolotskaia O, eds. Maine Printing Co, Portland, 1996;7.01.01–7.01.06.
7. Lagrand WK, Visser CA, Hermens WT, et al. C-reactive protein as a cardiovascular risk factor: more than an epiphenomenon? Circulation 1999;100:96–102.
8. Reynolds GD, Vance RP. C-reactive protein immunohistochemical localization in normal and atherosclerotic human aortas. Arch Pathol Lab Med 1987;111:265–269.
9. Liuzzo G, Biasucci LM, Gallimore JR, et al. The prognostic value of C-reactive protein and serum amyloid A protein in severe unstable angina. N Engl J Med 1994;331:417–424.
10. Liuzzo G, Biasucci LM, Gallimore JR, et al. Enhanced inflammatory response in patients with preinfarction unstable angina. J Am Coll Cardiol 1999;34:1696–1703.
11. Berk B, Weintraub W, Alexander W. Elevation of C-reactive protein in "active" coronary artery disease. Am J Cardiol 1990;65:168–172.
12. Biasucci LM, Vitelli A, Liuzzo G, et al. Elevated levels of interleukin-6 in unstable angina. Circulation 1996;94:874–877.
13. Morrow DA, Rifai N, Antman EM, Weiner DL, McCabe CH, Cannon CP, Braunwald E. C-reactive protein is a potent predictor of mortality independently and in combination with

troponin T in acute cornary syndromes: a TIMI 11A substudy. J Am Coll Cardiol 1998;31: 1460–1465.

14. Milazzo D, Biasucci LM, Luciani N, et al. Elevated levels of C-reactive protein before coronary artery bypass grafting predict recurrence of ischemic events. Am J Cardiol 1999;84: 459–461.
15. Buffon A, Liuzzo G, Biasucci LM, et al. Preprocedural serum levels of C-reactive protein predict early complications and late restenosis after coronary angioplasty. J Am Coll Cardiol 1999;34:1512–1521.
16. Ridker PM, Hennekens CH, Burins JE, Rifai N. C-reactive protein and other markers of inflammation in the prediction of cardiovascular disease in women. N Engl J Med 2000; 342:836–843.
17. Ridker PM, Cushman M, Stampfer MJ, Tracy RP, Hennekens CH. Inflammation, aspirin, and the risk of cardiovascular disease in apparently healthy men. N Engl J Med 1997;336: 973–979.
18. Köenig W, Sund M, Fröhlich M, et al. C-reactive protein, a sensitive marker of inflammation, predicts future risk of coronary heart disease in initially healthy middle-aged men. Results from the MONICA (Monitoring Trends and Determinants in Cardiovascular Disease) Augsburg cohort study, 1984-1992. Circulation 1999;99:237–242.
19. Kuller LH, Tracy RP, Shaten J, Meilahn EN. Relationship of C-reactive protein and coronary heart disease in the MRFIT nested case-control study: multiple risk factor intervention trial. Am J Epidemiol 1996;144:537–547.
20. Danesh J, Whincup P, Walker M, et al. Low grade inflammation and coronary heart disease: prospective study and updated meta-analyses. Br Med J 2000;321:199–204.
21. Ridker PM, Glynn RJ, Hennekens CH. C-reactive protein adds to the predictive value of total and HDL cholesterol in determining risk of first myocardial infarction. Circulation 1998;97:2007–2011.
22. Hokama Y, Nakamura RM. C-reactive protein: current status and future perspectives. J Clin Lab Anal 1987;1:15–27.
23. Rifai N, Ridker PM. Proposed cardiovascular risk assessment algorithm using high-sensitivity c-reactive protein and lipid screening. Clin Chem 2001;47:28–30.
24. Köenig W. C-reactive protein and cardiovascular risk: has the time come for screening the general population? Clin Chem 2001;1:9–10.
25. Chambers JC, Eda S, Bassett P, et al. C-reactive protein, insulin resistance, central obesity, and coronary heart disease risk in Indian Asians for the UK compared with European whites. Circulation 2001;104:145–150.
26. Wener MH, Dawn PR, McQuillan GM. The influence of age, sex and race on the upper reference limit of serum C-reactive protein concentration. J Rheumatol 2000;27:2351–2359.
27. Ledue TB, Weiner DL, Sipe JD, Poulin SE, Collins MF, Rifai N. Analytical evaluation of particle-enhanced immunonephelometric assays for C-reactive protein, serum amyloid A and mannose-binding protein in human serum. Ann Clin Biochem 1998;35:745–753.
28. Erlandsen EJ, Randers E. Reference interval for serum C-reactive protein in healthy blood donors using the Dade Behring N latex C-reactive protein mono assay. Scand J Clin Lab Invest 2000;60:37–44.
29. Hutchinson WL, Köenig W, Fröhlich M, Sund M, Lowe GDO, Pepys MB. Immunoradiometric assay of circulating C-reactive protein: age-related values in the adult general population. Clin Chem 2000;46:934–938.
30. Crawford VLS, Sweeney O, Coyle PV, Halliday IM, Stout RW. The relationship between elevated fibrinogen and markers of infection: a comparison of seasonal cycles. Q J Med 2000;93:745–750.
31. Ockene IS, Matthews CE, Rifai N, Ridker PM, Reed G, Stanek E. Variability and classification accuracy of serial high-sensitivity C-reactive protein measurements in healthy adults. Clin Chem 2001;47:444–450.

32. Clark GH, Graser CG. Biological variation of acute phase protein. Ann Clin Biochem 1993; 30:373–376.

33. Macy EM, Hayes TE, Tracy RP. Variability in the measurement of C-reactive protein in healthy subjects: implications for reference intervals and epidemiological applications. Clin Chem 1997;43:52–58.

34. Kluft C, deMaat MPM. Determination of the habitual low blood level of C-reactive protein in individuals. Ital Heart J 2001;2:172–180.

35. deMaat MPM, Kluft C. Determinants of C-reactive protein concentration in blood. Ital Heart J 2001;2:189–195.

36. Chakraborti S, Batabyal SK. Study of high altitude stress on some acute phase protein in plasma of humans. Clin Chim Acta 1997;347:347–349.

37. Watts DH, Krohn MA, Wener MA, Eschenbach DA. C-reactive protein in normal pregnancy. Obstet Gynecol 1991;77:176–180.

38. Weight CM, Alexander D, Jacobs P. Strenuous exercise: analogous to the acute phase response? Clin Sci 1991;81:677–683.

39. Danesh J, Muir J, Wong Y-K, Ward M, Gallimore JR, Pepys MB. Risk factors for coronary heart disease and acute-phase proteins. Eur Heart J 1999;20:954–959.

40. Lowe G, Yarnell W, Rumley A, Bainton D, Sweetnam P. C-reactive protein, fibrin D-dimer, and incident ischemic heart disease in the Speedwell study: Are inflammation and fibrin turnover linked to pathogenesis? Arterioscler Thromb Vasc Biol 2001;4:603–610.

41. Mendall MA, Patel P, Ballam L, Strachan D, Northfield TC. C-reactive protein and its relation to cardiovascular risk factors: a population based cross sectional study. Br Med J 1996; 312:1061–1065.

42. Padham AD, Manson JE, Rifai N, Buring JE, Ridker PM. C-reactive protein, interleukin-6, and risk of developing type 2 diabetes mellitus. JAMA 2001;286:327–334.

43. Visser M, Bouter LM, McQuillan GM, Wener MH, Harris TB. Elevated C-reactive protein levels in overweight and obese adults. JAMA 1999;282:2131–2135.

44. Yudkin JS, Stehouwer CDA, Emeis JJ, Coppack SW. C-reactive protein in healthy subjects associated with obesity, insulin resistance, and endothelial dysfunction. A potential role for cytokines originates from adipose tissue? Arterioscler Thromb Vasc Biol 1999;19:972–978.

45. Tracy RP, Psaty BM, Macy E, Bovill EG, Cushman M, Cornell ES, Kuller LH. Lifetime smoking exposure affects the association of C-reactive protein with cardiovascular disease risk factors and subclinical disease in healthy elderly subjects. Arterioscler Throm Vasc Biol 1997;17:2167–2176.

46. Macy E, Meilahn E, Declerck P, Tracy R. Sample preparation for plasma measured of plasminogen activator inhibitor-1 antigen in large population studies. Arch Pathol Lab Med 1993; 117:67–70.

47. Bovill E, Landesman M, Busch S, Gregeau G, Mann K, Tracy R. Studies on the measurement of protein s in plasma. Clin Chem 1991;37:1708–1714.

48. Cook GD, Mendall MA, Whincup PH, et al. C-reactive protein concentration in children: relationship to adiposity and other cardiovascular risk factors. Atherosclerosis 2000;149: 139–150.

49. Doggen CJM, Berckmans RJ, Stuck A, Cats VM, Rosendaal FR. C-reactive protein, cardiovascular risk factors and the association with myocardial infarction in men. J Intern Med 2000;248:406–414.

50. Kallner A, Blomquist L. Effect of heavy drinking and alcohol withdrawal on markers of carbohydrate metabolism. Alcohol Alcoholism 1991;26:425–429.

51. Cushman M, Leault C, Banett-Connor E, et al. Effect of postmenopausal hormones on inflammation-sensitive proteins: the postmenopausal estrogen/progestin intervention (PEPI) study. Circulation 1999;100:717–722.

52. Ridker PM, Hennekens CH, Rifai N, Buring JE, Manson JE. Hormone replacement therapy and increased plasma concentration of C-reactive protein. Circulation 1999;100:713–716.

53. Ledue TB, Rifai N. High sensitivity immunoassays for C-reactive protein: promises and pitfalls. Clin Chem Lab Med 2001;39:1171–1176.
54. Gudewell S, Pollmächer T, Veder H, Schreiber W, Fassbender K, Holsboer F. Nocturnal plasma levels of cytokines in healthy men. Eur Arch Psychiatry Clin Neurosci 1992;242: 53–56.
55. Young MR, Matthews JP, Kanabrocki EL, Sothem RB, Roitman-Johnson B, Scheving LE. Circadian rhythmometry of serum interleukin-2, interleukin-10, tumor necrosis factor-α, and granulocyte-macrophage colony-stimulating factor in adult men. Chronobiol Int 1995; 12:19–27.
56. Meier-Ewert HK, Ridker PM, Rifai N, Price N, Dinges DF, Mullington JM. Absence of diurnal variation of C-reactive protein circulation in healthy human subjects. Clin Chem 2001;47:426–430.
57. Kebler A, Grünert C, Wood WC. The limitation and usefulness of C-reactive protein and elastase-α_1 proteinase inhibitor complexes as analytes in the diagnosis and followup of sepsis in newborns and adults. Eur J Clin Chem Biochem 1994;32:365–368.
58. Wilkins J, Gallimore JR, Moore LG, Pepys MB. Rapid automated high sensitivity enzyme immunoassay of C-reactive protein. Clin Chem 1998;44:1358–1361.
59. Roberts WL, Moulton L, Law TC, et al. Evaluation of nine automated high-sensitivity C-reactive protein methods: implications for clinical and epidemiological applications. Part 2. Clin Chem 2000;47:418–425.
60. Roberts WL, Sedrick R, Moulton L, Spencer A, Rifai N. Evaluation of four automated high-sensitivity C-reactive protein methods: implications for clinical and epidemiological applications. Part 1. Clin Chem 2000;46:461–468.
61. Devleeschouwer N, Libeer JC, Chapelle JP, et al. Factors influencing between-laboratory variability of C-reactive protein results as evidenced by the Belgian external quality assessment (EQA) scheme. Scand J Clin Lab Invest 1994;54:435–440.
62. WHO Expert Committee on Biological Standardization. WHO Expert Committee on Biological Standardization 37th report. WHO Technical Report Series 760. Geneva: WHO. 1987:21–22.
63. Whicher JT, Ritchie RF, Johnson AM, et al. New international reference preparation for proteins in human serum (RPPHS). Clin Chem 1994;40:934–948.
64. Baudner S, Bienvenu J, Blirup-Jensen S, et al. The certification of a matrix reference material for immunochemical measurement of 14 human serum proteins. CRM 470. Brussels: Community Bureau of Reference, Commission of the European Communities, 1993:1–172.
65. Johnson AM, Whicher JT, Ledue TB, Carlström A, Itoh Y, Petersen PH. Effect of a new international reference preparation for proteins in human serum (certified reference material 470) on results of the College of American Pathologists Surveys for Plasma Proteins. Arch Pathol Lab Med 2000;124:1296–1501.
66. Lauder I. United Kingdom External Quality Assurance Schemes, Annual Report, 10th edit., 1991. London: Department of Health.

20

Fatty Acid Binding Protein as an Early Plasma Marker of Myocardial Ischemia and Risk Stratification

Jan F. C. Glatz, Roy F. M. van der Putten, and Wim T. Hermens

INTRODUCTION

Biochemical markers of myocardial injury are universally accepted as important determinants for the diagnosis of patients with suspected acute myocardial infarction (AMI), especially in those cases in which electrocardiographic (ECG) changes are equivocal or absent *(1,2)*. In the last decade, interest in these biochemical markers has increased for two reasons. First, the introduction of new therapeutic strategies has called for earlier and more appropriate diagnosis of patients admitted to the emergency room with chest pain, so as to begin the proper therapy as early as possible. Second, several new plasma markers have been introduced, and some (e.g., cardiac troponin T [eTnT]) allow for the assessment of patients with not only MI but also unstable angina and prolonged chest pains, and even provide prognostic value *(3)*.

Fatty acid binding protein (FABP) has similarly been proposed as an early plasma marker of acute coronary syndromes (ACS). In this chapter we describe some relevant features of this protein and summarize the studies that have investigated its application as marker of myocardial injury. The release and plasma kinetics of FABP closely resemble those of myoglobin, but the relatively low plasma reference concentration of FABP makes it superior to myoglobin for the monitoring of myocardial injury.

BIOCHEMISTRY AND BIOLOGICAL FUNCTION OF FABP

In the soluble cytoplasm of almost all tissue cells, a relatively small (14–15 kDA) protein is found that can reversibly and noncovalently bind long-chain fatty acids, and is therefore called (cytoplasmic) FABP. At least nine distinct types of FABP occur, and these are generally named after the tissue in which they were first identified and/or mainly occur, for example, H(heart)-FABP, L(liver)-FABP, I(intestinal)-FABP. Subsequent

Portions of this chapter were published in Markers in Cardiology: Current and Future Clinical Applications. Adams JE III, Apple FS, Jaffe AS, and Wu AHB, eds., Futura, Armonk, NY.

From: *Cardiac Markers, Second Edition*
Edited by: Alan H. B. Wu @ Humana Press Inc., Totowa, NJ

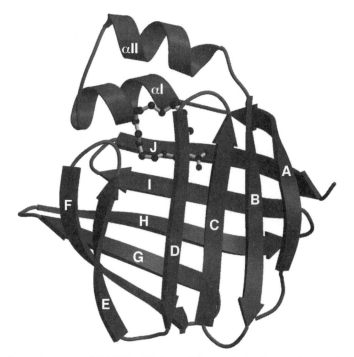

Fig. 1. A schematic view of FABP with bound long-chain fatty acid. A ribbon diagram is shown for human H-FABP, highlighting two short α-helical domains (αI and αII), and 10 β-strands (βA–βJ) forming two so-called β-sheets in between which the fatty acid ligand (in this case, oleate) is bound in a U-shaped conformation. (Figure created using data from refs. *6* and *7*. Courtesy of Dr. C. Lücke, Frankfurt, Germany.)

studies revealed the presence of L-FABP also in small intestine, and that of H-FABP also in skeletal muscle, in distal tubule cells of the kidney, and in some parts of the brain *(4)*. The FABPs are relatively abundant in tissues with an active fatty acid metabolism, such as liver, adipose tissue, and heart, which each show a tissue content of 0.5–1 mg FABP per gram wet weight of tissue *(4)*.

The FABPs belong to a multigene family of intracellular lipid-binding proteins that also includes the cellular retinoid-binding proteins *(4,5)*. These proteins each contain 126–137 amino acid residues (molecular mass 14–15 kDa) and show a similar tertiary structure that resembles that of a clam shell (Fig. 1) *(5)*. The lipid ligand is bound in between the two halves of the clam by interaction with specific amino acid residues within the binding pocket, a so-called β-barrel, of the protein. Human H-FABP contains 132 amino acid residues (14.5 kDa), and is an acidic protein (pI 5) *(8,9)*.

The FABPs appear to be stable proteins, exhibiting an intracellular turnover with a half-life of approx 2–3 d *(4)*. Their cellular expression is regulated primarily at the transcriptional level. In general, the FABP expression is responsive to changes in lipid metabolic activity as induced by various (patho)physiological and pharmacological stimuli *(4)*. For instance, the H-FABP content of heart and skeletal muscles increases by endurance training *(10)*, and is also higher in the diabetic state *(11)*, but is slightly decreased in the hypertrophied heart *(12,13)*.

The primary biological function of the FABPs is their facilitation of the cytoplasmic translocation of long-chain fatty acids, which is normally hampered by the very low solubility of these compounds in aqueous solutions *(14)*. Therefore, FABP can be regarded as an intracellular counterpart of plasma albumin. Definite proof of this function was obtained recently, when it was found that cardiac myocytes isolated from mice lacking the H-FABP gene showed a markedly lower (approx −50%) rate of fatty acid uptake and oxidation *(15)*. Other postulated functions for H-FABP and other types of FABP include a participation in signal transduction pathways such as fatty acid regulation of gene expression *(16,17)*, and the protection of myocytes against the adverse (detergent-like) effects of long-chain fatty acids *(4)*. The latter function would be of special importance for the ischemic heart because the tissue accumulation of fatty acids and their derivatives occurring in this condition have been associated with arrhythmias, increased myocardial infarct size, and depressed myocardial contractility *(18)*. The presence of H-FABP then may be crucial to sequester accumulating fatty acids and thus prevent tissue injury. However, currently available evidence for such a role for H-FABP remains inconclusive *(4)*.

IMMUNOCHEMICAL ASSAY OF FABP IN PLASMA

Because FABP is a nonenzymatic protein, its detection and quantification must be performed with an immunochemical assay. A large number of immunoassays for H-FABP have been described, mostly enzyme-linked immunosorbent assays (ELISA) of the antigen capture type *(19–22)*, but also a competitive immunoassay *(23)*, and an immunofluorometric assay *(24)*. In most cases monoclonal antibodies are used, and these show virtually no cross-reactivity with other FABP types *(7,25)*. Recombinant H-FABP appears immunochemically equivalent to the tissue-derived protein and therefore is now commonly applied as standard in the immunoassay *(7,19)*.

These assays have been used successfully for retrospective analyses of plasma FABP in patient samples. However, the implication of these tests for clinical decision making in the case of suspected AMI is hampered by the fact that the reported fastest immunoassay *(19)* still takes 45 min to complete. Therefore, more rapid FABP immunoassays are being developed. To date, these include a microparticle-enhanced turbidimetric assay to be performed on a conventional clinical chemistry analyzer (performance time 10 min) *(26)*, an automated sandwich immunoassay (performance time 23 min) *(27,28)*, and an electrochemical immunosensor (performance time 20 min) *(29–31)*. The electrochemical immunosensor is based on screen-printed graphite electrodes and uses an immunosandwich procedure and an amperometric detection system *(30)*. Measurements of plasma samples from patients with AMI with this immunosensor and with an ELISA show an excellent correlation *(30,32)*. More recently, a new principle for rapid immunoassay of proteins based on *in situ* precipitate-enhanced ellipsometry was presented and applied for assay of FABP *(33)*. This technique enables the development of a one-step ELISA with a performance time of less than 10 min. Finally, the development was described of a whole blood panel test for FABP using a one-step immunochromatography technique *(34)*. This panel test, which is completed in 15 min and is meant for point-of-care testing, identifies blood samples with an FABP concentration exceeding 6 ng/mL. With the exception of the ELISA assays, calibrated with recombinant FABP, these new techniques still require further evaluation and standardization.

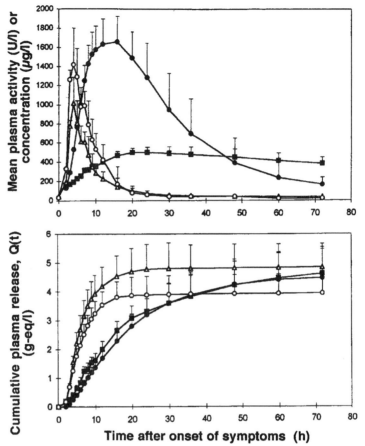

Fig. 2. Mean plasma concentration or activities (**top**) and mean cumulative release expressed in gram-equivalents (g-eq) of healthy myocardium per liter of plasma of FABP (multiplied by 10, O), myoglobin (□), CK activity (●), and LDH isoenzyme-1 (■) as function of time after onset of symptoms in 15 patients after AMI. Data refer to means ± SEM. (Adapted from ref. *37.*)

Release and Elimination of FABP on Muscle Injury

The release of H-FABP from injured muscle was first demonstrated in 1988 with isolated working rat hearts *(35),* and indicated the potential use of FABP as a plasma marker of myocardial injury in humans. Subsequently, several groups reported the release of FABP into plasma of patients with AMI *(20,21,23,36).* The characteristics of the release of FABP from injured myocardium closely resemble those of myoglobin. As an example, Fig. 2 shows mean plasma release curves of FABP and of several other plasma marker proteins for 15 AMI patients (treated with thrombolytic therapy) from whom blood samples were obtained frequently during the first 72 h of hospitalization *(37).* In patients treated with standard thrombolytic therapy after AMI, peak plasma concentrations of FABP and myoglobin were reached already at about 4 h after first symptoms, whereas for creatine kinase (CK) or the MB isoenzyme of CK (CK-MB) this took about 12 h, and for lactate dehydrogenase (LDH) about 20 h. Furthermore, plasma FABP and myoglobin returned to their respective reference values already within 24 h after AMI (Fig. 2),

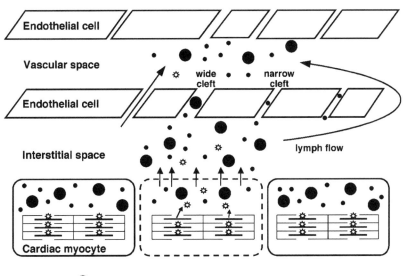

● = CK, LDH • = FABP, myoglobin ✿ = TnT

Fig. 3. Schematic presentation of the possible transport routes of protein released from damaged cardiac myocytes to the plasma compartment. Proteins can either directly cross the endothelial cell barrier (predominant route for small proteins such as FABP and myoglobin) or they can be transported through lymph drainage (predominant route for larger proteins such as creatine kinase MB [CK] and lactate dehydrogenase [LDH]). Structurally bound proteins (such as TnT) first must be dissociated from the myofibrillar structures before they can be released into the interstitial space. (Adapted from ref. *41*, with permission.)

indicating the usefulness of both markers particularly for the assessment of a recurrent infarction *(38)*. However, for AMI patients not treated with thrombolytics, peak levels are reached approx 8 h after AMI, and elevated plasma FABP and myoglobin concentrations are found up to 24–36 h after the onset of chest pain *(38)*. The release of the myofibrillar proteins cTnT and cardiac troponin I (cTnI) from injured myocardium follows a different pattern with elevated plasma concentrations occurring from approx 8 h up to more than 1 wk after infarction *(3,39)*. Hence, the so-called diagnostic window of the various marker proteins differs considerably.

The marked differences in the time course of plasma concentrations or activities among the cytoplasmic proteins (CK-MB, LDH, FABP, and myoglobin) are caused by (1) a more rapid washout of the smaller proteins (FABP, myoglobin) from the interstitium to the vascular compartment (Fig. 3), and (2) differences among the proteins in their rate of elimination from plasma *(40)*. Studies of isolated cardiac myocytes subjected to simulated ischemia showed that protein release from the damaged myocytes is independent of molecular mass *(42)*. This indicates that during the protein-release phase the sarcolemma does not act as a selective sieve through which small proteins are preferentially lost. The fact that smaller proteins can be detected in blood plasma earlier after muscle injury than can larger proteins therefore relates to a greater permeability of the endothelial barrier for smaller proteins (Fig. 3) *(40)*.

With respect to protein elimination from plasma, FABP and myoglobin, unlike the larger cardiac enzymes, are removed from the circulation predominantly by renal clearance

Table 1
Comparison of Relevant Characteristics
for FABP and Myoglobin as Markers of Myocardial Injury

Protein	Molecular mass (kDa)	Cardiac muscle content (mg/g)	Skeletal muscle content[a] (mg/g)	Reference conc. (ng/mL)
FABP	14.5	0.57	0.04–0.14	1.8
Myoglobin	17.6	2.7	2.2–6.7	34

Data obtained from refs. *13,19,38,45,46.*
[a]Range given for muscles of different fiber type composition.

(20,21,36,40). This explains not only their rapid clearance from plasma after AMI (Fig. 2) but also the maintenance of relatively low plasma concentrations of these proteins in healthy individuals. The plasma concentrations in healthy individuals are determined mainly by the release of protein from skeletal muscle because its total mass far exceeds that of cardiac muscle. Because the skeletal muscle FABP content is relatively low compared with that of myoglobin, the plasma reference concentration of FABP also is relatively low (Table 1) *(19,43–46).* This notion is also reflected in the ratio of the concentrations of myoglobin and FABP in plasma from healthy subjects (myoglobin/FABP ratio approx 20) *(45),* which resembles the ratio in which these proteins occur in skeletal muscle (myoglobin/FABP ratio 20:70) (*see* below).

The role of the kidney in the clearance of FABP and myoglobin from plasma further indicates that increased plasma concentrations of these proteins are likely to be found in case of renal insufficiency. Indeed, it has been reported that patients with chronic renal failure and normal heart function show several-fold increased plasma concentrations of both FABP and myoglobin *(47,48).* In addition, Kleine et al. *(21)* reported a patient with AMI and severe renal insufficiency in whom the plasma FABP concentration remained markedly elevated for at least 25 h after infarction.

DISCRIMINATION OF CARDIAC FROM SKELETAL MUSCLE INJURY

A potential drawback of the use of FABP as plasma marker for monitoring myocardial injury is its presence in significant quantities not only in heart muscle but also in skeletal muscle cells (Table 1). A proper diagnosis of AMI thus may be hampered in case of extensive skeletal muscle injury such as multiorgan failure, postoperative states, or vigorous exercise., This problem can be overcome, however, by the combined measurement of myoglobin and FABP concentrations in plasma and expressing the ratio of these, because this plasma ratio is a reflection of the ratio in which these proteins occur in the affected tissue cells and it differs between heart muscle (myoglobin/FABP ratio 4 to 5) and skeletal muscles (myoglobin/FABP ratio 20 to 70, depending on type of muscle) (Table 1) *(3,38,46).*

This finding is illustrated in Fig. 4 for patients after AMI in whom the plasma myoglobin/FABP ratio was approx 5 during the entire period of elevated plasma concentrations (upper panels), and for patients who underwent aortic surgery, which causes no-flow ischemia of the lower extremities, in whom the plasma myoglobin/FABP ratio was approx 45 (lower panels). In addition, van Nieuwenhoven et al. *(38)* described a patient who was defibrillated shortly after AMI, a treatment that most likely resulted in injury of inter-

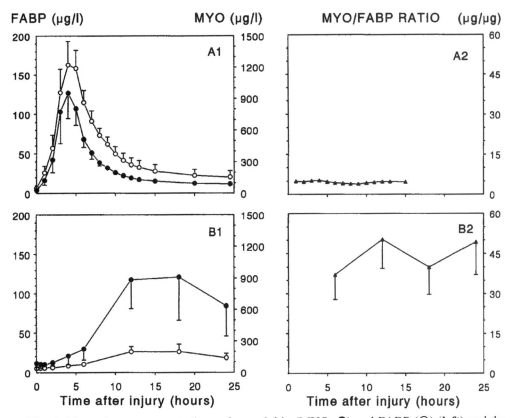

Fig. 4. Mean plasma concentrations of myoglobin (MYO; ●) and FABP (O) (**left**) and the myoglobin/FABP ratio (▲) (**right**) in nine patients after AMI (and receiving thrombolytic therapy) (**A**), and in nine patients after aortic surgery (**B**). Data refer to means ± SEM. (Adapted from ref. *38.*)

costal pectoral muscles, and in whom the plasma myoglobin/FABP ratio increased from 8 to 60 during the first 24 h after AMI. Finally, in situations where AMI patients show a second increase of plasma concentrations of marker proteins, the ratio may be of help to delineate whether this second increase was caused either by a recurrent infarction or by the occurrence of additional skeletal muscle injury. In the former case, the ratio will remain unchanged *(38)*.

EARLY DIAGNOSIS OF AMI

The application of FABP especially for the early diagnosis of ACS is already indicated from (1) its rapid release into plasma after myocardial injury, and (2) its relatively low plasma reference concentration. Several studies have now firmly established that FABP is an excellent plasma marker for the early differentiation of patients with and those without AMI, and that it even performs better than myoglobin. A selection of these studies is discussed here.

Retrospective analyses of various marker proteins in plasma samples from patients with AMI revealed that the diagnostic sensitivity for detection of AMI is better for FABP than for myoglobin or CK-MB, especially in the early hours after the onset of symptoms.

For example, in a study including blood samples from 83 patients with confirmed AMI, taken immediately upon admission to the hospital (<6 h after chest pain onset), the diagnostic sensitivity was significantly greater for FABP (78%, CI: 67–87%) than for myoglobin (53%, CI: 40–64%) or for CK-MB activity (57%, CI: 43–65%) ($p < 0.05$) *(44)*.

In the last few years, larger studies have been done that allow for the proper assessment of both the sensitivity and the specificity of FABP for AMI diagnosis. In a (single-center) study with 165 patients admitted 3.5 h (median value) after the onset of chest pain, Ishii et al. *(43)* found in admission blood samples diagnostic sensitivities and specificities for FABP (>12 ng/mL) of 82% and 86%, respectively, and for myoglobin (>105 ng/mL) of 73% and 76%, respectively (FABP vs myoglobin significantly different; $p < 0.05$). A similar superior performance of FABP over myoglobin, in terms of both sensitivity and specificity of AMI diagnosis, was also observed in a prospective multicenter study consisting of four European hospitals and including 312 patients admitted 3.3 h (median value; range 1.5–8 h) after the onset of chest pain suggestive of AMI (EURO-CARDI Multicenter Trial) *(49,50)*. For instance, specificities >90% were reached for FABP at 10 µg/L and for myoglobin at 90 ng/mL. Using these upper reference concentrations in the subgroup of patients admitted within 3 h after onset of symptoms ($n = 148$), the diagnostic sensitivity of the first blood sample taken was 48% for FABP and 37% for myoglobin, whereas for patients admitted 3–6 h after AMI ($n = 86$), the sensitivity was 83% for FABP and 74% for myoglobin *(49,50)*. In addition, the areas under the receiver operating characteristic (ROC) curves, constructed for the admission blood samples from all patients, were 0.901 for FABP and 0.824 for myoglobin (significantly different; $p < 0.001$) (Fig. 5). This better performance of FABP over myoglobin for the early diagnosis of AMI has also been reported in other smaller studies *(27,51,52)*.

More recently, Okamoto et al. *(53)* confirmed the above findings by demonstrating, in a single-center study consisting of 189 patients admitted to hospital within 12 h after the onset of symptoms, that the area under the ROC curve of FABP was 0.921, which was significantly ($p < 0.05$) greater than that of myoglobin (0.843) and CK-MB activity (0.654). In addition, a multicenter study consisting of three North American hospitals and including 460 consecutive patients, reported by Ghani et al. *(28)*, also revealed a better diagnostic performance of FABP over myoglobin during the first 4 h after admission, the areas under the ROC curves being 0.80 for FABP and 0.73 for myoglobin. Strikingly, the area under the ROC curve of CK-MB mass was 0.79, and that of cTnI was 0.91 *(28)*, which caused the authors to conclude that in their study neither FABP nor myoglobin show the sensitivity and specificity necessary to detect AMI significantly earlier than do the existing markers. This conclusion seemingly contradicts the well-documented poor diagnostic performance of CK-MB mass and cTnT or cTnI in the very early hours after infarction (cf. Fig. 6) *(13,39)*. The discrepancy is explained by the fact that the hospital delay time, which was not given, has to be added to the admission time. When assuming a hospital delay of 3–4 h, the study results would apply to the period up to 7 or 8 h after the onset of symptoms, whereas FABP and myoglobin are useful especially in the preceding hours.

In some of these above-mentioned studies, investigators evaluated whether the diagnostic performance of FABP as early plasma marker of myocardial injury could further improve when the criterion of a plasma myoglobin/FABP ratio <10 (or <14), that

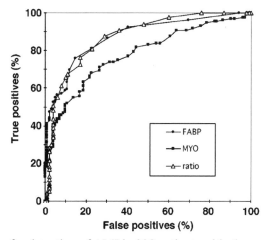

Fig. 5. ROC curves for detection of AMI in 238 patients with chest pain suggestive of AMI, and admitted to hospital within 6 hours from the onset of symptoms, comparing the concentrations of FABP (●) and myoglobin (■), and the myoglobin/FABP ratio (△) in the admission blood sample. ROC curves were constructed by plotting the sensitivity (% true positives) for the confirmed AMI group (135 patients) against 100 − specificity (% false positives) for the non-AMI group (103 patients). The areas under the ROC curves are 0.874 for FABP, 0.780 for myoglobin, and 0.870 for the myoglobin/FABP ratio (FABP vs myoglobin, and FABP vs the ratio significantly different; $p < 0.001$). (Data obtained from the EUROCARDI Multicenter Trial *[49,50]*.)

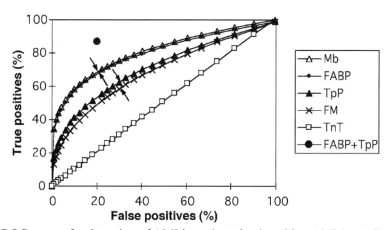

Fig. 6. ROC curves for detection of AMI in patients having either AMI ($n = 15$) or unstable angina pectoris (UAP; $n = 10$), comparing selected markers of muscle necrosis (FABP, myoglobin [Mb], and TnT) and markers of activated blood coagulation (fibrin monomers [FM] and TpP). Median hospital delay was 2.8 h (range 0.8–6 h). ROC curves were obtained from double-logarithmic plots. Lack of discrimination by TnT is apparent from its coincidence with the line of identity. *Arrows* indicate optimal cutoff values. For a combined test, that is when either FABP > 6 ng/mL or TpP >7 mg/L as diagnostic for AMI, the sensitivity was 87% and the specificity 80%. (Adapted from Hermens et al. *[67]*.)

is, the exclusion of skeletal muscle as source of FABP, is taken as an additional parameter *(28,43,50,52)*. In each of these study populations, there were a few cases in which both myoglobin and FABP were elevated in the admission plasma sample, but in which the myoglobin/FABP ratio was >10 (or >14). Without this latter result, these patients would be falsely diagnosed as having had myocardial injury. However, because the prevalence of skeletal muscle injury in these study populations was very low (<1% of cases), this additional parameter did not significantly alter the ROC curve for FABP (Fig. 5). Therefore, the routine measurement of the myoglobin/FABP ratio in samples from patients suspected for MI does not seem justified because it does not add value to the measurement of FABP alone. In addition, the myoglobin/FABP ratio cannot provide absolute cardiac specificity *(3)*.

At first sight it may be surprising that FABP appears as an earlier marker for AMI detection than does myoglobin, even though the two proteins show similar plasma release curves. However, these findings can be explained when realizing that the myocardial content of FABP (0.57 mg/g wet wt) is four- to fivefold lower than that of myoglobin (2.7 mg/g wet wt), yet the plasma reference concentration of FABP (1.8 ng/mL) is 19-fold lower than that of myoglobin (34 ng/mL) (Table 1). This means that after injury the tissue to plasma gradient is almost fivefold steeper for FABP than for myoglobin, making plasma FABP rise above its upper reference concentration at an earlier point after AMI onset than does plasma myoglobin, thereby permitting an earlier diagnosis of AMI.

It is now firmly documented that the subgroup of patients with unstable angina pectoris who show a significantly increased plasma concentration of cTnT (>0.2 ng/mL) have a prognosis as serious as do patients with definite AMI *(54,55)*. This observation most likely relates to the presence of minor myocardial cell necrosis. In those patients in whom unstable angina pectoris is in fact acute minor MI, the advantage of FABP for early assessment of injury may be used. Recently, Katrukha et al. *(56)* measured FABP and cTnI in serial plasma samples from 31 patients with unstable angina and showed that in the admission sample cTnI was elevated (cutoff value 0.2 ng/mL) in 13% and FABP (cutoff value 6 ng/mL) in 54% of patients, whereas at 6 h after admission cTnI was elevated in 58% and FABP in 52% of patients. Importantly, all patients who had an elevated FABP concentration at 6 h showed an elevated cTnI value at 12 h after admission *(56)*. These preliminary data suggest that FABP may identify (acute) minor MI with similar sensitivity as cTnI, but at an earlier point after admission of the patient.

EARLY ESTIMATION OF MYOCARDIAL INFARCT SIZE

Myocardial infarct size is commonly estimated from the serial measurement of cardiac proteins in plasma and calculation of the cumulative release over time (plasma curve area), taking into account the elimination rate of the protein from plasma *(57)*. This approach requires that the proteins are completely released from the heart after AMI and recovered quantitatively in plasma. Complete recovery is well documented for CK, LDH, and myoglobin (but does not apply for the structural proteins cTnT and cTnI *[39]*), and could also be shown for FABP *(37,58)*. Figure 2 (lower panel) presents the cumulative release patterns of these four proteins, expressed in gram-equivalents (g-eq) of healthy myocardium per liter of plasma (i.e., infarct size). The release of FABP and myoglobin is completed much earlier than that of either CK or LDH, but despite this kinetic difference for each of the proteins, the released total quantities yield comparable estimates of the mean extent of myocardial injury when evaluated at 72 h after the onset of AMI (Fig. 2).

This method to estimate infarct size has proven its value when applied to the evaluation of early thrombolytic therapy in patients with AMI (59). With the (classically used) enzymatic markers, the method has the drawback that the data on infarct size in the individual patient become available relatively late (72 h), that is, too late to have an influence on acute care (60). For the more rapidly released markers FABP and myoglobin, infarct size estimation for individual patients is hampered by the fact that these proteins are cleared by the kidneys, and the patients often suffer from renal insufficiency, which would lead to overestimation of infarct size. De Groot et al. (61) recently suggested the use of individually estimated clearance rates for FABP and myoglobin to measure myocardial infarct size within 24 h. These individual clearance rates are calculated using glomerular filtration rates (estimated from plasma creatinine concentrations and corrected for age and gender) and plasma volume (corrected for age and gender). This implies that a reliable estimate of myocardial infarct size becomes available when the patient is still in the acute care department, if frequent blood samples are taken and analyzed rapidly.

FABP AS REPERFUSION MARKER

The application of FABP as a plasma marker for the early detection of successful coronary reperfusion in patients with AMI has been investigated by three groups (62–64). Ishii et al. (62) studied 45 patients treated with intracoronary thrombolysis or direct percutaneous transluminal coronary angioplasty (PTCA), in whom coronary angiography was performed every 5 min to identify the onset of reperfusion. Both plasma FABP and myoglobin were found to rise sharply after the onset of reperfusion, and the relative first-hour increase rates of both markers showed a predictive accuracy of >93%. Subsequently, in a study consisting of 58 patients, de Lemos et al. (63) also demonstrated that following successful reperfusion plasma FABP and myoglobin rise sharply, whereas in patients with failed reperfusion these markers rise at a much slower rate. In this study the patency of the infarct-related artery was determined from a single-point angiogram, and could be predicted from either plasma FABP or myoglobin with a sensitivity of approx 60% and a specificity of approx 80%. This minor performance of the markers in this study when compared with that of Ishii et al. (62) may be explained by the strict inclusion criteria in the latter.

In a multicenter study consisting of 115 patients with confirmed AMI and receiving thrombolytic agents, and who underwent coronary angiography within 120 min of the start of thrombolysis, de Groot et al. (64) also observed that FABP and myoglobin perform equally well as markers to discriminate between reperfused and nonreperfused patients. Similar to the study of de Lemos et al. (63), these investigators found relatively low sensitivities and specificities (approx 70%), which, however, could be improved (to approx 80%) by normalization to infarct size (64). These data indicate the equal suitabilities of FABP and myoglobin as noninvasive reperfusion markers, especially in retrospective studies in which infarct size is known.

NEW APPROACHES TO INCREASE
FURTHER THE DIAGNOSIC PERFORMANCE OF FABP

A limitation of the use of markers of cell necrosis for assessment of tissue injury is the time lag between the onset of necrosis and the appearance of the marker proteins in plasma. This explains why up to 2–3 h after the onset of AMI, the performance of such markers generally is insufficient for clinical decision making. Therefore, approaches have been presented to increase further the diagnostic performance of the plasma markers in these early hours after AMI.

To circumvent the problem of the upper reference concentration that is defined for populations and used for individual cases, it has been suggested to collect two (or more) serial blood samples during the first hours after admission and express the difference in marker concentration or activity in these samples. This approach has been applied especially to identify low-risk patients who would show no ECG abnormalities as well as two negative results for protein markers (hence, no significant change with time), and for whom early discharge would be a safe option *(65)*. In a second EUROCARDI Multicenter Trial, we studied whether in patients admitted for suspected AMI without ECG changes, AMI can be ruled out by assay of FABP, myoglobin, or CK-MB mass in two serial blood samples, collected on admission and 1–3 h thereafter, respectively. For comparison, cTnT was measured in a third sample taken 12–36 h after admission. Preliminary results from this study revealed that two negative marker concentrations within 3 h from admission ruled out AMI with very high negative predictive values (>90%) with the highest value found for FABP (negative predictive value 98%), being similar to that of cTnT elevation (≥0.1 ng/mL) in the sample taken 12–36 h after admission (B. Haastrup et al., *unpublished data*, 1999). A similar conclusion was also reached in a subsequent single-center study consisting of 130 patients admitted for suspected AMI with no significant ST-segment elevation *(66)*. These data indicate the excellent utility of FABP for early triage and risk stratification of patients with chest pain.

Another approach to increase further the diagnostic performance of FABP in the early hours after onset of chest pain is its use in combination with markers of activated blood coagulation *(67)*. Because intracoronary formation of blood clots on ruptured arteriosclerotic plaques is considered the main cause of AMI, detection of activated blood coagulation potentially allows for the early diagnosis of AMI *(68)*. Various (small-size) studies have indicated that in the very early hours (0–3 h) after AMI onset, coagulation markers show a higher sensitivity and specificity for AMI detection than necrosis markers *(69, 70)*. In addition, a tendency toward higher marker concentrations was observed for shorter hospital delays, a finding related to the fact that the acute thrombotic event precedes coronary occlusion and muscle necrosis. In a pilot study consisting of 25 patients with either AMI or unstable angina pectoris, we showed that combining a marker of muscle cell necrosis (FABP) and a marker of activated blood coagulation (thrombus precursor protein [TpP]) yielded a markedly higher sensitivity and specificity for AMI detection than either of the markers alone (Fig. 6) *(67)*. Moreover, the performance of such a combined test is expected to be relatively insensitive to hospital delay because TpP will perform better in patients who are admitted earlier, whereas FABP will perform better in patients who are admitted later *(38,70)*. At present, we are investigating other markers of activated blood coagulation, a.o. tissue factor and soluble fibrin, which, in combination with FABP, could bridge the diagnostic time gap of the first few hours after onset of symptoms in patients with ACS *(71)*. A general problem in this field of research is that the tight physiological control of blood coagulation, required to prevent thrombolysis, is affected by a large number of feedback mechanisms and inhibitors that may easily obscure the relationship between the extent of prothrombolytic activation and the concentrations of activated products in plasma.

OTHER APPLICATIONS OF THE PLASMA MARKER FABP

FABP was also found to be useful for the early detection of postoperative myocardial tissue loss in patients undergoing coronary bypass surgery *(3,72–74)*. In these patients, myocardial injury may be caused by global ischemia/reperfusion and, in addition, by postoperative MI. In our study, we found that in such patients, plasma CK, myoglobin, and FABP are already significantly elevated 0.5 h after reperfusion. In the patients who developed postoperative MI, a second increase was observed for each plasma marker protein, but a significant increase was recorded earlier for FABP (4 h after reperfusion) than for CK or myoglobin (8 h after reperfusion) *(72)*. These data suggest that FABP would allow for an earlier exclusion of postoperative MI, thus permitting the earlier transfer of these patients from the intensive care unit to the ward. Recently, both Hayashida et al. *(73)* and Petzold et al. *(74)* also reported that FABP is an early and sensitive marker for the diagnosis of myocardial injury in patients undergoing cardiac surgery.

Antibodies directed against FABP have been shown to be useful for the immunohistochemical detection of very recent MIs *(75–77)*. Partial depletion of FABP was observed in cardiomyocytes with a post-infarction interval of <4 h *(75)*, indicating that FABP immunostaining can confirm the clinical diagnosis or suspicion of early MI in routine autopsy pathology.

Finally, besides the application of FABP in early diagnosis of myocardial injury in patients, the marker is now also applied for evaluating MI after coronary artery ligation and for estimating infarct size in experimental animals such as mice and rats *(78–81)*.

CONCLUSION

The early diagnosis of ACS is important because it may improve patient treatment and reduce complications. Biochemical markers of myocardial cell damage continue to be important tools for differentiating patients with AMI from those without AMI, because specific ST-segment changes in the admission ECG remain absent in a great number of patients with AMI *(1,3)*. FABP is a novel biochemical marker that shows release characteristics from injured myocardium and elimination rates from plasma that are similar to those of myoglobin, which at present is regarded as the preferred early plasma marker of cardiac injury *(82–85)*. Experimental studies indicate that this resemblance relates to the similar molecular masses of FABP (14.5 kDa) and myoglobin (17.6 kDa). Several clinical studies with patients suspected of having AMI reveal a superior performance of FABP over myoglobin (as well as other marker proteins) for the early detection of AMI. This finding most likely relates to marked differences in tissue contents of FABP and myoglobin in cardiac and skeletal muscles that result in a relatively low upper reference concentration in plasma for FABP compared with that for myoglobin. These differences in tissue contents are also reflected in the plasma concentrations of these proteins after either cardiac or skeletal muscle injury, in such a manner that the ratio of the plasma concentrations of myoglobin and FABP can be applied to discriminate myocardial from skeletal muscle injury.

Limitations of the use of FABP as a diagnostic plasma marker in the clinical setting include (1) the relatively small diagnostic window, which extends to only 24–30 h after the onset of chest pain, and (2) its elimination from plasma mainly by renal clearance, possibly causing falsely high values in case of kidney malfunction. These drawbacks can, however, be overcome by the simultaneous measurement in plasma of a late marker such as cTnT or cTnI and assay of plasma creatinine to identify patients with renal insufficiency and to calculate a corrected FABP concentration. It is important to note that these same limitations also apply to myoglobin, which is now recommended by both the National Academy of Clinical Biochemistry (NACB) Committee on Standards of Laboratory Practice *(82)* and the International Federation of Clinical Chemistry (IFCC) Committee on Standardization of Markers of Cardiac Damage *(83)* as preferred early marker of MI, to be used in combination with cTnT or cTnI. In spite of the recognition that, to date, relatively few centers have investigated the performance of FABP for early diagnosis of AMI, the uniformly observed superiority of FABP over myoglobin indicates that the optimal set of biochemical markers of muscle necrosis for assessment of ACS may be FABP together with cTnT or cTnI *(86)*.

ACKNOWLEDGMENTS

Work in the authors' laboratory was supported by grants from the Netherlands Heart Foundation (D90.003, 95.189 and 98.063), the Ministry of Economic Affairs (StiPT/MTR 88.002 and BTS 97.188), and the European Community (BMH1-CT93.1692 and CIPD-CT94.0273).

ABBREVIATIONS

ACS, Acute coronary syndrome(s); AMI, acute myocardial infarction; CK, creatine kinase; CK-MB, MB isoenzyme of CK; cTnI, cTnT, cardiac troponins I and T; ECG, electrocardiogram; ELISA, enzyme-linked immunosorbent assay; FABP, fatty acid binding protein; H-FABP, heart FABP; I-FABP, intestinal FABP; LDH, lactate dehydrogenase; L-FABP, liver FABP; PTCA, percutaneous transluminal coronary angioplasty; ROC, receiver operating characteristics; TpP, thrombus precursor protein.

REFERENCES

1. Adams JE, Abendschein DR, Jaffe AS. Biochemical markers of myocardial injury. Is MB creatine kinase the choice for the 1990s? Circulation 1993;88:750–763.
2. Christenson RH, Azzazy HME. Biochemical markers of the acute coronary syndromes. Clin Chem 1998;44:1855–1864.
3. Mair J. Progress in myocardial damage detection: new biochemical markers for clinicians. Crit Rev Clin Lab Sci 1997;34:1–66.
4. Glatz JFC, Van der Vusse GJ. Cellular fatty acid-binding proteins. Their function and physiological significance. Prog Lipid Res 1996;35:243–282.
5. Banaszak L, Winter N, Xu Z, et al. Lipid binding proteins: a family of fatty acid and retinoid transport proteins. Adv Protein Chem 1994;45:89–151.

6. Young AC, Scapin G, Kromminga A, et al. Structural studies on human muscle fatty acid binding protein at 1.4 A resolution: binding interactions with three C18 fatty acids. Structure 1994;2:523–534.

7. Lücke C, Rademacher M, Zimmerman AW, et al. Spin-system heterogeneities indicate a selected-fit mechanism in fatty acid binding to heart-type fatty acid-binding protein (H-FABP). Biochem J 2001;354:259–266.

8. Schaap FG, Specht B, Van der Vusse GJ, et al. One-step purification of rat heart-type fatty acid-binding protein expressed in *Escherichia coli*. J Chromatogr 1996;B 679:61–67.

9. Schreiber A, Specht B, Pelsers MMAL, et al. Recombinant human heart-type fatty acid-binding protein as standard in immunochemical assays. Clin Chem Lab Med 1998;36: 283–288.

10. Van Breda E, Keizer HA, Vork MM, et al. Modulation of fatty acid-binding protein content of rat heart and skeletal muscle by endurance training and testosterone treatment. Eur J Physiol 1992;421:274–279.

11. Glatz JFC, Van Breda E, Keizer HA, et al. Rat heart fatty acid-binding protein content is increased in experimental diabetes. Biochem Biophys Res Commun 1994;199:639–646.

12. Vork MM, Trigault N, Snoeckx LHEH, Glatz JFC, Van der Vusse GJ. Heterogeneous distribution of fatty acid-binding protein in the hearts of Wistar Kyoto and spontaneously hypertensive rats. J Mol Cell Cardiol 1992;24:317–321.

13. Kragten JA, Van Nieuwenhoven FA, Van Dieijen-Visser MP, et al. Distribution of myoglobin and fatty acid-binding protein in human cardiac autopsies. Clin Chem 1996;42:337–338.

14. Glatz JFC, Storch J. Unravelling the significance of cellular fatty acid-binding proteins. Curr Opinion Lipidol 2001;12:267–274.

15. Schaap FG, Binas B, Danneberg H, et al. Impaired long-chain fatty acid utilization by cardiac myocytes isolated from mice lacking the heart-type fatty acid binding protein gene. Circ Res 1999;85:329–337.

16. Glatz JFC, Börchers T, Spener F, et al. Fatty acids in cell signalling: modulation by lipid binding proteins. Prostagland Leukotr Essen Fatty Acids 1995;52:121–127.

17. Van der Lee KAJM, Vork MM, De Vries JE, et al. Long-chain fatty acid-induced changes in gene expression in neonatal cardiac myocytes. J Lipid Res 2000;41:41–47.

18. Van der Vusse GJ, Glatz JFC, Stam HCG, et al. Fatty acid homeostasis in the normoxic and ischemic heart. Physiol Rev 1992;72:881–940.

19. Wodzig KWH, Pelsers MMAL, Van der Vusse GJ, et al. One-step enzyme-linked immunosorbent assay (ELISA) for plasma fatty acid-binding protein. Ann Clin Biochem 1997;34: 263–268.

20. Tanaka T, Hirota Y, Sohmiya K, et al. Serum and urinary human heart fatty acid-binding protein in acute myocardial infarction. Clin Biochem 1991;24:195–201.

21. Kleine AH, Glatz JFC, van Nieuwenhoven FA, et al. Release of heart fatty acid-binding protein into plasma after acute myocardial infarction in man. Mol Cell Biochem 1992;116: 155–162.

22. Ohkaru Y, Asayama K, Ishii H, et al. Development of a sandwich enzyme-linked immunosorbent assay for the determination of human heart type fatty acid-binding protein in plasma and urine by using two different monoclonal antibodies specific for human heart fatty acid-binding protein. J Immunol Methods 1995;178:99–111.

23. Knowlton AA, Burrier RE, Brecher P. Rabbit heart fatty acid-binding protein. Isolation, characterization, and application of a monoclonal antibody. Circ Res 1989;165:981–988.

24. Katrukha A, Bereznikova A, Filatov V, et al. Development of sandwich time-resolved immunofluorometric assay for the quantitative determination of fatty acid-binding protein (FABP) (abstract). Clin Chem 1997;43:S106.

25. Roos W, Eymann E, Symannek M, et al. Monoclonal antibodies to human heart fatty acid-binding protein. J Immunol Methods 1995;183:149–153.

26. Robers M, Van der Hulst FF, Fischer MAJG, et al. Development of a rapid microparticle-enhanced turbidimetric immunoassay for plasma fatty acid-binding protein, an early marker of acute myocardial infarction. Clin Chem 1998;44:1564–1567.
27. Sanders GT, Schouten Y, De Winter RJ, et al. Evaluation of human heart type fatty acid-binding protein assay for early detection of myocardial infarction (abstract). Clin Chem 1998;44:A132.
28. Ghani F, Wu AHB, Graff L, et al. Role of heart-type fatty acid-binding protein in early detection of acute myocardial infarction. Clin Chem 2000;46:718–719.
29. Siegmann-Thoss C, Renneberg R, Glatz JFC, et al. Enzyme immunosensor for diagnosis of myocardial infarction. Sensors Actuators 1996;B30:71–76.
30. Schreiber A, Feldbrügge R, Key G, et al. An immunosensor based on disposable electrodes for rapid estimation of fatty acid-binding protein, an early marker of myocardial infarction. Biosens Bioelectr 1997;12:1131–1137.
31. Renneberg R, Cheng S, Kaptein WA, et al. Novel immunosensors for rapid diagnosis of acute myocardial infarction: a case report. Adv Biosens 1999;4:241–272.
32. Key G, Schreiber A, Feldbrügge R, et al. Multicenter evaluation of an amperometric immunosensor for plasma fatty acid-binding protein: an early marker for acute myocardial infarction. Clin Biochem 1999;32:229–231.
33. Robers M, Rensink IJAM, Hack CE, et al. A new principle for rapid immunoassay of proteins based on in situ precipitate-enhanced ellipsometry. Biophys J 1999;76:2769–2776.
34. Watanabe T, Ohkubo Y, Matsuoka H, et al. Development of a simple whole blood panel test for detection of human heart-type fatty acid-binding protein. Clin Biochem 2001;34:257–263.
35. Glatz JFC, Van Bilsen M, Paulussen RJA, et al. Release of fatty acid-binding protein from isolated rat heart subjected to ischemia and reperfusion or to the calcium paradox. Biochim Biophys Acta 1988;961:148–152.
36. Tsuji R, Tanaka T, Sohmiya K, et al. Human heart-type cytoplasmic fatty acid-binding protein in serum and urine during hyperacute myocardial infarction. Int J Cardiol 1993;41:209–217.
37. Wodzig KWH, Kragten JA, Hermens WT, et al. Estimation of myocardial infarct size from plasma myoglobin or fatty acid-binding protein. Influence of renal function. Eur J Clin Chem Clin Biochem 1997;35:191–198.
38. van Nieuwenhoven FA, Kleine AH, Wodzig KWH, et al. Discrimination between myocardial and skeletal muscle injury by assessment of the plasma ratio of myoglobin over fatty acid-binding protein. Circulation 1995;92:2848–2854.
39. Kragten JA, Hermens WT, Van Dieijen-Visser MP. Cardiac troponin T release into plasma after acute myocardial infarction: only fractional recovery compared with enzymes. Ann Clin Biochem 1996;33:314–223.
40. Hermens WT. Mechanisms of protein release from injured heart muscle. Dev Cardiovasc Med 1998;205:85–98.
41. Van Nieuwenhoven FA. Heart fatty acid-binding proteins. Role in cardiac fatty acid uptake and marker for cellular damage. Thesis, Maastricht University, 1996;65–71.
42. Van Nieuwenhoven FA, Musters RJP, Post JA, et al. Release of proteins from isolated neonatal rat cardiac myocytes subjected to simulated ischemia or metabolic inhibition is independent of molecular mass. J Mol Cell Cardiol 1996;28:1429–1434.
43. Ishii J, Wang JH, Naruse H, et al. Serum concentrations of myoglobin vs human heart-type cytoplasmic fatty acid-binding protein in early detection of acute myocardial infarction. Clin Chem 1997;43:1372–1378.
44. Glatz JFC, Van der Vusse GJ, Simoons M, et al. Fatty acid-binding protein and the early detection of acute myocardial infarction. Clin Chim Acta 1998;272:87–92.

45. Pelsers MMAL, Chapelle JP, Knapen M, et al. Influence of age and sex and day-to-day and within-day biological variation on plasma concentrations of fatty acid-binding protein and myoglobin in healthy subjects. Clin Chem 1999;45:441–443.
46. Yoshimoto K, Tanaka T, Somiya K, et al. Human heart-type cytoplasmic fatty acid-binding protein as an indicator of acute myocardial infarction. Heart Vessels 1995;10:304–309.
47. Górski J, Hermens WT, Borawski J, et al. Increased fatty acid-binding protein concentration in plasma of patients with chronic renal failure. Clin Chem 1997;43:193–195.
48. Nayashida N, Chihara S, Tayama E, et al. Influence of renal function on serum and urinary heart fatty acid-binding protein levels. J Cardiovasc Surg 2001;42:735–740.
49. Kristensen SR, Haastrup B, Hørder M, et al. Fatty acid-binding protein: a new early marker of AMI (abstract). Scand J Clin Lab Invest 1996;56(Suppl)225:36–37.
50. Glatz JFC, Haastrup B, Hermens WT, et al. Fatty acid-binding protein and the early detction of acute myocardial infarction: the EUROCARDI multicenter trial (abstract). Circulation 1997;96:I–215.
51. Panteghini M, Bonora R, Pagani F, et al. Heart fatty acid-binding protein in comparison with myoglobin for the early detection of acute myocardial infarction (abstract). Clin Chem 1997;43:S157.
52. Abe S, Saigo M, Yamashita T, et al. Heart fatty acid-binding protein is useful in early and myocardial-specific diagnosis of acute myocardial infarction (abstract). Circulation 1996; 94:I–323.
53. Okamoto F, Sohmiya K, Ohkaru Y, et al. Human heart-type cytoplasmic fatty acid-binding protein (H-FABP) for the diagnosis of acute myocardial infarction. Clinical evaluation of H-FABP in comparison with myoglobin and creatine kinase isoenzyme MB. Clin Chem Lab Med 2000;38:231–238.
54. Hamm CW, Ravkilde J, Gerhardt W, et al. The prognostic value of serum troponin T in unstable angina. N Engl J Med 1992;327:146–150.
55. Ravkilde J, Hørder M, Gerhardt W. Diagnostic performance and prognostic value of serum troponin T in suspected acute myocardial infarction. Scand J Clin Lab Invest 1993;53: 677–683.
56. Katrukha A, Bereznekiva A, Filatov V., et al. Improved detection of minor ischemic cardiac injury in patients with unstable angina by measurement of cTnI and fatty acid binding protein (FABP) (abstract). Clin Chem 1999;45:A139.
57. Hermens WT, Van der Veen FH, Willems GM, et al. Complete recovery in plasma of enzymes lost from the heart after permanent coronary occlusion in the dog. Circulation 1990;81: 649–659.
58. Glatz JFC, Kleine AH, Van Nieuwenhoven FA, et al. Fatty acid-binding protein as a plasma marker for the estimation of myocardial infarct size in humans. Br Heart J 1994;71:135–140.
59. Simoons ML, Serruys PW, Van den Brand M, et al. Early thrombolysis in acute myocardial infarction: limitation of infarct size and improved survical. J Am Coll Cardiol 1986;7: 717–728.
60. van der Laarse A. Rapid estimation of myocardial infarct size. Cardiovasc Res 1999;44: 247–248.
61. de Groot MJM, Wodzig KWH, Simoons ML, et al. Measurement of myocardial infarct size from plasma fatty acid-binding protein or myoglobin, using individually estimated clearance rates. Cardiovasc Res 1999;44:315–324.
62. Ishii J, Nagamura Y, Nomura M, et al. Early detection of successful coronary reperfusion based on serum concentration of human heart-type cytoplasmic fatty acid-binding protein. Clin Chim Acta 1997;262:13–27.
63. de Lemos JA, Antman EM, Morrow D, et al. Heart-type fatty acid binding protein as a marker of reperfusion after thrombolytic therapy. Clin Chim Acta 2000;298:85–97.

64. de Groot MJM, Muijtjens AMM, Simoons ML, et al. Assessment of coronary reperfusion in patients with myocardial infarction using fatty acid binding protein concentrations in plasma. Heart 2001;85:278–285.

65. Noble MIM. Can negative results for protein markers of myocardial damage justify discharge of acute chest pain patients after a few hours in hospital? Eur Heart J 1999;20:925–927.

66. Haastrup B, Gill S, Kristensen SR, et al. Biochemical markers of ischaemia for the early identification of acute myocardial infarction without ST segment elevation. Cardiology 2000; 94:254–261.

67. Hermens WT, Pelsers MMAL, Mullers-Boumans ML, et al. Combined use of markers of muscle necrosis and fibrinogen conversion in the early differentiation of myocardial infarction and unstable angina. Clin Chem 1998;44:890–892.

68. Jesse RL, Kontos MC. Evaluation of chest pain in the emergency department. Curr Prob Cardiol 1997;22:149–236.

69. Merlini PA, Bauer KA, Oltrona L, et al. Persistent actvation of coagulation mechanism in unstable angina and myocardial infarction. Circulation 1994;90:61–68.

70. Carville DGM, Dimitrijevic N, Walsh M, et al. Thrombus precursor protein (TpP): marker of thrombosis early in the pathogenesis of myocardial infarction. Clin Chem 1996;42: 1537–1541.

71. van der Putten RFM, Hermens WT, Giesen PLA, et al. Plasma tissue factor in the early differentiation of myocardial infarction and unstable angina (abstract). In: Abstract Book of the European Meeting on Biomarkers of Organ Damage and Dysfunction, Cambridge UK, April 3–7, 2000:116.

72. Fransen EJ, Maessen JG, Hermens WT, Glatz JF. Demonstration of ischaemia-reperfusion injury separate from postoperative infarction in CABG patients. Ann Thoracic Surg 1998; 65:48–53.

73. Hayashida N, Chihara S, Akasu K, et al. Plasma and urinary levels of heart fatty acid-binding protein in patients undergoing cardiac surgery. Jpn Circ J 2000;64:18–22.

74. Petzold T, Feindt P, Sunderdiek U, et al. Heart-type fatty acid binding protein (hFABP) in the diagnosis of myocardial damage in coronary artery bypass grafting. Eur J Cardiothor Surg 2001;19:859–864.

75. Kleine AH, Glatz JFC, Havenith MG, et al. Immunohistochemical detection of very recent myocardial infarctions in man with antibodies against heart type fatty acid-binding protein. Cardiovasc Pathol 1993;2:63–69.

76. Watanabe K, Wakabayashi H, Veerkamp JH, et al. Immunohistochemical distribution of heart-type fatty acid-binding protein immunoreactivity in normal human tissues and in acute myocardial infarct. J Pathol 1993;170:59–65.

77. Ortmann C, Pfeiffer H, Brinkmann B. A comparative study on the immunohistochemical detection of early myocardial damage. Int J Legal Med 2000;113:215–220.

78. Knowlton AA, Apstein CS, Saouf R, et al. Leakage of heart fatty acid binding protein with ischemia and reperfusion in the rat. J Mol Cell Cardiol 1989;21:577–583.

79. Volders PGA, Vork MM, Glatz JFC, et al. Fatty acid-binding proteinuria diagnosis myocardial infarction in the rat. Mol Cell Biochem 1993;123:185–190.

80. Sohmiya K, Tanaka T, Tsuji R, et al. Plasma and urinary heart-type cytoplasmic fatty acid-binding protein in coronary occlusion and reperfusion induced myocardial injury model. J Mol Cell Cardiol 1993;25:1413–1426.

81. Aartsen WM, Pelsers MMAL, Hermens WT, et al. Heart fatty acid binding protein and cardiac troponin T plasma concentrations as markers for myocardial infarction after coronary artery ligation in mice. Eur J Physiol 2000;439:416–422.

82. Wu AHB, Apple FA, Gibler WB, et al. National Academy of Clinical Biochemistry Standards on Laboratory Practice: recommendations for the use of cardiac markers in coronary artery diseases. Clin Chem 1999;45:1104–1121.

83. Panteghini M, Apple FS, Christenson RH, et al. Use of biochemical markers in acute coronary syndromes. IFCC Scientific Division, Committee on Standardization of Markers of Cardiac Damage. Clin Chem Lab Med 1999;37:687–693.
84. Storrow AB, Gibler WB. The role of cardiac markers in the emergency department. Clin Chim Acta 1999;284:187–196.
85. Alpert JS, Thygesen K, Antman E, et al. Myocardial infarction redefined—a consensus document of The Joint European Society of Cardiology/American College of Cardiology Committee for the redefinition of myocardial infarction. J Am Coll Cardiol 2000;36:959–969.
86. Wu AH. Analytical and clinical evaluation of new diagnostic tests for myocardial damage. Clin Chim Acta 1998;272:11–21.

21

Oxidized Low-Density Lipoprotein and Malondialdehyde-Modified Low-Density Lipoprotein in Patients with Coronary Artery Disease

Paul Holvoet

INTRODUCTION

Increased low-density lipoprotein (LDL) oxidation is associated with coronary artery disease (CAD). The predictive value of circulating oxidized LDL is additive to the Global Risk Assessment Score for cardiovascular risk prediction based on age, gender, total and high-density lipoprotein (HDL) cholesterol, diabetes, hypertension, and smoking. Circulating oxidized LDL does not originate from extensive metal ion induced oxidation in the blood but from mild oxidation in the arterial wall by cell-associated lipoxygenase and/or myeloperoxidase. The increase of circulating oxidized LDL is most probably independent of plaque instability. Indeed, plasma levels of oxidized LDL are very similar among patients with stable CAD and patients with acute coronary syndromes (ACS).

Endothelial ischemia induces increased prostaglandin synthesis and platelet adhesion/ activation. These processes are associated with the release of aldehydes, which induce oxidative modification of the protein moiety of LDL in the absence of lipid oxidation and thus in the generation of malondialdehyde (MDA)-modified LDL. Levels of MDA-modified LDL are higher among patients with ACS. The release of MDA-modified LDL is independent of necrosis of myocardial cells.

Our data suggest that oxidized LDL is a marker of coronary atherosclerosis whereas MDA-modified LDL is a marker of plaque instability.

OXIDATIVE MODIFICATION OF LDL

Figure 1 summarizes different possible mechanisms of oxidative modification of LDL. Endothelial cells, monocytes, macrophages, lymphocytes, and smooth muscle cells are all capable of enhancing the rate of oxidation of LDL *(1)*. During inflammation, several cell types synthesize and secrete phospholipase A$_2$. Myeloperoxidase, a heme protein secreted by activated phagocytes, oxidizes L-tyrosine to a tyrosyl radical that is a physiological catalyst for the initiation of lipid oxidation in LDL. In striking contrast to other cell-mediated mechanisms for LDL oxidation, the myeloperoxidase-catalyzed reaction is independent of free metal ions *(2)*. Lipid oxidation results in the generation of aldehydes that substitute lysine residues in the apolipoprotein B-100 moiety of LDL and causes its fragmentation. The resulting oxidatively modified LDL is generally referred

From: *Cardiac Markers, Second Edition*
Edited by: Alan H. B. Wu @ Humana Press Inc., Totowa, NJ

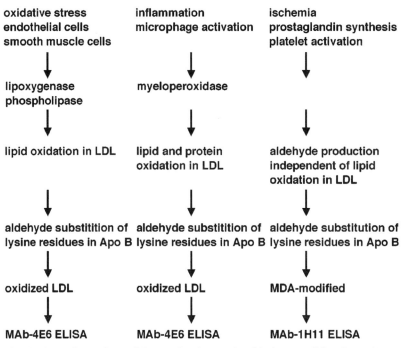

Fig. 1. Overview of possible mechanisms of oxidative modification of LDL.

to as oxidized LDL. A monoclonal antibody (MAb)-4E6 based competition enzyme-linked immunosorbent assay (ELISA) can be used for the measurement of oxidized LDL in plasma *(3)*. The C_{50} values, concentrations that are required to obtain 50% inhibition of antibody binding in the ELISA, are 25 mg/dL for native LDL and 0.25 mg/dL for oxidized LDL with at least 60 aldehyde-substituted lysines per apolipoprotein B-100.

Oxidative stress in endothelial cells and platelet activation are associated with the oxidation of arachidonic acid to aldehydes. These interact with lysine residues in the apolipoprotein B-100 moiety of LDL resulting in oxidative modification of the protein part of LDL in the absence of lipid oxidation *(4–6)*. The resulting oxidatively modified LDL is generally referred to as MDA-modified LDL. A MAb-1H11-based competition ELISA may be used for the measurement of MDA-modified LDL in plasma *(7,8)*. The C_{50} values are 0.25 mg/dL for MDA-modified LDL with at least 60 aldehyde-substituted lysines per apolipoprotein B-100 compared to 25 mg/dL for native LDL and oxidized LDL.

OXIDIZED LDL IS A MARKER OF CAD

The association of oxidative modification of LDL and stable angina and ACS has been studied *(3)*. Table 1 shows characteristics of controls and patients with angiographically confirmed CAD. CAD patients were older; more often male and smokers; and had more frequently hypertension, diabetes, and hypercholesterolemia. CAD patients had higher levels of total and LDL cholesterol and of triglycerides, lower levels of HDL cholesterol, and 2.6-fold higher levels of oxidized LDL. Receiver operating characteristic (ROC) curve analysis revealed that oxidized LDL had a higher sensitivity for CAD than

Table 1
Characteristics of Controls and CAD Patients

Characteristic	Control (n = 246)	CAD (n = 106)	p Value
Age, yr (mean ± SD)	44 ± 16	65 ± 9.1	<0.001
Gender (male/female)	92/154	68/38	<0.001
Hypertension (%)	21	39	<0.001
Diabetes type 2 (%)	19	28	NS
Hypercholesterolemia (%)	19	50	<0.001
Treated with statins (%)	2.4	19	<0.001
Treated with fibrates (%)	3.3	6.6	NS
Smokers (%)	26	46	<0.001
BMI (height/weight^2)	28 ± 8.5	27 ± 5.1	0.26
Total cholesterol (mg/dL)	168 ± 34	185 ± 40	<0.001
LDL cholesterol (mg/dL)	96 ± 31	112 ± 32	<0.001
Triglycerides (mg/dL)	121 ± 89	156 ± 91	<0.001
HDL cholesterol (mg/dL)	47 ± 14	42 ± 15	0.0028
Oxidized LDL (mg/dL)	1.11 ± 0.82	2.91 ± 1.15	<0.001

The p values were determined by nonparametric multiple comparisons test or by chi-square analysis. BMI, Body mass index; other abbreviations as in text.

the total cholesterol to HDL cholesterol (Tot-C/HDL-C) ratio. The area under the curve (AUC) was 0.93 (95% CI: 0.91–0.94) for oxidized LDL compared to 0.68 (0.65–0.71) for the Tot-C/HDL-C ratio (p < 0.0001). Plasma levels of oxidized LDL were very similar among patients with stable CAD and patients with ACS *(3)*.

Major independent risk factors for CAD are advancing age, elevated blood pressure, elevated serum total and LDL cholesterol, low serum HDL cholesterol, diabetes mellitus, and cigarette smoking *(9–11)*. The Framingham Heart Study has elucidated the quantitative relationship between these risk factors and CAD. It showed that the major risk factors are additive in predictive power. Accordingly, the total risk of a person can be estimated by a summing of the risk imparted by each of the major risk factors. Recently, the American Heart Association and the American College of Cardiology issued a scientific statement that assessed the Global Risk Assessment Scoring (GRAS) as a guide to primary prevention *(12)*. GRAS is based on age, total cholesterol, HDL cholesterol, systolic blood pressure, diabetes mellitus, and smoking. Predisposing factors such as obesity, physical inactivity, and family history of premature CAD are not included in GRAS.

We have compared the diagnostic value of circulating oxidized LDL for CAD with that of established risk factors in a subsequent and independent study *(13)*. A total of 304 subjects were included: 178 patients with angiographically proven CAD (mean age 59 yr) and 126 age-matched (mean age 60 yr) subjects without clinical evidence of cardiovascular disease. CAD patients had higher levels of circulating oxidized LDL (p < 0.001), higher Tot-C/HDL-C ratio, and higher GRAS (p < 0.001) than controls (Table 2). GRAS was calculated on the basis of age, total and HDL cholesterol, blood pressure, diabetes mellitus, and smoking.

ROC analysis revealed that oxidized LDL had a higher sensitivity for CAD than the Tot-C/HDL-C ratio and GRAS, respectively. The AUC was 0.91 (95% CI: 0.87–0.94)

Table 2
Comparison of Tot-C to HDL-C Ratio, GRAS, and Circulating
Oxidized LDL (OxLDL) in Controls and CAD Patients

Characteristics	($n = 126$)	Control ($n = 178$)	CAD p Value
Tot-C/HDL-C	4.03 ± 1.51	4.80 ± 1.54	<0.001
GRAS	6.13 ± 5.00	8.65 ± 3.41	<0.001
OxLDL (mg/dL)	1.30 ± 0.88	3.11 ± 1.19	<0.001

The p values were determined by nonparametric multiple comparisons test or by chi-square analysis.

for oxidized LDL compared to 0.71 (0.66–0.76) for the Tot-C/HDL-C ratio ($p < 0.0001$) and 0.82 (0.77–0.86) for GRAS ($p < 0.0001$) (Fig. 2).

Logistic regression analysis revealed that the predictive value of oxidized LDL was additive to that of GRAS ($p < 0.001$). Ninety-four percent of subjects with high (exceeding the 90th percentile of distribution in controls) circulating oxidized LDL and high GRAS had CAD (94% of men and 100% of women). Thus, addition of circulating oxidized LDL to the established risk factors can improve cardiovascular risk prediction (Table 3) *(13)*.

Table 4 shows the relationship of CAD with age, sex, hypertension, diabetes type 2, hypercholesterolemia, dyslipidemia, smoking, body mass index, and circulating oxidized LDL. Inclusion of circulating oxidized LDL in the multivariate model resulted in an increase of r^2 value from 0.22 to 0.67. Overall 72% of subjects were predicted correctly by the multivariate model containing established cardiovascular risk factors and oxidized LDL, compared to 40% by a model that did not include oxidized LDL *(13)*.

Recently, two other groups have developed and used assays for circulating oxidized LDL to study the relationship between oxidation of LDL and CAD. Nagai's group *(14, 15)* developed a test based on an antioxidized phosphatidylcholine monoclonal antibody and an anti-human apolipoprotein B antibody. Levels of oxidized LDL were 1.8-fold higher for CAD patients than for subjects without clinical evidence of CAD. The sensitivity of the assay for CAD was 79% with a specificity of 75%. Ehara et al. *(16)* used an ELISA based on another antioxidized phosphatidylcholine MAb. Compared to controls, levels of circulating oxidized LDL were 1.5- to 3.4-fold higher in CAD patients independent of differences in serum levels of total and LDL and HDL cholesterol.

MDA-MODIFIED LDL IS A MARKER OF ACS

We have collected plasma samples of 64 patients with angiographically confirmed stable CAD, 42 patients with unstable angina pectoris, and 62 patients with acute myocardial infarction (AMI) (Table 5) *(8)*. Plasma levels of MDA-modified LDL were similar for controls and patients with stable angina pectoris, were 3.6-fold higher ($p < 0.001$) for patients with unstable angina pectoris, and were 3.1-fold higher ($p < 0.001$) for AMI patients. C-reactive protein (CRP) levels were similar for controls and patients with stable CAD, were 3.7-fold higher for unstable angina patients, and were 6.5-fold higher

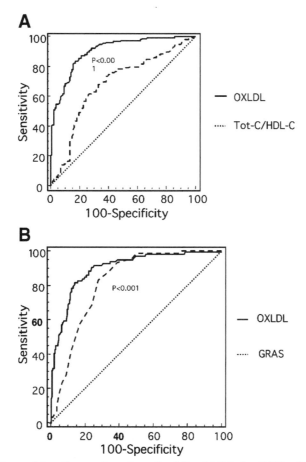

Fig. 2. Comparison of the diagnostic value of oxidized LDL for CAD with that of the Tot-C to HDL-C (**A**) or the GRAS (**B**). The AUC was 0.91 (95% CI: 0.87–0.94) for oxidized LDL compared to 0.71 (0.66–0.76) for the Tot-C to HDL-C ($p < 0.0001$) and 0.82 (0.77–0.86) for the GRAS ($p < 0.0001$).

Table 3
Prediction of CAD with GRAS and Circulating Oxidized LDL

	Odds ratio (95% CI)	p	Predictive value (%)
Men (*n* = 174)			
GRAS	1.2 (1.1–1.4)	<0.001	43
GRAS	1.2 (1.0–1.4)	0.027	
+			94
oxidized LDL	3.9 (2.4–6.1)	<0.001	
Women (*n* = 130)			
GRAS	1.2 (1.1–1.3)	<0.001	60
GRAS	1.2 (1.1–1.4)	<0.001	
+			98
oxidized LDL	7.5 (3.7–14)	0.0010	

Classification cutoff was 0.9.

Table 4
Logistic Regression Analysis of the Relationship
Between CAD and Potential Cardiovascular Risk Factors

Covariate	χ^2	p	Odds ratio (95% CI)
Multivariate model 1			
Male sex	15	<0.001	3.1 (1.8–5.6)
Dyslipidemia	8.2	0.0042	2.6 (1.4–5.0)
Age	6.1	0.013	1.1 (1.0–1.1)
Hypercholesterolemia	4.3	0.037	1.9 (1.0–3.4)
Multivariate model 2			
Oxidized LDL	59	<0.001	7.0 (4.3–11)
Dyslipidemia	6.0	0.014	3.0 (1.3–7.4)
Male sex	6.2	0.013	3.1 (1.3–7.7)
Age	4.3	0.038	1.1 (1.0–1.1)

The multivariate model 1 contained age, sex, hypertension, diabetes type 2, hypercholesterolemia, dyslipidemia, smoking, and body mass index as covariates. The r^2 value of this model was 0.22. Overall 40% of patients were predicted correctly at a classification cutoff of 0.9. The multivariate model 2 contained levels of circulating oxidized LDL and all other covariants included in the first model. The r^2 value of this model was 0.67. Overall 72% of patients were predicted correctly at a classification cutoff of 0.9.

for AMI patients ($p < 0.001$). Plasma levels of CRP were higher ($p < 0.05$) for AMI patients than for patients with unstable angina. Cardiac troponin I levels were similar for controls and patients with stable CAD, were 5.4-fold higher for patients with unstable angina ($p < 0.001$), and were 19-fold higher for AMI patients ($p < 0.001$) than for controls. AMI patients had 3.6-fold higher plasma cTnI level than patients with unstable angina ($p < 0.001$). D-dimer levels were similar for controls and for patients with chronic stable angina or unstable angina pectoris and were 4.4-fold higher for AMI patients (8).

Logistic regression analysis revealed an association of clinically diagnosed ACS with CRP ($p < 0.0001$), cTnI ($p < 0.0001$), and MDA-modified LDL ($p = 0.0003$). ROC curve analysis revealed that MDA-modified LDL ($p = 0.0014$), but not cTnI or CRP, could discriminate between stable CAD and unstable angina. In contrast, cTnI ($p = 0.0007$), but neither MDA-modified LDL nor CRP, discriminated between unstable angina and AMI. Both MDA-modified LDL ($p = 0.0001$) and cTnI ($p = 0.021$), but not CRP, discriminated between stable CAD and AMI. At a cutoff value of 10 mg/dL (value exceeding the 95th percentile of distribution for patients with stable angina), the sensitivity of CRP was 19% for unstable angina and 42% for AMI, whereas the specificity was 95%. At a cutoff value of 0.05 ng/mL (value exceeding the 95th percentile of distribution for patients with stable angina), the sensitivity of cTnI was 38% for unstable angina and 90% for AMI, whereas the specificity was 95%. At a cutoff value of 0.70 mg/dL (value exceeding the 95th percentile of distribution for patients with stable angina), the sensitivity of MDA-modified LDL was 95% for unstable angina and 95% for AMI, whereas the specificity was 95%.

Table 5
Characteristics of Controls and CAD Patients

	Stable angina (n = 64)	Unstable angina (n = 42)	AMI (n = 62)
Age	65 ± 10^b	72 ± 12^a	63 ± 12
Male/female ratio	53/11	28/14	45/17
TC (mg/dL)	177 ± 35	174 ± 37	178 ± 44
LDL-C (mg/L)	115 ± 30	109 ± 33	112 ± 40
HDL-C (mg/dL)	38 ± 13	45 ± 16	39 ± 12
TG (mg/dL)	123 ± 46	100 ± 55	128 ± 67
OxLDL (mg/dL)	2.65 ± 1.36^c	2.84 ± 0.91^c	3.44 ± 1.5^c
MDA-modified LDL (mg/dL)	0.46 ± 0.20	1.33 ± 0.49^c	1.14 ± 0.46^c
cTnI (ng/mL)	0.035 ± 0.075	0.19 ± 0.44^c	0.68 ± 1.2^c
CRP (mg/dL)	5.30 ± 6.89	12.48 ± 23.50^b	22 ± 35^c
D-dimer (μg/dL)	30 ± 28	37 ± 44^a	57 ± 75^c

Quantitative data represent means ± SD. The *p* values were determined by nonparametric multiple comparisons test except for male/female ratios, which were compared by chi-square analysis.
[a]$p < 0.05$.
[b]$p < 0.01$.
[c]$p < 0.001$.

CONCLUSIONS

Our studies show that plasma levels of oxidized LDL are significantly elevated in CAD patients. These levels are very similar for patients with stable CAD and patients with ACS, suggesting that their increase is independent of plaque instability. The similar ROC values of oxidized LDL for CAD in two independent studies (0.93 and 0.91, respectively) demonstrate that the assay for circulating oxidized LDL is indeed valid for studying the relationship between oxidation of LDL and CAD.

The sensitivity of oxidized LDL for CAD was higher than that of the total to HDL cholesterol ratio and of the GRAS. Logistic regression analysis revealed that the predictive value of oxidized LDL was additive to that of GRAS ($p < 0.001$). Ninety-four percent of subjects with high (exceeding the 90th percentile of distribution in controls) circulating oxidized LDL and high GRAS had CAD (94% of men and 100% of women) CAD. Thus, circulating oxidized LDL is a sensitive marker of CAD.

Our prospective study in heart transplant patients showed that baseline levels of oxidized LDL predicted the development of transplant CAD independent of levels of LDL and HDL cholesterol and of pretransplant history of ischemic heart disease *(17)*. Thus, the level of oxidized LDL in the blood is an independent predictor of the development of transplant CAD that was associated with a further increase of plasma levels of oxidized LDL. Although the study identifies oxidized LDL as a prognostic marker of transplant CAD it does not prove that oxidized LDL has an active role in the development of CAD. Our recent finding of increased plasma levels of oxidized LDL in obese and type 2 diabetes patients, who are at increased risk for CAD even before there is any clinical evidence of CAD, suggests that this may be the case. Oxidized LDL may contribute to the progression of atherosclerosis by enhancing endothelial injury, by inducing foam cell generation and smooth muscle proliferation.

Intervention trials are required to evaluate the active role of oxidized LDL in the development of CAD in general. Interventions may aim at a further decrease of LDL cholesterol, at an increase of levels of antioxidants in LDL, and/or at an increase of HDL that contain enzymes such as paraoxonase and platelet-activating factor acetylhydrolase that may prevent the oxidation of LDL or may degrade oxidized phospholipids in LDL.

Levels of MDA-modified LDL are dependent on the ischemic syndromes for patients with unstable angina pectoris or AMI. The association between MDA-modified LDL and cTnI, a marker of ischemic syndromes, further supports this hypothesis.

In conclusion, oxidized LDL is a marker of coronary atherosclerosis whereas MDA-modified LDL is a marker of plaque instability.

ACKNOWLEDGMENTS

This work was supported in part by a grant from the Fonds voor Geneeskundig Wetenschappelijk Onderzoek-Vlaanderen (FWO) (Projects 7.0022.98 and 7.0033.98) and by the Interuniversitaire Attractiepolen (Program 4/34). The patient studies were performed at the University Hospital of the Katholieke Universiteit Leuven, Belgium, in collaboration with Prof. Dr. Désiré Collen of the Center for Molecular and Vascular Biology, Prof. Dr. Erik Muls of the Department of Endocrinology, and Prof. Dr. Frans Van de Werf of the Department of Cardiology.

ABBREVIATIONS

ACS, Acute coronary syndrome(s); AMI, acute myocardial infarction; AUC, area under the curve; C, cholesterol; CAD, coronary artery disease; CRP, C-reactive protein; cTnI, cardiac troponin I; ELISA, enzyme-linked immunosorbent assay; GRAS, Global Risk Assessment Scoring; HDL, high-density lipoprotein; LDL, low-density lipoprotein; MAb, monoclonal antibody; MDA, malondialdehyde; ROC, receiver operating characteristic; Tot-C, total cholesterol.

REFERENCES

1. Steinbrecher UP, Parthasarathy S, Leake DS, Witztum JL, Steinberg D. Modification of low density lipoprotein by endothelial cells involves lipid peroxidation and degradation of low density lipoprotein phospholipids. Proc Natl Acad Sci USA 1984;81:3883–3887.
2. Farber HW, Barnett HF. Differences in prostaglandin metabolism in cultured aortic and pulmonary arterial endothelial cells exposed to acute and chronic hypoxia. Circ Res 1991; 68:1446–1457.
3. Holvoet P, Vanhaecke J, Janssens S, Van de WF, Collen D. Oxidized LDL and malondi-aldehyde-modified LDL in patients with acute coronary syndromes and stable coronary artery disease. Circulation 1998;98:1487–1494.
4. Farber HW, Barnett HF. Differences in prostaglandin metabolism in cultured aortic and pulmonary arterial endothelial cells exposed to acute and chronic hypoxia. Circ Res 1991; 68:1446–1457.
5. Lynch SM, Morrow JD, Roberts LJ, Frei B. Formation of non-cyclooxygenase-derived prostanoids (F2-isoprostanes) in plasma and low density lipoprotein exposed to oxidative stress in vitro. J Clin Invest 1994;93:998–1004.

6. Laskey RE, Mathews WR. Nitric oxide inhibits peroxynitrite-induced production of hydroxy-eicosatetraenoic acids and F2-isoprostanes in phosphatidylcholine liposomes. Arch Biochem Biophys 1996;330:193–198.
7. Holvoet P, Perez G, Zhao Z, Brouwers E, Bernar H, Collen D. Malondialdehyde-modified low density lipoproteins in patients with atherosclerotic disease. J Clin Invest 1995;95: 2611–2619.
8. Holvoet P, Collen D, Van de WF. Malondialdehyde-modified LDL as a marker of acute coronary syndromes. JAMA 1999;281:1718–1721.
9. Wilson PW. Established risk factors and coronary artery disease: the Framingham Study. Am J Hypertens 1994;7(7 Pt 2):7S–12S.
10. Grundy SM, Balady GJ, Criqui MH, et al. Primary prevention of coronary heart disease: guidance from Framingham: a statement for healthcare professionals from the AHA Task Force on Risk Reduction. American Heart Association. Circulation 1998;97:1876–1887.
11. Wilson PW, D'Agostino RB, Levy D, Belanger AM, Silbershatz H, Kannel WB. Prediction of coronary heart disease using risk factor categories. Circulation 1998;97:1837–1847.
12. Grundy SM, Pasternak R, Greenland P, Smith S Jr, Fuster V. Assessment of cardiovascular risk by use of multiple-risk-factor assessment equations: a statement for healthcare professionals from the American Heart Association and the American College of Cardiology. Circulation 1999;100:1481–1492.
13. Holvoet P, Mertens A, Verhamme P, et al. Circulating oxidized LDL is a useful marker for identifying patients with coronary artery disease. Arterioscler Thromb Vasc Biol 2001;21: 844–848.
14. Kohno H, Sueshige N, Oguri K, et al. Simple and practical sandwich-type enzyme immunoassay for human oxidatively modified low density lipoprotein using antioxidized phosphatidylcholine monoclonal antibody and antihuman apolipoprotein-B antibody. Clin Biochem 2000;33:243–253.
15. Toshima S, Hasegawa A, Kurabayashi M, et al. Circulating oxidized low density lipoprotein levels. A biochemical risk marker for coronary heart disease. Arterioscler Thromb Vasc Biol 2000;20:2243–2247.
16. Ehara S, Ueda M, Naruko T, et al. Elevated levels of oxidized low density lipoprotein show a positive relationship with the severity of acute coronary syndromes. Circulation 2001;103: 1955–1960.
17. Holvoet P, Van Cleemput J, Collen D, Vanhaecke J. Oxidized low density lipoprotein is a prognostic marker of transplant-associated coronary artery disease. Arterioscler Thromb Vasc Biol 2000;20:698–702.

Part V
Cardiac Markers
of Congestive Heart Failure

22
Pathophysiology of Heart Failure

Johannes Mair

INTRODUCTION

Heart failure (HF) has become a public health issue that is so important that it has been named a "new epidemic of cardiovascular disease," and its prognosis is poor. The 5-yr mortality rate in patients with mild HF is approx 50%; the annual mortalities depend on disease severity and range from <5% in asymptomatic patients to 30–80% in endstage disease, with 10% in mild HF and 20–30% in moderate HF *(1)*. Today, HF is the single most frequent cause of hospitalization in persons 65 yr of age or older *(1)*. HF becomes more common with increasing age. The increase in the aging of the population and the growing number of people surviving myocardial infarctions are important reasons why the prevalence of HF has been rising steadily. Fortunately, during the last three decades substantial improvements in the diagnosis, management, and treatment of patients with HF have been achieved. Drugs have become available that have been demonstrated unequivocally to delay death, enable patients to avoid hospitalization, and improve the quality of life assessed by exercise capacity and symptoms questionnaires. In the 1970s HF was perceived as a disease with symptoms that were closely allied to hemodynamic disequilibrium. This hemodynamic model suggested that increased ventricular wall stress is the principal cause of HF. It was thought that these abnormalities can be rectified by the use of vasodilating drugs that lead to afterload reduction. These drugs in fact lowered left atrial pressure and increased cardiac output, and acute HF symptoms are rapidly improved by the use of drugs such as diuretics, vasodilators, and morphine. This response relates largely to changes in central hemodynamics. However, it was soon realized that the administration of some of these afterload-reducing drugs was not associated with any clinical benefit on patients' outcomes even after improvement in hemodynamic status had been achieved. The origin of symptoms in chronic HF (CHF) is not related in a simple manner to hemodynamic findings as well *(2)*. These discoveries led to the formulation of the neurohormonal hypothesis of the progression of HF *(3)*. In recent years much has been learned about the pathophysiology of HF, and HF is today regarded as a hemodynamic disorder due to impaired pump function with reduced cardiac output and subsequent venous congestion. Complex neurohormonal activation is aimed at improving the mechanical environment of the heart, and circulating and local hormones as well as proinflammatory cytokines play an important role in disease progression. In fact, in

From: *Cardiac Markers, Second Edition*
Edited by: Alan H. B. Wu @ Humana Press Inc., Totowa, NJ

recent years the most important developments in the treatment of HF have been the introduction of first the angiotensin converting enzyme (ACE) inhibitors and then β-blockers, which resulted in an almost 50% decrease in mortality in the last decade in therapeutic trials. The great benefits of these drugs on delaying the progression of HF are mainly attributable to their neurohumoral effects with beneficial effects on the remodeling of the failing heart. This chapter focuses on the complex neurohormonal changes in HF with their diagnostic implications.

DEFINITION

HF is a difficult disease to define, and this complex multisystem disorder has been defined in several ways, but none is completely adequate and entirely satisfactory. Braunwald *(4)* defined this complex syndrome as a pathological state in which an abnormality of cardiac function is responsible for failure of the heart to pump blood at a rate commensurate with the requirements of the metabolizing tissues, or can do so only from an elevated filling pressure. A simple objective definition of CHF is also currently impossible as there is no cutoff value of ventricular dysfunction or change in flow, pressure, dimension, or volume that can be used reliably to identify all patients with HF. HF diagnosis is therefore based on clinical judgment, history, physical examination, and appropriate objective investigations. It is easy to recognize HF in its moderate or severe version where the patient has pronounced symptoms and signs. However, the problem of defining and diagnosing HF arises in its milder forms. None of the signs and symptoms is heart specific. To overcome the various difficulties in defining HF, guidelines for its diagnosis have been developed by the cardiological societies *(5)*. Essential features are the presence of clinical signs and symptoms of HF (e.g., exertional dyspnea, breathlessness, fatigue, low arterial blood pressure, ankle swelling, pulmonary edema) and objective evidence for cardiac dysfunction, for example, by echocardiography. In equivocal cases a response to treatment directed toward HF is helpful in establishing the diagnosis. At a pragmatic level the clinician has to answer two major questions: (1) Are the symptoms of cardiac origin? (2) If so, what kind of cardiac disease (systolic, diastolic dysfunction, or valve disease) is producing these symptoms?

ETIOLOGY

Any kind of cardiac disorder that impairs the ability of the heart to eject blood leads to HF. CHF usually develops from myocardial failure due to loss of a critical amount of functioning myocardium after damage to the heart (e.g., myocardial ischemia and infarction that alter regional function, and myocarditis, dilated, toxic, or metabolic cardiomyopathies that alter global function) or due to chronically persisting hemodynamic changes leading to pressure or volume overload (e.g., heart valve diseases, systemic or pulmonary hypertension) which lead to hypertrophy and dilation of the chamber (*see* Table 1). Today, the most common causes of CHF in industrialized countries are coronary artery disease (CAD, approx 60% of HF cases) and hypertension. Heart valve diseases and cardiomyopathies are comparably rare causes. HF should be distinguished from other pathophysiological conditions without a primary cardiac cause of a disturbed integrity of the arterial circulation or reduced tissue oxygenation (e.g., anemia, hypovolemia, hypoxia, low peripheral arterial resistance in sepsis).

Table 1
Causes of Heart Failure

1. Loss of myocardium
    Myocardial infarction
    Myocarditis
    Cardiomyopathies
2. Hemodynamic changes
    Pressure overload
      Systemic hypertension
      Pulmonary hypertension
      Heart valve disease
        (e.g., valvular aortic stenosis)
      Congenital heart diseases or diseases of the aorta
    Volume overload
      Heart valve diseases
        (e.g., valvular aortic regurgitation)
      Left-to-right shunts
        (e.g., congenital heart or vascular diseases, arteriovenous fistula)
    Abnormal heart rate
      Tachycardia
      Bradycardia

DESCRIPTIVE TERMS IN HEART FAILURE

Acute vs Chronic Heart Failure

The description of CHF was given above. Acute HF is characterized by acute cardiac dyspnea with signs of pulmonary congestion including pulmonary edema or by cardiogenic shock, a syndrome characterized by a low arterial pressure, oliguria, and a cool periphery.

Systolic vs Diastolic Heart Failure

HF can result from any cardiac disorder that impairs the heart's ability to fill and/or relax or empty, and the syndrome of HF consists of two entities, namely, systolic and diastolic dysfunction. Both can lead to HF and ultimately death. Inability to fill and relax the left ventricle is diastolic dysfunction, defined as an elevated end-diastolic pressure in a normal-sized ventricle. Difficulty emptying the left ventricle is systolic dysfunction, represented by a reduced ejection fraction. Almost one third of all HF patients have normal systolic function but abnormal left ventricular diastolic function. Diastolic ventricular relaxation is an energy-requiring process and not just simple passive elastic recoil. Normal ventricular filling is a prerequisite for normal ventricular emptying. It is important to differentiate between systolic and diastolic dysfunction because treatment is different for systolic and diastolic dysfunction. Frequently both systolic and diastolic dysfunction are found in HF patients. These functional abnormalities of the left ventricle are important contributors to HF symptoms and play a critical role in sodium retention that leads to congestion in the pulmonary circulation and edema in the systemic circulation.

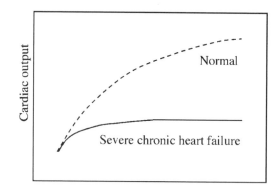

Pulmonary capillary wedge pressure

Fig. 1. Frank–Starling's law of the heart. Relationship between filling pressure and cardiac output in the normal (*dashed line*) and the failing heart (*solid line*).

Other Descriptive Terms in Heart Failure

The clinical value of other descriptive terms in HF has yet to be determined. Right and left HF refer to syndromes presenting predominantly with congestion of the systemic or pulmonary veins, respectively. These terms do not necessarily indicate which ventricle is most severely damaged. Isolated right or left ventricular HF are rare disorders, and usually both ventricles are affected in CHF. Forward and backward HF are other descriptive terms still occasionally in use. The symptoms of HF are predominantly shortness of breath and fatigue, and breathlessness was believed to be largely attributable to a raised left atrial pressure (the so-called "backward failure") and fatigue attributable to a low cardiac output (so-called "forward failure"). Usually CHF patients show the symptoms of both forward and backward failure. Forward failure is sometimes also called "low-output" failure. The so-called "high-output" failure must be distinguished from HF because cardiac dysfunction is not the cause of arterial underfilling or tissue hypoxia. As mentioned above this pathophysiological condition is found in other diseases, such as anemia, hypovolemia, or sepsis, in which the heart tries to compensate for other causes of reduced tissue oxygenation or in patients with hyperthyroidism.

HEMODYAMIC CHANGES IN HEART FAILURE

The heart has a number of hemodynamic adaptive mechanisms for maintenance of its pumping function. The relationship between diastolic filling and contractile function of the heart is described by Frank–Starling's law. Accordingly, any reduction of filling pressure of the heart should result in a reduction of cardiac output. After acute myocardial damage, an increase in cardiac filling pressure helps to maintain a sufficient cardiac output. This observation in healthy cardiac muscle is, however, not true in CHF patients (*see* Fig. 1). In severe HF, the relationship between filling pressure and cardiac output is no longer increasing; instead the curve tends to run parallel to the abscissa or may even down-slope *(6)*. Therefore, the dilation of the ventricle is of no benefit in chronic HF; instead it further increases wall stress and mitral regurgitation and worsens ejection efficiency. Therefore, a reduction of filling pressures (preload), for example, by treatments

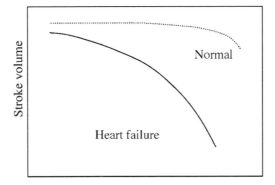

Peripheral vascular resistance

Fig. 2. Stroke volume–peripheral vascular resistance relationship of the heart. Relationship between stroke volume and peripheral vascular resistance in the normal (*dashed line*) and the failing heart (*solid line*).

with diuretics, in these patients does not decrease cardiac output but, in the long run, may even increase it because of the benefits of a reduced myocardial wall stress.

Similarly, there are substantial differences in the relationships between stroke volume and vascular resistance of the normal and failing heart (Fig. 2). The stroke volume of a normal heart is almost constant over a broad range of increasing peripheral vascular resistance. By contrast, the failing heart demonstrates a pronounced decrease in stroke volume with increasing peripheral vascular resistance. Thus, a decrease in vascular resistance may lead to a strong increase in the stroke volume of CHF patients. All in all, in contrast to normal hearts a simultaneous decrease in pre- and afterload may drastically improve stroke volume.

Even in the presence of myocardial hypertrophy and increased mitochondrial density, molecular and structural changes in the chronically failing human heart (*see* below) lead to an intrinsic contractile defect, that is, a reduction in the velocity of shortening at any level of tension development. In addition, the force–frequency relationship, that is, in normal hearts myocardial force development increases with heart rate (Bowditch effect), is altered in human heart failure *(7)*. The initial injury to the heart leads to low output with subsequent arterial underfilling. These hemodynamic changes are sensed by vascular baroreceptors. High-pressure receptors are located in the left ventricle, carotid sinus, aortic arch, and renal afferent arterioles and respond to decreases in arterial blood pressure, peripheral vascular resistance, or renal perfusion. They activate the vaso-motor center in the medulla oblongata (*see* Fig. 3), and the sympathetic nervous system (SNS), renin–angiotensin–aldosterone system (RAAS), and vasopressin (VP) are the activated principal neurohumoral effectors *(8)*. The immediate effects are tachycardia, increased myocardial contractility, vasoconstriction with increased cardiac pre- and afterload, and stimulation of thirst. Salt and water retention occur with a delay of several days. These hemodynamic mechanisms and baroreceptor-mediated reflexes are of clear benefit during the acute phase (acute HF) and initially compensate for the failing heart and maintain perfusion of the brain and heart in the presence of severe reduction in cardiac output, but, as outlined below, long-term neurohormonal activation is largely

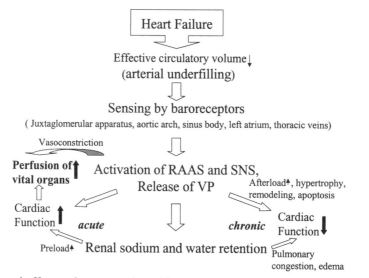

Fig. 3. Sensor and effector elements activated in response to arterial underfilling in heart failure.

maladaptive and exacerbates the hemodynamic abnormalities by a vicious cycle or causes myocyte hypertrophy and exerts a direct toxic effect on the myocardium (Fig. 3).

Although central hemodynamic changes are by definition the initiating pathophysiological event in HF, it has been shown that the degree of left ventricular dysfunction in CHF does not correlate with exercise tolerance or symptoms. There is no simple relationship between pulmonary capillary pressure and exercise performance. Abnormalities of pulmonary diffusion, respiratory skeletal muscles and blood flow in peripheral skeletal muscles, and cardiac deconditioning contribute importantly to the sensation of breathlessness. Similarly, there is also no simple relationship between right heart pressure and peripheral edema. Capillary permeability for fluid and small proteins and reduced physical activity are additional important factors for the development of peripheral edema. These mismatches are explained by the complex interplay among central hemodynamic factors, pulmonary factors, and peripheral circulation, as well as—as discussed in detail below—by neuroendocrine adaptation.

MYOCARDIAL ADAPTIONS IN CHRONIC HEART FAILURE

It is now clear that structural change in the heart often precedes the functional alterations that result in the typical HF symptoms (Table 2). Typical macroscopic findings are chamber dilation and myocardial hypertrophy. The hemodynamic benefit of dilation is that it initially makes possible to eject a similar stroke volume despite a reduced ejection fraction than a normal-sized ventricle with a normal ejection fraction. Myocardial hypertrophy initially helps to reduce ventricular wall tension and unloads individual muscle fibers, but in the long term it is a maladaptive process and increases myocardial oxygen demand. This change in focus to the endogenous factors that alter long-term structure of the myocardium and vasculature has revolutionized HF treatment. Activation of neurohormonal systems play an important role in the alterations in ventricular

Table 2
Myocardial Changes in CHF

Molecular changes within cardiomyocytes
  Calcium homeostasis
    Sarcoplasmatic reticulum calcium content ↓, SERCA 2a activity ↓, plasmalemmal Na^+/Ca^{2+}
    exchanger activity ↑
  β-adrenergic responsiveness
    Receptor density ↓, impaired signal transduction
  Contractile and regulatory proteins
    Myosin and troponin T isoform shifts, myosin ATPase activity ↓
  Energetics
    CK activity ↓, CK-MB ↑, creatine phosphate and ATP ↓
Structural changes (cardiac remodeling)
  Hypertrophy
  Dilatation
  Fibrosis
  Progressive loss of cardiomyocytes
    Necrosis or apoptosis

CK, creatine kinase, CK-MB, MB isoenzyme of CK.

architecture that occurs during the development of HF (cardiac remodeling). Therapies that have been effective in reducing HF mortality have been associated with a reduction in chamber remodeling. This structural process is in the long-term maladaptive, and it is therefore a key component of the progressive nature of HF *(9)*.

Ventricular remodeling involves the myocytes and interstitial myocardial components including collagen. HF is characterized by a number of neurohormonal abnormalities. In addition to its vasoconstrictor effect, angiotensin II is an important mediator of cardiomyocyte hypertrophy. Increased local and circulating norepinephrine contributes to myocardial hypertrophy either directly or secondarily by activating the RAAS. Similarly, circulating aldosterone increases the production of collagen by fibroblasts and thereby the deposition of interstitial collagen in the failing ventricle (cardiac fibrosis). The structural changes in the myocyte cannot occur in the absence of a remodeling of the collagen framework (matrix remodeling with degradation and replacement fibrosis) that surrounds individual myocytes and fiber bundles *(10)*. Proliferation of the extracellular matrix with interstitial fibrosis may reduce chamber dilation. Both angiotensin II and aldosterone play a major role in the genesis of myocardial fibrosis. Aldosterone is released systemically by the adrenal glands and locally in the myocardium. The whole aldosterone synthesis pathway is present in the myocardium and probably controlled by pathways similar to those of adrenocortical cells (tissue ACE system). The initial beneficial effect of angiotensin II is an increase in myocardial contractility. Interstitial myocardial fibrosis increases myocardial stiffness, reduces diastolic ventricular compliance, and is therefore important in the development of HF, in particular diastolic dysfunction. With increasing myocardial fibrosis capillary density decreases and diffusion distances from the capillaries to the cardiomyocytes increase. In addition, the cardiomyocytes are abnormally integrated into this newly formed extracellular matrix,

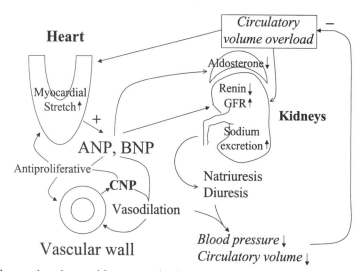

Fig. 4. The natriuretic peptide system in the regulation of circulatory homeostasis. GFR, Glomerular filtration rate; other abbreviations as defined in text.

which leads to slippage of myocytes *(10)*. The naturally occurring antagonists of cardiovascular remodeling are the natriuretic peptides (NPs), which limit the myocardial proliferative or hypertrophic and fibrotic response to damage and the remodeling of vessels (*see* Fig. 4). The clinical efficacy of ACE inhibitors is closely related to their inhibition of ventricular remodeling by lowering angiotensin II and aldosterone. ACE inhibitors also express their effect by increasing bradykinin- and kinin-mediated prostaglandin synthesis, which also modulates cardiomyocyte hypertrophy. At the receptor level angiotensin II receptor blockers and aldosterone receptor blockers (spironolactone) modulate the remodeling of the failing ventricle. β-blockers modify the hypertrophic and directly toxic effects of norepinephrine on the cardiomyocyte and also decrease the rate of apoptosis in HF. It is also recognized that myocyte loss or apoptosis may occur in the setting of HF and such myocyte disappearance also must be accompanied by collagen remodeling. It is likely that the cardiomyocytes and fibroblasts maintain some form of interactive communications. The degree of cardiac remodeling is influenced by left ventricular hemodynamic load, which is significantly influenced by the structural remodeling of the vasculature to alter compliance and resistance (afterload). Therefore, the link between hypertension and HF may be explained by the interaction of ventricular–vascular coupling, that is, the hemodynamic load imposed on the heart by the vascular remodeling in hypertension and the hormonal load imposed on the vasculature by the neurohormonal activation in HF.

Myocardial cell death is an important mechanism of HF. There are two principal causes: apoptosis and necrosis. As a consequence of cell dropout the load on the remaining cardiomyocytes is increased. Neurohormonal–cytokine abnormalities cause apoptosis, which usually occurs in a spotty manner throughout the ventricles. Ischemic necrosis usually causes more localized myocardial scarring. By contrast, myocardial hibernation (sometimes also called chronic stunning or prolonged ischemic left ventricular dysfunction) is a relatively common form of potentially reversible ischemic HF. The myocardium is hypoperfused with impaired contraction but still viable *(11)*.

MOLECULAR CHANGES
IN CARDIOMYOCYTES OF THE FAILING HEART

Familial cardiomyopathies are rare diseases that are based on genetically determined mutations of cardiac contractile and regulatory proteins, such as myosin and troponin isoforms *(12,13)*. However, important molecular changes at the levels of energetics, contractile responsiveness to SNS stimulation, and electromechanical coupling occur in all types of CHF, which finally lead to depressed myocardial contractility (Table 2).

In ventricular dysfunction, ventricular hypertrophy, and other cardiac pathologies with chronic hemodynamic pressure or volume overload, cardiomyocytes undergo phenotypic modifications and reexpress several fetal genes (Table 2), which may be energy-sparing *(9,12,13)*. In contrast to the growing fetal heart, the fetal expression pattern of sarcomeric proteins (e.g., myosin, troponin T) and the proteins of the calcium-handling machinery in cardiomyocytes of failing hearts leads to impairment of myocardial contraction and relaxation as well as cardiac dilation. The myosin heavy and light chain isoform shift leads to a reduced myosin ATPase activity. Calcium plays a central role in the regulation of myocardial contraction and relaxation. A reduced activity or expression of sarcoplasmic SERCA-2a, which mediates diastolic calcium reuptake by the sarcoplasmic reticulum, the calcium-release channel, and voltage-dependent calcium channel as well as an increased activity of the plasmalemmal Na–Ca transporter have been reported in failing hearts *(14)*. These changes lead to diastolic calcium overload with impaired relaxation and reduced sarcoplasmic reticulum calcium content with reduced systolic calcium release from the sarcoplasmic reticulum and reduced extracellular calcium influx and consequently impaired myocardial contractility, particularly with higher heart rates. In addition, abnormalities of the cytoskeletal proteins are found in CHF *(10)*.

β_1-Adrenergic receptors are down-regulated or have abnormalities in signal-transduction activity, which leads to an impaired responsiveness of the failing heart to sympathetic nerve stimulation or circulating norepinephrine with a decrease in contractility *(15)*.

Total high-energy phosphate stores (creatine phosphate, adenosine triphosphate) are also depressed in the failing heart. Creatine kinase activity is reduced; the expression of creatine kinase subunit B is up-regulated. Mitochondrial function is altered, and myocardial substrate utilization switches from free fatty acid to glucose. This imbalance between myocardial energy supply and demand impairs both cardiac contraction and relaxation *(11)*.

THE HEART AS AN ENDOCRINE ORGAN

The heart functions not only as a pump, but also as an endocrine organ. Twenty years ago, de Bold and co-workers *(16)* demonstrated the existence of the long-predicted natriuretic factor and the endocrine function of the heart. This discovery finally led to the characterization of a whole family of structurally similar but genetically distinct peptides, the NPs *(17)*. These looped peptides are the main hormones in the body's defense against volume overload and hypertension. Two members of the NP family, atrial natriuretic peptide (ANP) and brain natriuretic peptide (BNP), are mainly released in response to myocardial stretch induced by volume expansion and pressure overload of the heart (*see* Fig. 4). In addition, neurohormones activated in CHF, such as VP, phenylepinephrine, and endothelin, stimulate NP gene expression and release after binding to G-protein-coupled receptors. The NP system is up-regulated and activated to its highest degree in CHF. ANP and BNP are broadly involved in the regulation of blood pressure, blood volume, and sodium balance (Fig. 4). A third member of the family, C-type natriuretic peptide (CNP), is produced by the vascular endothelium and may be important as a paracrine factor in the regulation of vascular tone, its exact role in CHF remains unclear. NPs are the naturally occurring antagonists of the hormones of the RAAS and the SNS. NPs inhibit the secretion of VP and corticotropin, and inhibit salt appetite and water drinking as well as sympathetic tone in the central nervous system, and peripherally they increase glomerular filtration rate and natriuresis to protect the heart from acute volume loads. The hemodynamic effects of NP comprise a decrease in systemic and pulmonary vascular resistance, systemic and pulmonary arterial pressure (afterload), plasma volume, venous return and right atrial, pulmonary capillary wedge and left-ventricular end-diastolic pressures (preload), and dilation of coronary arteries with increased coronary blood flow. As a result the cardiac output increases and diastolic function improves. Besides their natriuretic, diuretic, vasodilatory, and renin as well as aldosterone inhibitory effects, NPs exert antimitotic and antifibrotic effects on cardiovascular tissues. NPs also lower the activation threshold of vagal efferents, thereby suppressing reflex tachycardia and vasoconstriction. Under physiological conditions ANPs and BNPs are mainly expressed in and released from atrial myocardium. In left ventricular hypertrophy or CHF, both NPs are highly up-regulated in ventricles and ventricular myocardium becomes the main source of circulating NPs, particularly BNP *(17,18)*.

NEUROHORMONAL ADAPTIVE MECHANISMS IN CHF

Understanding CHF has moved from a hemodynamic concept into accepting the importance of neuroendocrine pathophysiological changes in the progression of HF *(11)*. Baroreceptor dysfunction is an important link between vasomotor and neuroendocrine dysfunction. The SNS and RAAS are activated; VP is released nonosmotically (Fig. 3). The clinical signs and symptoms of CHF largely result from neurohormonal activation leading to vasoconstriction and renal salt and water retention. Low-pressure baroreceptors that are located in the atria react to volume expansion or increasing stretch by enhancing NP release from the heart. However, in overt CHF high-pressure baroreceptors override the low-pressure receptors, as sodium and water retention occur despite elevated atrial pressures. The association between elevation of levels of circulating effector hormones of the RAAS and the progression of CHF is now irrefutable, and all members of this system are increased in blood in patients with advanced HF. In the CONSENSUS study the improved prognosis associated with enalapril was accompanied by a reduction in plasma concentrations of aldosterone, angiotensin II, and renin *(19)*.

The Sympathetic Nervous System

The SNS activation is a hallmark of acute or chronic HF (Fig. 3). Besides its direct cardiovascular effects, which in the long term increase myocardial oxygen demand by increasing heart rate, myocardial wall tension, and contractility, the SNS is an important promotor of sodium and water retention through renal vasoconstriction, stimulation of the RAAS, and direct effects on the proximal convoluted tubule and exerts direct toxic effects on the myocardium (*see* above). There are complex interactions between the SNS and RAAS in HF. The activation of the renal SNS promotes renin release, and angiotensin II also potentiates SNS drive by direct stimulation and impairing its control by baroreceptors *(8)*.

The Renin–Angiotensin–Aldosterone System

Aldosterone plays a crucial pathophysiological role in CHF *(20)*. It is a steroid hormone synthesized from cholesterol in the mitochondria of the zona glomerulosa of the adrenal glands' cortex. Recent research demonstrated extraadrenal sites of aldosterone production, such as in cardiovascular tissue (*see* above). Adrenal glands do not store aldosterone but are capable of rapidly synthesizing it. Angiotensin II is the most important stimulus to aldosterone synthesis. Renin converts angiotensinogen, which is formed mainly in the liver and to a lesser extent in the kidneys and vascular endothelium, into angiotensin I. ACE is the major pathway that converts angiotensin I into angiotensin II. As a negative feedback, aldosterone and angiotensin II inhibit renin release. Apart from aldosterone secretion angiotensin II stimulates VP release and norepinephrine release. It is also a potent vasoconstrictor.

In CHF the decrease in renal blood flow and the increase in sympathetic tone promote aldosterone formation. Adrenal corticotropin, a stress hormone, and hyperkalemia also stimulate aldosterone synthesis. There are also several minor stimulators of aldosterone synthesis, such as endothelin, VP, catecholamines, prostaglandins, and nitric oxide, all of which are also affected by the process of HF. A potent inhibitor of aldosterone synthesis is ANP. Aldosterone is metabolized primarily in the liver. Hepatic blood flow and metabolism within the hepatocytes are potentially impaired in HF by congestion, and aldosterone clearance from the blood is reduced in advanced HF. Secondary hyperaldosteronism in HF has deleterious effects and worsens hemodynamic conditions, because an escape from the sodium-retaining action does not occur in CHF (*see* below). It perpetuates congestion by promoting renal sodium reabsorption and triggers hypokalemia and magnesium depletion with subsequent electrical instability and the risk for potentially life-threatening arrhythmias. Today, it is clear that aldosterone contributes to the progression of CHF not only via the classical renal mineralocorticoid effect, but also by a direct effect on the heart (fibrosis, remodeling; *see* above) and arterial vasculature (fibrosis and remodeling with decreased vascular compliance, endothelial dysfunction), and by blunting the baroreflex, which aggravates an imbalance in autonomic tone leading to a further increase in sympathetic tone.

Nonosmotic Release of Vasopressin

The neurohypophyseal hormone VP or antidiuretic hormone is crucial for the regulation of water conservation in the body, and under physiological conditions it plays little role in the control of vascular resistance and blood pressure *(21)*. VP and thirst are jointly involved in maintaining body fluid balance. An increase as small as 2% in plasma osmolality stimulates thirst and secretion of VP. VP is synthesized in specific neurons of the supraoptic and paraventricular nuclei and stored in the neurohypophysis. It is secreted in response to either increases in plasma osmolality detected by special osmoreceptor neurons in the hypothalamus (very sensitive stimulus) or as in HF to arterial underfilling detected by pressure-sensitive receptors in atria, aorta, and carotid sinus (less-sensitive stimulus). VP causes antidiuresis by activating peritubular V2 receptors in the collecting duct, which increases water permeability in the whole collecting duct (increased synthesis and shuttling of aquaphorin-2 water channels), urea permeability in the distal collecting duct, and sodium reabsorption in most of the collecting duct. Via binding to V1a receptors VP reduces blood flow to inner medulla without affecting blood flow to outer medulla. All these actions concur to increase urine osmolality.

Activation of carotid baroreceptors during arterial underfilling in CHF is essential for nonosmotic VP release and overrides activation of atrial receptors. VP is highly increased and sufficient to induce general systemic V1a receptor mediated vasoconstriction, which is crucial in attempting to limit the fall in blood pressure and includes a fall in kidney perfusion and glomerular filtration rate. Consequently, in patients with HF and hyponatremia, hypoosmolality, which inhibits the release of VP in normal subjects, is associated with persistently high plasma concentrations of VP *(21)*. ANP as its physiological inhibitor inhibits VP release in the neurohypophysis and its effect on water and ion transport in the collecting duct. Nonpeptide VP receptor antagonists have been developed and are currently being tested in first clinical studies as a new approach in CHF treatment *(22)*.

Endothelial Autocrine and Paracrine Factors

Prostacyclin and prostaglandin E are vasodilating factors produced from arachidonic acid in many cells, including the vascular endothelium. Catecholamines and angiotensin II are potent stimuli for their synthesis. These vasodilatory prostaglandins may counterbalance the neurohormone-induced systemic and renal vasoconstriction and are important for maintaining diuresis in HF patients.

Nitric oxide is an even more potent vasodilator than prostaglandins. The activity of the constitutive nitric oxide synthase is decreased in the endothelium of CHF patients, which is an important contribution to endothelial dysfunction observed in CHF. Similarly, endomyocardial nitric oxide gene expression is lower in patients with advanced CHF. Reduced myocardial nitric oxide content could lower ventricular diastolic distensibility and contribute to diastolic dysfunction *(23)*.

Adrenomedullin is a 52-amino-acid vasodilatory peptide that was originally isolated from human pheochromocytoma *(24)*. This autocrine or paracrine peptide, which belongs to the calcitonin, calcitonin-gene-related peptide, amylin family, is highly expressed in endothelial cells, and appears to be more than simply a vasodilator. It is unclear whether increased plasma adrenomedullin in disease states in a compensatory response to cardiovascular changes reflects an overflow from local sites of production and action or decreased clearance. In CHF a progressive increase in plasma adrenomedullin with disease severity has been reported, and in CHF there is also evidence for increased myocardial production of adrenomedullin *(24)*.

Endothelin-1 is another peptide secreted by the vascular endothelium. It is one of the most potent vasoconstrictors, has inotropic and mitogenic actions, modulates salt and water homeostasis, and plays an important role in the maintenance of vascular tone and blood pressure *(25)*. Endothelin-1 contributes to the systemic and renal vasoconstriction associated with severe HF, and it is also involved in cardiovascular remodeling (*see* above).

Plasma endothelin concentrations are increased in some HF patients and indicate a poor prognosis *(25)*. In failing hearts also an activation of the endothelin system is found; tissue concentrations and receptor density are increased. Up-regulation of the myocardial endothelin system may be beneficial in the short-term due to positive inotropic action, but in the long term it is harmful due to increased afterload and the induction of remodeling. Endothelin receptor antagonists showed beneficial effects in experimental heart failure animal models, and first clinical data in the treatment of HF patients are promising *(25)*.

Urotensin-II is another potent vasoconstrictor expressed within the human cardiovasculature that seems to be involved in the aberrant vasoconstriction found in CHF *(26)*.

In summary, these adaptive mechanisms of the endothelium in CHF patients result in vasoconstriction and endothelial dysfunction, which is characterized by an attenuated ischemia and exercise-induced vasodilation in the extremities.

Neurohormones in Asymptomatic Left Ventricular Dysfunction

NPs have an important role in maintaining the compensated state of HF and delaying the progression to overt HF by opposing vasoconstriction and renal sodium retention. NPs are important for maintenance of renal perfusion and urine flow in HF. NP activation is a beneficial humoral response in asymptomatic left ventricular dysfunction (LVD) and increased plasma concentrations of NP are frequently found in asymptomatic LVD. Although the activity of the SNS is increased, plasma levels of norepinephrine are within reference limits during this stage of the disease. Catecholamines are increased only in severe HF. Similarly the plasma concentrations of the hormones of the RAAS system are not increased in untreated patients with asymptomatic LVD because this system is completely suppressed by the NP. However, they may be increased secondarily by treatment of patients with diuretics, and loop diuretic treatment seems to be the main cause of increased plasma renin and angiotensin II in CHF. It is important to note that the tissue RAAS in the myocardium may be activated during compensated HF at a time when activity of the circulating system can be relatively normal. In summary, through a combination of ventricular dilation and hypertrophy, and the activation of vasoconstrictor and vasodilator forces, a delicate hemodynamic and neurohormonal balance is achieved, which restores cardiac function toward that before myocardial damage at minimum energetic cost (Figs. 3 and 4, Table 3). Vasoconstrictive and sodium retentive actions by the RAAS, SNS, VP, thromboxane, and endothelin are completely counter-regulated by NPs, nitric oxide, bradykinin, adrenomedullin, and prostaglandins. In addition to the important actions of endogenous NPs, pharmacological inhibition of the RAAS and SNS by ACE inhibitors and β-blockers slows HF progression.

Neurohormones in Symptomatic LVD

Overt HF develops when the compensatory hemodynamic and neurohormonal mechanisms are overwhelmed or exhausted. With the progression of the disease to overt HF, the NP cannot sufficiently counteract and suppress the SNS and RAAS. NP receptor down-regulation does not seem to be of great importance in the development of NP resistance in HF, because therapeutically administered NPs in decompensated HF patients are still effective and lead to an improved central hemodynamics with an increase in stroke volume *(17)*. Short-term infusions of NPs also decrease plasma renin and aldosterone

Table 3
Neurohormonal Systems Activated in CHF

Vasoconstrictors and promoters of renal sodium and water retention	Vasodilators and promotors of natriuresis and diuresis
Sympathetic nervous system (epinephrine, norepinephrine)	Natriuretic peptides
Renin–angiotensin–aldosterone system	Other vasodilators (prostaglandins, kallikrein-kinin system, calcitonin-gene-related peptide, adrenomedullin, nitric oxide)
Vasopressin	
Endothelin	
Urotensin-II	

concentrations and increase sodium and water excretion. Vasoconstrictor effects and salt and water retention predominate with the progression of CHF, which leads to development of the clinical signs and symptoms of HF and further deteriorates cardiac function. In overt HF also the hormones of the RAAS and norepinephrine are increased in plasma. In addition to these circulating factors there is an increased release of locally active vasoconstrictors produced by the vascular endothelium, for example, endothelin. In severe HF circulating NP, norepinephrine, renin, aldosterone, and endothelin are powerful prognostic markers and may be even helpful in the tailoring of CHF therapy *(18)*.

THE KIDNEYS AS THE MAIN EFFECTORS OF SODIUM AND WATER RETENTION IN CHF

The renal excretion of sodium and water normally parallels sodium and water intake, so that an increase in intravascular fluid volume is associated with increased renal sodium and water excretion. In CHF sodium and water are paradoxically retained. From 1940 through 1960 HF was thought to result primarily from renal hypoperfusion, and also in the current HF model the kidneys are the main effectors of sodium and water retention in CHF *(11,27)*. When, irrespective of the CHF etiology, cardiac output or effective circulating volume falls below physiologically acceptable limits, extrarenal and renal baroreceptors sense arterial underfilling (Fig. 2), which sets in motion a vicious cycle through a continuous stimulation of the RAAS. Arterial underfilling triggers the release of catecholamines, angiotensin II, endothelin, and VP. Subsequently, renal vascular resistance rises and renal plasma flow is reduced relatively more than the glomerular filtration rate, which leads to an increase in the filtration fraction. The basis for this is that angiotensin II, norepinephrine, endothelin, and VP constrict the efferent glomerular arteriole more than the afferent. An increase in the filtration fraction leads to an increase in the sodium reabsorption in the proximal tubule. In addition, the SNS and angiotensin II directly enhance proximal tubular sodium reabsorption. As a consequence, sodium delivery to the distal tubule and collecting duct is diminished. This stimulates renal renin release, which in turn causes increased production of angiotensin II. Angiotensin II is also the major stimulus for aldosterone secretion in the adrenal glands, and aldosterone enhances sodium reabsorption in the distal renal tubule. In patients who are dependent on angiotensin II mediated efferent arterial vasoconstriction, such as individuals with renal artery stenosis, to maintain glomerular capillary pressure and filtration rate, ACE inhibitors or angiotensin II receptor blockers compromise renal function.

In a counter-regulatory effort to maintain plasma volume homeostasis, the NP system is highly activated in CHF. In the kidneys NPs stimulate the dilation of afferent renal arterioles and the constriction of efferent arterioles, leading to increased pressure in glomerular capillaries with an increase in glomerular filtration. NPs relax mesangial cells and thereby increase the effective surface area for filtration. ANP redistributes blood flow to the renal outer medullary region, thereby promoting diuresis. NPs also increase natriuresis by direct tubular actions, that is, inhibition of sodium reabsorption in the collection duct. They inhibit renal renin release from the macula densa and aldosterone release from the zona glomerulosa. NPs inhibit tubular water transport by antagonizing the action of VP. With the progression of HF the glomerular filtration rate decreases, and there is increased sodium reabsorption in the proximal tubule with decreased sodium delivery to the collecting duct, the place of action of NP. This explains NP resistance and the lack of escape from secondary hyperaldosteronism in advanced HF *(28)*. Finally, in CHF the natriuretic and diuretic systems cannot sufficiently suppress the sodium- and water-retaining systems. Consequently, the kidneys retain sodium, and HF patients develop pulmonary congestion and peripheral edema.

CYTOKINES IN HF

Several peptide growth factors and inflammatory cytokines appear to be involved in HF. These growth factors may mediate the structural changes in the failing heart. Activation of various cytokines may also contribute to cardiac dysfunction and to the clinical syndrome and disease progression by direct toxic effects on the heart and circulation ("cytokine hypothesis" of CHF), particularly in more advanced stages. Cytokines and nitric oxide may contribute to the reversible myocardial depression by mediating alterations in excitation–contraction coupling and β-adrenergic desensitization. It has now been well established that patients with HF exhibit elevated plasma concentrations of proinflammatory mediators, such as tumor necrosis factor-alpha (TNF-α), interleukin (IL)-1, or IL-6 *(29–31)*. Many aspects of CHF can be explained by the known biological effects of TNF-α, for example, TNF-α depresses myocardial function and induces apoptosis. Increased tissue TNF-α concentrations have also been reported in failing human hearts in the absence of a demonstrable inflammatory infiltrate, and TNF-α may play a role in the process of ventricular remodeling *(29)*. ILs (e.g., IL-1β, IL-6) also appear to be involved in the pathophysiology of HF, and IL-6 and related cytokines are involved in the regulation of cardiomyocyte hypertrophy and apoptosis. IL-6 and TNF-α plasma concentrations are independent prognostic markers of mortality in CHF patients *(29,30)*. Thus, the activation of cytokines along with angiotensin II, norepinephrine, and other neurohormones appears to play an important role in the progressive deterioration of CHF. There is now a growing body of evidence that suggests that modulating cytokine levels may represent a new therapeutic option in patients with CHF.

CONCLUSIONS

The traditional view of HF was to consider HF as a hemodynamic derangement of the left ventricle. This traditional concept of this common disease has now undergone a major revision. Instead HF is a progressive structural process altering the shape and volume of the chamber of the left ventricle, the cellular composition of the ventricular wall, and the structure of the vasculature into which the left ventricle must empty. Improvement in the contraction of the left ventricle is no longer the sole focus of CHF treatment. Attention must be directed also to the progressive structural processes that lead to adverse events and disease progression. Complex activation of neurohormonal systems is crucial for disease progression, and pharmacotherapy in CHF should aim at antagonizing the detrimental effects of neurohumoral activation. Arterial underfilling is sensed by renal and extrarenal baroreceptors, which activate neurohormonal effectors, such as SNS, RAAS, VP, and endothelin. Sodium and water retention is induced by reduced renal plasma flow, constriction of the efferent glomerular arteriole, enhanced proximal and distal tubular sodium reabsorption, increased renal water reabsorption, and increased renin as well as aldosterone release. Over the long term, these neurohormonal reflexes have deleterious effects. In asymptomatic HF vasoconstriction and fluid retention are counter-regulated by activation of vasodilatory and natriuretic substances, such as NPs, prostaglandin, nitric oxide, and adrenomedullin. In advanced HF vasoconstriction and sodium and water retention predominate. Newer drugs on the horizon for HF treatment include the neuropeptidase inhibitors, such as omapatrilat, which block the RAAS system and at the same time decrease the degradation of NPs *(32)*. Neurohormonal markers also gained attention as diagnostic and prognostic markers in HF patients. Recently, it was demonstrated that neurohormones are useful markers for treatment guidance. Of all neurohormonal parameters the NPs, in particular BNP and N-terminal-proBNP, proved to be the most promising markers for these purposes, and measurement of these NPs has already been included into recent guidelines on the diagnosis of HF *(5,18)*.

ABBREVIATIONS

ACE, Angiotensin converting enzyme; ANP, BNP, CNP, atrial, brain, and C-type natriuretic peptide; CAD, coronary artery disease; CHF, chronic heart failure; HF, heart failure; IL, interleukin; LVD, left ventricular dysfunction; RAAS, renin–angiotensin–aldosterone system; SNS, sympathetic nervous system; TNF-α, tissue necrosis factor-α; VP, vasopressin.

REFERENCES

1. Sharpe N, Doughty R. Epidemiology of heart failure and left ventricular dysfunction (review). Lancet 1998;352(Suppl I):3–7.
2. Poole-Wilson PA, Buller NP. Causes of symptoms in chronic congestive heart failure and implications for treatment (review). Am J Cardiol 1988;62:31A–34A.
3. Packer M. The neurohormonal hypothesis: a theory to explain the mechanism of disease progression in heart failure. J Am Coll Cardiol 1992;20:248–254.
4. Colucci WS, Braunwald E. Pathophysiology of heart failure. In: Heart Disease. Braunwald E, ed. Philadelphia: WB Saunders, 1997, pp. 394–444.
5. Task Force for the Diagnosis and Treatment of Chronic Heart Failure, European Society of Cardiology. Guidelines for the diagnosis and treatment of chronic heart failure. Eur Heart J 2001;22:1527–1560.
6. Schwinger RH, Bohm M, Koch A, et al. The failing human heart is unable to use the Frank–Starling mechanism. Circ Res 1994;74:959–969.
7. Mulieri LA, Hasenfuss G, Leavitt B, Allen PD, Alpert NR. Altered myocardial force-frequency relation in human heart failure. Circulation 1992;85:1743–1750.

8. Schrier RW, Abraham WT. Hormones and hemodynamics in heart failure (review). N Engl J Med 1999;341:577–585.
9. Gerdes AM, Capasso JM. Structural remodeling and mechanical dysfunction of cardiac myocytes in heart failure. J Mol Cell Cardiol 1995;27:849–856.
10. Jane-Lise S. The extracellular matrix and cytoskeleton in heart hypertrophy and failure (review). Heart Fail Rev 2000;5:239–250.
11. Braunwald E. Congestive Heart failure: a half century perspective. Eur Heart J 2001;22: 825–836.
12. Miyata S, Minobe WA, Bristow MR, Leinwand LA. Myosin heavy chain isoform expression in the failing and non-failing human heart. Circ Res 2000;86:386–390.
13. Anderson PA, Malouf NN, Oakeley AE, Pagani ED, Allen PD. Troponin T isoform expression in humans. A comparison among normal and failing adult heart, fetal heart, and adult and fetal skeletal muscle. Circ Res 1991;69:1226–1233.
14. Hasenfuss G. Alterations in calcium-regulatory proteins in heart failure (review). Cardiovasc Res 1998;37:279–289.
15. Brodde OE, Michel MC, Zerkowski HR. Signal transduction mechanisms controlling cardiac contractility and their alterations in heart failure. Cardiovasc Res 1995;30:570–584.
16. de Bold AJ, Borenstein HB, Veress AT, Sonnenberg H. A rapid and potent natriuretic response to intravenous injection of atrial myocardial extracts in rats. Life Sci 1981;28:89–94.
17. Vesely DL. Atrial natriuretic peptides in pathophysiological diseases (review). Cardiovasc Res 2001;51:647–658.
18. Mair J, Hammerer-Lercher A, Puschendorf B. The impact of cardiac natriuretic peptide determination on the diagnosis and management of heart failure (review). Clin Chem Lab Med 2001;39:571–588.
19. Swedberg K, Eneroth P, Kjekshus J, Snapinn S. Effects of enalapril and neuroendocrine activation on prognosis in severe congestive heart failure (follow-up of the CONSENSUS trial). CONSENSUS trial study group. Am J Cardiol 1990;66:44D–45D.
20. Ferrari R. The harmful effects of aldosterone in heart failure (review). Eur Heart J Supplements 2000;2(Suppl A):A6–A12.
21. Bankir L. Antidiuretic action of vasopressin: quantitative aspects and interactions between V1a and V2 receptor-mediated effects (review). Cardiovasc Res 2001;51:372–390.
22. Wong LL, Verbalis JG. Vasopressin V2 receptor antagonists (review). Cardiovasc Res 2001; 51:391–402.
23. Paulus WJ. The role of nitric oxide in the failing heart (review). Heart Fail Rev 2001;6: 105–118.
24. Hinson JP, Kapas S, Smith DM. Adrenomedullin, a multifunctional regulatory peptide (review). Endocr Rev 2000;21:138–167.
25. Giannesi D, Del Ry S, Vitale RL. The role of endothelins and their receptors in heart failure (review). Pharmacol Res 2001;43:111–126.
26. Douglas SA, Ohlstein EH. Human urotensin-II, the most potent mammalian vasoconstrictor identified to date, as a therapeutic target for the management of cardiovascular disease (review). Trends Cardiovasc Med 2000;10:229–237.
27. Hess B. Chronic heart failure: pathophysiology and therapeutic approaches–why is the kidney so important (review)? Eur Heart J Suppl 2001;3(Suppl G):G3–G7.
28. Inoue T, Nonoguchi H, Tomita K. Physiological effects of vasopressin and atrial natriuretic peptide in the collecting duct (review). Cardiovasc Res 2001;51:470–480.
29. Mann DL. Recent insights into the role of tumor necrosis factor in the failing heart (review). Heart Fail Rev 2001;6:71–90.
30. Wollert KC, Drexler H. The role of interleukin-6 in the failing heart (review). Heart Fail Rev 2001;6:95–103.
31. Long CS. The role of interleukin-1 in the failing heart (review). Heart Fail Rev 2001;6:81–94.
32. Sagnella GA. Atrial natriuretic peptide mimetics and vasopeptidase inhibitors (review). Cardiovasc Res 2001;51:416–428.

23

B-Type Natriuretic Peptide

Biochemistry and Measurement

Jeffrey R. Dahlen

BIOCHEMISTRY OF BNP

Identification

In 1988, Sudoh and co-workers first isolated a novel peptide from porcine brain and designated the peptide "brain natriuretic peptide," or BNP, based on its similarity to atrial natriuretic peptide (ANP) *(1)*. BNP also was isolated from the cardiac tissue of pigs, rats, and humans *(2–5)*. Owing to its presence in cardiac tissue, the designation "brain natriuretic peptide" is a misnomer. Hence, the designation "B-type natriuretic peptide" is currently used. Subsequent immunological studies identified the cardiac ventricle as the major source of circulating BNP in humans *(6)*. Additional studies indicated that the left ventricle is the major source of circulating BNP and that the release of BNP into the circulation is stimulated by increased ventricular wall tension and volume overload *(7–11)*.

Synthesis and Structure

The BNP gene is located in tandem with the ANP gene on the short arm of chromosome 1 in humans *(12)*. The gene is composed of three exons separated by two introns, and the majority of the BNP gene product is encoded by the second exon *(11)*. BNP messenger RNA, unlike ANP, contains a series of adenosine and uridine nucleotide repeat units, AUUUA, in the 3' untranslated region. This conserved sequence is known to destabilize mRNA by directing removal of the poly(A) tail, which may result in a shorter half-life of the BNP message *(13–15)*. BNP mRNA synthesis occurs at basal levels and is induced by angiotensin II and mechanical strain, which are reflective of volume overload and hemodynamic stress *(16–18)*.

BNP is synthesized as an inactive 134-amino-acid precursor molecule, preproBNP, that is composed of a 26-amino-acid signal peptide and a 108-amino-acid precursor molecule, proBNP. PreproBNP is converted to proBNP through cleavage of the signal peptide during BNP synthesis. ProBNP is subsequently cleaved in the cardiac myocyte to produce an active 32-amino-acid 3.5-kDa BNP neurohormone and an inactive 76-amino-acid peptide, amino- (N)-terminal proBNP (NT-proBNP). BNP, like ANP, has a 17-amino-acid ring structure produced by a cysteine disulfide bond, and extensions on the N-terminal and carboxy- (C)-terminal ends of nine and six amino acids, respectively

From: *Cardiac Markers, Second Edition*
Edited by: Alan H. B. Wu @ Humana Press Inc., Totowa, NJ

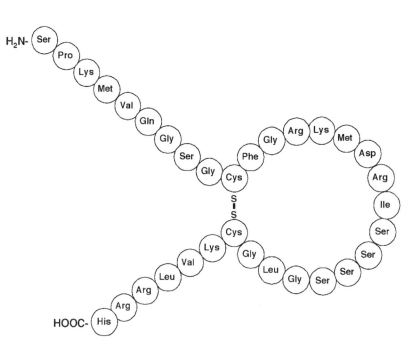

Fig. 1. Structure of the BNP molecule.

(Fig. 1). The ring structures of BNP and ANP share a high degree of sequence homology, differing by only five amino acid residues *(11)*. Although the mechanism of BNP production from proBNP is unclear, the cleavage site has the sequence Arg[73]–Ala[74]–Pro[75]–Arg[76] immediately preceding the cleavage site. This sequence conforms to the minimal sequence, Arg–Xaa–Xaa–Arg, required for efficient processing by the archetypical prohormone convertase furin, a ubiquitously expressed membrane-bound calcium-dependent serine endoproteinase that cleaves a wide variety of proteins in the exocytic and endocytic pathways *(19,20)*. Selective inhibition of furin in cultured rat cardiocytes suppressed the liberation of active BNP from proBNP, suggesting that furin is involved in the processing of proBNP in vivo *(21)*. Immunocytochemical studies have localized intracellular BNP to the cardiac secretory granules, and BNP release from cardiac tissue is stimulated by a stretch-pressure mechanism *(8,9)*.

Mechanism of Action and Metabolism

BNP has potent natriuretic, diuretic, and vasorelaxant effects primarily through its counteraction of the renin–angiotensin–aldosterone system (RAAS). The physiological actions of BNP are mediated through its binding to natriuretic peptide receptor A (NPR-A), a transmembrane receptor found in various tissues, including the vasculature and the heart *(22,23)*. Three transmembrane NPRs have been identified: NPR-A, NPR-B, and NPR-C. The NPR-A and NPR-B receptors are similar in size, structure, and sequence, and both contain intracellular guanylate cyclase and kinase-like domains *(11)*. NPR-C, unlike NPR-A and NPR-B, does not have guanylate cyclase activity, and has a short 37-amino-acid intracellular component. NPR-A and NPR-B mediate the biological activity of the natriuretic peptides through the intracellular production of the second messenger cGMP, and NPR-C appears to function mainly as a clearance receptor. NPR-A is

Table 1
Specificity of Natriuretic Peptide Receptors

Receptor	Specificity
NPR-A	ANP ≥ BNP >> CNP
NPR-B	CNP > ANP ≥ BNP
NPR-C	ANP > CNP > BNP

expressed in lung, kidney, adrenal, heart, adipose tissue, pituitary, cerebellum, and eye *(9,13)*. NPR-B is expressed in the adrenal medulla, pituitary, heart, and cerebellum *(9, 11)*, and NPR-C is expressed in the sympathetic trunk, vasculature, kidney, adrenal, heart, brain, and pituitary *(11)*. NPR-A selectively binds ANP and BNP; NPR-B selectively binds C-type natriuretic peptide (CNP); and NPR-C exhibits broad specificity to ANP, BNP, and CNP *(9,11)*. The relative rank order of NPR specificity is described in Table 1. To date, no specific BNP receptor has been identified.

BNP has a metabolic clearance rate in humans similar to that of ANP and CNP (approx 6 L/min), but has a longer half-life (approx 20 min vs approx 3 min for ANP and CNP) *(9,11,13,24)*. The N-terminal portion of the proBNP molecule, NT-proBNP, has a longer half-life, estimated to be 60–120 min *(25)*. The clearance of BNP from the circulation appears to be controlled by receptor-mediated endocytosis by NPR-C and proteolytic degradation by the zinc-containing neutral endopeptidase 24.11 (NEP) *(9)*. NEP was initially cloned and sequenced from a human placenta cDNA library, and it is expressed in numerous tissues, including vascular smooth muscle, kidney, and skeletal muscle *(26)*. NEP has broad specificity for the natriuretic peptides, with preference for CNP, followed by ANP, and then BNP. NEP is a membrane-bound enzyme that cleaves BNP between Met^{80} and Val^{81} near the N-terminus *(27)*. Regulation of NEP activity is thought to be achieved through control of the amount of NEP on cell surfaces. The tissue distribution of NEP and NPR-C suggests that these unique mechanisms for BNP metabolism play a role not only in the clearance of BNP, but also in modulating the local concentration and effects of BNP.

MEASUREMENT OF BNP IN CLINICAL SPECIMENS

A wealth of scientific literature exists that establishes the relevance of BNP measurements in assisting the diagnosis and management of patients with congestive heart failure (CHF) (for reviews *see 28–31*). Furthermore, there is evidence that BNP measurements in patients with acute coronary syndromes (ACS) within the first few days after onset are of prognostic significance *(32)*. Early analysis of BNP in clinical specimens was performed using an immunoradiometric assay *(33)*. Shionogi & Co., Ltd. (Osaka, Japan) produces the Shionoria BNP test, an immunoradiometric assay that quantifies the amount of BNP in ethylenediaminetetraacetic acid (EDTA)-anticoagulated plasma, that is available in the United States not for diagnostic purposes, but for research use only *(34)*. The Shionoria BNP test procedure is completed in approx 24 h. The test measures BNP molecules sandwiched between a bead-coated mouse monoclonal anti-BNP antibody specific

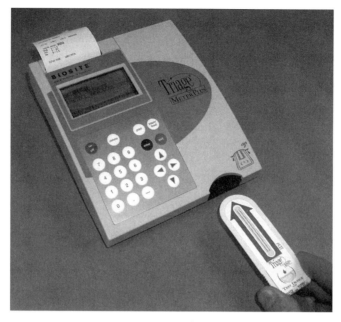

Fig. 2. The Triage® BNP Test.

to the C-terminal portion of BNP, and a mouse monoclonal anti-BNP antibody labeled with radioactive ^{125}I that is specific to the ring portion of BNP. After its release in Europe in 1999, Biosite® Incorporated introduced the Triage® BNP Test into the U. S. marketplace in the year 2000, the first test cleared by the U.S. Food and Drug Administration for use as an aid in the diagnosis of CHF (Fig. 2). The Triage BNP Test has been adopted for diagnostic use in clinical practice and also is used for clinical research. The Triage BNP Test is safer to use because it does not contain radioactive ingredients, and has the added benefits of producing rapid results (approx 15 min), performing accurate measurements in whole blood or plasma, and requiring fewer procedural steps *(35,36)*. Furthermore, the Triage BNP Test is portable, making it ideal for use in a point-of-care setting.

Triage BNP Test

The Triage BNP Test is a fluorescence immunoassay used to quantify the BNP concentration in EDTA-anticoagulated human whole blood or plasma. The test is performed by adding a small volume of specimen to a small test device or "protein chip." The protein chip contains all the reagents necessary to perform the test. The protein chip is then placed into the Triage Meter, which measures and displays the BNP concentration automatically after the reaction is completed, in approx 15 min.

Triage® BNP Test Procedure

The test is performed by first adding several drops (approx 250 μL) of EDTA-anticoagulated whole blood or plasma to the Triage BNP protein chip. After addition of a blood sample to the sample port of the protein chip, the red blood cells are separated from the plasma via a filter. A predetermined quantity of plasma moves by microcapillary action into a reaction chamber and is allowed to react with fluorescent antibody conjugates within the reaction chamber to form a reaction mixture. The fluorescent antibody conjugates contain a mouse polyclonal antibody that specifically binds the BNP molecule. After an incubation period, the reaction mixture flows through the protein array detection microcapillary. Complexes of the analyte and fluorescent antibody conjugates are captured on discrete zones on the protein array. The BNP–fluorescent antibody conjugate complexes are captured by murine monoclonal antibodies directed to the ring portion of the BNP molecule. Excess plasma washes the unbound fluorescent antibody conjugates from the protein array microcapillary into a waste reservoir. The Triage Meter is a portable fluorometer that quantifies the amount of fluorescence bound to the discrete zones on the protein array. The concentration of the analyte in the specimen is calculated and displayed automatically by the Triage Meter using an internal reagent lot-specific calibration curve, and is proportional to the fluorescence bound to the detection lane *(36)*. BNP measurements on whole blood and plasma are equivalent; the correlation is $y = 0.925x + 13.439$, $r = 0.9878$.

Diagnostic Utility

The diagnostic utility of the Triage BNP Test was determined through an analysis of BNP measurements on a population of more than 800 individuals with CHF and more than 1200 individuals without CHF *(36)*. The area under the receiver operating characteristic (ROC) curve was 0.955 ± 0.005. These data validate the results previously described in the scientific literature that indicate a high degree of separation in the distributions of BNP concentrations in individuals with and without CHF. The most appropriate decision threshold, or cutoff, for the diagnosis of CHF using the Triage BNP Test was determined by calculating the 95th percentile of BNP concentration in individuals without CHF who were age 55 and older, since it is within this population that CHF is most prevalent *(37)*. The absence of CHF in this population was confirmed through an analysis of echocardiography data. Using a cutoff of 100 pg/mL, the Triage BNP Test has an overall sensitivity and specificity for the diagnosis of CHF across all ages and both genders of 80.6% and 98.0%, respectively. In patients with CHF, increases in BNP concentration were significantly associated with the New York Heart Association classification of CHF. IN addition, BNP concentrations were significantly increased in CHF patients with preserved systolic function, or diastolic dysfunction, and separated from the distribution of BNP concentrations in individuals without CHF, with an area under the ROC curve of 0.934 ± 0.012 *(38)*.

NT-proBNP has been identified as an alternative marker for CHF, as it, like BNP, is significantly elevated in association with CHF *(39)*. While the extent of published reports on the effectiveness of NT-proBNP is significantly less than the reports on the effectiveness of BNP, it appears that the utility of NT-proBNP approaches and is, at best, equivalent to the utility of BNP in diagnosing left ventricular dysfunction *(40)*. However, because the clearance rate of NT-proBNP appears to be at least three times slower than that of BNP, BNP may be more effective as a marker of current ventricular status. Furthermore, because NT-proBNP appears to be renally cleared, the presence of renal dysfunction may adversely affect the clinical utility of NT-proBNP. Measurements of NT-proBNP were not able to detect acute changes in preload during hemodialysis and were less useful than BNP measurements in detecting ventricular hypertrophy and functional cardiac impairment *(41)*.

Comparison Between the Triage BNP and the Shionoria BNP Tests

The Triage BNP and Shionoria BNP tests have a similar assay range, 5–5000 pg/mL for Triage BNP and 4–2000 pg/mL for Shionoria BNP *(33,35)*. Two independent published studies have described the correlation between these two methods *(42,43)*. Both reports indicate a nearly identical correlation coefficient ($r = 0.96$, $n = 145$ and $r = 0.94$, $n = 70$), and similar linear slopes of approx 1.5, although the slope has been reported to be as low as 0.93 with a similar correlation coefficient ($r = 0.93$, $n = 83$) *(44)*. Although the two methods use different antibodies, the primary differences are in the detection method and procedure. The Shionoria BNP test requires the use of a gamma scintillation counter to measure bound radioactivity. The amount of bound radioactivity is converted to concentration using a calibration curve that must be generated with each batch of samples that are analyzed *(34)*. The Shionoria BNP test also requires extensive manipulation of reagents during the test procedure. The test requires addition and aspiration of reagents to the reaction vessel, and results are obtained in approx 24 h *(34)*. In contrast, the Triage BNP Test is a self-contained portable immunoassay that uses fluorescence-based detection to measure the BNP concentration *(36)*. There is no requirement for manipulation of reagents during the test procedure, and the test is completed in approx 15 min *(36)*.

BNP Stability

There have been various reports on the stability of BNP in whole blood and plasma. Various studies indicate that BNP is stable in EDTA-anticoagulated whole blood or plasma specimens at room temperature for at least 24 h, and the stability is prolonged through refrigerated storage *(45–49)*. However, it is recommended that BNP measurements using the Triage BNP Test be performed within 4 h of specimen collection *(36)*. The presence of the proteinase inhibitor aprotinin may be useful in prolonging the stability of BNP in specimens frozen at –20°C *(49)*. It has been reported that the stability of BNP is enhanced when the blood specimen is collected in plastic polyethylene terephthalate collection tubes *(34,50)*. Although the selection of blood collection tube type does not significantly affect BNP measurements within the first 4 h after blood sampling, it appears that the stability of BNP in whole blood specimens may be enhanced by collecting the blood specimen in plastic tubes *(50)*.

SUMMARY

BNP is a potent natriuretic, diuretic, and vasorelaxant neurohormone that is secreted mainly from the cardiac ventricles in response to increased ventricular stretch and pressure. BNP, like other neurohormones, is synthesized as an inactive precursor molecule, proBNP, that is subsequently proteolytically processed to yield the active BNP hormone and the inactive NT-proBNP peptide. BNP elicits its physiological effects primarily through binding to NPR-A, and its removal from the circulation is controlled through receptor-mediated endocytosis and proteolytic degradation by NPR-C and NEP, respectively. BNP measurements have been demonstrated to have utility in the assisting diagnosis and management of patients with CHF, and also have prognostic significance when measured shortly after the onset of ACS. The Triage BNP Test is a rapid, accurate, and reliable method for the quantification of BNP in EDTA-anticoagulated whole blood and plasma specimens. The test can be performed either at the point-of-care or in the clinical laboratory. Furthermore, the test has a clinically validated benefit in assisting physicians with diagnostic decisions.

ABBREVIATIONS

ACS, Acute coronary syndrome(s); ANP, BNP, CNP, A-type, B-type, and C-type natriuretic peptides; CHF, congestive heart failure; EDTA, ethylenediaminetetraacetic acid; NEP, neutral endopeptidase; NPR, natriuretic peptide receptor; NT-proBNP, amino-terminal proBNP; RAAS, renin–angiotensin–aldosterone system; ROC, receiver operating characteristic.

REFERENCES

1. Sudoh T, Kangawa K, Minamino N, Matsuo H. A new natriuretic peptide in porcine brain. Nature 1988;332:78–81.
2. Saito Y, Nakao K, Itoh H, et al. Brain natriuretic peptide is a novel cardiac hormone. Biochem Biophys Res Commun 1989;158:360–368.
3. Itoh H, Nakao K, Kamhayashi Y, et al. Occurrence of a novel cardiac natriuretic peptide in rats. Biochem Biophys Res Commun 1989;161:732–739.
4. Kamhayashi Y, Nakao K, Itoh H, et al. Isolation and sequence determination of rat cardiac natriuretic peptide. Biochem Biophys Res Commun 1989;163:233–240.
5. Kamhayashi Y, Nakao K, Mukoyama M, et al. Isolation and sequence determination of human brain natriuretic peptide in human atrium. FEBS Lett 1990;259:341–345.
6. Mukoyama M, Nakao K, Hosoda K, et al. Brain natriuretic peptide as a novel cardiac hormone in humans. J Clin Invest 1991;87:1402–1412.
7. Yasue H, Yoshimura M, Sumida H, et al. Localization and mechanism of secretion of B-type natriuretic peptide in comparison with those of A-type natriuretic peptide in normal subjects and patients with heart failure. Circulation 1994;90:195–203.
8. McDowell G, Shaw C, Buchanan KD, Nicholls DP. The natriuretic peptide family. Eur J Clin Invest 1995;25:291–298.
9. Davidson NC, Struthers AD. Brain natriuretic peptide. J Hypertens 1994;12:329–336.
10. de Bold AJ, Bruneau BG, Kuroski de Bold ML. Mechanical and neuroendocrine regulation of the endocrine heart. Cardiovasc Res 1996;31:7–18.
11. Yandle TG. Biochemistry of natriuretic peptides. J Intern Med 1994;235:561–576.
12. Tamura N, Ogawa Y, Yasoda A, et al. Two cardiac natriuretic peptide genes (atrial natriuretic peptide and brain natriuretic peptide) are organized in tandem in the mouse and human genomes. J Mol Cell Cardiol 1996;28:1811–1815.
13. Espiner EA, Richards AM, Yandle TG, Nicholls MG. Natriuretic hormones. Endocrinol Metab Clin North Am 1995;24:481–509.
14. Wilson T, Treisman R. Removal of poly(A) and consequent degradation of c-fos mRNA facilitated by 3' AU-rich sequences. Nature 1988;336:396–399.
15. Shaw G, Kamen R. A conserved AU sequence from the 3' untranslated region of GM-CSF mRNA mediates selective mRNA degradation. Cell 1986;46:659–667.
16. Liang F, Wu J, Garam M, Gardner DG. Mechanical strain increases expression of the brain natriuretic peptide gene in rat cardiac myocytes. J Biol Chem 1997;272:28050–28056.
17. Magga J, Vuolteenaho O, Tokola H, et al. B-type natriuretic peptide: a myocyte-specific marker for characterizing load-induced alterations in cardiac gene expression. Ann Med 1998;30(Suppl 1):39–45.
18. Weise S, Breyer T, Dragu A, et al. Gene expression of brain natriuretic peptide in isolated atrial and ventricular human myocardium. Circulation 2000;102:3074–3079.

19. Molloy SS, Bresnahan PA, Leppla SH, et al. Human furin is a calcium-dependent serine endoprotease that recognizes the sequence Arg–X–X–Arg and efficiently cleaves anthrax toxin protective antigen. J Biol Chem 1992;267:16396–16402.

20. Dahlen JR, Jean F, Thomas G, et al. Inhibition of soluble recombinant furin by human proteinase inhibitor 8. J Biol Chem 1998;273:1851–1854.

21. Sawada Y, Suda M, Yokoyama H, et al. Stretch-induced hypertrophic growth of cardiocytes and processing of brain-type natriuretic peptide are controlled by proprotein-processing endoprotease furin. J Biol Chem 1997;272:20545–20554.

22. Lin X, Hanze J, Heese F, et al. Gene expression of natriuretic peptide receptors in myocardial cells. Circ Res 1995;77:750–758.

23. Matsukawa N, Grzesik WJ, Takahashi N, et al. The natriuretic peptide clearance receptor locally modulates the physiological effects of the natriuretic peptide system. Proc Natl Acad Sci USA 1999;96:7403–7408.

24. Holmes SJ, Espiner EA, Richards AM, et al. Renal, endocrine, and hemodynamic effects of human brain natriuretic peptide in normal man. J Clin Endocrinol Metab 1993;76:91–96.

25. Mair J, Friedl W, Thomas S, Puschendorf B. Natriuretic peptides in assessment of left-ventricular dysfunction. Scan J Clin Lab Invest 1999;59 (Suppl 230):132–142.

26. Malfroy B, Kuang WJ, Seeburg PH, et al. Molecular cloning and amino acid sequence of human enkephalinase (neutral endopeptidase). FEBS Lett 1988;229:206–210.

27. Kenny AJ, Bourne A, Ingram J. Hydrolysis of human and pig brain natriuretic peptides, urodilatin, C-type natriuretic peptide and some C-receptor ligands by endopeptidase 24.11. Biochem J 1993;291:83–88.

28. Maisel A. B-type natriuretic peptide in the diagnosis and management of congestive heart failure. Cardiol Clin 2001;19:557–571.

29. Mair J, Hammerer-Lercher A, Puschendorf B. The impact of cardiac natriuretic peptide determination on the diagnosis and management of heart failure. Clin Chem Lab Med 2001; 39:571–588.

30. Sagnella GA. Measurement and significance of circulating natriuretic peptides in cardiovascular disease. Clin Sci 1998;95:519–529.

31. de Lemos JA, Morrow DA, Bentley JH, et al. The prognostic value of B-type natriuretic peptide in patients with acute coronary syndromes. N Engl J Med 2001;345:1014–1021.

32. Mair J, Friedl W, Thomas S, Puschendorf B. Natriuretic peptides in assessment of left-ventricular dysfunction. Scand J Clin Lab Invest Suppl 1999;230:132–142.

33. Tateyama H, Hino J, Minamino N, et al. Characterization of immunoreactive brain natriuretic peptide in human cardiac atrium. Biochem Biophys Res Commun 1990;166:1080–1087.

34. Shionoria BNP package insert. Shionogi & Co., Osaka, Japan.

35. Peacock WF. The B-type natriuretic peptide assay: a rapid test for heart failure. Cleve Clin J Med 2002;69:243–251.

36. Triage® BNP Test package insert. Biosite, San Diego, CA.

37. 2001 Heart and Stroke Statistical Update, American Heart Association.

38. Data on file, Biosite.

39. Campbell DJ, Mitchelhill KI, Schlicht SM, Booth RJ. Plasma amino-terminal pro-brain natriuretic peptide: a novel approach to the diagnosis of cardiac dysfunction. J Cardiac Fail 2000;6:130–139.

40. Hammerer-Lercher A, Neubauer E, Muller S, et al. Head-to-head comparison of N-terminal pro-brain natriuretic peptide, brain natriuretic peptide and N-terminal pro-atrial natriuretic peptide in diagnosing left ventricular dysfunction. Clin Chim Acta 2001;310:193–197.

41. Clerico A, Caprioli R, Del Ry S, Giannessi D. Clinical relevance of cardiac natriuretic peptides measured by means of competitive and non-competitive immunoassay methods in patients with renal failure on chronic hemodialysis. J Endocrinol Invest 2001;24:24–30.

42. Fischer Y, Filzmaier K, Stiegler H, et al. Evaluation of a new, rapid bedside test for quantitative determination of B-type natriuretic peptide. Clin Chem 2001;47:591–594.

43. Vogeser M, Jacob K. B-type natriuretic peptide (BNP)—validation of an immediate response assay. Clin Lab 2001;47:29–33.
44. Del Ry S, Giannessi D, Clerico A. Plasma brain natriuretic peptide measured by fully-automated immunoassay and by immunoradiometric assay compared. Clin Chem Lab Med 2001; 39:446–450.
45. Buckley MG, Marcus NJ, Yacoub MH. Cardiac peptide stability, aprotinin and room temperature: importance for assessing cardiac function in clinical practice. Clin Sci (Lond) 1999; 97:689–695.
46. Buckley MG, Marcus NJ, Yacoub MH, Singer DR. Prolonged stability of brain natriuretic peptide: importance for non-invasive assessment of cardiac function in clinical practice. Clin Sci (Lond) 1998;95:235–239.
47. Murdoch DR, Byrne J, Morton JJ, et al. Brain natriuretic peptide is stable in whole blood and can be measured using a simple rapid assay: implications for clinical practice. Heart 1997;78:594–597.
48. Evans MJ, Livesey JH, Ellis MJ, Yandle TG. Effect of anticoagulants and storage temperatures on stability of plasma and serum hormones. Clin Biochem 2001;34:107–112.
49. Gobinet-Georges A, Valli N, Filliatre H, et al. Stability of brain natriuretic peptide (BNP) in human whole blood and plasma. Clin Chem Lab Med 2000;38:519–523.
50. Shimizu H, Aono K, Masuta K, et al. Stability of brain natriuretic peptide (BNP) in human blood samples. Clin Chim Acta 1999;285:169–172.

24

B-Type Natriuretic Peptide in the Diagnoses and Management of Congestive Heart Failure

Ramin Tabbibizar and Alan Maisel

INTRODUCTION

Congestive heart failure (CHF) imposes significant diagnostic and therapeutic challenges in cardiovascular medicine. Despite the recent advances in our understanding of the complex pathophysiology, both the diagnosis of heart failure and the assessment of therapeutic approaches remain difficult. The incidence and prevalence of heart failure have increased in the general population. CHF affects 1% of the population as a whole and up to 10% of individuals over 75 yr of age. In addition, morbidity and mortality remain high, with 65% of patients expiring within 5 yr from the time of diagnosis with CHF *(1–4)*. Medical expenses due to heart failure are staggering, accounting for 1–2% of total health care expenditures (the direct cost of heart failure exceeds $38 billion dollars annually), and it represents one of the major reasons for emergency hospital admissions *(5–7)*. Thus, it is clear that we must continue our search to improve diagnostic and therapeutic measures, while striving to enhance our understanding of the underlying pathophysiology.

B-TYPE NATRIURETIC PEPTIDE (BNP)

BNP was originally cloned in extracts of porcine brain *(8,9)*. Its name has become a misnomer, as the protein is synthesized, stored, and released mainly in the ventricular myocardium (10). It is also found in the human brain and amnion *(11–14)*. Whereas atrial natriuretic peptide (ANP) is contained in storage granules in the atria and ventricles, and even minor stimuli such as exercise may trigger a significant release of ANP into the bloodstream *(15,16)*, only small amounts of BNP are colocalized in atrial granules. Instead, the stimulus for BNP secretion is in response to changes in left ventricular (LV) wall stretch and volume overload. This suggests that BNP may be a "distress hormone," more specific for ventricular disorders than other members of the natriuretic peptide family *(17–19)*.

Biochemistry and Molecular Biology

Human proBNP consists of 108 amino acids (Fig. 1). Processing of proBNP produces a mature B-type natriuretic peptide, which consists of 32 amino acids and an amino-(N)-terminal BNP. Both polypeptides, proBNP and mature BNP, circulate in plasma. BNP contains a 17-amino-acid ring with a cysteine–cysteine disulfide crosslink, which

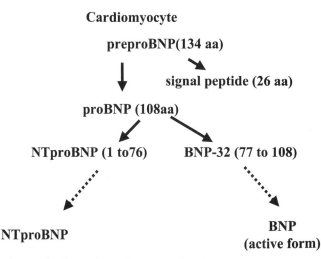

Fig. 1. The formation of BNP (active form) from preproBNP.

is present in all natriuretic peptides *(20,21)*. Eleven amino acids in the ring are homologous among all members of the natriuretic peptide family. BNP DNA has a 3'-untranslated region that is rich in an adenosine–thiamine sequence. This sequence destabilizes the mRNA molecule and causes it to have a short half-life *(22,23)*. This TATTAT sequence is absent in ANP DNA.

BNP expression in myocytes is induced with rapid kinetics of the primary response gene *(24)*. The rapid induction of transcription can be achieved by molecules that increase the half-life of mRNA. One of these molecules is an α-adrenergic receptor agonist that stabilizes BNP mRNA and induces its expression *(24)*. In addition, BNP mRNA is inducible via ventricular wall tension or stretch *(25–27)*. As a result, changes in BNP expression may represent myocardial ischemia, necrosis, damage, and local mechanical stress on ventricular myocytes, even when the global hemodynamic parameters remain unchanged *(17)*.

Mechanism of Action

The natriuretic peptides incite their action through binding to high-affinity receptors mainly on endothelial cells, vascular smooth muscle cells, and other target cells. Three distinct natriuretic peptide receptors (NPRs) have been identified in mammalian tissues: NPR-A, -B, and -C *(28)*. NPR-A and -B are structurally similar, with a 44% homology in the ligand-binding domain *(29,30)*. A single membrane-spanning portion bridges the intracellular and extracellular segments of these receptors. Both types of receptors utilize a cGMP signaling cascade *(28)*. NPR-B is mostly found in the brain, whereas NPR-A is more commonly located in large blood vessels *(28)*. Both receptor types are also found in the adrenal glands and kidneys. NPR-A binds preferentially to ANP, but also binds to BNP. On the other hand, CNP is the natural ligand for B receptors *(28)*.

BNP is removed from plasma through two distinct mechanisms: endocytosis and enzymatic degradation by endopeptidases *(31)*. NPR-C binds to all members of natriuretic peptide family with equal affinity. When a ligand–receptor complex forms, the complex undergoes receptor-mediated endocytosis. The C-type receptors are recycled to the cellular membrane, and the various natriuretic peptides are degraded to building blocks.

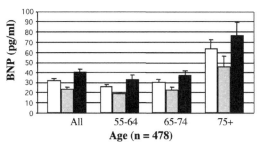

Fig. 2. Age- and gender-related changes in BNP concentrations. (Data adapted from Wierzorek et al. Am Heart J 2002;144(5):834–839.) *White bars*: all subjects, *dotted bars*: males, *black bars*: females.

The second mechanism to remove natriuretic peptides from plasma involves zinc-containing endopeptidases. These enzymes are present in renal tubules and vascular endothelial cells. They chew and degrade natriuretic peptides among other proteins.

Physiological Effects of BNP

BNP is a potent natriuretic, diuretic, and vasorelaxant peptide. It coordinates fluid and electrolyte homeostasis through its activity in the central nervous system (CNS) and peripheral tissue. BNP promotes vascular relaxation and lowers blood pressure, particularly in states of hypervolemia. It inhibits sympathetic tone, the renin–angiotensin axis, and synthesis of vasoconstrictor molecules such as catecholamines, angiotensin II, aldosterone, and endothelin-1 *(28)*. An improvement in central hemodynamics, including the cardiac index, in patients with chronic heart failure is achieved through suppression of myocyte proliferation, cardiac growth, and compensatory hypertrophy of the heart *(28)*. Its renal effects include increasing the glomerular filtration rate and enhancing sodium excretion. BNP does not cross the blood–brain barrier, yet it reaches areas of CNS that are not protected by the barrier. Its action in the CNS complements that in the periphery. BNP reinforces the diuretic effects through suppressing centers for salt appetite, and it counteracts sympathetic tone via its action in the brain stem *(28)*.

BNP Concentrations in Normals and in Patients with CHF

As can be seen in Fig. 2, BNP concentrations rise with age, likely because the LV appears to stiffen over time, offering up a stimulus to BNP production. Females without CHF tend to have somewhat higher BNP concentrations than do males of the same age group. Patients with lung disease may have somewhat higher concentrations of BNP than patients without lung disease, in part because many patients with end-stage lung disease have concomitant right ventricular dysfunction, another source of BNP.

Using BNP to Diagnose CHF: What Is the Appropriate Cut Point?

Receiver operating characteristic (ROC) curves (Fig. 3) suggest a BNP cut point of 100 pg/mL using the Biosite Triage. This gives a 95% specificity for the diagnosis of CHF (area under the curve [AUC] = 0.91). This concentration allows for increased concentrations seen with advancing age and provides an excellent ability to discriminate patients with CHF from patients without CHF. This concentration shows a sensitivity from 82% for all CHF to >99% in New York Heart Association (NYHA) class IV.

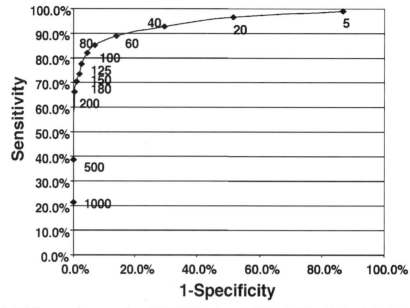

Fig. 3. ROC curve for normal vs CHF BNP values (NYHA I–IV). AUC = 0.971 (0.96–0.99) (*p* < 0.001). The box-and-whiskers plot shows the range and 25th percentile/median/75th percentile (*box*) for the BNP and control groups. The *dashed line* is the diagnostic threshold of 100 pg/mL. (Adapted from Wierzorek et al. Am Heart J 2002;144(5):834–839.)

Although 100 pg/mL is the approved cutoff for separating CHF from no CHF, most patients presenting with acute heart failure will have values far higher than this. The negative predictive value of concentrations <100 pg/mL is also excellent. But there are certain situations in which 100 pg/mL might not be sensitive enough, for example, screening asymptomatic patients for LV dysfunction. Lower concentrations (20–40 pg/mL) would sacrifice specificity but would give the needed sensitivity and negative predictive value in screening situations.

BNP as a Prognostic Marker in CHF

Because BNP concentrations correlate with elevated end-diastolic pressure, and because end-diastolic pressure correlates closely with the chief symptom of CHF, dyspnea, it is not surprising that BNP concentrations correlate with the NYHA classification (Fig. 4). Although NYHA classification is used as the main prognosticator in CHF, its subjective nature engenders doubt as to its usefulness in many patients, especially those who are relatively immobile because of arthritis, chronic obstructive pulmonary disease, and so forth. BNP gives objective values for functional class.

Several algorithms incorporating various hemodynamic variables or symptomatic indexes have been developed in an attempt to assess an individual heart failure patient's prognosis *(32,33)*. However, most of single variable markers are characterized by unsatisfactory discrimination of patients with and without increased heart failure mortality risk *(32)*.

BNP has been shown to be a powerful marker for prognosis and risk stratification in the setting of heart failure. In a recent study of 78 patients referred to a heart failure clinic,

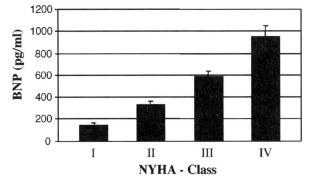

Fig. 4. BNP concentrations in patients with CHF.

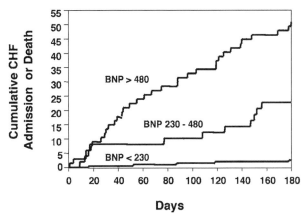

Fig. 5. Reverse Kaplan Meier plot showing cumulative risk of any hospitalization or death from CHF, stratified by BNP concentrations at the time of initial visit to the emergency department. Higher BNP concentrations are associated with progressively worse prognosis. Patients with BNP concentrations >480 pg/mL had a 6-mo cumulative probability of CHF admission or death of 42%. Patients with BNP concentrations <230 pg/mL had only a 2% probability of an event.

BNP showed a significant correlation with the heart failure survival score *(34)*. In addition, changes in plasma BNP concentrations were significantly related to changes in limitations of physical activities and were a powerful predictor of the functional status deterioration. Harrison et al. followed 325 patients for 6 mo after an index visit to the emergency department for dyspnea *(35)*. Higher BNP concentrations were associated with a progressively worse prognosis (Fig. 5). The relative risk of 6-mo CHF death in patients with BNP concentrations >230 pg/mL was 24 to 1.

Risk stratification of congestive heart failure is confounded by the fact that CHF is a multisystem disease involving altered regulation of neurohormonal systems and altered function of other systems such as renal and skeletal muscle *(36)*. Yet CHF trials have suggested that up to 50% of deaths may be due to an arrhythmia rather than deterioration of pump function. Although other markers of hemodynamic status might help assess severity of disease, BNP may be the first marker that also reflects the physiologic attempt

Table 1
Factors that Can Account for High BNP Concentrations

Age
Sex
Renal failure
Myocardial infarction
Acute coronary syndrome
Lung disease with right-sided failure
Acute, large pulmonary embolism

to compensate for the pathophysiologic alterations and restore circulatory homestasis *(37)*. Hence, BNP might be expected to influence both mechanical dysfunction and arrhythmic instability as the mechanisms most commonly involved in heart failure mortality. Berger et al. followed 452 patients with ejection fractions <35% for up to 3 yr and found that the BNP concentration was the only independent predictor of sudden death *(38)*. Their cutoff value of 130 pg/mL was similar to the 80 pg/mL used by Dao et al. *(39)* and the 100 pg/mL cutoff of the Triage rapid assay.

The significance of Berger et al.'s findings is underscored by the renewed interest in preventing sudden cardiac death by use of implantable cardiaoverter defibrillators (ICDs) *(40)*. To achieve maximum benefit of these costly devices, one needs to be able to prognosticate which patients will do better with an ICD. This study showed that BNP allowed specification of a patient group with a much higher risk of sudden death, suggesting it is an additional simple method to help identify patients who might benefit from ICD implantation.

Factors Other than Heart Failure that Can Raise BNP

Table 1 lists those factors that can account for high BNP concentrations. BNP is increased in late (predialysis) stages of renal failure, and in virtually every patient on dialysis *(41)*. This is in part related to the decreased renal clearance secondary to down-regulation of the NPR clearance receptor, as well as the accompanying increased intravascular volume. Some of this increase may be secondary to fluid overload, borne out by the fact that post-dialysis, although still increased, there are significant drops of BNP concentrations *(41)*.

Both BNP and N-terminal BNP are increased early in the course of acute myocardial infarction (AMI). A second peak of BNP measured 2–4 d after MI is associated with remodeling of the heart and is a strong predictor of subsequent LV dysfunction and mortality *(42,43)*.

In a trial of more than 2000 patients presenting with acute coronary syndrome, a BNP concentration >80 pg/mL was an independent prognosticator of death, CHF, and recurrent MI *(44)*. While the cause is not known, it is possible in this setting that BNP represents acute diastolic dysfunction from increased area of myocardium at risk.

Heart Failure with Normal BNP Concentrations

Heart failure can occur in several settings where the BNP concentration is normal (Table 2). It is estimated that in the setting of flash pulmonary edema, at least 1 h is

Table 2
Heart Failure with Low BNP Concentrations

Flash pulmonary edema
CHF secondary to causes upstream from the left ventricle:
    Acute mitral regurgitation
    Mitral stenosis
    Atrial myxoma
Stable NYHA class I patients with low ejection fractions

necessary to produce increases in BNP concentrations. It is speculated that this early release may be preformed BNP located in the atrium. CHF occurring upstream from the LV is most commonly seen with acute mitral regurgitation. These patients often present with acute CHF, yet LV function is not yet compromised.

USING BNP IN THE CLINICAL SETTING

BNP Concentrations for Patients Presenting to the Emergency Department with Dyspnea

For the acutely ill patient presenting to the emergency department, a misdiagnosis could place the patient at risk for both morbidity and mortality *(45)*. Therefore, the emergency department diagnosis of CHF needs to be rapid and accurate. Unfortunately, the signs and symptoms of CHF are nonspecific *(46)*. A helpful history is not often obtainable in an acutely ill patient, and dyspnea, a key symptom of CHF, may also be a nonspecific finding in the elderly or obese patient in whom comorbidity with respiratory disease and physical deconditioning are common *(47)*. Routine laboratory values, electrocardiograms, and X-rays are also not accurate enough to always make the appropriate diagnosis *(46–48)*. Thus, it is difficult for clinicians to differentiate patients with CHF from other diseases such as pulmonary disease on the basis of routinely available laboratory tests.

Echocardiography has limited availability in acute care settings. Dyspneic patients may be unable to remain motionless long enough for an echocardiographic study, and others may be difficult to image secondary to comorbid factors such as obesity or lung disease. Therefore, even in settings where emergency department echocardiography is available, an accurate, sensitive, and specific blood test for heart failure would be useful addition to the currently existing tools available to the physician.

For diagnostic screening tests to be useful in acute care, a test should have a high negative predictive value, allowing clinicians to rapidly rule out serious disorders *(49)*, and facilitating efficient use of valuable resources. BNP was first used in the evaluation of dyspnea by Davis et al., who measured the natriuretic hormones ANP and BNP in 52 patients presenting with acute dyspnea. They found that admission plasma BNP concentrations more accurately reflected the final diagnosis than did ejection fraction or concentration of plasma ANP *(50)*. As intriguing as those results were, it was not until a rapid assay became available that BNP testing could be applied in the urgent care or clinic setting.

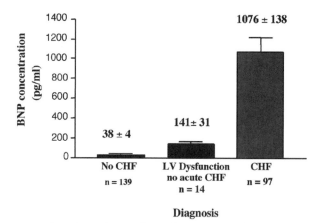

Fig. 6. BNP concentrations in patients whose dyspnea was due to CHF, non-CHF causes, or non-CHF causes with baseline LV dysfunction.

Dao et al. were the first to use the rapid assay in evaluating 250 patients presenting to the San Diego Veterans Administration Healthcare Urgent Care Center with dyspnea as their chief complaint *(39)*. Physicians assigned to the emergency department were asked to make an assessment of the probability of the patient having CHF as the cause of his or her symptoms, blinded to the results of BNP measurements. To determine a patient's actual diagnosis, two cardiologists reviewed all medical records pertaining to the patient and made independent initial assessments of the probability of each patient having CHF (high or low, or low plus baseline LV dysfunction), blinded to the patient's BNP concentration. While blinded to ED physicians' diagnosis, cardiologists had access to the emergency department data sheets, as well as to any additional information that later became available.

Patients diagnosed with CHF ($n = 97$) had a mean BNP concentration of 1076 ± 138 pg/mL, while the non-CHF group ($n = 139$) had a mean BNP concentration of 38 ± 4 pg/mL (Fig. 6). The group of 14 identified as baseline ventricular dysfunction without an acute exacerbation had a mean concentration of 141 ± 31 pg/mL. Of crucial importance was that patients with the final diagnosis of pulmonary disease had lower BNP values (86 ± 39 pg/mL) than those with a final diagnosis of CHF (1076 ± 138 pg/mL, $p < 0.001$). This is perhaps the key differential in patients who present with acute dyspnea.

BNP at a cut point of 80 pg/mL was found to be highly sensitive (98%) and highly specific (92%) for the diagnosis of CHF. The negative predictive value of BNP values <80 pg/mL was 98% for the diagnosis of CHF. Multivariate analysis revealed that after all useful tools for making the diagnosis were taken into account by the emergency department physician, BNP concentrations continued to provide meaningful diagnostic information not available from other clinical variables.

The above study set the stage for the recently completed multinational Breathing Not Properly study *(51)*. In this unique large-scale study, 1586 patients with acute shortness of breath were examined. Not only was BNP able to differentiate CHF from non-CHF causes of dyspnea (area under ROC curve = 0.91,) with good specificity and high negative predictive values, but a single BNP concentration was more accurate than both the National Health and Nutrition Examination Survey (NHANES) and Framingham crite-

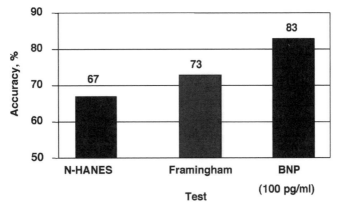

Fig. 7. Accuracy of a single BNP concentration (>100 pg/mL) in diagnosing CHF compared to established criteria of NHANES and Framingham. (Adapted from Maisel et al. *[51].*)

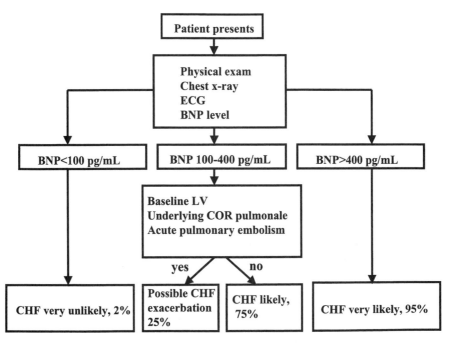

Fig. 8. Diagnostic algorithm for patients presenting with dyspnea.

ria, arguably the two most commonly used criteria to diagnose CHF (Fig. 7). In this trial, the physicians were required to give a probability from 0 to 100% on the likelihood the patient had CHF. Forty-three percent of the time physicians were only 20–80% sure of the diagnosis. A BNP concentration in this setting of >100 pg/mL reduced the indecision by 74% to 11%.

Based on one of the authors' experience (AM), an algorithm for CHF diagnosis in the emergency department is presented in Fig. 8. When a patient comes to the emergency department with acute shortness of breath, an electrocardiogram, a chest X-ray, and a BNP concentration are obtained. CHF is usually absent at BNP concentrations <100 pg/mL and usually present in patients with BNP concentrations >400 pg/mL. Those patients with BNP concentrations between 100 and 400 have several other diagnostic possibilities that need to be considered. First, patients may have known LV dysfunction. BNP concentrations are often >100 in these cases, but if their cause of dyspnea is something other than acute exacerbation, the concentrations are usually <400 pg/mL. Morrison et al. were recently able to show that rapid testing of BNP could help differentiate pulmonary from cardiac etiologies of dyspnea *(52)*. Some types of pulmonary disease, however, such as cor pulmonale, lung cancer, and pulmonary embolism have elevated BNP concentrations, but these are not usually elevated to the extent as in patients with acute LV dysfunction. Thus, clinical judgment needs to be used in these cases. Often times, patients present with both pulmonary and cardiac disease, as one often begets the other, again calling for clinical acumen and further tests. Finally, a pulmonary embolism large enough to raise the pulmonary artery pressure due to right ventricular strain may raise BNP concentrations. If the above can be ruled out, then it is much more likely that BNP concentrations between 100 and 400 pg/mL represent CHF.

Thus, the measurement of the BNP concentration in blood appears to be a sensitive and specific test for identification of patients with CHF in acute care settings. If the results of this study are borne out in subsequent ones, BNP concentrations may replace chest X-ray (and perhaps even echocardiography) as the test of choice in differential diagnosis of dyspnea in acute care settings. At the minimum, it is likely to be a potent, cost-effective addition to the diagnostic armamentarium of acute care physicians.

BNP as a Screen of LV Dysfunction

BNP has been used to a limited extent as a screening procedure in primary care settings and in this venue has been shown to be a useful addition in the evaluation of possible CHF *(6,53–55)*. In a community-based study in which 1653 subjects underwent cardiac screening, the negative predictive value of BNP of 18 pg/mL was 97% for LV systolic dysfunction *(54)*. In a study of 122 consecutive patients with suspected new heart failure referred by general practitioners to a rapid-access heart failure clinic for diagnostic confirmation, a BNP concentration of 76 pg/mL, chosen for its negative predictive value of 98% for heart failure, had a sensitivity of 97%, a specificity of 84%, and a positive predictive value of 70% *(6)*.

Maisel et al. characterized patients who had both echocardiography and BNP concentrations *(56)*. Figure 9 is a breakdown of all patients referred for echocardiography, based on the presence or absence of history of CHF. Among the patients with no documented history of CHF and no past determination of LV function, 51% had abnormal echocardiographic findings. In this group BNP concentrations were significantly higher (328 ± 29 pg/mL) than the 49% of patients with no history of CHF and a normal echocardiogram (30 ± 3 pg/mL, $p < 0.001$). In patients with a known history of CHF, with preciously documented LV dysfunction, all had abnormal findings ($n = 102$), with elevated BNP concentrations (545 ± 45 pg/mL).

The ability of BNP to detect abnormal cardiac function (systolic or diastolic) was recently assessed with ROC analysis *(57)* (Fig. 10). The area under the ROC curve using BNP to detect any abnormal echocardiographic finding was 0.952. A BNP value of 75 pg/mL had a sensitivity of 85%, specificity of 97% and an accuracy of 90% for predicting LV dysfunction. The ability of BNP independently to predict abnormal systolic function (as compared to all other patients) or abnormal diastolic function (as compared to all

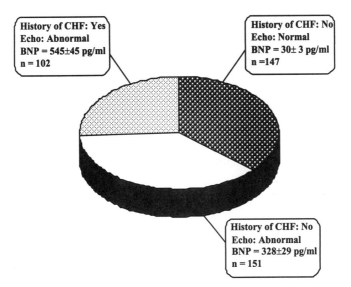

History of CHF: Yes
Echo: Abnormal
BNP = 545±45 pg/ml
n = 102

History of CHF: No
Echo: Normal
BNP = 30± 3 pg/ml
n =147

History of CHF: No
Echo: Abnormal
BNP = 328±29 pg/ml
n = 151

Fig. 9. BNP concentrations in patients referred for echocardiography for evaluation of ventricular dysfunction. Data based on the presence or absence of CHF history.

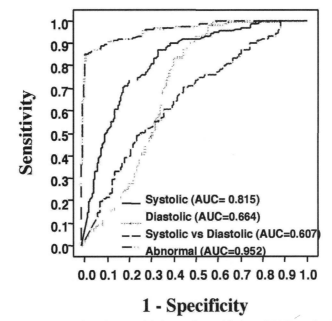

1 - Specificity

Fig. 10. ROC curve comparing the sensitivity and specificity of BNP and echocardiographic diagnosis of ventricular dysfunction (any abnormal—systolic or diastolic), systolic dysfunction (vs normal and diastolic), diastolic dysfunction (vs normal and systolic), and systolic vs diastolic (normals excluded).

other patients) was not as good. Although BNP concentrations were still able to detect both isolated systolic dysfunction (independent of normal overall function or pure diastolic dysfunction), and diastolic dysfunction (independent of normal overall function or pure systolic dysfunction), the accuracy was less than that when predicting any echocardiographic abnormality. In analyzing just the patients with abnormal LV function, BNP concentrations were not able to differentiate those with systolic dysfunction from those with diastolic dysfunction.

Yamamoto et al. recently compared the predictive characteristics of BNP with a five-point clinical score in 466 patients referred for echocardiography because of symptoms of CHF *(58)*. BNP was sensitive and specific for detection of systolic dysfunction, with an area under the ROC curve of 0.79.

The above findings suggest that BNP may be a useful screen for patients with LV dysfunction, with accuracies similar to that of prostate-specific antigen for prostate cancer detection which had an AUC of 0.94, and superior to those of Papanicolaou smears and mammography (AUC = 0.70 and 0.85, respectively) *(59–61)*.

BNP and Diastolic Dysfunction

The European Society of Cardiology recently published its recommendations regarding the diagnosis of isolated diastolic heart failure, which included the presence of symptoms, presence of normal or mildly reduced systolic function, and evidence of abnormal LV relaxation and filling, diastolic distensibility, and diastolic stiffness *(62)*. Redfield et al. studied 657 subjects with normal systolic function and found that BNP concentrations were higher than those with isolated diastolic dysfunction *(62)*. Recently, Lubien et al. studied 294 patients referred for echocardiography to evaluate ventricular function were studied *(63)*. Patients with abnormal systolic function were excluded. BNP concentrations were blinded from cardiologists making the assessment of LV function. Patients with a restrictive filling pattern ($n = 37$) had higher BNP concentrations (428 pg/mL) than patients with impaired relaxation (230 pg/mL). The area under the ROC curve for BNP to detect diastolic dysfunction by echocardiography in patients with CHF and normal systolic function was 0.958. A BNP value of 71 pg/mL was 96% accurate in the prediction of diastolic dysfunction in this setting. BNP concentrations <57 pg/mL gave a negative predictive value of 100% for the detection of clinically significant diastolic dysfunction. In addition, multivariate analysis showed that in patients with clinical CHF and normal LV function, BNP was the strongest predictor of diastolic abnormalities seen on echocardiography.

Thus, although BNP concentrations cannot by themselves differentiate between systolic and diastolic dysfunction, a low BNP concentration in the setting of normal systolic function by echocardiography can likely rule out clinically significant diastolic dysfunction. On the other hand, an elevated BNP concentration in patients with clinical CHF and normal systolic function appears to substantiate the diagnosis of diastolic dysfunction.

Potential Uses for BNP Concentrations to Diagnose LV Dysfunction

Table 3 presents other possible areas in which BNP might potentially be of use as a screening tool to monitor either the development of LV function in at-risk patients or to monitor progression of established disease.

THE FUTURE FOR BNP USE IN CHF: MODULATING THERAPY

Inpatient Monitoring

There are approx 1 million hospital admissions annually in the United States for CHF. Although patients who are admitted to the hospital with decompensated heart failure

Table 3
Potential Uses for BNP to Screen for LV Dysfunction

Patients receiving cardiotoxic drugs
Assess need for surgery in patients with valvular heart disease
LV dysfunction in diabetes
Screening for transplant rejection
Adult respiratory distress syndrome
Screening for hypertrophic cardiomyopathy

often have improvement in symptoms with the various treatment modalities available, there has been no good way to evaluate the long-term effects of the short-term treatment. Readmission after hospitalization for heart failure is surprisingly common, estimated at 44% at 6 mo within the Medicare population *(64)*. Considering that hospitalization is the principal component of the cost for patient care (70–75%) of the total direct costs *(65)*, a reduction in heart failure hospitalizations is an appropriate goal for whatever treatment modalities are in place.

Because BNP is a volume-sensitive hormone with a short half-life (18–22 min), there may be a future use for BNP concentrations in guiding diuretic and vasodilator therapy on presentation with decompensated CHF. Cheng et al. found that patients who were not readmitted in the following 30 d after discharge could be characterized by falling BNP concentrations during hospitalization *(66)*. On the other hand, patients who were readmitted or died in the following 30 d had no such decrease in BNP concentrations on their index hospitalization, despite their overall "clinical" improvement. In a study by Kazenegra et al., patients undergoing hemodynamic monitoring had changes in wedge pressures that were strongly correlated with dropping BNP concentrations and clinical improvement *(67)*. Thus, in the future it may be possible that titration of vasodilators will no longer require Swan–Ganz catheterization, but rather the use of a BNP concentration as a surrogate for wedge pressure.

Recently, a new vasodilator, Nesiritide, has been approved by the U.S. Food and Drug Administration for treatment of decompensated heart failure. The drug is human B-type natriuretic peptide and possesses many of the characteristics of an ideal agent for treating acute decompensated heart failure. The question as to why exogenous BNP would be administered when endogenous concentrations are also high has not been fully explained. It is probably analogous to giving insulin for insulin resistance. Endogenous BNP may be released as a "distress hormone" and that exogenously provided BNP may overwhelm the dampened system, perhaps up-regulating the renal natriuretic peptide clearance receptor and clearing BNP. In preliminary studies by one of the authors (AM) it appears that within 6 h after cessation of Natrecor infusion, endogenous BNP concentrations are 20–30% lower than baseline.

Outpatient Treatment

The correlation between the drop in BNP concentration and the patient's improvement in symptoms (and subsequent outcome) during hospitalization suggests that BNP-guided treatment might make "tailored therapy" more effective in an outpatient setting

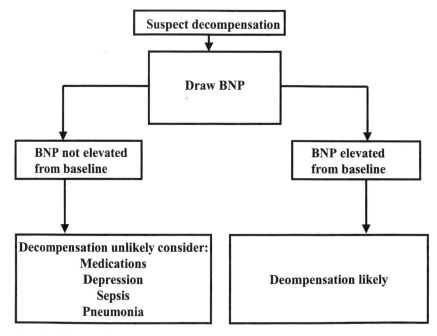

Fig. 11. Algorithm to detect decompensation in patients with established heart failure and with baseline BNP values.

such as a primary care or cardiology clinic. The Australia–New Zealand Heart Failure Group analyzed plasma neurohormones for prediction of adverse outcomes and response to treatment in 415 patients with LV dysfunction randomly assigned to receive Carvedilol or placebo *(68)*. They found that BNP was the best prognostic predictor of success or failure of Carvedilol use. Recently, Troughton et al. randomized 69 patients to N-terminal BNP guided treatment vs symptom-guided therapy *(69)*. Patients receiving N-terminal BNP guided therapy had lower N-BNP concentrations along with reduced incidence of cardiovascular death, readmission, and new episodes of decompensated CHF.

Although BNP concentrations may be helpful in guiding therapy in the outpatient setting, delineating the magnitude of fluctuations of BNP concentrations in an individual patient over time needs to be ascertained before BNP concentrations can be used to titrate drug therapy.

BNP has been shown to be a powerful marker for prognosis and risk stratification in the setting of ambulatory heart failure *(34)*. Our own experience is shown in Fig. 11. Because most patients with heart failure at our institution have baseline "euvolemic" BNP concentrations recorded in their medical records, when they present with symptoms that could be exacerbation of heart failure, a new BNP concentration is obtained. In our experience if the BNP concentration has not increased, there is little chance that this is CHF exacerbation. On the other hand, increases of BNP concentrations >50% of baseline often turn out to be worsening CHF.

Perhaps patients who have high BNP concentrations that do not respond to treatment should be considered for other more invasive types of therapies such as cardiac transplantation or use of ventricular assist devices. In a recent trial of patients who received ventricular assist devices for end-stage heart failure, BNP concentrations appeared to fall as remodeling of the heart occurred, and an early decrease in BNP plasma concentration was indicative of recovery of cardiac function during mechanical circulatory support *(70)*.

CONCLUSIONS

Finding a simple blood test that would aid in the diagnosis and management of patients with CHF should clearly have a favorable impact on the staggering costs associated with the disease. BNP, which is synthesized in the cardiac ventricles and correlates with LV pressure, amount of dyspnea, and the state of neurohormonal modulation, makes this peptide the first potential "white count" for heart failure. Data now strongly puts BNP testing as the biggest advancement in diagnosing heart failure since the advent of echocardiography 20 yr ago. Depending on the prevalence of disease and the age of the population, BNP should prove to be a good screening tool in high-risk patients. Finally, the role of BNP in the outpatient cardiac or primary care clinic may be one of critical importance in titration of therapies as well as in assess the state of neurohormonal compensation of the patient.

ABBREVIATIONS

AMI, Acute myocardial infarction; ANP, BNP, atrial and B-type natriuretic peptides; AUC, area under the curve; CHF, congestive heart failure; CNS, central nervous system; ICD, implantable cardioverter-defibrillator; LV, left ventricular; NHANES, National Health and Nutrition Examination Survey; NPR, natriuretic peptide receptor; NYHA, New York Heart Association; ROC, receiver operating characteristic.

REFERENCES

1. Adams KF. Post hoc subgroup analysis and the truth of a clinical trial. Am Heart J 1998; 136:751–758.
2. Drumholz HM, Douglas PS, Goldman L, Waksmonski C. Clinical utility of transthoracic two-dimensional and Doppler echocardiography. J Am Coll Cardiol 1994;24:125–131.
3. Rich MW, Freedland KE. Effect of DRGs on three month readmission rate of geriatric patients with heart failure. Am J Publ Health 1988;78:680–882.
4. Stevenson LW, Braunwald E. Recognition and Management of Patients with Heart Failure. Primary Cardiology. Philadelphia: WB Saunders, 1998, pp. 310–329.
5. American Journal of Cardiology/Advisory Council to Improve Outcomes Nationwide in Heart Failure. Consensus Recommendations for the Management of Chronic Heart Failure. Am J Cardiol 1999;83:1A–38A.
6. Cowie MR, Struthers AD, Wood DA, et al. Value of natriuertic peptides in assessment of patients with possible new heart failure in primary care. Lancet 1997;350:1449–1453.
7. O'Connell JB, Bristow M. Economic impact of heat failure in the United States: a time for a different approach. J Heart Lung Transplant 1993;13:S107–S112.
8. Sudoh T, Minamino N, Kangawa K, Matsuo H. A new natriuretic peptide in human brain. Nature 1988;332:78–81.
9. Stein BC, Levin RI. Natriuretic peptides: physiology, therapeutic potential, and risk stratification in ischemic heart disease. Am Heart J 1998;135:914–923.
10. Dries DL, Stevenson LW. Brain natriuretic peptide as bridge to therapy for heart failure. Lancet 2000;355:1112–1113.
11. Mukoyama M, Nakao K, Hosoda K, et al. Brain natriuretic peptide as a novel cardiac hormone in humans. Evidence for an exquisite dual natriuretic peptide system, atrial natriuretic peptide and brain natriuretic peptide. J Clin Invest 1991;87:1402–1412.

12. Troughton RW, Frampton CM, Yandle TG, et al. Treatment of heart failure guided by plasma aminoterminal brain natriuretic peptide (N-BNP) concentrations. Lancet 2000;355:1126–1130.

13. Kinnunen P, Vuolteenaho O, Ruskoaho H. Mechanisms of atrial and brain natriuretic peptide release from rat ventricular myocardium: effects of stretching. Endocrinology 1993; 132:1961–1970.

14. Magga J, Vuolteenaho O, Tokola H, et al. B-type natriuretic peptide: a myocyte-specific marker for characterizing load-induced alterations in cardiac gene expression. Ann Med 1998;20(Suppl 1):39–45.

15. Richards AM, Crozier IG, Yandle TG, et al. Brain natriuretic factor: regional plasma concentrations and correlations with haemodynamic state in cardiac disease. Br Heart J 1993; 69:414–417.

16. Nagagawa O, Ogawa Y, Itoh H, et al. Rapid transcriptional activation and early mRNA turnover of BNP in cardiocyte hypertrophy. Evidence for BNP as an "emergency" cardiac hormone against ventricular overload. J Clin Invest 1995;96:1280–1287.

17. Tsutamoto T, Wada A, Maeda K, et al. Attenuation of compensation of endogenous cardiac natriuretic peptide system in chronic heart failure: prognostic role of plasma brain natriuretic peptide concentration in patients with chronic symptomatic left ventricular dysfunction. Circulation 1997;96:509–516.

18. Struthers AD. Prospects for using a blood sample in diagnosis of heart failure. Q J Med 1995;88:303–306.

19. Cheung BMY, Kumana CR. Natriuretic peptides—relevance in cardiac disease. JAMA 1998; 280:1983–1984.

20. Stein BC, Levin RI. Natriuretic peptides: physiology, therapeutic potential, and risk stratification in ischemic heart disease. Am Heart J 1998;135:914–923.

21. Porter JG, Arestem A, Palasi T, et al. Cloning of cDNA encoding porcine brain natriuretic peptide. J Biol Chem 1989;264:6689–6692.

22. Wallen T, Landahl S, Hedner T, et al. Brain natriuretic peptide predicts mortality in the elderly. Heart 1997;77:264–267.

23. Hanford DS, Glembotski CC. Stabilization of the b-type natriuretic peptide mRNA in cardiac myocytes by alpha-adrenergic receptor activation: potential roles for protein kinase C and mitogen-activated protein kinase. Mol Endocrinol 1996;10:1719–1727.

24. Kojima M, Minamino M, Kangawa K, Matsuo H. Cloning and sequence analysis of cDNA encoding a precursor for rat brain natriuretic peptide. Biochem Biophys Res Commun 1989; 159:1420–1426.

25. Nakao K, Mukoyama M, Hosoda K, et al. Biosynthesis, secretion, and receptor selectivity of human brain natriuretic peptide. Can J Physiol Pharmacol 1991;87:1402–1412.

26. Hama N, Itoh H, Shirakami G, et al. Rapid ventricular induction of brain natriuretic peptide gene expression in experimental acute myocardial infarction. Circulation 1995;92:1558–1564.

27. Richards AM. The renin–angiotensin–aldosterone system and the cardiac natriuretic peptides. Heart 1996;76(S3):36–44.

28. Levin ER, Gardner DG, Samson WK. Mechanisms of disease: natriuretic peptides. N Engl J Med 1998;339:321–328.

29. Koller KJ, Goeddel DV. Molecular biology of the natriuretic peptides and their receptors. Circulation 1992;86:1081–1088.

30. Davidson NC, Naas AA, Hanson JK, et al. Comparison of atrial natriuretic peptide, b-type natriuretic peptide, and N-terminal proatrial natriuretic peptide as indicators of left ventricular systolic dysfunction. Am J Cardiol 1996;77:828–831.

31. Ming Ng S, Krishnaswamy P, Morissey R, Clopton P, Fitzgerald R, Maisel AS. Ninety minute accelerated critical pathway for chest pain evaluation Am J Cardiol 2001;86:611–617.

32. Cohn JN. Prognositc factors in heart failure: poverty amidst a wealth of variables. J Am Coll Cardiol 1989;14:571–572.

33. Kelly TL, Cremo R, Nieosen C, Shabetai. Prediction of outcome in late-stage cardiomyopathy. Am Heart J 1990;119:1111–1121.
34. Koglin J, Pehlivanli S, Schwaiblamir M, Vogeser M, Cremer P, von Scheidt W. Role of brain natriuretic peptide in risk stratification of patients with congestive heart failure. J Am Coll Cardiol 2001;38:1934–1940.
35. Harrison A, Morrison LK, Krishnaswamy P, et al. B-type natriuretic peptide (BNP) predicts future cardiac events in patients presenting to the emergency department with dyspnea. Ann Emerg Med 2002;39:131–138.
36. Schrier RW, Abraham WT. Hormones and hemodynamics in heart failure. N Engl J Med 1999;341:577–585.
37. Levin ER, Gardner DG, Samson WK. Natriuretic peptides. N Engl J Med 1998;339:321–328.
38. Berger R, Huelsman M, Stecker K, et al. B-type natriuretic peptide predicts sudden death in patients with chronic heart failure. Circulation 2002;105:2392–2397.
39. Dao Q, Krishnaswamy P, Kazanegra R, et al. Utility of B-type natriuretic peptide (BNP) in the diagnosis of CHF in an urgent care setting. J Am Coll Cardiol 2001;37:379–385.
40. Connolly SJ, Hallstrom AP, Cappato R, et al. Meta analysis of the implantable cardioverter defibrillator secondary prevention trials. AVID, CASH, CIDS studies. Eur Heart J 2000;21:2071–2078.
41. Haug C, Metzele A, Steffgen J, Kochs M, Hombach V, Grunert A. Increased brain natriuretic peptide and atrial peptide plasma concentration in dialysis-dependent chronic renal failure and in patients with elevated left ventricular filling pressure. Clin Invest 1994;72:430–434.
42. OmLand T, Bonarjee VVS, Lie RT, Caidahl K. Neurohumoral measuremnnts as indicators of long term prognosis after acute myocardial infarction. Am J Cardiol 1995;76:230–235.
43. Richards AM, Nicholls MG, Yandle TH, et al. Neuroendocrine prediction of left ventricular function and heart failure after acute myocardial infarction. Heart 1999;81:114–120.
44. de Lemos JA, Morrow DA, Bentley JH, et al. The prognostic value of B-type natriuretic peptide in patients with acute coronary syndromes. N Engl J Med 2001;345:1014–1020.
45. Wuerz RC, Meador SA. Effects of prehospital medications on mortality and length of stay in CHF. Ann Emerg Med 1992;21:669–674.
46. Stevenson LW. The limited availability of physical signs for estimating hemodynamics in chronic heart failure. JAMA 1989;261:884–888.
47. Deveraux RB, Liebson PR, Horan MJ. Recommendations concerning use of echocardiography in hypertension and general population research. Hypertension 1987;9:97–104.
48. Davie AP, Francis CM, Love MP, Caruana L, Starkey IR, Shaw TR. Value of the electrocardiogram in identifying heart failure due to left ventricular systolic dysfunction. Br Med J 1996;312:222
49. Vinson JM, Rich MW, Sperry JC, Shah AS, McNamara T. Early readmission of elderly patients with heart failure. J Am Geriatr Soc 1990;38:1290–1295.
50. Davis M, Espiner E, Richards G, et al. Plasma brain natriuretic peptide in assessment of acute dyspnea. Lancet 1994;343:440–444.
51. Maisel AM, Krishnaswamy P, Nowak R, et al. Bedside B-type natriuretic peptide in the emergency diagnosis of heart failure: primary results from the Breathing Not Properly (BNP) Multinational study. Presented at ACC meeting, Atlanta, 2002.
52. Morrison KL, Harrison A, Krishnaswamy P, Kazanegra R, Clopton P, Maisel AS. Utility of a rapid B-natriuretic peptide (BNP) assay in differentiating CHF from lung disease in patients presenting with dyspnea. J Am Coll Cardiol 2002;39:202–209.
53. McDonagh TA, Robb SD, Murdoch DR, et al. Biochemical detection of left-ventricular systolic dysfunction. Lancet 1998;351:9–13.
54. McDonagh TA, Morrison CE, Lawrence A, et al. Symptomatic and asymptomatic left-ventricular systolic dysfunction in an urban population. Lancet 1997;350:829–833.

55. Muders F, Kromer EP, Griese DP, et al. Evaluation of plasma natriuretic peptides as markers for left ventricular dysfunction. Am Heart J 134:442–449.
56. Maisel AS, Koon J, Krishnaswamy P, et al. Utility of B-natriuretic peptide (BNP) as a rapid, point-of-care test for screening patients undergoing echocardiography for left ventricular dysfunction. Am Heart J 2001;141:367–374.
57. Krishnaswamy P, Lubien E, Clopton P, et al. Utility of B-natriuretic peptide levels identifying patients with left ventricular systolic or diastolic dysfunction. Am J Med 2001;111: 274–279.
58. Yamamoto K, Burnett J Jr, Bermudez EA, Jougasaki M, Bailey KR, Redfield MM. Clinical criteria and biochemical markers for the detection of systolic dysfunction. J Cardiac Fail 2000;6:194–200.
59. Fahey MT, Irwig L, Macaskill P. Meta-analysis of Pap test accuracy. Am J Epidemiol 1995; 141:680–689.
60. Jacobsen SJ, Bergstralh EJ, Guess HA, et al. Predictive properties of serum prostate-specific antigen testing in a community-based setting. Arch Intern Med 1996;156:2462–2468.
61. Tsutamoto T, Wada A, Maeda K, et al. Attenuation of compensation of endogenous cardiac natriuretic peptide system in chronic heart failure: prognostic role of plasma brain natriuretic peptide concentration in patients with chronic symptomatic left ventricular dysfunction. Circulation 1997;96:509–516.
62. Anonymous. How to diagnose diastolic heart failure. Eur Heart J 1998;19:990–1003.
63. Lubien E, DeMaria A, Krishnaswamy P, et al. Utility of B-natriuretic peptide in detecting diastolic dysfunction. Comparison with Doppler velocity recordings. Circulation 2002;105: 595–601.
64. Krumholz HM, Parent EM, Tu N, et al. Readmission after hospitalization for congestive heart failure among Medicare beneficiaries. Arch Intern Med 1997;157:99–104.
65. Konstam MA, Kimmelstiel CD. Economics of heart failure. In: Exercise and Heart Failure. Balady GJ, Pina IL, eds. Armonk, NY: Futura, 1997, pp. 19–28.
66. Cheng VL, Kazanegra R, Garcia A, et al. A rapid bedside test for B-type natriuretic peptide predicts treatment outcomes in patients admitted with decompensated heart failure. J Am Coll Cardiol 2001;37:386–391.
67. Kazanagra R, Chen V, Garcia A, et al. A rapid test for B-type natriuretic peptide (BNP) correlates with falling wedge pressures in patients treated for decompensated heart failure: a pilot study. J Cardiac Fail 2001;7:21–29.
68. Richardson AM, Doughty R, Nicholls MG, et al. Neurohumoral predictors of benefit from Carvedilol in ischemic left ventricular dysfunction. Circulation 1999;99:786–797.
69. Troughton RW, Frampton CM, Yandle TG, Espiner EA, Nicholls MG, Richards AM. Treatment of heart failure guided by plasma amino terminal brain natriuretic peptide (N-BNP) concentrations. Lancet 2000;355:1126–1130.
70. Sodian R, Loebe M, Schmitt C, et al. Decreased plasma concentrations of brain natriuretic peptide as a potential indicator of cardiac recovery in patients supported by mechanical circulatory assist systems. J Am Coll Cardiol 2001;38:1942–1949.

25

Monitoring Efficacy of Treatment with Brain Natriuretic Peptide

Emil D. Missov and Leslie W. Miller

INTRODUCTION

Congestive heart failure (CHF) is a major health problem. Its incidence and prevalence are increasing because of the aging of the population and improved treatment and outcomes *(1)*. Hospital admissions for CHF increased dramatically from 377,000 in 1979 to 970,000 in 1998 according to the National Hospital Discharge Survey *(2)*. Despite advances in treatment, mortality from CHF remains high, especially in patients with more advanced disease.

The challenges in the diagnosis, treatment, and management of patients with CHF are threefold: (1) making a definite diagnosis of heart failure; (2) staging of the disease and assessing its severity, extent, and progression; and (3) monitoring efficacy of treatment. It has become apparent that the natriuretic peptides are important biomarkers in CHF. The natriuretic peptide family consists of several naturally occurring peptide hormones synthesized by the myocardium. In vitro studies have shown that the ventricles are the major source of cardiac brain natriuretic peptide (BNP), which is released into the circulation largely in response to increased intracardiac pressure. Secretion of atrial natriuretic peptide (ANP) from the atria is determined by increases in atrial transmural pressure as well as intraatrial pressure *(3)*. This chapter focuses on monitoring the efficacy of treatment for heart failure using BNP, which has emerged as the most reliable diagnostic and prognostic tool among all natriuretic peptides *(4)*. The use of BNP in clinical conditions other than heart failure or unrelated to left ventricular (LV) dysfunction is also covered as they represent fields where the use of BNP could provide meaningful pathophysiological and hemodynamic information. Finally, the authors' personal approach and experience are briefly outlined. The diagnostic and prognostic issues related to the use of natriuretic peptides are covered elsewhere in this book.

ROLE OF BNP IN MONITORING OF PHARMACOTHERAPY FOR HEART FAILURE

Although it is unlikely that the diagnosis of the complex pathophysiological syndrome of heart failure will ever rely on a single clinical or biological variable, the use of BNP as an aid in the diagnosis of heart failure to support the clinical impression would certainly be a meaningful approach. The major clinical applications of the natriuretic

From: *Cardiac Markers, Second Edition*
Edited by: Alan H. B. Wu @ Humana Press Inc., Totowa, NJ

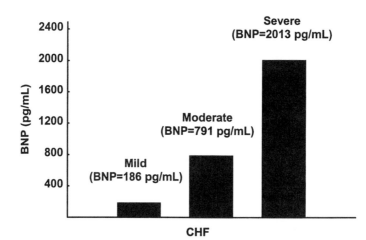

Fig. 1. Levels of BNP increase proportionally to CHF severity. Note the more than 10-fold increase in BNP levels in patients with severe heart failure compared to patients with mild symptoms. (Adapted from ref. *5.*)

peptides, in general, and of BNP, in particular, would be to guide therapeutic interventions and strategies, and possibly identify patients at high risk for rehospitalizations and subsequent cardiovascular events.

The goal of pharmacological treatment of heart failure is primarily to improve symptomatology. However, the chronic monitoring of patients with heart failure has been substantially inaccurate as it relies on clinical assessment of symptoms. This approach is neither structured nor standardized and therapies guided by invasive hemodynamic measurements have provided a more objective way to guide treatment and document its efficacy in CHF. An interesting substitute for hemodynamic measurements might be BNP. It has been shown that BNP levels increase proportionally to New York Heart Association (NYHA) functional class, CHF severity (Fig. 1), and magnitude of hemodynamic failure; they decline after successful treatment of the disease, reflecting *de facto* hemodynamic improvement *(5)*. Kazanegra et al. reported on the ability of changes in BNP levels to reflect accurately changes in pulmonary capillary wedge pressure during treatment of an acute episode of decompensated heart failure (Fig. 2) *(6)*. Out of the 20 patients with NYHA functional class III/IV heart failure undergoing therapy, 15 responded with a substantial decrease in wedge pressure during the first 24 h. These patients were noted to have a significant decrease in BNP levels by 55%, compared to an 8% decrease in BNP levels in patients who did not experience the same decline in wedge pressure. The authors also report that those patients who died within 30 d of enrollment also had higher levels of BNP compared to the rest of the study population (1078 ± 123 vs 701 ± 107 pg/mL, respectively). The data from this study suggest that BNP may be used as an effective means to monitor hemodynamic improvement in patients with an acute episode of heart failure and help guide therapy according to a decrease in BNP levels. A similar study by Sasaki et al. *(7)* found that treatment with pimobendan resulted in a significant decrease in plasma concentration of BNP and improvement of LV ejection fraction in patients with nonischemic mild to moderate heart failure. After 1 yr of

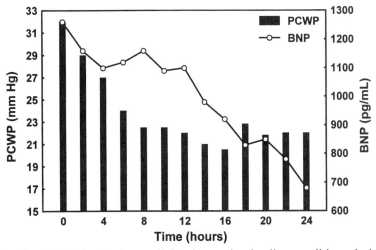

Fig. 2. Levels of BNP decline in parallel to improving loading conditions during treatment of an episode of acute heart failure. PCWP, Pulmonary capillary wedge pressure. (Adapted from ref. *6.*)

follow-up, patients treated with pimobendan also improved their NYHA functional class, which was paralleled by a reduction in LV end-diastolic diameter. In a recently published study, Dao et al. *(8)* documented the feasibility of near-patient BNP testing with a point of care device in an urgent care setting. The results show that the mean BNP concentration in patients with heart failure (1076 ± 138 pg/mL) was higher than it was in patients without signs and symptoms of heart failure (38 ± 4 pg/mL, $p < 0.001$). The authors also found that a cutoff limit of 80 pg/mL of BNP concentration was an accurate predictor of the presence of heart failure, while values below 80 pg/mL increased the negative predictive value of the test. In an immediate follow-up to this study, the same group was able to show that in patients admitted with decompensated heart failure changes in BNP levels during aggressive medical management were not only strong predictors of mortality and early readmission, but also provided an objective guide to treatment of patients admitted for decompensated heart failure. The authors suggest that therapy tailored to BNP test results may reduce the need for invasive hemodynamic monitoring in selected patients, therefore reducing to some degree the high cost associated with the management of heart failure *(9).*

In the study by Murdoch et al. *(10),* the authors sought to determine the benefit of oral therapy tailored to BNP test results in CHF. Patients with mild to moderate symptoms of heart failure on stable, conventional therapy, including an angiotensin converting enzyme (ACE) inhibitor, were assigned to titration of the ACE inhibitor dosage according to serial measurement of plasma BNP concentration or to optimal empirical ACE inhibitor therapy. The results show that at the end of the 8-wk follow-up period, the BNP-guided approach was associated with a significant 42% reduction in plasma BNP concentrations compared to only a 12% decrease in the empirical group. The study also concludes that plasma BNP concentration is chronically reduced by sustained vasodilator therapy in heart failure, which is also associated with more profound inhibition of the renin–angiotensin– aldosterone system in patients being treated according to BNP levels when compared with the empiric treatment group of patients. The study by Troughton et al. *(11)* reports fewer cardiovascular events of death and hospital admission or heart failure decompensation in patients receiving therapy guided by plasma BNP levels compared to patients in whom adjustment of treatment relied on clinical assessment. During the 6-mo follow-up period, only 27% of patients in the BNP guided group experienced a cardiovascular event compared to as much as 53% of the patients in the clinical group. However, there was no difference in terms of quality of life, LV function, and renal function between the BNP and the clinically guided treatment group. The study also emphasizes that circulating levels of BNP can be reduced by aggressive drug therapy. This might be even more important for patients who have the highest elevations of BNP levels.

β-Adrenergic receptor blocking agents are now part of the current recommendations for treatment of heart failure. It has been suggested that the patients most likely to benefit from the use of β-blockers are those with the highest circulating levels of BNP. Therefore, neurohumoral profiling may be useful in identifying high-risk patients who might benefit from more aggressive treatment options. A study by Stanek et al. *(12)* assessed the value of neurohumoral profiling in patients with advanced LV dysfunction during treatment with the β-blocking agent atenolol. The study shows that treatment with the β-blocking agent decreased ANP after 6 mo of treatment and BNP levels after 6, 12, and 24 mo of treatment. Treatment with placebo did not change significantly any of the natriuretic peptide levels in this study. LV ejection fraction increased from 18% to 30% in the atenolol group, which was paralleled by a fall in BNP levels. The study clearly supports a potential role for BNP levels not only for the purposes of diagnosis and prognosis of CHF, but also as a tool for therapeutic monitoring of patients receiving complete neurohumoral blocking therapy.

Appropriate patient selection and accurate prediction of which patient would benefit most from interventions with ACE inhibitors and β-blocking agents, or from any other form of intervention remains unclear. The Australia–New Zealand heart failure study was specifically designed to address the issue of the efficacy of carvedilol in patients with ischemic LV dysfunction. Plasma neurohormones, including ANP and BNP, and norepinephrine levels were used as tools for prediction of adverse outcomes and response to treatment in 415 patients randomly assigned to receive carvedilol or placebo *(13)*. In this study, treatment with carvedilol reduced mortality rates and the incidence of heart failure in those patients who presented with higher pretreatment levels of BNP, but lesser activation of plasma norepinephrine. Furthermore, high norepinephrine levels did not predict additional benefit from carvedilol. The Australia–New Zealand heart failure study presents conclusive data showing that neurohumoral profiling in patients with heart failure may be a valuable tool to guide the use of β-blocking agents and objectively assess their efficacy. In a similar analysis of the clinical use of natriuretic peptides, the same group reported recently that the plasma concentrations of amino- (N)-terminal (NT)-proBNP and adrenomedullin were independent predictors of mortality and heart failure in patients with ischemic cardiomyopathy *(14)*. Importantly, treatment with the β-blocker carvedilol reduced both the mortality and the incidence of heart failure in those patients who presented with higher pretreatment plasma levels of NT proBNP and adrenomedullin. The study by Kawai et al. *(15)* also added to the growing body of evidence showing that treatment of CHF patients can be monitored using BNP levels. In a study of 30 patients with idiopathic dilated cardiomyopathy of measurements of plasma BNP levels provided accurate information regarding LV function and structure during β-blocker therapy. Treatment with carvedilol significantly reduced the LV end-diastolic dimension from 65 ± 8 mm to 61 ± 8 mm after 6 mo and improved LV ejection fraction from 34 ± 13% to 43 ± 12% in these patients. Carvedilol also decreased BNP levels in these patients from an average of 127 pg/mL to an average of 69 pg/mL. Interestingly, norepinephrine levels did not change significantly in this patient population.

In a study of 37 patients with stable NYHA functional class II or III heart failure and an ejection fraction of 45% or less, Tsutamoto et al. *(16)* sought to evaluate the effects of the aldosterone receptor antagonist spironolactone on neurohumoral factors and LV remodeling. Their findings indicate that treatment with spironolactone improves LV volume and mass, as documented by a decrease in LV end-diastolic volume index in the spironolactone group (192 ± 11 vs 178 ± 10 mL/m^2), while there were no changes in placebo-treated patients (169 ± 15 vs 170 ± 17 mL/m^2). LV mass index was also reduced in spironolactone-treated patients compared to placebo (158 ± 7.8 vs 147 ± 7.5 g/m^2). Treatment with spironolactone also resulted in markedly decreased levels of both BNP and ANP. The study suggests that spironolactone has a clear role in the process of LV remodeling in patients with nonischemic cardiomyopathy and that its efficacy can be documented using BNP.

The study by Ishikawa et al. *(17)* provides further evidence that efficacy of treatment can be documented using measurements of natriuretic peptides. In a population of 85 patients diagnosed with Duchenne's muscular dystrophy, 11 patients presented with dilated cardiomyopathy. Neuroendocrine monitoring with BNP and ANP was helpful in establishing the diagnosis of the underlying cardiomyopathy and in providing evidence for the efficacy of drug therapy with ACE inhibitors and β-adrenergic blocking agents. Treatment of these patients resulted in a significant decrease in neuroendocrine activation with a decline in BNP levels from 524 ± 439 to 59 ± 24 pg/mL, reversal of symptoms and signs of heart failure, and improvement of LV diastolic dimensions.

Because most patients with heart failure receive a standardized treatment, it has been hypothesized that pharmacotherapy guided by the levels of BNP would be more effective than pharmacotherapy guided by traditional assessment based on clinical symptoms. The available body of information supports this hypothesis and clearly suggests that measurements of BNP can be used for neurohumoral profiling in heart failure patients and as an indicator of efficacy of treatment regardless of the etiology of the disease. BNP levels may obviate the need for invasive hemodynamic monitoring; the concept of BNP guided treatment algorithms for heart failure may prove useful if they are adequately documented by well-designed studies. However, neurohumoral profiling is not intended as a substitute for routine clinical examination or other diagnostic studies. The natriuretic peptides in heart failure should be perceived only as a useful clinical tool, which may improve and facilitate the management of patients with heart failure by triggering additional and/or more aggressive management strategies.

MONITORING CHEMOTHERAPY

Doxorubicin is an anthracycline antibiotic used clinically in the treatment of leukemias, lymphomas, and solid tumors. The major side effect of doxorubicin is its cardiotoxicity, which ultimately leads to dilated cardiomyopathy with clinical signs and symptoms of heart failure. Measurement of radionuclide LV ejection fraction has been the gold standard for monitoring cardiac function in patients receiving chemotherapy. However, this technique is not sensitive enough and measurable changes in LV ejection fraction are usually indicative of an already significant amount of myocardial damage.

Several clinical studies have attempted to use the natriuretic peptides to monitor doxorubicin cardiotoxicity. In a study of 30 adult patients who received 8–10 cycles of cyclophosphamide, doxorubicin, vincristine, and prednisone to a cumulative doxorubicin dose of 400–500 mg/m^2 of body surface area for non-Hodgkin's lymphoma, Nousiainen et al. *(18)* sought to determine the value of serial measurements of the natriuretic peptides for the early detection of doxorubicin-induced cardiomyopathy. LV ejection fraction decreased early in these patients, at a cumulative doxorubicin dose of 200 mg/m^2 of body surface area. However, ANP, NT-proANP, and BNP levels increased significantly when compared to prechemotherapy values only when the total cumulative dose of doxorubicin was achieved and LV function was reduced significantly from 58.0 ± 1.3% to 49.6 ± 1.7%. There was a significant correlation between the increase in ANP and the decrease in LV ejection fraction and a trend toward significance between the increase in NT-proANP and the decrease in LV ejection fraction. From a clinical perspective, the serial measurements of three different natriuretic peptides—ANP, NT-proANP, and BNP —did not accurately predict early enough the degree of impairment of myocardial performance in patients receiving chemotherapy for non-Hodgkin's lymphoma. This observation provides an important insight into the pathophysiological sequence of events leading to natriuretic peptide hormone secretion during chemotherapy. It suggests that the compensatory capability of the myocardium is exceeded first as a result of exposure to chemotherapy, leading consequently to atrial and ventricular chamber dilation with upregulation of the synthesis of natriuretic peptides and their release into the circulation.

Meinardi et al. *(19)* provide several levels of evidence for early onset of subclinical cardiotoxicity in a prospective study of patients receiving epirubicin in the adjuvant treatment of advanced breast cancer followed by locoregional radiotherapy. The results of the study show a decrease in LV ejection fraction from 0.61 before treatment to 0.54 at the end of therapy. Seventeen percent of the patients had a LV ejection fraction of 0.50 or less and 28% of the population had a decline of 0.10 units. Increasing levels of BNP from 2.9 pmol/L to 5.1 pmol/L and ANP from 237 pmol/L to 347 pmol/L paralleled this decline in ejection fraction. The authors also report increased duration of the time-corrected QT interval but no changes in different indices of diastolic function. The changes reported in the study were observed after low cumulative doses of epirubicin and are thought to represent subclinical myocardial damage. This may indicate a long-term risk for the development of late-onset refractory heart failure because of cumulative exposure to both chemotherapy and radiotherapy. Snowden et al. *(20)* have used a similar approach in a study designed to document the value of serial plasma BNP levels for detecting signs of heart failure in patients undergoing cytotoxic conditioning for hemopoietic stem cell transplantation. Three of the 15 patients originally included into the study developed clinical signs of heart failure paralleled by a significant release of BNP. There was an association between BNP levels and the presence of high-dose cyclophosphamide in the preoperative regimen. The authors conclude that BNP levels accurately identified patients at risk for the development of subsequent CHF and that BNP levels may be helpful for monitoring cytotoxic conditioning before stem cell transplantation.

In a study of patients diagnosed with acute leukemia receiving a daunorubicin-based chemotherapy protocol, three out of the 13 patients included into the study developed clinical signs of CHF after completion of chemotherapy, while five patients were diagnosed with subclinical heart failure *(21)*. The plasma levels of BNP in these patients increased above the prechemotherapy levels while patients who did not develop signs and symptoms of heart failure did not have an increase in BNP levels, even though a total accumulative dose of daunorubicin of >700 mg/m^2 of body surface area was reached. These observations suggest that BNP may be a useful marker for risk statification, early indication of anthracycline-induced cardiotoxicity and a sensitive tool for monitoring chemotherapy in adult patients. Similarly, in a study of pediatric patients who had previously received doxorubicin-based chemotherapy, LV dysfunction was detected by echocardiography in almost 24% of the children *(22)*. Measurements of BNP and ANP were increased in these patients compared to children with normal cardiac function and healthy controls. The levels of BNP and ANP correlated closely with LV systolic dysfunction but not with indices of diastolic dysfunction in this patient population.

Small cell lung cancer is clinically notorious for its ability to induce a paraneoplastic syndrome by synthesizing different biologically active substances. An interesting observation at the basic science level was made by Ohsaki et al. *(23)*, who demonstrates that small cell lung cancer cells have the ability to also synthesize BNP. The study shows that small cell lung cancer cells have detectable BNP mRNA and display BNP immunoreactivity. Whether these cells have the capability to produce final BNP protein in quantities large enough to cause potential analytical interferences with the measurement of BNP released from the myocardium in response to the toxic insult from chemotherapy requires further investigation.

The overall evidence suggests that monitoring of natriuretic peptide levels during the course of chemotherapy may provide a useful tool for identifying patients with asymptomatic LV dysfunction or patients at high risk for the development of significant chemotherapy-induced cardiomyopathy. One potential monitoring strategy would include obtaining baseline BNP levels and then repeating the measurement at every subsequent cycle of chemotherapy. This strategy will also allow the evaluation of protective regimens designed to minimize the side effects of doxorubicin-based protocols. It may also provide an opportunity to evaluate the cardiotoxic effects of new chemotherapeutic agents or combination of such agents. However, these applications remain speculative and require further testing in clinical studies.

TREATMENT OF ARTERIAL HYPERTENSION

Natriuretic peptides are increased in patients with LV hypertrophy, above-normal LV mass index, and LV diastolic dysfunction. Therefore, measurements of natriuretic peptides in hypertensive patients would not permit an accurate differentiation between the pathophysiological mechanisms known to cause elevations of natriuretic peptides in arterial hypertension *(24)*. Despite these limitations, Kato et al. *(25)* have reported that both ANP and BNP were significantly increased in patients with essential and malignant hypertension when compared to normotensive controls. These levels significantly declined after the patients received adequate antihypertensive treatment. It has also been shown that regression of LV mass is paralleled by a significant decline in plasma BNP levels in hypertensive patients. An interesting study by Minami et al. *(26)* in obese hypertensive patients shows that a dietary intervention using a standard diet of 2000 kcal/d followed by a hypocaloric diet of 850 kcal/d was associated with reduction in body weight, decrease in blood pressure, and a significant decrease in both BNP and ANP levels. Case reports in the literature also have shown the feasibility of using plasma levels of BNP as a tool to monitor efficacy of antihypertensive therapy *(27)*.

TREATMENT OF ARRHYTHMIAS AND MONITORING OF ELECTRICAL TREATMENT OPTIONS FOR CHF

Little attention has been directed at cardiac arrhythmias and their treatment from the perspective of natriuretic peptides. Cardiac arrhythmias are frequently associated with asynchronous contraction of atrial and ventricular chambers, which leads to chamber overload and dilation. At the myocyte level, this translates into a powerful stretch-mediated signal for the production and release of natriuretic peptides. In a study by Ohta et al. *(28),* patients who required cardioversion for rapid atrial fibrillation had significantly higher BNP levels compared to a group of healthy control subjects. More important, in the group of patients who experienced atrial fibrillation and had documented structural heart disease, BNP levels were further increased compared to patients who had atrial fibrillation, but in whom structural heart disease could not be identified. The results of this study also show that successful cardioversion and restoration of normal sinus rhythm reduced plasma BNP levels in patients with atrial fibrillation, suggesting that elevations of BNP occur as a result of the combination of volume imbalance and underlying heart disease. Furthermore, plasma ANP and BNP levels have been found to be increased in patients with nonphysiological VVI pacing compared to patients with physiological DDD and AAI pacing modes, suggesting that secretion of natriuretic peptides is also influenced by pacing mode and its consequences *(29)*.

MONITORING OF ACUTE CARDIAC ALLOGRAFT REJECTION IN HEART TRANSPLANT RECIPIENTS

There is a strong interest in the use of natriuretic peptides in clinical heart transplantation *(30,31)*. However, much of the information gathered in earlier studies has been descriptive and primarily focused on ANP *(32)*. The complexity of clinical transplantation is related to many factors, including recipient- and donor-related issues and pathologies, hemodynamic support and volume status during transplantation, and postoperative course. Adding to this complexity is the fact that many heart transplant recipients will experience episodes of high-grade acute cellular rejection, which usually requires aggressive immunosuppressive treatment. An interesting concept is the use of the natriuretic peptides to document acute rejection and/or predict the occurrence of future episodes of rejection. This approach would have the potential to decrease the number of serial endomyocardial biopsies and the risks and cost associated with these procedures. An interesting study by Masters et al. *(33)* reports a significant and selective increase in plasma BNP levels in heart transplant recipients with high-grade 3A acute cellular rejection. All rejection episodes that necessitated additional immunosuppressive treatment were usually accompanied by a significant increase in BNP plasma levels >400 pg/mL.

The authors also report that increasing BNP levels preceded overt rejection as assessed by histopathological criteria. Particularly noteworthy, ANP levels did not correlate with BNP levels in this study. The authors suggest that the up-regulation and secretion of different natriuretic peptides in heart transplant recipients follows different stimuli and signal transduction pathways. They further speculate that BNP plasma levels could theoretically provide the basis for a noninvasive screening test to document acute cardiac allograft rejection and the efficacy of anti-rejection treatment in patients who experience multiple acute rejection episodes.

PERSONAL EXPERIENCE WITH BNP

Heart Failure Secondary to LV Dysfunction

Tumor necrosis factor-α (TNF-α) is a pleiotropic cytokine with potent negative inotropic effects. There is evidence to suggest that inhibition of the TNF-α signaling pathway may improve the clinical status of patients with heart failure. We used BNP levels to assess the efficacy of a novel treatment strategy in CHF and the effect of TNF-α inhibition by a soluble TNF receptor fusion protein *(34)*. We obtained BNP levels at baseline and after 3 mo of treatment in patients with NYHA functional class III or IV *(35)*. These patients were randomly allocated to receive placebo or the TNF-α receptor fusion protein at a dose of 5 mg/m^2 or 12 mg/m^2 administered subcutaneously twice a week. Measurement of NYHA functional class, LV ejection fraction, and levels of the proinflammatory cytokine interleukin (IL)-6 and the antiinflammatory cytokine IL-10 were part of the protocol. Not surprisingly, BNP levels correlated with LV ejection fraction but the strength of the correlation was modest ($r = -0.33$, $p = 0.04$). There was a positive correlation between BNP levels and IL-6 levels at baseline ($r = 0.42$, $p = 0.01$). After 3 mo of treatment, BNP levels appeared to be lower in the group of patients receiving 12 mg/m^2 of the TNF receptor fusion protein. However, the amplitude of decrease in BNP levels (median change from baseline, -1.15 pg/mL) was modest. Importantly, patients in the placebo group showed an increase in BNP levels (median change from baseline, 1.88 pg/mL), which nearly achieved statistical significance ($p = 0.06$). At 3 mo of follow-up, decreased levels of BNP were associated with increased levels of the anti-inflammatory cytokine IL-10 ($r = -0.40$, $p = 0.02$). BNP levels also tended to be lower in patients with improved clinical outcomes as documented by a change in the clinical composite score based on death, hospitalization, NYHA functional class, and quality of life. These findings suggest that BNP levels correlate with markers of disease severity in patients with stable signs and symptoms of heart failure, and with improved clinical status and suppressed inflammatory response after 3 mo of treatment with a soluble TNF-α receptor fusion protein. However, the amplitude of the response to treatment was modest. The reason for this limited decrease in BNP levels after 3 mo of treatment is interesting to analyze. Two hypotheses should be considered. The first would suggest that the BNP assay used in the study (Biosite Diagnostics, San Diego, CA) was not sensitive enough and failed to detect any further improvement in patients' clinical status. The alternative explanation would be that the assay was adequately sensitive and objectively documented the lack of clinical response to active treatment. This implies lack of efficacy of the TNF-α receptor fusion protein in patients with stable heart failure symptoms.

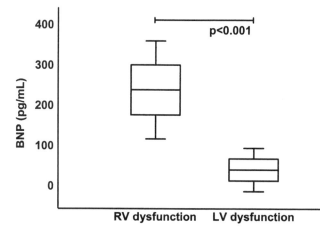

Fig. 3. Box and whisker plots of BNP levels in patients with RV and LV dysfunction. The *line* within the box is the mean value, the *upper* and *lower* box values represent ± 1 times the standard error, and the whiskers in the plot are defined as the mean ± 1.96 times the standard error. (E. Missov, *unpublished data*.)

Heart Failure Secondary to Right Ventricular (RV) Dysfunction

The right ventricle has a limited ability to respond to pressure and volume overload. The increased afterload in pulmonary arterial hypertension rapidly leads to remodeling, hypertrophy, and failure. In a study of 23 patients with pulmonary hypertension and a normal LV ejection fraction of 0.61 ± 0.02, we obtained BNP levels at baseline and 3 mo after initiating intravenous prostacyclin therapy. BNP values as high as 1190 pg/mL at baseline and 1390 pg/mL at follow-up were recorded in some patients. The most consistent correlations were found between BNP levels and invasive hemodynamic indices. Baseline and follow-up BNP measures showed a positive correlation with right atrial pressure and a negative correlation with cardiac index. However, the baseline values and values after 3 mo of therapy with prostacyclin, on average 245 pg/mL and 274 pg/mL, respectively were substantially equivalent. (E. Missov, *unpublished data*). These observations led basically to two conclusions: (1) that BNP levels can be increased in clinical conditions associated with RV dysfunction in the absence of LV failure; and (2) that more frequent serial measurements of BNP may be necessary for the monitoring of individual response to therapy in selected patients.

The combined analysis of our experience with BNP measurements in patients with LV dysfunction and isolated RV dysfunction shows higher values in patients in RV dysfunction (245 ± 62 vs 46 ± 27 pg/mL, $p < 0.001$) and suggests an interesting pathophysiological difference. Patients with pulmonary hypertension and a normal LV ejection fraction, as those described in our study, present with RV dysfunction secondary to pressure overload while patients with classic LV dysfunction usually are more volume overloaded. Although based on a relatively small number of observations, these data suggest a selective response of BNP synthesis to pressure vs volume overload stimuli. These differences are presented in Fig. 3 and will necessitate confirmation in a larger series as well as with the use of ANP and newer BNP assays.

Heart Transplant Recipients

The major long-term complication of heart transplantation is the development of transplant-related vasculopathy, which usually manifests as heart failure or its complications. Transplant-related vasculopathy has been the focus of intense research at the basic science and clinical level. Its incidence is rising as the number of long-term heart transplant survivors increases largely because of the availability of new and more effective immunosuppressive regimens. We have previously reported that lactate dehydrogenase isoenzyme profiling in endomyocardial biopsy tissue samples provided accurate diagnostic and prognostic information in long-term heart transplant survivors *(36)*. BNP levels have not been described in long-term heart transplant survivors nor have they been systematically linked to results from coronary angiography, intravascular ultrasound analysis, and magnetic resonance imaging. Preliminary data from our laboratory show that heart transplant recipients may have average BNP levels of 1280 pg/mL while being completely asymptomatic and free of acute rejection. In a study of more than 80 patients who received a heart transplant between 1985 and 2001, BNP levels ranged from normal at 76 pg/mL to as high as 12,000 pg/mL, with values in the 2500–5000 pg/mL range being frequently observed. These values are typical for heart failure patients with advanced disease or during an acute episode of decompensation. The clinical significance and potential implications of these findings are being currently investigated (E. Missov, *unpublished data*).

SUMMARY

BNP is a useful adjunct to the diagnosis of heart failure. It also provides useful prognostic information. Here, we have summarized some of the data on what will probably become the most important clinical utilization of BNP—monitoring of the efficacy of therapy. CHF promises to be the most significant field of application for BNP but any clinical condition associated with pressure or volume overload from any etiology, or any form of hemodynamic dysfunction, will most likely benefit from the pathophysiological information derived from the measurement of BNP. Few markers have matured the way BNP has—from a research tool to a widely accepted and useful in routine clinical practice assay.

ABBREVIATIONS

ACE, Angiotensin converting enzyme; ANP, BNP, atrial and B-type natriuretic peptides; CHF, congestive heart failure; LV, left ventricular; NT, amino (N)-terminal; NYHA, New York Heart Association; RV, right ventricular; TNF-α, tumor necrosis factor-α.

REFERENCES

1. Miller L, Missov E. Epidemiology of heart failure. Cardiol Clin 2001;19:547–555.
2. Haldeman G, Croft J, Giles W, et al. Hospitalization of patients with heart failure: National Hospital Discharge Survey, 1985 to 1995. Am Heart J 1999;137:352–360.
3. Espiner E. Physiology of natriuretic peptides. J Intern Med 1994;235:527–541.
4. Mair J, Friedl W, Thomas S, et al. Natriuretic peptides in assessment of left ventricular dysfunction.scand J Clin Lab Invest 1999;59:132–142.
5. Maisel A. B-type natriuretic peptide in the diagnosis and management of congestive heart failure. Cardiol Clin 2001;19:557–571.

6. Kazanegra R, Cheng V, Garcia A, et al. A rapid test for b-type natriuretic peptide correlates with falling wedge pressures in patients treated for decompensated heart failure: a pilot
   study. J Cardiac Fail 2001;7:21–29.

7. Sasaki T, Kubo T, Komamura K, Nishikimi T. Effects of long-term treatment with pimobendan on neurohumoral factors in patients with non-ischemic chronic moderate heart
   failure. J Cardiol 1999;33:317–325.

8. Dao Q, Krishnaswamy P, Kazanegra R, et al. Utility of B-type natriuretic peptide in the
   diagnosis of congestive heart failure in an urgent-care setting. J Am J Coll Cardiol 2001;
   37:379–385.

9. Cheng V, Kazanagra R, Garcia A, et al. A rapid bedside test for b-type peptide predicts
   treatment outcomes in patients admitted for decompensated heart failure: a pilot study.
   J Am Coll Cardiol 2001;37:386–391.

10. Murdoch DR, McDonagh TA, Byrne J, et al. Titration of vasodilator therapy in chronic
    heart failure according to plasma brain natriuretic peptide concentration: randomized com-
    parison of the hemodynamic and neuroendocrine effects of tailored versus empirical ther-
    apy. Am Heart J 1999;138:1126–1132.

11. Troughton RW, Frampton CM, Yandle TG, et al. Treatment of heart failure guided by plasma
    aminoterminal brain natriuretic peptide (N-BNP) concentrations. Lancet 2000;355:1126–1130.

12. Stanek B, Frey B, Hülsmann, et al. Prognostic evaluation of neurohumoral plasma levels
    before and during beta-blocker therapy in advanced left ventricular dysfunction. J Am Coll
    Cardiol 2001;38:436–442.

13. Richards AM, Doughty R, Nicholls MG, et al. Neurohumoral prediction of benefit from
    carvedilol in ischemic left ventricular dysfunction. Circulation 1999;99:786–792.

14. Richards AM, Doughty R, Nicholls MG, et al. Plasma N-terminal pro-brain natriuretic pep-
    tide and adrenomedullin: prognostic utility and prediction of benefit from carvedilol in
    chronic ischemic left ventricular dysfunction. J Am Coll Cardiol 2001;37:1781–1787.

15. Kawai K, Hata K, Takaoka H, et al. Plasma brain natriuretic peptide as a novel therapeutic
    indicator in idiopathic dilated cardiomyopathy during beta-blocker therapy: a potential of
    hormone-guided treatment. Am Heart J 2001;141:925–932.

16. Tsutamoto T, Wada A, Maeda K, et al. Effect of spironolactone on plasma brain natriuretic
    peptide and left ventricular remodeling in patients with congestive heart failure. J Am Coll
    Cardiol 2001;37:1228–1233.

17. Ishikawa Y, Bach JR, Minami R. Cardioprotection for Duchenne's muscular dystrophy.
    Am Heart J 1999;137:895–902.

18. Nousiainen T, Jantunen E, Vanninen E, et al. Natriuretic peptides as markers of cardiotox-
    icity during doxorubicin treatment for non-Hodgkin's lymphoma. Eur J Haematol 1999;62:
    135–141.

19. Meinardi MT, van Veldhuisen DJ, Gietema JA, et al. Prospective evaluation of early cardiac
    damage induced by epirubicin-containing adjuvant chemotherapy and locoregional radio-
    therapy in breast cancer patients. J Clin Oncol 2001;19:2746–2753.

20. Snowden JA, Hill GR, Hunt P, et al. Assessment of cardiotoxicity during haemopoietic
    stem cell transplantation with plasma brain natriuretic peptide. Bone Marrow Transplant
    2000;26:309–313.

21. Okumura H, Iuchi K, Yoshida T, et al. Brain natriuretic peptide is a predictor of anthracy-
    cline-induced cardiotoxicity. Acta Haematol 2000;104:158–163.

22. Hayakawa H, Komada Y, Hirayama M, et al. Plasma levels of natriuretic peptides in rela-
    tion to doxorubicin-induced cardiotoxicity and cardiac function in children with cancer.
    Med Pediatr Oncol 2001;37:4–9.

23. Ohsaki Y, Gross AJ, Le PT, Oie H, Johnson BE. Human small cell lung cancer cells pro-
    duce brain natriuretic peptide. Oncology 1999;56:155–159.

24. Mair J, Hammerer-Lercher A, Puschendorf B. The impact of cardiac natriuretic peptide determination on the diagnosis and management of heart failure. Clin Chem Lab Med 2001; 39:571–588.

25. Kato J, Kitamura K, Matsui E, et al. Plasma adrenomedullin and natriuretic peptides in patients with essential or malignant hypertension. Hypertens Res1999;22:61–65.

26. Minami J, Nishikimi T, Ishimitsu T, et al. Effect of a hypocaloric diet on adrenomedullin and natriuretic peptides in obese patients with essential hypertension. J Cardiovasc Pharmacol 2000;36(Suppl 2):S83–S86.

27. Nishikimi T, Matsuoka H, Ishikawa K, et al. Antihypertensive therapy reduces increased plasma levels of adrenomedullin and brain natriuretic peptide concomitant with regression of left ventricular hypertrophy in a patient with malignant hypertension. Hypertens Res 1996; 19:97–101.

28. Ohta Y, Shimada T, Yoshitomi H, et al. Drop in plasma brain natriuretic peptide levels after successful direct current cardioversion in chronic atrial fibrillation. Can J Cardiol 2001;17: 415–420.

29. Horie H, Tsutamoto T, Ishimoto N, et al. Plasma brain natriuretic peptide as a biochemical marker for atrioventricular sequence in patients with pacemakers. Pacing Clin Electrophysiol 1999;22:282–290.

30. Master R, Davies R, Keon W, et al. Neuroendocrine response to cardiac transplantation. Can J Cardiol 1993;9:609–617.

31. El Gamel A, Yonan N, Keevil B, et al. Significance of raised natriuretic peptides after bicaval and standard cardiac transplantation. Ann Thorac Surg 1997;63:1095–1100.

32. Farge D, Perrier P, Viossat I, et al. Elevation of plasma natriuretic factor after cardiac transplantation in rats. Transplantation 1990;50:167–170.

33. Masters RG, Davies RA, Veinot JP, et al. Discoordinate modulation of natriuretic peptides during acute cardiac allograft rejection in humans. Circulation 1999;100:287–291.

34. Lisman K, Stetson S, Koerner M. Managing heart failure with immunomodulatory agents. Cardiol Clin 2001;19:547–555.

35. Missov E, Wieczorek S, Wu A, et al. Brain natriuretic peptide levels are associated with improved clinical status in patients with chronic heart failure after treatment with Enbrel (etanerept, TNF receptor) (abstract). Circulation 2000;102:II–532.

36. Missov E, Boularan AM, Bonifacj C, et al. Prognostic value of myocardial lactate dehydrogenase subunit ratio in heart transplant recipients. J Heart Lung Transplant 1998;17:959–968.

26

N-Terminal pro-B-Type Natriuretic Peptide

Torbjørn Omland and Christian Hall

INTRODUCTION

Historical Background, Biochemistry, and Physiology

The demonstration of specific granules in atrial muscle cells *(1)* and of the potent natriuretic, diuretic, and hypotensive response elicited by intravenous injection of atrial myocardial extract in rats *(2)* represent seminal, landmark findings in the era of cardiac natriuretic peptide research. During the past 20 yr remarkable scientific progress has been made, and by 2002 measurement of natriuretic peptides has been established as a valuable diagnostic and prognostic tool in clinical cardiology. Atrial or A-type natriuretic peptide (ANP) was purified, sequenced, and synthesized in the early 1980s *(3,4)*, and the first report showing a natriuretic, diuretic, and vasodilatory effect of infusion of synthetic ANP in humans was published in 1985 *(5)*. Within a short period of time several research groups reported that elevated plasma concentrations of ANP were found in patients with congestive heart failure (CHF) *(6,7)*. Moreover, a positive correlation between circulating ANP concentrations and atrial pressures was observed *(8,9)*.

Brain or B-type natriuretic peptide (BNP) was first identified in porcine brain in 1988 *(10)*, but subsequently found to be present in ventricular myocardium, the main source of circulating BNP *(11)*. ANP and BNP share structural and physiological features. Although encoded by separate genes, the two peptides show a high degree of primary structure homology and share a common ring structure. Through binding to guanylyl cyclase coupled, high-affinity natriuretic peptide-A (NPA) receptors on target cells, intracellular levels of cGMP are increased. This second messenger mediates the main physiological actions of ANP and BNP, including vasodilation, natriuresis, diuresis, and inhibition of renin release and aldosterone production. Accordingly, these peptides may be regarded as endogenous, functional antagonists of the renin–angiotensin–aldosterone system *(12)*.

The main secretory stimulus for both ANP and BNP appears to be stretch of cardiomyocytes *(13,14)*, and both ANP and BNP have therefore been proposed as potentially useful, noninvasive indicators of hemodynamic status and ventricular function. Because of the combined ventricular and atrial origin and the very low circulating concentrations found in the normal state, BNP has been considered a more sensitive and specific indicator of left ventricular (LV) function than ANP, which is predominantly secreted from the atria. Indeed, in most comparative studies BNP has been shown to reflect LV function more accurately than ANP.

From: *Cardiac Markers, Second Edition*
Edited by: Alan H. B. Wu @ Humana Press Inc., Totowa, NJ

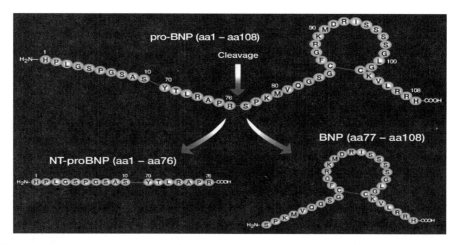

Fig. 1. Schematic presentation of the human proBNP precursor. ProBNP 1–108 is cleaved into BNP-32 and an N-terminal fragment.

Like most peptide hormones, ANP and BNP are synthesized as longer precursor peptides or prohormones, which are subsequently split into biologically active and inactive fragments. The 126-amino-acid ANP prohormone is cleaved on secretion into a biologically active, 28-amino-acid, carboxy- (C)-terminal fragment (proANP 99–126) and a biologically inactive amino- (N)-terminal fragment (proANP 1–98). NT-proANP circulates predominantly as a 98-amino-acid peptide *(15),* but there is some evidence to suggest further subdivision into smaller fragments that may possess biological activity *(16).* Although the N- and C-terminal fragments are secreted in a 1:1 fashion, circulating levels may differ because of different clearance characteristics. Accordingly, the in vivo plasma half-life of NT-proANP is much longer than that of the ANP (slow component 55 min vs 13 min in the rat) *(17),* and the circulating concentrations in humans are correspondingly higher *(15,18).*

The processing of proBNP to NT-proBNP and the 32-amino-acid, biologically active BNP is less well defined. A family of peptides is derived from the BNP gene. In human cardiac tissue BNP appears to be found predominantly in the 32-amino-acid form, but a significant amount is also stored as the intact 108-amino-acid precursor peptide, proBNP *(11).* In contrast to proANP, proBNP is only partially stored in granules, and the regulation of BNP synthesis and secretion appears to take place at the level of gene expression *(12,14).* In human plasma both the biologically active 32-amino-acid C-terminal fragment (BNP or proBNP 77–108), the 76-amino-acid NT fragment (NT-proBNP or proBNP 1–76), and other high-molecular-weight fragments, possibly intact proBNP 1–108, are found circulating *(19–23).* The processing of proBNP to NT-proBNP and BNP probably occurs both intracellularly and in the circulation. The amino acid sequences of proBNP and of the C- and N-terminal fragments are illustrated in Fig. 1.

HEART FAILURE

The Magnitude of the Problem

In spite of a significant reduction in the incidence of acute myocardial infarction (AMI) in Western societies during the last decades, the prevalence of chronic symptomatic and

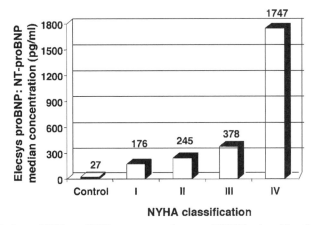

Fig. 2. Correlation of NT-proBNP concentrations to NYHA classification of heart failure. (Data from Roche Diagnostics, Elecsys proBNP package insert.)

asymptomatic LV systolic dysfunction has been increasing *(24)*. The rising prevalence has been ascribed to an increase in the proportion of elderly in the population and to therapeutic advances in the care of patients with AMI and chronic heart failure, notably the use of thrombolytic agents, aspirin, angiotensin converting enzyme (ACE) inhibitors, and β-adrenergic antagonists *(25)*. In the United States the prevalence of chronic symptomatic LV systolic dysfunction has been estimated to be approx 2% of the adult population *(26)*.

The public health importance of chronic heart failure is attributable not only to its high prevalence, but also to the markedly reduced quality of life and shortened life expectancy associated with its diagnosis. Because patients with symptomatic chronic heart failure commonly require frequent and prolonged hospitalizations, health care expenditure attributed to this patient group is significant. In addition to being a major cause of morbidity, particularly in the elderly, chronic heart failure is associated with a grave prognosis. In the United States the death of about 200,000 patients is attributed to chronic heart failure annually.

The Diagnosis of Heart Failure and LV Dysfunction

The clinical diagnosis of heart failure may represent a considerable challenge, particularly in the obese, in women, and in the elderly *(27)*. Because contemporary heart failure therapy has been shown to reduce significantly mortality and the number of hospital readmissions, an early and correct diagnosis is crucial. The cost and potential side effects associated with heart failure therapy also mean that overtreatment should best be avoided.

The clinical syndrome of CHF failure is often the end stage of progressive LV dysfunction and is often preceded by an asymptomatic "latent" phase. Asymptomatic LV dysfunction may in fact be as common as the symptomatic form *(28)*. Importantly, the asymptomatic phase may be prolonged by proper medical therapy, including ACE inhibitors *(29)*. As mentioned in the preceding, the diagnostic value of natriuretic peptides as indicators of LV dysfunction and the prognostic value in patients with AMI and chronic heart failure have been evaluated in a large number of studies. All cardiac natriuretic peptide fragments, including NT-proBNP, increase in proportion to the severity of symptoms, as expressed by the New York Heart Association (NYHA) functional class (Fig. 2).

Early Studies of NT-proBNP in Heart Failure

Using an antiserum raised in rabbits to a synthetic human NT-proBNP fragment (proBNP 1–13), the Christchurch Cardioendocrine Research Group in 1995 for the first time reported the presence of circulating NT-proBNP (proBNP 1–76) in human plasma *(20)*. Not unexpectedly, given the previous studies of BNP in heart failure, circulating concentrations of NT-proBNP were higher in patients with CHF than in healthy subjects. Interestingly, the ratio between plasma NT-proBNP and BNP in healthy subjects ranged from 1.9 to 3.0:1, whereas in patients with CHF this ratio ranged from 3.0 to 9.2:1. The more pronounced increments in circulating NT-proBNP from the healthy to the diseased state suggested enhanced discriminatory ability for NT-proBNP compared to BNP. The observation that circulating concentrations of NT-proBNP exceed those of BNP is suggestive of a slower clearance rate for NT-proBNP than for BNP. The in vivo plasma half-life of BNP has been estimated to be approx 21 min *(11)*. Studies in humans have yet to be performed to calculate the circulating half-life of NT-proBNP, but investigations indicate that in sheep the half-life may be as long as 70 min *(30)*.

NT-proBNP as a Diagnostic Test
for LV Systolic Dysfunction in High-Risk Individuals

In a study of 249 consecutive patients referred for echocardiography (195 inpatients) because of clinical suspicion of heart failure, current treatment for heart failure (ACE inhibitors, diuretics, digoxin), a history of ischemic heart disease (prior MI or angina, presence of pathological Q waves), a history of hypertension, or a history of shortness of breath in the absence of chronic airways disease, NT-proBNP was measured and related to an echocardiographic LV wall motion score *(31)*. Ninety-six out of the 243 patients with analyzable echocardiograms were diagnosed with LV dysfunction, defined as a wall motion score ≤ 1.2. The concentration of NT-proBNP was significantly higher in patients with LV dysfunction than in those with a wall motion score > 1.2. Moreover, an inverse relationship between plasma NT-proBNP levels and the wall motion score was observed ($r = -0.62$; $p < 0.001$). In a multivariate regression model, NT-proBNP was a better predictor of LV dysfunction than any other single factor, including age, gender, and diuretic and ACE inhibitor use, and the predictive ability of the model improved only marginally by including these covariables. A plasma NT-proBNP concentration > 275 pmol/L predicted LV dysfunction with a sensitivity of 94%, a specificity of 55%, a positive predictive value of 58%, and a negative predictive value of 93%. The area under the receiver operating characteristic (ROC) curve was 0.85 (Fig. 3), meaning that a subject with LV dysfunction would have a higher plasma NT-proBNP level than subjects without LV dysfunction in 85 out of 100 cases.

In a recent article, the diagnostic performance of NT-proBNP as an indicator of LV dysfunction was compared in a head-to-head fashion with two other natriuretic peptide fragments, BNP and NT-proANP *(32)*. Fifty-seven patients with stable, NYHA class I–III chronic heart failure were studied. LV ejection fraction was determined by three-dimensional echocardiography and radionuclide ventriculography. Areas under ROC curves for detection of an ejection fraction $< 40\%$ were 0.83, 0.79, and 0.65 for BNP, NT-proBNP, and NT-proANP, respectively. The difference between BNP and NT-proBNP was not statistically significant, suggesting that in practical terms the diagnostic accuracy

Area under ROC curve = 0·8539

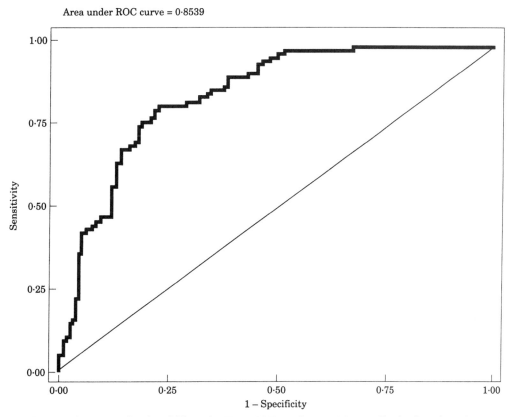

Fig. 3. ROC curve for the ability of NT-proBNP to detect LV systolic dysfunction. See text for details. (Talwar S, et al. Eur Heart J 1999:20:1740.)

of the two fragments is similar. However, the statistical power of a study this size to detect differences in diagnostic accuracy is quite limited.

NT-proBNP as a Screening Test
for LV Systolic Dysfunction in the General Population

The diagnostic value of NT-proBNP as a screening test for symptomatic and asymptomatic LV dysfunction in a population-based study has also been investigated *(33)*. Using an enzyme-linked immunosorbent assay (ELISA) method, NT-proBNP plasma concentrations were determined in 1209 men and women aged 25–74 yr. LV ejection fraction was assessed by two-dimensional echocardiography. An ejection fraction <30%, considered significant LV dysfunction, was detected in 3.2% of the study subjects. A NT-proBNP concentration of 86 pg/mL had a sensitivity of 69% and a specificity of 92% for detecting LV dysfunction. The diagnostic value of NT-proBNP > 86 pg/mL (odds ratio [95% CI] of 7.3 [3–18]) tended to be slightly better than that of BNP > 12.9 pg/mL (odds ratio [95% CI 5.6 [2–17]). However, this difference was not statistically significant, again suggesting that the predictive ability of BNP and NT-proBNP is comparable.

In another preliminary report, a Danish group evaluated the diagnostic accuracy of NT-proBNP as indicators of clinical heart failure and/or LV systolic dysfunction in an age-controlled sample of the general population *(34)*. NT-proBNP concentrations were assessed in 683 subjects who, after having filled in a heart failure questionnaire, were examined clinically and had an electrocardiogram and echocardiography performed. LV dysfunction, defined as an ejection fraction < 55%, was diagnosed in 11% of study subjects. The inverse correlation between NT-proBNP and ejection fraction was relatively modest ($r = -0.33$), but highly significant. In a multivariate analysis, the presence of an abnormal electrocardiogram and NT-proBNP were the only independent markers of LV dysfunction across all gender and age groups, and NT-proBNP emerged as the single most powerful marker of LV dysfunction.

NT-proBNP-Guided Therapy in Heart Failure

Although investigators in the field have for some time raised the possibility that BNP determination might represent a useful tool in guiding therapy in patients with chronic CHF, not until recently have data become available supporting such a concept. In a landmark paper in *The Lancet*, the Christchurch group demonstrated that in a small group of patients with systolic LV dysfunction and symptomatic chronic heart failure ($n = 69$), treatment guided by measurement of NT-proBNP resulted in significantly fewer total cardiovascular events (death, hospital admissions, or heart failure decompensations) than treatment guided by clinical assessment (Fig. 4) *(35)*. Despite the intriguing results, the clinical consequences of the study are somewhat unclear due to some important study limitations: (1) the sample size was modest, (2) the study was conducted prior to widespread use of β-blockers in chronic heart failure, and (3) as the reference guide to therapy, the Framingham criteria, originally constructed as a tool for diagnosing heart failure in the setting of an epidemiological study, were used. However, the data are very intriguing, and attempts to reproduce the findings in large-scale studies employing modern, commercially available, rapid assays are clearly warranted.

The Prognostic Value of NT-proBNP in the General Population

The prognostic value of natriuretic peptide determination in the general population has been examined by the North Glasgow Monitoring Trends and Determinants in Cardiovascular Disease (MONICA) study group *(36)*. In a random geographical sample of 1209 men and women aged 25–74 yr, baseline plasma NT-proBNP levels, as assessed by an ELISA, were significantly related to all-cause mortality at 4 yr. The median plasma concentration in survivors (22 pg/mL) was significantly lower than the median concentration in those who died (62 pg/mL). When the prognostic value of BNP (cut-off value 13 pg/mL) and NT-proBNP (cutoff value 86 pg/mL) were directly compared in a Cox proportional hazards regression model, BNP did not provide additional prognostic value to that obtained from N-BNP alone. Moreover, the univariate hazard ratio point estimates were somewhat higher for NT-proBNP (3.0 [95% CI: 1.6–5.3]) than that for BNP (2.0 [95% CI: 1.1–3.6]). However, the confidence intervals did overlap, suggesting that the difference was not statistically significant.

The Prognostic Value of NT-proBNP in Chronic LV Dysfunction

The prognostic value of NT-proBNP in patients with chronic LV dysfunction has been examined in a substudy of the Australia–New Zealand Heart Failure Group Carvedilol

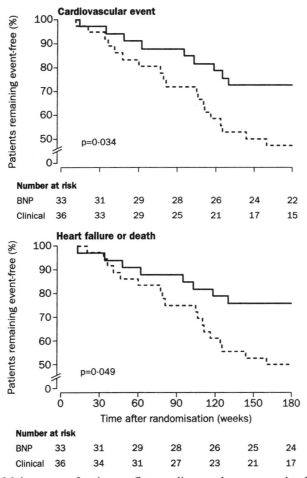

Fig. 4. Kaplan–Meier curves for time to first cardiovascular event and to heart-failure event or death in patients randomized to NT-proBNP guided (*solid line*) vs clinically guided (*dashed line*) heart failure therapy (see text for details). (Reprinted with permission from Elsevier Science, Troughton RW, et al. Lancet 2000;355:1126–1130.)

Trial *(37)*. Plasma NT-proBNP concentrations were determined in 297 patients with chronic, stable heart failure and a LV ejection fraction < 45%, who were followed for 18 mo. A baseline NT-proBNP value greater than the median was associated with a significantly increased risk of mortality (risk ratio [95% CI] 4.7 [2.0–10.9]) and hospital admissions for heart failure (4.7 [2.2–10.3]). These relationships remained significant after adjustment for age, NYHA functional class, LV ejection fraction, a history of previous myocardial infarction, and previous admissions for heart failure. Interestingly, the β-adrenoceptor blocker carvedilol reduced the risk of death or heart failure in patients with supramedian plasma levels of NT-proBNP to rates not significantly different from those with inframedian plasma levels. These results underscore the great prognostic power of NT-proBNP and raise the possibility that future heart failure therapy may be tailored according to the neurohormonal profile of the patient.

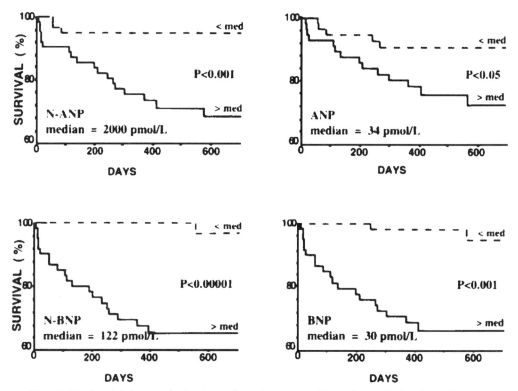

Fig. 5. Kaplan–Meier survival curves for subgroups with early postinfarction plasma peptide (NT-proANP [N-ANP], ANP, NT-proBNP [N-BNP], and BNP) concentrations above (*solid line*) and below (*dashed line*) the group median in 121 patients with MI. (Richards AM, et al. Circulation 1998;97:1921–1929, with permission from Lippincott Williams & Wilkins.)

ISCHEMIC HEART DISEASE

Plasma levels of NT-proBNP are raised in AMI in proportion to the degree of LV dysfunction *(38–40)* and have recently been shown to provide important prognostic information *(38,41)*. Following anterior AMI, a biphasic pattern has been observed with plasma level peaks at 14–48 h and 121–192 h. In general, patients with anterior wall myocardial infarction appear to reach higher plasma levels than those with inferior wall infarctions *(40)*. Moreover, in-hospital plasma levels correlate significantly with the in-hospital echocardiographic or radionuclide LV ejection fraction *(38,39)* and wall motion score index *(40),* and were predictive of death or LV dysfunction at 6 wk *(40)*. A strong relationship between plasma levels of NT-proBNP, obtained in the subacute phase, and long-term, all-cause mortality, as well as the rate of readmissions for heart failure after MI, has been convincingly demonstrated (Fig. 5) *(38)*.

Until recently, sparse information has been available regarding the natriuretic peptide system in patients with unstable angina and non-ST-segment elevation MI. In a small-scale, cross-sectional study, patients with unstable angina had significantly higher circulating NT-proBNP concentrations than patients with stable angina *(42)*. No significant difference was observed between patients with stable angina and healthy control subjects. The prognostic value of NT-proBNP in patients with non-ST-segment elevation acute coronary syndromes (unstable angina or non-ST-segment elevation MI) has

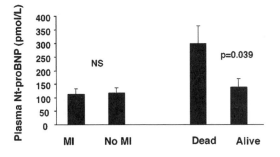

Fig. 6. Plasma NT-proBNP concentrations (mean ± SEM) in patients with non-ST-segment elevation acute coronary syndromes (ACS) who subsequently had a nonfatal MI or died within 43 d of admission, and in age- and sex-matched control subjects who did not die or progress to nonfatal MI (i.e., ACS patient with no MI). (Reprinted from Omland T, et al. Am J Cardiol 2002;89:463–465, with permission from Excerpta Medica Inc.)

recently been evaluated in a substudy of the Thrombolysis in Myocardial Infarction (TIMI) 11B trial. Circulating NT-proBNP levels were significantly associated with death within 43 d and provided complementary prognostic information to conventional risk markers, including cardiac troponin I *(41)* (Fig. 6). These findings challenge the view that substantial and irreversible reduction in LV function is required to produce increments in NT-proBNP levels of sufficient magnitude to provide prognostic information.

VALVULAR HEART DISEASE

Aortic stenosis is associated with LV hypertrophy, LV relaxation abnormalities, and may in some cases eventually progress to LV systolic dysfunction. The progression of aortic stenosis is routinely monitored by serial Doppler echocardiographic examinations, permitting noninvasive estimates of the transvalvular gradient and aortic valve orifice area. Recently, the relationship between NT-proBNP plasma levels and indices of cardiac function and structure has been examined in patients with aortic stenosis *(43,44)*. NT-proBNP was found to be a sensitive marker of mild LV hypertrophy *(44)*. In contrast, more advanced LV hypertrophy was required to induce elevation in circulating N-terminal proANP. Interestingly, calculation of the area under the ROC curves suggested that NT-proBNP was superior as an indicator of LV mass, whereas NT-proANP was a more sensitive marker of increased in left atrial pressure *(44)*. NT-proBNP levels have also been found to correlate significantly with the transvalvular pressure gradient *(43)*.

Mitral regurgitation, secondary to LV dilation, is common in patients with chronic heart failure. Moreover, mitral regurgitation is commonly associated with increased left atrial pressure. Given the associations with LV volumes and atrial pressure, it is not surprising that in patients with LV dysfunction, the severity of mitral regurgitation is predictive of circulating NT-proBNP levels *(31)*.

CONFOUNDING FACTORS

Several factors, cardiac and noncardiac, may influence the circulating levels of NT-proBNP and potentially confound the relationship to indices of cardiac function, thereby

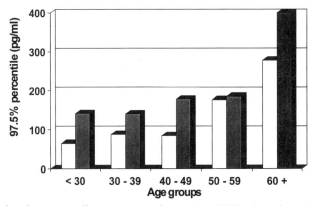

Fig. 7. Normal values according to age and sex (*n* = 2980; data from Roche Diagnostics, Elecsys proBNP package insert). Open bar, males; shaded bar, females.

reducing the diagnostic and prognostic accuracy. Age has been shown to be an important determinant of circulating natriuretic peptide levels, including NT-proBNP *(23,45)*. Both increased release and decreased clearance may contribute to elevated circulating levels of NT-proBNP in advanced age, but the exact mechanisms remain to be elucidated. Subclinical reduction in renal function, increased LV mass, and LV diastolic dysfunction are factors that may be essential for the observed increments in BNP and NT-proBNP levels with age. Recent population based studies from the Augsburg MONICA MI register and the Framingham Heart Study and have convincingly shown that BNP and NT-proBNP levels increase not only with age, but are also significantly higher in women than in men *(45,46)*. Accordingly, to reduce the confounding effect of age and gender upon the relationship between BNP/NT-proBNP and cardiac function, age-, and gender-specific normal values should probably be used. Figure 7 illustrates the effect of these confounding factors.

Other factors that may significantly affect circulating levels of NT-proBNP (although in most cases not to levels seen in advanced heart failure) include renal impairment *(31,45),* cardiac arrhythmias, including atrial fibrillation, myocardial ischemia *(42),* valvular heart disease *(42,43),* hypertension, and LV hypertrophy *(45,47).* These observations suggest that a normal NT-proBNP concentration with a high degree of diagnostic accuracy may rule out the presence of heart failure. On the other hand, a mildly to moderately increased NT-proBNP value is a nonspecific finding and implies that further investigations, including an echocardiogram in most cases, are required to obtain a definite diagnosis.

ASSAYS

The first assays used to measure NT-proBNP in plasma were competitive radioimmunoassays with or without prior chromatographic extraction *(20–23).* The analytic performance of different antibodies vary, and the results obtained depend critically on the antibody used. For instance, in two studies comparing different cardiac natriuretic peptides as indicators of LV dysfunction, the predictive value of proBNP (amino acid sequence 22–46) was markedly lower than that of BNP, ANP, and NT-proANP *(48,49).* However, the commercial antibody used in both studies appears to show limited recognition of endogenous immunoreactive NT-proBNP, explaining the poor diagnostic performance *(50)*.

Other methods used to measure NT-proBNP include immunoluminometric assays *(51)* and enzyme-linked immunoassays *(52,53)*. Recently, Roche Diagnostics introduced an electrochemiluminescence immunoassay (Elecsys proBNP) for automated determination of NT-proBNP on the Roche Elecsys 1010/2010 and Modular Analytics E170 (Elecsys module) immunoassay analyzers *(54)*. The Elecsys proBNP assay contains polyclonal antibodies that recognize epitopes located on the N-terminal part of proBNP. Both serum and plasma samples may be used and the total duration of the assay is 18 min. Clearly, a high-quality, rapid test, such as the Elecsys proBNP assay, is a prerequisite for the propagation of NT-proBNP measurement in clinical routine.

IN VITRO STABILITY

In general terms, the apparent in vitro stability of a given peptide will depend on the type of assay and the characteristics of the antibodies used. Although the plasma half-life of NT-proBNP remains to be determined in humans, the in vitro stability of this peptide in plasma and full blood samples stored at room temperature has been investigated *(23,55)*. In one study, using an immunoluminometric assay with antibodies directed at the middle and C-terminal portions of NT-proBNP, EDTA and aprotinin plasma samples showed no significant difference in immunoreactive peptide levels between samples centrifuged immediately and stored at −70°C or kept at room temperature or on ice for 24 or 48 h *(55)*. In contrast, using a competitive radioimmunoassay with a polyclonal antibody directed at the N-terminal fragment (amino acid sequence 1–21) of NT-proBNP, plasma concentrations were stable after storage at room temperature for 3 and 6, but not for 24 or 72 h *(23)*. Two freeze–thaw cycles did not affect NT-proBNP immunoreactivity *(23)*.

CONCLUSIONS

Only 7 yr have passed from the first publication demonstrating the presence of NT-proBNP in human plasma. During this period a number of clinical studies have been published, documenting the usefulness of NT-proBNP measurements in the diagnosis of heart failure and LV dysfunction, and as a prognostic tool in acute coronary syndromes and in chronic LV dysfunction. With the introduction of rapid, automated assays, NT-proBNP determination will find an important place in the diagnostic armamentarium of the clinical cardiologist. It should still be emphasized that NT-proBNP, like other natriuretic peptides, are sensitive but unspecific markers of ventricular dysfunction. Although correlated to various indices of cardiac function, NT-proBNP should not be regarded as a surrogate for a single cardiac index (e.g., ejection fraction or end-diastolic pressure). Rather, circulating NT-proBNP (and BNP) levels are increased in a variety of cardiac conditions characterized by increased myocardial wall stress and increased intracardiac pressure *(45,56)*. The powerful independent prognostic information obtained from peptide measurements is probably related to this lack of diagnostic specificity, that is, many of the conditions associated with increased NT-proBNP levels may be associated with increased risk. Although remarkable progress has been made during recent years, further studies are required. To document the usefulness of natriuretic peptide measurements in the serial follow-up of heart failure patients in a large-scale trial, is one example of a study that is needed in the current era of evidence-based medicine.

ABBREVIATIONS

ACE, Angiotensin converting enzyme; AMI, acute myocardial infarction; ANP, atrial and BNP, B-type natriuretic peptide; CHF, congestive heart failure; ELISA, enzyme-linked immunosorbent assay; LV, left ventricular; MONICA, Monitoring Trends and Determinants in Cardiovascular Disease; NPA, natriuretic peptide A; NT, amino- (N)-terminal; NYHA, New York Heart Association; ROC, receiver operating characteristic; TIMI, Thrombolysis in Myocardial Infarction.

REFERENCES

1. Jamieson JD, Palade GE. Specific granules in atrial muscle cells. J Cell Biol 1964;23:151–172.
2. de Bold AJ, Borenstein HB, Veress AT, Sonnenberg H. A rapid and potent natriuretic response to intravenous injection of atrial myocardial extract in rats. Life Sci 1981;28:89–94.
3. Atlas SA, Kleinert HD, Camargo MJ, et al. Purification, sequencing, and synthesis of natriuretic and vasoactive rat atrial peptide. Nature 1984;309:717–719.
4. Kangawa K, Matsuo H. Purification and complete amino acid sequence of α-human atrial natriuretic polypeptide (α-hANP). Biochem Biophys Res Commun 1984;118:131–139.
5. Richards AM, Nicholls MG, Ikram H, Webster MW, Yandle TG, Espiner EA. Renal, haemodynamic, and hormonal effects of human alpha atrial natriuretic peptide in healthy volunteers. Lancet 1985;1:545–549.
6. Sugawara A, Nakao K, Morii N, et al. Alpha-human atrial natriuretic polypeptide is released from the heart and circulates in the body. Biochem Biophys Res Commun 1985;129:439–446.
7. Lang RE, Tholken H, Ganten D, Luft FC, Ruskoaho H, Unger T. Atrial natriuretic factor—a circulating hormone stimulated by volume loading. Nature 1985;314:264–266.
8. Raine AEG, Erne P, Bürgisser E, et al. Atrial natriuretic peptide and atrial pressure in patients with congestive heart failure. N Engl J Med 1986;315:533–537.
9. Burnett JC Jr, Kao PC, Hu DC, et al. Atrial natriuretic peptide elevation in congestive heart failure in the human. Science 1986;231:1145–1147.
10. Sudoh T, Kangawa K, Minamino N, Matsuo H. A new natriuretic peptide in porcine brain. Nature 1988;332:78–81.
11. Mukoyama M, Nakao K, Hosoda K, et al. Brain natriuretic peptide as a novel cardiac hormone in humans: evidence for an exquisite dual natriuretic peptide system, atrial natriuretic peptide and brain natriuretic peptide. J Clin Invest 1991;87:1402–1412.
12. Levin ER, Gardner DG, Samson WK. Natriuretic peptides (review). N Engl J Med 1998; 339:321–328.
13. Edwards BS, Zimmerman RS, Schwab TR, Heublein DM, Burnett JC Jr. Atrial stretch, not pressure, is the principal determinant controlling the acute release of atrial natriuretic factor. Circ Res 1988;62:191–195.
14. Magga J, Vuolteenaho O, Tokola H, Marttila M, Ruskoaho H. B-type natriuretic peptide: a myocyte-specific marker for characterizing load-induced alterations in cardiac gene expression (review). Ann Med 1998;30(Suppl 1):39–45.
15. Sundsfjord JA, Thibault G, Larochelle P, Cantin M. Identification and plasma concentrations of the N-terminal fragment of proatrial natriuretic factor in man. J Clin Endocrinol Metabol 1988;66:605–610.
16. Vesely D, Douglass MA, Dietz JR, et al. Three peptides from the atrial natriuretic factor prohormone amino terminus lower blood pressure and produce diuresis, natriuresis, and/or kaliuresis in humans. Circulation 1994;90:1129–1140.

17. Thibault G, Murthy K, Gutkowska J, et al. NH$_2$-terminal fragment of rat pro-atrial natriuretic factor in the circulation: identification, radioimmunoassay and half-life. Peptides 1988; 9:147–153.

18. Mathisen P, Hall C, Simonsen S. Comparative study of atrial peptides ANF (1–98) and ANF (99–126) as diagnostic markers of atrial distension in patients with cardiac disease. Scand J Clin Lab Invest 1991;53:41–49.

19. Yandle TG, Richards AM, Gilbert A, Fisher S, Holmes S, Espiner EA. Assay of brain natriuretic peptide (BNP) in human plasma: evidence for high molecular weight BNP as a major plasma component in heart failure. J Clin Endocrinol Metab 1993;76:832–838.

20. Hunt PJ, Yandle TG, Nicholls MG, Richards AM, Espiner EA. The amino-terminal portion of pro-brain natriuretic peptide (pro-BNP) circulates in human plasma. Biochem Biophys Res Commun 1995;214:1175–1183.

21. Hunt PJ, Espiner EA, Nicholls MG, Richards AM, Yandle TG.. The role of the circulation in processing pro-brain natriuretic peptide (proBNP) to amino-terminal BNP and BNP-32. Peptides 1997;18:1475–1481.

22. Hunt PJ, Espiner EA, Nicholls MG, Richards AM, Yandle TG. Immunoreactive amino-terminal pro-brain natriuretic peptide (NT-proBNP): a new marker of cardiac impairment. Clin Endocrinol (Oxf) 1997;47:287–296.

23. Schulz H, Langvik TÅ, Lund Sagen E, Smith J, Ahmadi N, Hall C. Radioimmunoassay for N-terminal probrain natriuretic peptide in human plasma. Scand. J Clin Lab Invest 2001;61: 33–42.

24. Cowie MR, Mosterd A, Wood DA, et al. The epidemiology of heart failure. Eur Heart J 1997; 18:208–225.

25. Dargie H J, McMurray JJ, McDonagh TA. Heart failure—implications of the true size of the problem. J Intern Med 1996;239:309–315.

26. Schocken DD, Arrieta MI, Leaverton PE, Ross EA. Prevalence and mortality rate of congestive heart failure in the United States. J Am Coll Cardiol 1992;20:301–306.

27. Remes J, Miettinen H, Reunanen A, Pyorala K. Validity of clinical diagnosis of heart failure in primary health care. Eur Heart J 1991;12:315–321.

28. McDonagh TA, Morrison CE, Lawrence A, et al. Symptomatic and asymptomatic left-ventricular systolic dysfunction in an urban population. Lancet 1997;350:829–833.

29. The SOLVD Investigators. Effect of enalapril on mortality and the development of heart failure in asymptomatic patients with reduced left ventricular ejection fractions. N Engl J Med 1992;327:685–691.

30. Pemberton CJ, Johnson ML, Yandle TG, Espiner EA. Deconvolution analysis of cardiac natriuretic peptides during acute volume overload. Hypertension 2000;36:355–359.

31. Talwar S, Squire IB, Davies JE, Barnett DB, Ng LL. Plasma N-terminal pro-brain natriuretic peptide and the ECG in the assessment of left-ventricular systolic dysfunction in a high risk population. Eur Heart J 1999;20:1736-1744.

32. Hammerer-Lercher A, Neubauer E, Müller S, Pachinger O, Puschendor B, Mair J. Head-to-head comparison of N-terminal pro-brain natriuretic peptide, brain natriuretic peptide and N-terminal pro-atrial natriuretic peptide in diagnosing left ventricular dysfunction. Clin Chim Acta 2001;310:193–197.

33. McDonagh TA, Morton JJ, Baumann M, Trawinski J, Dargie HJ. N-terminal pro BNP: role in the diagnosis of left ventricular dysfunction in a population-based study (abstract). J Cardiac Fail 2000;6(Abstr Suppl 2):23.

34. Grønning BA, Raymond I, Pedersen F, et al. N-terminal pro brain natriuretic peptide concentrations in the diagnosis of heart failure in the general population (abstract). Eur J Heart Fail 2000;3(Suppl 1):Abstr 95.

35. Troughton RW, Frampton CM, Yandle TG, Espiner EA, Nicholls MG, Richards AM. Treatment of heart failure guided by plasma aminoterminal brain natriuretic peptide (N-BNP) concentrations. Lancet 2000;355:1126–1130.

36. McDonagh TA, Baumann M, Trawinski J, Morton JJ, Dargie HJ. N-terminal pro BNP and prognosis of left ventricular dysfunction in a population-based study (abstract). Circulation 2000;102(Abstr Suppl):II–845.

37. Richards AM, Doughty R, Nicholls MG, et al. Plasma N-terminal pro-brain natriuretic peptide and adrenomedullin: prognostic utility and prediction of benefit from carvedilol in ischemic left ventricular dysfunction. J Am Coll Cardiol 2001;37:1781–1787.

38. Richards AM, Nicholls MG, Yandle TG, et al. Plasma N-terminal pro-brain natriuretic peptide and adrenomedullin. New neurohormonal predictors of left ventricular function and prognosis after myocardial infarction. Circulation 1998;97:1921–1929.

39. Omland T, Samuelsson A, Richards AM, et al. Plasma N-terminal pro-brain natriuretic peptide in acute myocardial infarction. In: Proceedings of the XIII World Congress of Cardiology, Rio de Janeiro, Brasil, 1998, pp. 181–185.

40. Talwar S, Squire IB, Downie PF, et al. Profile of plasma NT-proBNP following acute myocardial infarction. Correlation with left ventricular dysfunction. Eur Heart J 2000;21:1514–1521.

41. Omland T, de Lemos JA, Morrow DA, et al. Prognostic value of N-terminal pro-atrial and pro-brain natriuretic peptide in patients with acute coronary syndromes. Am J Cardiol 2002; 89:463–465.

42. Talwar S, Squire IB, Downie PF, Davies JE, Ng LL. Plasma N terminal pro-brain natriuretic peptide and cardiotrophin-1 are raised in unstable angina. Heart 2000;84:421–424.

43. Talwar S, Downie PF, Squire IB, Davies JE, Barnett DB, Ng LL. Plasma N-terminal proBNP and cardiotrophin-1 are elevated in aortic stenosis. Eur J Heart Fail 2001;3:15–19.

44. Qi W, Mathisen P, Kjekshus J, et al. Natriuretic peptides in patients with aortic stenosis. Am Heart J 2001;142:725–732.

45. Luchner A, Hengstenberg C, Lowell H, et al. N-terminal pro-brain natriuretic peptide after myocardial infarction. A marker of cardio-renal function. Hypertension 2002;39:99–104.

46. Wang TJ, Levy D, Leip EP, et al. Determinants of natriuretic peptide levels in a healthy population and derivation of reference limits (abstract). Circulation 2001;104(Abstr Suppl): II–189.

47. Talwar S, Siebenhofer A, Williams B, Ng LL. Influence of hypertension, left ventricular hypertrophy, and left ventricular systolic dysfunction on plasma N-terminal proBNP. Heart 2000;83:278–282.

48. Muders F, Eckhard EP, Griese DP, et al. Evaluation of plasma natriuretic peptides as markers for left ventricular dysfunction. Am Heart J 1997;134:442–449.

49. Daggubati S, Parks JR, Overton RM, Cintron G, Schocken DD, Vesely DL. Adrenomedullin, endothelin, neuropeptide Y, atrial, brain, and C-natriuretic prohormone peptides compared as early heart failure indicators. Cardiovasc Res 1997;36:246–255.

50. Yandle T, Fisher S, Espiner E, Richards AM, Nicholls G. Validating aminoterminal BNP assays: a word of caution. Lancet 1999;353:1068.

51. Hughes D, Talwar S, Squire IB, Davies JE, Ng LL. An immunoluminometric assay for N-terminal pro-brain natriuretic peptide: development of a test for left ventricular dysfunction. Clin Sci (Colch) 1999;96:373–380.

52. Karl J, Borgya A, Galluser A, et al. Development of a novel, N-terminal proBNP (NT-proBNP) assay with a lower detection limit. Scand J Clin Lab Invest 1999;59:177–181.

53. Missbichler A, Hawa G, Woloszczuk W, Schmal N, Hartter E. Enzyme immunoassays for proBNP fragments (8–29) and (32–57). J Lab Med 1999;23:241–244.

54. http://www.roche.com/ diagnostics/news/2002/020128.html

55. Downie PF, Talwar S, Squire IB, Davies JE, Barnett DB, Ng LL. Assessment of the stability of N-terminal pro-brain natriuretic peptide in vitro: implications for assessment of left ventricular dysfunction. Clin Sci (Colch) 1999;97:255–258.

56. Nakamura M, Endo H, Nasu M, Arakawa N, Segawa T, Hiramori K. Value of plasma B type natriuretic peptide measurement for heart disease screening in a Japanese population. Heart 2002;87:131–135.

Part VI

Role of Infectious Diseases and Genetics in Heart Disease

27

Infectious Diseases in the Etiology of Atherosclerosis and Acute Coronary Syndromese

Focus on Chlamydia pneumoniae

Martin Möckel

INTRODUCTION

Several infectious agents including *Herpes simplex virus*, *Cytomegalovirus, Helicobacter pylori,* and *Chlamydia pneumoniae* have been investigated with respect to their role in the genesis of atherosclerosis. Although the increasing number of articles published on this issue suggests a causal role of infectious agents, the matter is far from settled and yet not proven.

The fascination of the "infection hypothesis" of atherosclerosis has been stimulated by the recognition of *H. pylori* (*HP*) playing a causal role in the pathogenesis of peptic ulcers. Owing to the possibility of eradication of HP by antibiotic treatment, the disease has been changed completely during the last years. Earlier reviews by Libby et al. *(1)* and Danesh et al. *(2)* in 1997 have summarized the evidence at that time that infectious agents may initiate, propagate, and complicate atherosclerosis. During the last 5 yr several new works have been published on this topic. The data on *C. pneumoniae* as an infectious agent that potentially plays a causal role in the development and progression of atherosclerosis in general and especially coronary artery disease seem to be most compelling. Another important cause for the focus on *C. pneumoniae* is that a cheap and well-tolerated antibiotic therapy is available.

DIFFERENT INFECTIOUS AGENTS STUDIED WITH RESPECT TO ATHEROSCLEROSIS AND MYOCARDIAL INFARCTION

The different agents studied mostly were *Cytomegalovirus, H. pylori,* and *C. pneumoniae.*

Cytomegalovirus

Cytomegalovirus has been recognized as a possible cause of atherosclerosis. Published studies have been summarized by Danesh et al. *(2)* and Libby et al. *(1)* in 1997. Recent studies led to the cumulation of evidence that *Cytomegalovirus* does not play a crucial role in atherosclerosis *(3–5)*.

Analysis of blood samples from the Physicians' Health Study with respect to antibodies against *H. simplex virus* and *Cytomegalovirus* showed no increase of atherothrombotic risk in individuals with positive titers *(3)*. A clear argument against a significant role of

From: *Cardiac Markers, Second Edition*
Edited by: Alan H. B. Wu @ Humana Press Inc., Totowa, NJ

Cytomegalovirus in the development of myocardial infarction comes from the study of Hernandez et al. *(5)* in patients after renal transplantation. It is well known that patients under immunosuppression are prone to viral infections and therefore have a higher incidence of new infection and reactivation of *Cytomegalovirus*. In this population, incident cases of myocardial infarction should be in some way related to *Cytomegalovirus*, if this agent would play a causative role for atherosclerosis. In fact, that is not the case. Hernandez and colleagues clearly show that despite of a high event rate (11.6%) and a high rate of *Cytomegalovirus* disease (around one third of the 1004 consecutive patients) this was no significant risk factor *(5)*.

Helicobacter pylori

As early as 1997, the study overview of Danesh et al. *(2)* showed only a weak association of *H. pylori* with atherosclerosis and myocardial infarction. This has been confirmed by data from the Physicians' Health Study *(6)*. Recently, two reports have re-emphasized the role of *H. pylori*. Hoffmeister et al. found an altered, atherogenic lipid profile in current *H. pylori* but not in *C. pneumoniae* or *Cytomegalovirus* seropositivity *(7)*. This study concludes that "proof of principle" has been shown but did not report any association between *H. pylori* and incident ischemic events in patients. *H. pylori* "infection" has been determined by $[^{13}C]$urea breath test in this study. A positive breath test is not strictly associated with local or systemic infection but could reflect local colonization only. Therefore, the reported associations of lipid profile changes and *H. pylori* positivity are perhaps not free of chance. The second study by Hara et al. *(8)* was a case control study in patients with acute or old myocardial infarction, stable or vasospastic angina, and age-matched controls. The main result is an odds ratio of 4.09 (95% CI 0.79–21.11) for 21 patients with elevated IgA levels and acute myocardial infarction versus the other patient groups. As the confidence limits include 1.0, the result did not show a clear association between *H. pylori* infection and acute myocardial infarction. In the light of other negative studies with more patients, the lack of animal models and a clear concept of principle, *H. pylori* cannot be considered to play definitely a causal role in atherosclerosis.

Chlamydia pneumoniae

The studies with respect to *C. pneumoniae* are numerous and have conflicting results. Danesh et al. have summarized evidence that *C. pneumoniae* may play a role in the development of atherosclerosis and myocardial infarction *(2)*. The same group presented data from 5661 British men aged 40–59 yr who provided blood samples during 1978–1980 *(9)*. The study results show an odds ratio of 1.7 comparing highest with lowest IgG titer tertiles with respect to incident ischemic heart disease. After adjustment for age, town, smoking, and social class, the odds ratio was still 1.6. The authors then additionally adjust for childhood social class, which reduced the odds ratio to 1.2. I believe with others *(10)* that Danesh et al. *(9)* did an "overadjustment" in this case and in some way "threw the baby out with the bathwater." As newer data suggest especially an association of *C. pneumoniae* with premature myocardial infarction *(11)*, early infection may play an causative role. In contrast to this positive study, the data of the Physicians' Health Study have negative results irrespective of the IgG titer *(12)*.

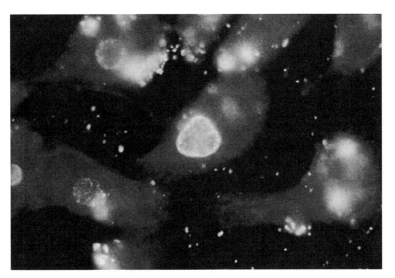

Fig. 1. Immunofluorescence stain reveals infection of Hep-2 host cells with replicating *C. pneumoniae* isolated from the occluded coronary artery of a 62-yr-old man (passage 15 after primary isolation). Multiple inclusions in the host cells are characteristic of *C. pneumoniae*. This cardiovascular strain is morphologically identical to the common respiratory isolates. (From Maass et al. *[34]* with permission.)

SEROEPIDEMIOLOGICAL STUDIES

Several seroepidemiological studies have been published with respect to the risk of atherothrombotic complications and *C. pneumoniae* seropositivity or infections with other infectious agents. Saikku et al. were the first to show an association between *C. pneumoniae* IgG titer of ≥32, chronic coronary heart disease (CCHD), and acute myocardial infarction (AMI). The authors reported on paired sera from 40 male patients with AMI, 30 male patients with CCHD, and 41 age- and sex-matched controls. The IgG titers were increased in 65% AMI patients, 50% CCHD patients, and 17% of controls *(13)*. Danesh et al. summarized the studies up to 1997 *(2)*. Table 1 gives an overview of the important studies published including the more recent articles.

It has to be mentioned that most of the studies were cross-sectional in design, and, because of the limited number of patients, control for all potential confounders was not possible. In addition, the different cutoff antibody titers make comparison of the studies difficult, and it seems unlikely that all of these cutoffs were prospectively defined. The study by Ridker et al. *(12),* which was longitudinal in design, could not show any association of CAD and previous *C. pneumoniae* infection. In summary, the studies show conflicting data on the association between CAD and past *C. pneumoniae* infection. More recent studies show a positive correlation with high antibody cutoffs *(21)* or premature AMI *(11)* as target variable. Prospective studies with other pathogens such as cytomegalovirus and Herpes simplex virus 1 + 2 showed an increased risk of MI or death with increased pathogen burden in a dose–response fashion *(22,23)*. Thus, the inconsistencies in the seroepidemiological data could be due to the broad spectrum of different disease intensities and missing differentiation between past and chronic persistent infection.

Table 1
Seroepidemiological Studies with Respect to Elevation
of *C. pneumoniae* IgG Antibody Titers and Risk of CAD or Complications

Source	No. of cases/controls	Titer cutoff	Results
Saikku et al. 1988 *(6)*	70/41 Age/sex matched	IgG ≥ 32	Titer positive in 68% of AMI and 50% of CCHD patients; 17% positivity in controls
Thom et al. 1991 *(7)*	461/95 Matched for age and sex; controls were angiography patients without CAD	IgG ≥ 64	Odds ratio for CAD (compared to subjects with low [less or equal than 1:8] antibody titer): 2.0, 95% CI: 1.0/4.0
Saikku et al. 1992 *(8)*	103/103 Patients from Helsinki Heart Study, matched for treatment, locality and time point	IgG ≥ 64	Odds ratio for the development of CHD: 2.3, 95% CI: 0.9/6.2
Thom et al. 1992 *(9)*	171/120 Adjustment for age, sex, and calender quarter of blood drawing	IgG ≥ 8	Odds ratio for CAD: 2.6, 95% CI: 1.4/4.8
Melnick et al. 1993 *(10)*	326/326 Matched by age, race, sex, examination period, field center (ARIC substudy)	IgG ≥ 8	Odds ratio for asymptomatic atherosclerosis: 2.0, 95% CI: 1.19/3.35
Dahlén et al. 1995 *(11)*	60/60 Sex matched	IgG ≥ 32	Odds ratio for angiographic CAD was 3.56, 95% CI: 0.99/16.10 with smoking as covariable
Ridker et al. 1999 *(4)*	343/343 (All male) Age/smoking matched	IgG ≥ 32	Relative risk 1.0 for future MI (12-yr follow-up)
Nieto et al. 1999 *(12)* multi-	246/550 3.3 yr ARIC follow up	IgG ≥ 64	Odds ratio for CHD: 1.6 ($p < 0.01$); not significant in multivariate analysis (1.2)
Siscovick et al. 2000 *(13)*	213/405 Controls matched for several variables including major risk factors	IgG ≥ 8	Odds ratio for risk of MI and CV death: 1.1, 95% CI: 0.7/1.8, adjusted for several matching factors
Chandra et al. 2001 *(14)*	830/-	IgG ≥ 1024	Odds ratio for ACS vs non-ACS: 1,62; unselected patients admitted to chest pain center
Gattone et al. 2001 *(15)*	120/120 Age matched; post AMI patients ≤ 50 Jahre	IgG ≥ 16	Odds ratios for premature AMI: 2.4, 95% CI: 1.3/4.6; additional smoking: 3.7; additional CMV infection: 12.5

AMI, (acute) (old) myocardial infarction; ACS, acute coronary syndrome; ARIC, Atherosclerosis Risk in Communities Study; CAD, coronary artery disease; (C)CHD, (chronic) coronary heart disease; CI, confidence interval; CV, cardiovascular.

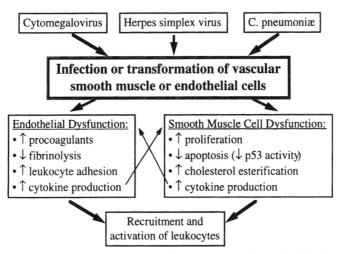

Fig. 2. Direct effects of infectious agents on intrinsic vascular wall cells. (Reproduced from Libby et al. *[1]* with permission.)

C. PNEUMONIAE IN ATHEROSCLEROTIC LESIONS

Although the matter of seroepidemiologic evidence has become more confusing due to several negative studies published in the last 3 yr, in the mid-1990s several research groups had been able to demonstrate *C. pneumoniae* antigen in atherosclerotic lesions and therefore added some evidence to the infectious hypothesis of atherosclerosis. In 1993, Kuo et al. were first to identify *C. pneumoniae* in atheromas of autopsy cases by use of the polymerase chain reaction (PCR; 43% positive) and immunocytochemistry (42% positive) *(24)*. Further studies confirmed these findings *(25–31)*. Except for a few studies using PCR only *(32)*, *C. pneumoniae* has been found in >50% and up to 100% of the lesions studied *(33)*. It must be emphasized that not only could the antigen be detected but also isolation of viable bacteria was possible *(34)*. Maass and co-workers were able to recover viable *C. pneumoniae* from 11 (16%) of 70 atheromas (from cardiovascular surgical procedures) investigated (from surgical procedures, see Fig. 1) *(34)*. Therefore, the association of *C. pneumoniae* and atherosclerosis appears to be established beyond a reasonable doubt. The significance of the association for the development of atherosclerosis, the disease progression, and complications remains uncertain.

POSSIBLE MECHANISMS OF ATHEROSCLEROSIS DEVELOPMENT DUE TO *C. PNEUMONIAE*

The mechanisms that are possibly involved in the development of atherosclerotic lesions due to infectious agents are summarized in Fig. 2 *(1)*. Atherosclerosis is becoming increasingly recognized as an inflammatory disease *(35)*. The process probably starts with endothelial dysfunction in distinct arteries *(36)*. In the progression of the disease "fatty streaks" appear in children and young adults *(37)*. In subsequent decades, the disease progresses depending on concomitant risk factors such as diabetes mellitus, arterial hypertension, smoking, and so on. The inflammatory process of atherosclerosis includes transformed macrophages ("foam cells") as important players *(35)*. Prior to the onset of complications such as acute coronary syndrome (ACS) or stroke, the atheromas fibrous cap undergoes thinning. The rupture of the fibrous cap can occur spontaneously or it is triggered by exhaustive exercise, extensive rise of blood pressure, or other factors.

Infectious agents may lead to a chronic inflammatory response with increased concentrations of proinflammatory cytokines and C-reactive protein (CRP) (35), which themselves contribute to a progression of the disease (38). Adhesion molecules may have an additional impact on ACS depending on the mode of therapy (39).

It has been demonstrated in recent studies that CRP is an independent risk factor for complications of CAD (40–43) and that antiinflammatory properties of cholesterol synthetic enzyme (CSE) inhibitors may be beneficial in these patients (44–47). Taking into consideration that CRP itself appears to contribute to atherosclerotic lesion formation (38), it could be hypothesized that chronic inflammation, for example, by *C. pneumoniae* or other infectious agents, therefore propagates the disease. This concept was supported further by a study that showed that an increased pathogen burden increases the risk of adverse events in CAD patients (23). Several cofactors are potentially involved in the disease progression by chronic *C. pneumoniae* infection including interleukin-1 gene polymorphism (48) and NF-κB-activation, induction of tissue factor, and plasminogen activator inhibitor (PAI)- 1 expression (49). Future studies will need to address further important cofactors and the exact molecular mechanisms of the atherosclerosis development and progression by infectious agents such as *C. pneumoniae*.

ANIMAL MODELS OF ATHEROSCLEROSIS DUE TO INFECTION

To determine an etiological role for *C. pneumoniae* for the development of atherosclerosis, some animal studies have been performed (50–53). In a rabbit model (New Zealand White rabbits), 11 animals were infected via the nasopharynx with *C. pneumoniae* (TWAR strain VR 1310). Animals were killed after 7, 14, 21, and 28 d. Atherosclerotic lesions were detected in two animals with fatty streaks at d 7 and an intermediate lesion at d 14 (51). In a second study with New Zealand White rabbits, animals were infected and reinfected after 3 wk. Of nine reinfected rabbits, six (67%) showed inflammatory changes of the aorta consisting of intimal thickening or fibroid plaques resembling atherosclerosis 2–4 wk after reinfection (50). The third study with these rabbits included treatment with azithromycin, a macrolide antibiotic known to be effective against *C. pneumoniae* and a modest cholesterol-enhanced diet. In this study, 20 animals were infected by three separate intranasal inoculations of *C. pneumoniae*. Ten animals served as controls. The infected animals were then divided into treatment and no treatment groups. The main result was an increased maximal intimal thickness (MIT) in infected and nontreated (0.55 mm) vs control animals (0.16 mm, $p = 0.009$). Infected rabbits receiving antibiotics had a significantly lower increase of MIT (0.20 mm, $p < 0.025$ vs both other groups). Chlamydial antigen was detected in two untreated, three treated, and no control animals (52).

Finally, Moazed et al. investigated the influence of *C. pneumoniae* infection on the aortic atherosclerotic areas in apolipoprotein E-deficient mice. They found at 16 wk of age, a 1.6-fold larger atherosclerotic area compared to uninfected controls (53). In conclusion, the animal models consistently suggest a pathogenetic role of *C. pneumoniae* in the development and progression of atherosclerosis. It is not clear which cofactors are necessary, which molecular mechanisms are involved, and if the results can be attributed to humans because no studies in primate models have been undertaken yet.

THERAPY TRIALS WITH ANTIBIOTICS AGAINST *C. PNEUMONIAE*

Another method for the determination of an etiologic role of *C. pneumoniae* in athero-sclerosis are secondary prevention studies in humans, using antibiotic treatment against *C. pneumoniae* with respect to complications and progression of atherosclerosis.

The first secondary prevention study by Gupta et al. *(54)* on 213 patients used azithromy-cin therapy in a subgroup of 60 out of 80 patients with high IgG titers (≥1:64). Patients were randomized to one or two 3-d courses of 500 mg of azithromycin/d or placebo. In this small study, patients with high antibody titers had a 4.2-fold risk for adverse cardio-vascular events after AMI compared to those with low titers. The risk for patients receiv-ing therapy with azithromycin was the same as in the control group. The results of this study have been criticized because of several flaws: (1) Twenty patients not randomized were added to the control group, (2) the event rate was unexpectedly high in both pla-cebo and untreated controls, and (3) there was a dramatic reduction of events after only a very short course of antibiotic therapy *(33)*.

In a second study called Randomized Trial of Roxithromycin in non-Q-wave Coro-nary Syndromes (ROXIS), 202 patients with unstable angina or non-Q-wave AMI were randomized to receive roxithromycin 150 mg twice daily or placebo for 30 d. In an early report on a 31-d follow-up, a significant reduction of the combined primary end point of cardiac ischemic death, MI, and severe recurrent ischemia was reported *(55)*. After 6 mo, this beneficial effect had waned *(56)*. Interestingly, IgG titers against *C. pneu-moniae* remained unchanged and only 64% of patients have completed the active treat-ment period.

The third and up to now largest study, again using azithromycin treatment (as in the study by Gupta et al. *[54]*), was conducted in 302 CAD patients. The individuals were randomized to receive either 500 mg/d of azithromycin for 3 d and then 500 mg/wk for 3 mo or placebo. The study did not show a significant reduction of the primary end point of cardiovascular death, resuscitated cardiac arrest, nonfatal MI, stroke, unstable angina, and unplanned coronary revascularization at 2 yr *(57)*. Nevertheless, the authors pointed out that a clinically worthwhile benefit of 20–30% risk reduction is possible but requires further large-scale studies to be detected.

Finally, a study by Neumann et al. investigated the effect of a 28-d treatment with 300 mg of roxithromycin/d on angiographic restenosis after successful coronary stenting in 1010 patients. There was no significant reduction of restenosis rate in the treatment group. A subgroup analysis resulted in a beneficial effect of treatment in patients with high (≥1:512) IgG antibody titers *(58)*.

A population-based case-control study including 1796 patients with AMI and 4882 age-, sex-, and event-year-matched controls investigated the association of past use of erythromycin, tetracycline, or doxycycline with the risk of first MI. No significant asso-ciation could be found *(59)*.

In summary, the studies published up to now show that the issue is far from settled and further studies are needed. There are now at least two large secondary prevention studies under way to determine the effect of prophylactic antibiotic treatment on coronary artery disease. The Weekly Intervention with Zithromax (azithromycin) for Atherosclerosis and its Related Disorders (WIZARD) trial, sponsored by Pfizer, is treating 3500 sub-jects with prior MI and *C. pneumoniae* IgG antibody titer ≥ 1:16 for 3 mo. The duration of the trial was determined to be 3 yr *(60)*. The Azithromycin Coronary Events study

(ACES), sponsored by the National Heart Lung and Blood Institute, will treat 4000 subjects with evidence of CAD, irrespective of antibody status, for 1 yr, with a planned 4-yr observation period *(33)*.

RECENT NEW ASPECTS, CONCLUSIONS, AND OUTLOOK

The implications of *C. pneumoniae* in the development of atherosclerosis and complications such as the acute coronary syndrome range from the initiation of the disease to the acceleration of complications. In summary of the above mentioned published data, it is still unclear if the occurrence of *C. pneumoniae* in the atherosclerotic plaque significantly influences the clinical course of the disease. At present, antimicrobial therapy for atherosclerosis is not advocated outside of well-controlled research settings *(61)*. Recently Gieffers et al. found that *C. pneumoniae* uses monocytes as transport system for systemic dissemination. In addition, the authors showed that the bacteria became less susceptible against otherwise effective antibiotic treatment *(62)*. This appears to be a good explanation of why the results of all treatment studies were in the end negative. The issue of *C. pneumoniae* in atherosclerosis must possibly be revisited by screening patients for monocytes infected by the agent and conducting a novel antibiotic therapy that covers resistant strains. While waiting for the results of the ongoing mega-trials WIZARD and ACES *(33)*, this should be another interesting and important field of research.

ABBREVIATIONS

ACES, Azithromycin Coronary Events Study; ACS, acute coronary syndrome(s); AMI, acute myocardial infarction; CAD, coronary artery disease; CCHD, chronic coronary heart disease; CRP, C-reactive protein; CSE, cholesterol synthesis enzyme, HP, *Helicobacter pylori*; IgG, immunoglo-bulin G; MIT, maximal intimal thickness; PCR, polymerase chain reaction; ROXIS, randomized trial of roxithromycin in non-Q-wave coronary syndromes; WIZARD, Weekly Intervention with Zithromax (azithromycin) for Atherosclerosis and its Related Disorders.

REFERENCES

1. Libby P, Egan D, Skarlatos S. Roles of Infectious Agents in Atherosclerosis and Restenosis: An Assessment of the Evidence and Need for Future Research. Circulation 1997;96:4095–4103.
2. Danesh J, Collins R, Peto R. Chronic infections and coronary heart disease: is there a link? Lancet 1997;350:430–436.
3. Ridker PM, Hennekens CH, Stampfer MJ, Wang F. Prospective Study of Herpes Simplex Virus, Cytomegalovirus, and the Risk of Future Myocardial Infarction and Stroke. Circulation 1998;98:2796–2799.
4. Borgia MC, Mandolini C, Barresi C, Battisti G, Carletti F, Capobianchi MR. Further evidence against the implication of active cytomegalovirus infection in vascular atherosclerotic diseases. Atherosclerosis 2001;157:457–462.
5. Hernandez D, Hanson E, Kasiske MK, Danielson B, Roel J, Kasiske BL. Cytomegalovirus disease is not a major risk factor for ischemic heart disease after renal transplantation1. Transplantation 2001;72:1395–1399.

6. Ridker PM, Danesh J, Youngman L, Collins R, Stampfer MJ, Peto R, Hennekens CH. A prospective study of Helicobacter pylori seropositivity and the risk for future myocardial infarction among socioeconomically similar U.S. men. Ann Intern Med 2001;135: 184–188.

7. Hoffmeister A, Rothenbacher D, Bode G, Persson K, Marz W, Nauck MA, Brenner H, Hombach V, Koenig W. Current infection with Helicobacter pylori, but not seropositivity to Chlamydia pneumoniae or cytomegalovirus, is associated with an atherogenic, modified lipid profile. Arterioscler Thromb Vasc Biol 2001;21:427–432.

8. Hara K, Morita Y, Kamihata H, Iwasaka T, Takahashi H. Evidence for infection with Helicobacter pylori in patients with acute myocardial infarction. Clin Chim Acta 2001;313:87–94.

9. Danesh J, Whincup P, Walker M, Lennon L, Thomson A, Appleby P, Wong Y, Bernardes-Silva M, Ward M. Chlamydia pneumoniae IgG titres and coronary heart disease: prospective study and meta-analysis. BMJ 2000; 321:208–213.

10. West R. Commentary: adjustment for potential confounders may have been taken too far. BMJ 2000; 321:213.

11. Gattone M, Iacoviello L, Colombo M, Castelnuovo AD, Soffiantino F, Gramoni A, Picco D, Benedetta M, Giannuzzi P. Chlamydia pneumoniae and cytomegalovirus seropositivity, inflammatory markers, and the risk of myocardial infarction at a young age. Am Heart J 2001;142:633–640.

12. Ridker PM, Kundsin RB, Stampfer MJ, Poulin S, Hennekens CH. Prospective Study of Chlamydia pneumoniae IgG Seropositivity and Risks of Future Myocardial Infarction. Circulation 1999;99:1161–1164.

13. Saikku P, Leinonen M, Mattila K, Ekman MR, Nieminen MS, Makela PH, Huttunen JK, Valtonen V. Serological evidence of an association of a novel Chlamydia, TWAR, with chronic coronary heart disease and acute myocardial infarction. Lancet 1988;2:983–986.

14. Thom DH, Wang SP, Grayston JT, Siscovick DS, Stewart DK, Kronmal RA, Weiss NS. Chlamydia pneumoniae strain TWAR antibody and angiographically demonstrated coronary artery disease. Arterioscler Thromb 1991;11:547–551.

15. Saikku P, Leinonen M, Tenkanen L, Linnanmaki E, Ekman MR, Manninen V, Manttari M, Frick MH, Huttunen JK. Chronic Chlamydia pneumoniae infection as a risk factor for coronary heart disease in the Helsinki Heart Study. Ann Intern Med 1992;116:273–278.

16. Thom DH, Grayston JT, Siscovick DS, Wang SP, Weiss NS, Daling JR. Association of prior infection with Chlamydia pneumoniae and angiographically demonstrated coronary artery disease. JAMA 1992;268:68–72.

17. Melnick SL, Shahar E, Folsom AR, Grayston JT, Sorlie PD, Wang SP, Szklo M. Past infection by Chlamydia pneumoniae strain TWAR and asymptomatic carotid atherosclerosis. Atherosclerosis Risk in Communities (ARIC) Study Investigators. Am J Med 1993; 95:499–504.

18. Dahlen GH, Boman J, Birgander LS, Lindblom B. Lp(a) lipoprotein, IgG, IgA and IgM antibodies to Chlamydia pneumoniae and HLA class II genotype in early coronary artery disease. Atherosclerosis 1995;114:165–174.

19. Nieto FJ, Folsom AR, Sorlie PD, Grayston JT, Wang SP, Chambless LE. Chlamydia pneumoniae infection and incident coronary heart disease: the Atherosclerosis Risk in Communities Study. Am J Epidemiol 1999;150:149–156.

20. Siscovick DS, Schwartz SM, Corey L, Grayston JT, Ashley R, Wang SP, Psaty BM, Tracy RP, Kuller LH, Kronmal RA. Chlamydia pneumoniae, herpes simplex virus type 1, and cytomegalovirus and incident myocardial infarction and coronary heart disease death in older adults : the Cardiovascular Health Study. Circulation 2000;102:2335–2340.

21. Chandra HR, Choudhary N, O'Neill C, Boura J, Timmis GC, O'Neill WW. Chlamydia pneumoniae exposure and inflammatory markers in acute coronary syndrome (CIMACS). Am J Cardiol 2001;88:214–218.

22. Rupprecht HJ, Blankenberg S, Bickel C, Rippin G, Hafner G, Prellwitz W, Schlumberger W, Meyer J. Impact of viral and bacterial infectious burden on long-term prognosis in patients with coronary artery disease. Circulation 2001;104:25–31.

23. Zhu J, Nieto FJ, Horne BD, Anderson JL, Muhlestein JB, Epstein SE. Prospective study of pathogen burden and risk of myocardial infarction or death. Circulation 2001;103:45–51.

24. Kuo CC, Shor A, Campbell LA, Fukushi H, Patton DL, Grayston JT. Demonstration of Chlamydia pneumoniae in atherosclerotic lesions of coronary arteries. J Infect Dis 1993; 167:841–849.

25. Kuo CC, Gown AM, Benditt EP, Grayston JT. Detection of Chlamydia pneumoniae in aortic lesions of atherosclerosis by immunocytochemical stain. Arterioscler Thromb 1993; 13:1501–1504.

26. Bauriedel G, Andrie R, Likungu JA, Welz A, Braun P, Welsch U, Luderitz B. Persistence of Chlamydia pneumoniae in coronary plaque tissue. A contribution to infection and immune hypothesis in unstable angina pectoris. Dtsch Med Wochenschr 1999;124:1408–1413.

27. Bauriedel G, Welsch U, Likungu JA, Welz A, Luderitz B. Chlamydia pneumoniae in coronary plaques: Increased detection with acute coronary syndrome. Dtsch Med Wochenschr 1999;124:375–380.

28. Blasi F, Denti F, Erba M, Cosentini R, Raccanelli R, Rinaldi A, Fagetti L, Esposito G, Ruberti U, Allegra L. Detection of Chlamydia pneumoniae but not Helicobacter pylori in atherosclerotic plaques of aortic aneurysms. J Clin Microbiol 1996;34:2766–2769.

29. Juvonen J, Laurila A, Juvonen T, Alakarppa H, Surcel HM, Lounatmaa K, Kuusisto J, Saikku P. Detection of Chlamydia pneumoniae in human nonrheumatic stenotic aortic valves. J Am Coll Cardiol 1997;29:1054–1059.

30. Juvonen J, Juvonen T, Laurila A, Alakarppa H, Lounatmaa K, Surcel HM, Leinonen M, Kairaluoma MI, Saikku P. Demonstration of Chlamydia pneumoniae in the walls of abdominal aortic aneurysms. J Vasc Surg 1997;25:499–505.

31. Ramirez JA. Isolation of Chlamydia pneumoniae from the coronary artery of a patient with coronary atherosclerosis. The Chlamydia pneumoniae/Atherosclerosis Study Group. Ann Intern Med 1996;125:979–982.

32. Jantos CA, Nesseler A, Waas W, Baumgartner W, Tillmanns H, Haberbosch W. Low prevalence of Chlamydia pneumoniae in atherectomy specimens from patients with coronary heart disease. Clin Infect Dis 1999;28:988–992.

33. Grayston JT. Antibiotic Treatment Trials for Secondary Prevention of Coronary Artery Disease Events. Circulation 1999;99:1538–1539.

34. Maass M, Bartels C, Engel PM, Mamat U, Sievers HH. Endovascular presence of viable Chlamydia pneumoniae is a common phenomenon in coronary artery disease. J Am Coll Cardiol 1998;31:827–832.

35. Ross R. Atherosclerosis—An Inflammatory Disease. N Engl J Med 1999;340:115–126.

36. Zeiher AM. Endothelial vasodilator dysfunction: pathogenetic link to myocardial ischaemia or epiphenomenon? Lancet 1996;348(Suppl 1):s10–s12.

37. Strong JP, Malcom GT, McMahan CA, Tracy RE, Newman WP, III, Herderick EE, Cornhill JF. Prevalence and extent of atherosclerosis in adolescents and young adults: implications for prevention from the Pathobiological Determinants of Atherosclerosis in Youth Study. JAMA 1999;281:727–735.

38. Torzewski M, Rist C, Mortensen RF, Zwaka TP, Bienek M, Waltenberger J, Koenig W, Schmitz G, Hombach V, Torzewski J. C-reactive protein in the arterial intima: role of C-reactive protein receptor-dependent monocyte recruitment in atherogenesis. Arterioscler Thromb Vasc Biol 2000;20:2094–2099.

39. Kerner T, Ahlers O, Reschreiter H, Buhrer C, Mockel M, Gerlach H. Adhesion molecules in different treatments of acute myocardial infarction. Crit Care 2001;5:145–150.

40. Koenig W, Sund M, Frohlich M, Fischer HG, Lowel H, Doring A, Hutchinson WL, Pepys MB. C-Reactive protein, a sensitive marker of inflammation, predicts future risk of coro-

nary heart disease in initially healthy middle-aged men: results from the MONICA (Monitoring Trends and Determinants in Cardiovascular Disease) Augsburg Cohort Study, 1984 to 1992. Circulation 1999;99:237–242.

41. Möckel M, Heller G, Jr., Müller C, Klefisch FR, Riehle M, Searle J, Frei U, Strachan DP. C-reactive protein as an independent marker of prognosis in acute coronary syndrome: comparison with troponin T. Z Kardiol 2000;89:658–666.

42. Heeschen C, Hamm CW, Bruemmer J, Simoons ML. Predictive value of C-reactive protein and troponin T in patients with unstable angina: a comparative analysis. CAPTURE Investigators. Chimeric c7E3 AntiPlatelet Therapy in Unstable angina REfractory to standard treatment trial. J Am Coll Cardiol 2000;35:1535–1542.

43. Biasucci LM, Liuzzo G, Grillo RL, Caligiuri G, Rebuzzi AG, Buffon A, Summaria F, Ginnetti F, Fadda G, Maseri A. Elevated levels of C-reactive protein at discharge in patients with unstable angina predict recurrent instability. Circulation 1999;99:855–860.

44. Ridker PM, Rifai N, Pfeffer MA, Sacks F, Braunwald E. Long-term effects of pravastatin on plasma concentration of C-reactive protein. The Cholesterol and Recurrent Events (CARE) Investigators. Circulation 1999;100:230–235.

45. Ridker PM, Rifai N, Clearfield M, Downs JR, Weis SE, Miles JS, Gotto AMJ. Measurement of C-reactive protein for the targeting of statin therapy in the primary prevention of acute coronary events. N Engl J Med 2001;344:1959–1965.

46. Ridker PM, Rifai N, Lowenthal SP. Rapid reduction in C-reactive protein with cerivastatin among 785 patients with primary hypercholesterolemia. Circulation 2001; 103(9):1191–1193.

47. Albert MA, Danielson E, Rifai N, Ridker PM. Effect of statin therapy on C-reactive protein levels: the pravastatin inflammation/CRP evaluation (PRINCE): a randomized trial and cohort study. JAMA 2001;286:64–70.

48. Momiyama Y, Hirano R, Taniguchi H, Nakamura H, Ohsuzu F. Effects of interleukin-1 gene polymorphisms on the development of coronary artery disease associated with Chlamydia pneumoniae infection. J Am Coll Cardiol 2001;38:712–717.

49. Dechend R, Maass M, Gieffers J, Dietz R, Scheidereit C, Leutz A, Gulba DC. Chlamydia pneumoniae infection of vascular smooth muscle and endothelial cells activates NF-kappaB and induces tissue factor and PAI-1 expression: a potential link to accelerated arteriosclerosis. Circulation 1999;100:1369–1373.

50. Laitinen K, Laurila A, Pyhala L, Leinonen M, Saikku P. Chlamydia pneumoniae infection induces inflammatory changes in the aortas of rabbits. Infect Immun 1997;65:4832–4835.

51. Fong IW, Chiu B, Viira E, Fong MW, Jang D, Mahony J. Rabbit model for Chlamydia pneumoniae infection. J Clin Microbiol 1997;35:48–52.

52. Muhlestein JB, Anderson JL, Hammond EH, Zhao L, Trehan S, Schwobe EP, Carlquist JF. Infection with Chlamydia pneumoniae accelerates the development of atherosclerosis and treatment with azithromycin prevents it in a rabbit model. Circulation 1998;97:633–636.

53. Moazed TC, Campbell LA, Rosenfeld ME, Grayston JT, Kuo CC. Chlamydia pneumoniae infection accelerates the progression of atherosclerosis in apolipoprotein E-deficient mice. J Infect Dis 1999;180:238–241.

54. Gupta S, Leatham EW, Carrington D, Mendall MA, Kaski JC, Camm AJ. Elevated Chlamydia pneumoniae antibodies, cardiovascular events, and azithromycin in male survivors of myocardial infarction. Circulation 1997;96:404–407.

55. Gurfinkel E, Bozovich G, Daroca A, Beck E, Mautner B. Randomised trial of roxithromycin in non-Q-wave coronary syndromes: ROXIS Pilot Study. ROXIS Study Group. Lancet 1997;350:404–407.

56. Gurfinkel E, Bozovich G, Beck E, Testa E, Livellara B, Mautner B. Treatment with the antibiotic roxithromycin in patients with acute non-Q-wave coronary syndromes. The final report of the ROXIS Study. Eur Heart J 1999;20:121–127.

57. Muhlestein JB, Anderson JL, Carlquist JF, Salunkhe K, Horne BD, Pearson RR, Bunch TJ, Allen A, Trehan S, Nielson C. Randomized secondary prevention trial of azithromycin in patients with coronary artery disease: primary clinical results of the ACADEMIC study. Circulation 2000;102:1755–1760.

58. Neumann F, Kastrati A, Miethke T, Pogatsa-Murray G, Mehilli J, Valina C, Jogethaei N, da Costa CP, Wagner H, Schomig A. Treatment of Chlamydia pneumoniae infection with roxithromycin and effect on neointima proliferation after coronary stent placement (ISAR-3): a randomised, double-blind, placebo-controlled trial. Lancet 2001;357:2085–2089.

59. Jackson LA, Smith NL, Heckbert SR, Grayston JT, Siscovick DS, Psaty BM. Past use of erythromycin, tetracycline, or doxycycline is not associated with risk of first myocardial infarction. J Infect Dis 2000;181(Suppl 3):S563–S565.

60. Dunne MW. Rationale and design of a secondary prevention trial of antibiotic use in patients after myocardial infarction: the WIZARD (weekly intervention with zithromax [azithromycin] for atherosclerosis and its related disorders) trial. J Infect Dis 2000;181(Suppl 3): S572–S578.

61. Möckel M. Persistence of Chlamydia pneumoniae in coronary plaque tissue. Dtsch Med Wochenschr 2000;125:645.

62. Gieffers J, Fullgraf H, Jahn J, Klinger M, Dalhoff K, Katus HA, Solbach W, Maass M. Chlamydia pneumoniae Infection in Circulating Human Monocytes Is Refractory to Antibiotic Treatment. Circulation 2001;103:351–356.

28
Polymorphisms Related to Acute Coronary Syndromes and Heart Failure

Potential Targets for Pharmacogenomics

Alan H. B. Wu

INTRODUCTION

The pathophysiology of many if not most human diseases is a combination of environmental and genetic risk factors. The balance between environment vs genetics can vary from diseases that are entirely environmentally influenced, such as in viral infections, to nearly 100% penetrance by genetic predisposition, such as Huntington's disease. In the area of coronary artery disease (CAD), the traditional notion is that environmental factors play the most important part in disease occurrence and progression. Cardiovascular risk factors such as smoking, obesity, diet, and the lack of exercise are environmental in nature and can be modified to reduce risk. However, the National Cholesterol Education Program (NCEP) has identified family history of premature heart disease (first-degree male relative <45 yr, female <55 yr) as a major risk factor *(1)*. NCEP has also identified the presence of diabetes, which has a definite genetic component, as a CAD risk factor. This chapter summarizes the large volume of relatively recent work devoted toward finding genetic polymorphisms that are linked to a higher incidence of acute coronary syndromes (ACS). The markers that have been examined are directed toward mutations in pathways that are implicated in the pathophysiology of ACS, that is, thrombosis, platelet dysfunction, and lipid and other biochemical metabolism.

The majority of the variances are the result of point mutations known as single nucleotide polymorphisms (SNPs). Detection of genotypes typically requires extraction of DNA from leukocytes of whole blood samples and amplification of the DNA using the polymerase chain reaction. From the known DNA sequence, specific forward and reverse primers are used to isolate the DNA sections containing the gene of interest. The amplified DNA is incubated with specific restriction site endonucleases to degrade the DNA into fragments. The resulting mixture of fragments is resolved using the polyacrylamide gel electrophoresis and visualized with ethidium bromide. Typical results are shown in Fig. 1 for Factor V Leiden.

GENES OF THROMBOTIC OR THROMBOLYTIC FUNCTION

The balance between thrombosis and thrombolysis is a complex balance between factors. Thrombosis is necessary to maintain loss of blood volume during injury and involves

From: *Cardiac Markers, Second Edition*
Edited by: Alan H. B. Wu @ Humana Press Inc., Totowa, NJ

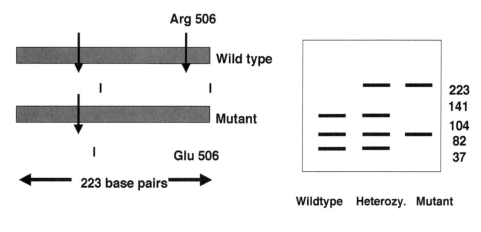

Gene   **RFLP gel**

Fig. 1. Representative restriction fragment length polymorphism (RFLP) analysis. The Factor V gene contains 223 basepairs. The wild-type has two restriction sites for *Mnl*I and produces three fragments (37, 82, and 104 bp). The substitution of an arginine for a glutamine results in loss of one restriction site in the mutation and produces two fragments (82 and 141 bp). The heterozygous genotype produces four bands.

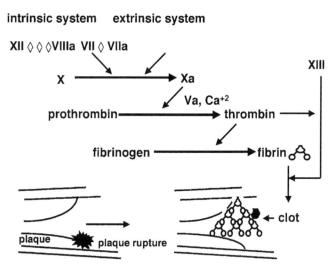

Fig. 2. Abbreviated summary of the intrinsic and extrinsic coagulation cascades. The end product of this system is the insoluble fibrin clot. Together with a platelet plug (not shown), the fibrin clot is formed following rupture of a coronary artery causing blockage.

the formation of a platelet clot and the conversion of fibrinogen to insoluble fibrin. Once the injury has been repaired, thrombolysis is necessary to remove the remaining elements of the clot so that a permanent block does not occur. There are two major activation pathways for thrombin formation. The intrinsic pathway begins when Factor XII is activated by binding to a negatively charged surface. This activates in sequence Factors XI, IX, VIII, and X. In the extrinsic pathway, tissue factor and ionized calcium activates Factor VII, which activates Factor X. As shown in Fig. 2, prothrombin (Factor II) is con-

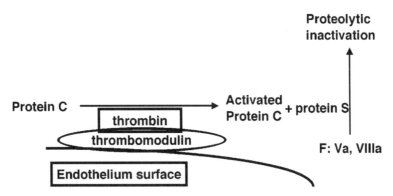

Fig. 3. Summary of the protein C and S pathways for the inactivation of Factor Va and VIIIa.

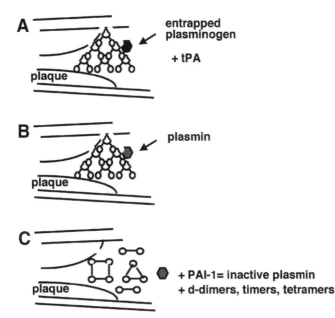

Fig. 4. Fibrinolysis. (**A**) Entrapped plasminogen binds to tPA. (**B**) Plasmin is formed. (**C**) The fibrin clot is degraded into degradation products including the D-dimer. The released plasmin is inactivated by PAI-1.

verted to thrombin by Factor Xa as activated from either pathway. Thrombin converts fibrinogen to soluble fibrin monomers, and activates Factor XIII. Together, soluble fibrin is converted to an insoluble fibrin clot. Alterations in the concentrations and function of these protein factors have the potential to disrupt the balance between clot formation and lysis.

An important part of the hemostasis balance is the role of protein C, S, and Factor V. Under normal conditions, protein C is activated by the complex of thrombin and thrombomodulin on the surface of endothelial cells (Fig. 3). Activated protein C (APC) combines with protein S and preferentially inactivates Factors Va and VIIIa. This ultimately limits the degree and extent of hemostasis.

Once the clot forms, it can be cleared by the fibrinolytic system. In the process of clot formation, plasminogen is entrapped (Fig. 4). In the presence of fibrin, plasminogen is converted by tissue plasminogen activator (tPA) to plasmin, a potent proteolytic enzyme that degrades the fibrin clot. The end products of fibrinolysis are fragments from the D domain of fibrinogen, which combine to form D-dimers, trimers, and tetramers. Measurement of D-dimers is an indicator of fibrinolysis. The activity of tissue plasminogen activator is controlled by the presence of plasminogen activator inhibitor-1 (PAI-1), protein C inhibitor, and α_2-antiplasmin.

Factors V and II

A single point mutation in the Factor V gene produces a factor that when activated is resistant to degradation by the activated protein C and S complex. A change from guanosine to adenine results in the substitution of arginine to glutamine in codon 506 of the untranslated 3' region (Table 1). This amino acid is at the site of cleavage by APC and the mutation is thought to be responsible for APC resistance. The prevalence for the mutation varies across racial populations. The allele frequency is about 5% among American Caucasians, 4% among Northern Europeans, 1.5% among Southern Europeans, and <1% among African blacks and Asians *(2)*. The mutation is referred to as "Factor V Leiden."

The majority of interest in Factor V Leiden comes from the finding that the mutation is positively associated with the presence of deep venous thrombosis. In the Physicians' Health Study, 121 cases of venous thromboembolism were identified over a 8.6-yr follow-up among 14,916 subjects. The prevalence of the mutation among men with venous thrombosis was almost double of those who were free of disease (11.6% vs 6.0%, respectively; odds ratio 2.7, 95% CI: 1.3–5.6) *(3)*. Routine testing for Factor V Leiden is recommended for patients at high risk for venous thrombosis, such as the presence of thrombosis at an early age of onset (<50 yr), recurrent thrombotic events, family history, and possibly after a complicated pregnancy *(4)*.

Given the important role of Factor V Leiden in venous thrombosis, studies were conducted to determine if this polymorphism is a risk factor for arterial thrombosis. Surprisingly, the data have consistently shown that the presence of Factor V Leiden is not associated with an increased incidence of CAD. In the Physician's Health Study, the odds ratio was not statistically significant for development of acute myocardial infarction (AMI), when all subjects were examined, or within various subgroups (i.e., age ≤60 yr, nonsmokers, and absence of familial history, hypercholesterolemia, or hypertension) *(5)*. A meta-analysis of 5431 CAD cases and controls from nine published studies confirmed these data (odds ratio: 1.24, 95% CI: 0.84–1.59) *(6)*.

Like Factor V, there is a common point mutation in nucleotide 20210 resulting in Factor II, resulting in a change of guanosine to adenine and the substitution of arginine to glutamine. This creates a site for endonuclease degradation by *Mnl*I. The prevalence of the Factor II A allele at 1–2% is lower than for Factor V Leiden, and very low among Africans and Asians. In terms of risk for venous thrombosis, Factor II A20210G polymorphism is a risk factor, although the odds ratios are lower than for Factor V Leiden *(6)*. The presence of both mutations, however, carries a significant risk that is greater than the sum of the two alone. In one study of patients with a mutation in either or both Factors II and V, the incidence of venous thrombosis was 5.7% for Factor II, 7.8% for Factor V, and 17.1% for both, as compared to 2.5% for noncarriers *(7)*. These individuals in particular would benefit from prophylactic anticoagulants (e.g., coumadin). Women with these mutations and who are on oral contraceptives are also at risk. In terms of

Table 1
Summary of Single Nucleotide Polymorphism
and Representative Restriction Endonuclease Used in Detection

Factor	Gene	SNP location	Endonuclease[a]
II	3' Untranslated region,	20210 G→A, Arg→Gln	*Hind*III
V	Leiden gene, exon 10	1691 G→A, Arg→Gln	*Mnl*I
VII	Catalytic region, exon 8	353 G→A, Arg→Gln	*Msp*I
	Hypervariable region, intron 7	37-bp repeat, VNTR	*Rsa*I
	5' F7, 5' promoter region	10-bp insertion	NA
Fibrinogen	β-Chain promoter region	−455 G→A	*Hae*III
PAI-1	Promoter region	−675, G insertion/deletion	NA
GP Ia	Coding region, intron 7	807 C→T, no sub.[a]	NA
	Coding region, intron 7	873 G→A, no sub.	NA
	Cation binding domain	1648G→A, Glu→Lys	*Mnl*I
GP Iba	Hpa-2, Ko polymorphism	434 C→T, Thr→Met	*Bsa*HI
	HPA-2	Variable no. tandem repeats, 39 bp	
	HPA-2, Kozak polymorphism	−5 from ATG start, T→C no sub.[b]	
GP IIb	HPA-3, heavy chain	843 T→G, Ile→Ser	*Bse*GI or *Fok*I
GP IIIa	HPA-1, exon 2	1565 C→T, Leu→Pro	*Nci*I
GP VI	Exon 5	13254 T→C, Ser→Pro	*Hpa*II
MTHFR	Encoding region	677 C→T, Ala→Val	*Hinf*I
Lipoprotein	Intron 8	495 T→G	*Hind*III
lipase	Intron 6	C→T	*Pvu*II
	Exon 9	447 C→G, Ser→Term	*Mnl*I
	Exon 2	9, G→A, Asp→Asn	*Bcl*I
	Exon 6	291 A→G Asn→Ser	*Rsa*I
Apo E	ε2	118, 158 Cys	*Hha*I
	ε3	118 Cys, 158 Arg	
	ε4	118, 158 Arg	
ACE	Intron 16	287-bp insertion/deletion	NA
Angiotensin Receptor	5' End of the 3' untranslated region	1166 A→C	*Dde*I
β₁	N-terminal of coding exon	145 A→G Ser[49]Gly	*Eco*0109I
	Transmembrane helix VII region	1165 G→C Arg[389]Gly	*Bcg*I
β₂	Fourth transmembrane-spanning domain	Arg[16]Gly	*Sty*1 or *Eco*130I
		Gln[27]Glu	*Fnu*4H1
		Thr[164]Ile	*Mnl*1

[a]Representative restriction endonuclease. Other appropriate ones may be used.
[b]No sub. Polymorphism does not result in an alteration in gene expression. NA, Not applicable.

arterial thrombosis, the G20210A polymorphism is not associated with an increased incidence of ACS. In a meta-analysis of 5607 CAD cases and controls, the odds ratio was 1.15 (95% CI: 0.84–1.59) *(5)*.

Factor VII

The rupture of a coronary artery results in the exposure of tissue factor to Factor VII in blood which becomes activated and initiates the extrinsic coagulation pathway. High plasma concentrations of Factor VII have been implicated as a risk factor for CAD *(8)*. There are several common polymorphisms in the gene for Factor VII. One of the more widely studied is the R353Q involving a substitution of glutamine for arginine in exon 8. The allele frequency is about 13% with a homozygous rate of about 2%. The allele frequency among Asians is lower at about 6%. The mutation results in the elimination in one of the two restriction sites by *Msp*I. Girelli et al. found that subjects with AA wild-type genotype had a higher Factor VIIa concentration (50.9 mU/mL) than subjects with the heterozygous AG (31.5 mU/mL) and the homozygous GG (14.0 mU/mL) genotypes *(9)*. The lower Factor VIIa concentration in subjects with the G allele would suggest that this mutation offers a protective effect against ACS. This has been demonstrated in several reports correlating the presence of Factor VII genotypes with incidence of ACS. Although many of the initial studies did not have the number of subjects to demonstrate statistical significance, a meta-analysis of 2574 CAD cases and controls produced an odds ratio of 0.78 (95% CI: 0.65–0.93) for the AG and GG genotypes *(5)*. Yet undeveloped therapies might be directed at lowering Factor VII concentrations in individuals with the AA genotype.

There are other mutations in Factor VII that have been identified. In intron 7, there is a size polymorphism due to the presence of a 37-basepair (bp) repeat. The endonuclease *Rsa*I enables this gene to be degraded into three fragments. The wild-type is the presence of replication of six repeat sequences. A less common allele is the presence of seven repeats, and a rare allele is the presence of five or eight repeat sequences. In one study, the allele frequencies were 66%, 33%, 0.7%, and <0.1% for the five to eight repeats, respectively *(9)*. There is an insertion polymorphism in the 5' F7 of the 5' promoter region, which corresponds to the addition of 10 bp. The allele frequency for the insertion mutation is about 18%. While the significance of these polymorphisms for CAD has not been thoroughly studied as yet, preliminary data do not suggest that there will be a major correlation with arterial thrombosis and determination of Factor VII plasma concentrations.

Fibrinogen

Fibrinogen is a large dimeric plasma protein with a molecular mass of 340 kDa. It is composed of six polypeptide chains: two Aα, two Bβ, and two γ chains. Each half of the molecule contains one each subunit linked together by disulfide bonds. Schematically, fibrinogen consists of a central nodular section known as the "E" domain, and two peripheral sections known as the "D" domain (Fig. 5). Thrombin removes two short peptides (fibrinopeptides A and B) from each Aα and Bβ chain within the E domain to form fibrin. This facilitates the polymerization of fibrin into an insoluble fibrin complex. Covalent crosslinks stabilizes the fibrin clot. The adult reference interval for plasma fibrinogen is 200–400 mg/dL. There is no fibrinogen in serum, as it is consumed in the formation of the clot.

Increased plasma fibrinogen concentrations are linked to CAD. In the Northwick Park Heart Study, an increase of 60 mg/dL confers an 84% increase in the risk of CAD over 5 yr *(8)*. Smoking also increases the fibrinogen concentration and is an established

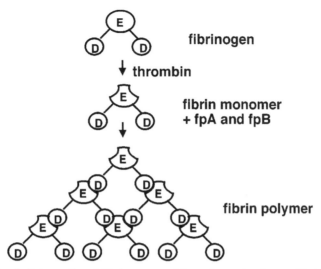

Fig. 5. Schematic of fibrinogen and its polymerization to fibrin.

environmental risk factor. Plasma fibrinogen concentrations and cardiovascular risk may also be linked to genetic factors. At least eight fibrinogen gene polymorphism have recently been described in the α, β, and γ chains *(10)*. The one most commonly studied is in the B-fibrinogen promoter region at position −455, where there is a change from a guanosine to adenine. Production of the B chain is the rate-limiting step in the formation of mature fibrinogen. The A allele frequency is 20%. The 455 A genotype is associated with an increased plasma fibrinogen concentration (370 mg/dL) vs the wild-type (G455, 320 mg/dL) as shown in one study *(11)*. However, other studies have rather consistently shown that there is no association of the fibrinogen polymorphism and presence of or risk for CAD *(12)*.

Plasminogen Activator Inhibitor-1

Interest in polymorphisms in PAI-1 stems in part from the observation that there is reduced fibrinolytic function and increased risk for CAD in the presence of increased concentrations of PAI-1 in blood, due to an accelerated inactivation of tPA, a natural agent for thrombolysis. Paradoxically, increased plasma tPA concentrations are also associated with risk for MI *(13)*. In the European Concerted Action on Thrombosis and Disabilities Angina Pectoris Study, the blood of 3043 patients with angina was analyzed for tPA and PAI-1. Patients who subsequently suffered MI or sudden coronary death had higher concentrations of PAI-1 and tPA (18.2 and 11.8 ng/mL, respectively) than those who did not suffer an event (14.8 and 10.0 ng/mL, respectively) *(14)*. It is possible that although tPA has a fibrinolytic role, it may also destabilize the atherosclerotic plaque.

A insertion/deletion polymorphism is known in the promoter region of the *PAI-1* gene whereby one allele sequence has four guanosines (4G) and the other has five (5G). Both alleles bind a transcriptional activator. However, the 5G allele also binds a repressor protein to an overlapping binding site, thereby reducing the level of transcription. As a consequence, the 4G allele has been related to higher PAI-1 concentrations in plasma *(15)*. The 5G allele frequency is about 48% among Caucasians and is slightly lower among Asians.

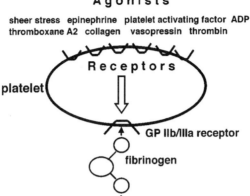

Fig. 6. Agonists of platelet aggregation. Activation stimulates the GP IIb/IIIa receptor to bind to fibrinogen where it can interact with another platelet to initiate aggregation. GP IIb/IIIa activation also leads to the binding of fibronectin and von Willebrand Factor, which causes adhesion of platelets to the subendothelium.

Studies on the role of PAI-1 polymorphism in ACS have been equivocal. Most studies, however, had low numbers (<1000) of enrolled subjects. In a meta-analysis, Iacoviello et al. combined results of nine studies on 3641 CAD cases and controls. A positive association between the 4G/4G allele for CAD vs controls was obtained (odds ratio: 1.30, 95% CI: 1.07–1.58) *(16)*. For most of the individual studies that were included, the odds ratio did not produce a statistically significant association for the 4G allele and CAD (i.e., a positive association observed only when studies were combined). For genetic risk assessment markers that may have only a borderline association, enrollment bias such as history of CAD may play a major role in the accuracy of results. For example, in an age-matched control population, how does the individual or investigator verify that silent ischemic disease had not occurred? As such, Ossei-Gerning et al. used coronary angiography as criteria for CAD, and found a positive association of the 4G genotype with the presence or absence of multivessel disease *(17)*. The final word on PAI-1 polymorphism has not yet been written.

PLATELET GLYCOPROTEINS

Platelets work in concert with coagulation factors to maintain hemostasis. In ACS, platelet activation plays a major role in the arterial thrombosis of coronary arteries. Whereas a fibrin clot dominates in patients with totally occluded ST-segment AMI, platelet clots are more responsible for the partial occlusions observed in non-ST-segment AMI and unstable angina *(18)*. There are several glycoprotein (GP) receptor complexes found on the platelet surface that facilitate the binding functions of platelets *(19)*. GP Ib-V–IX receptor binds to the von Willebrand factor receptor and is involved with the adhesion to platelets to the subendothelium, particularly under conditions of high sheer stress. GP Ia–IIa receptor binds to collagen and also stimulates platelet adhesion to endothelial surfaces. GP IIb/IIIa is the most abundant receptor and functions to bind fibrinogen. As shown in Fig. 6, sheer forces from systole and many different agonists can activate the GP IIb/IIIa receptor. Once activated, aggregation occurs by the binding of multiple platelets to the fibrinogen molecule (Fig. 6). The GP IIb/IIIa receptor is of particular interest for cardiologists, as inhibitors to the receptor are used to treat patients with ACS and as a prophylactic measure for patients undergoing percutaneous coronary intervention (PCI).

Specific mutations to either GP IIb or IIIa may result in a reduced or possibly enhanced binding of platelets to fibrinogen. A widely studied polymorphism is in the GPIIIa receptor, a change from cytosine to thymidine at nucleotide 1565, resulting in the substitution from a leucine to a proline. This polymorphism leads to the production of a second restriction site for *Ncl*I. The A2 allele frequency is 16% with a 2% incidence of homozygotes among Caucasians. The allele frequency at 7% is lower among Asians. This particular mutation has been implicated in immune-mediated platelet destruction, an allogen referred to as PI[A2]. As with other polymorphisms studied for arterial thrombosis, the literature contains contradictory findings *(20,21)*. Individual studies may be limited in the number of subjects who can be practically enrolled. If the relationship between the polymorphism and incidence of CAD is minimal, it will require large numbers of subjects to achieve statistical significance. This may be the case for the GP IIIa polymorphism, as a meta-analysis of nine studies on 7920 CAD cases and controls produced a modest odds ratio of 1.12, which barely reached statistical significance (95% CI: 1.01–1.24) *(5)*. A genetic marker with such minimal effect may have little clinical significance unless it is shown to be additive to other genetic and possibly environmental markers of cardiovascular risk.

Given the importance of GP IIb/IIIa receptor inhibitors as therapeutic agents in patients with ACS, it may be important to determine if GP IIb/IIIa polymorphisms affect the success of these drugs. This may be an important application in the relatively new field of pharmacogenomics, that is, the prediction of therapeutic success based on genotyping. There have been a few angioplasty studies that have attempted to correlate GP IIIa polymorphisms with clinical outcomes. Laule et al. *(22)* found no association of the A2 allele for the 30-d composite endpoints (target-vessel revascularization, AMI, and death) when 653 cases were examined. In contrast, Kastrati reported a higher restenosis rates at 6 mo for the A2 allele (odds ratio: 1.35, 95% CI: 1.07–1.70) among 1150 coronary angioplasty patients *(23)*. Unfortunately, the effects of GP IIIa polymorphisms on the success of GP IIb/IIIa inhibitor therapy were not examined as these inhibitors were not given to patients in either of these studies. Given the low rate of adverse events for patients given GP IIb/IIIa inhibitors, a fairly large clinical trial will be necessary to document the effect. Such a study is unlikely to be funded by pharmaceutical companies, as they may view such testing as a gate or hinderance for widespread use of these drugs.

There has been less attention in the measurement of polymorphisms in the other platelet glycoproteins. GP IIb is designated as the human platelet alloantigen-3 (HPA-3). A polymorphism exists at position 943 where there is a change from thymidine to guanosine resulting in the substitution of an isoleucine for a serine. The allele frequency for the mutation is about 40% with 12–15% homozygotes. Preliminary studies suggest that the HPA-3 polymorphism is not associated with the presence of CAD *(24)*.

GP Ia is part of the GP Ia/IIa heterodimer and functions to adhere platelets to injured vessel walls, and is designated as the human platelet allogen-5. There are two silent polymorphisms present in the *GP Ia* gene. At 807, there is a substitution of a cytosine for a thymidine, and at 873, guanosine for adenine. These polymorphisms are linked. In both cases, there is no change in the amino acid sequence. Although silent mutations do not result in the alteration of the actual GP product, they may be associated with mutations in regulatory regions, such as the gene promoter. Alternately, changes in the DNA sequence may influence the survival of mRNA such that the amount of protein produced is altered. The detection of these polymorphisms is achieved by use of allele-specific fluorescence probes.

Using flow cytometry and specific monoclonal antibodies, Kunicki et al. showed that individuals with the T807/A873 allele had a high density of the GP Ia–IIa receptor, while individuals with the C807/G873 allele had a low density of receptors *(25)*. The presence of a high density of receptors might correlate with a greater degree of platelet adhesion onto collagen and the endothelial wall, thereby stimulating a hyperthrombotic response.

Studies have been conducted to determine if GP Ia polymophorism is associated with an increased incidence of ACS or poor outcomes in patients treated with PCI. In a study of young patients (<49 yr) who survived MI, there was a significant association of the T807 allele of GP Ia *(26)*. It was hypothesized that this polymorphism is more effective as a risk factor among young patients, which might get "diluted" with the presence of other risk factors, e.g., as the age of the patient increases. GP Ia polymorphism was studied as a risk factor for patients undergoing angioplasty. Restenosis and the need for revascularization can be caused by stent placement, as it can activate platelets to form thrombosis, and promote the migration and growth of smooth muscle cells. However, von Beckerath et al. found no significant difference in the 30-d incidence of death, AMI, or urgent target vessel revascularization and polymorphisms among 1797 patients undergoing PCI *(27)*. The authors postulate that the mechanism of platelet activation following PCI may explain these findings. Stents are usually placed in high-grade lesions that contain more collagen-rich plaques as opposed to low-grade lesions, which are richer in platelet tissue factor. If the restenosis and other adverse events occurred in these low-grade areas, GP Ia polymorphism may not be a factor.

In contrast to these studies, there is another GP Ia polymorphism that may have more promise as a genetic marker for CAD. A change of glutamine for adenine at nucleotide 1648 results in the substitution of glutamine for lysine. This polymorphism is linked to the *C807T* gene, with the AA1648 found exclusively with CC807 and GG1648 with TT807. The incidence of the A1648 allele is approx 10% *(28)*. This frequency of this polymorphism is lower among Asians. In a study of 2163 Caucasian males, the presence of the A1648 allele was associated with an increased incidence of CAD when the analysis was restricted to low-risk subgroups. This association was independent of the C807T genotype. There was no statistical difference in genotype frequency and incidence of CAD when all patients were studied. It may be possible that the role of platelet polymorphism may be minimized or superceded by the presence of established CAD risk factors.

Polymorphisms also exist in the third of three platelet receptors, that is, GP-Ib-IX–V. GP Ib is associated with the HPA-2 alloantigen. The Ko polymorphism is an SNP at nucleotide 434 involving a change of a cytosine to thymidine, producing a substitution of a threonine to a methionine at codon position 145. The allele frequency for the 434T is 12% *(29)*. A variable number of tandem repeats of 39 bp is present in GP Ibα, resulting in the presence of a 13-amino-acid sequence that is repeated between one and four times *(30)*. Both of these polymorphisms have the potential to affect the structure of GP Ibα and appear to have strong linkage disequilibrium. The allele frequency is 8.3%,

78%, 13%, and 1% for the 1–4 repeats, respectively (labeled D, C, B, and A). The hypothesis is that an increased number of repeats pre-disposes the platelet receptor to binding to endothelial surfaces and thrombosis. The Kozak sequence polymorphism results in the change of a thymidine to a cytosine at position −5 from the ATG start codon. While this does not alter the mature GP, it may influence the extent of the gene expression. The frequency of the −5C allele is 15%.

As with the other studies on platelet polymorphisms, the incidence of CAD and complications following angioplasty and presence of GP Ibα genotypes is equivocal. Mikkelsson et al. found that the 145M genotype of HPA-2 was associated with the VNTR B (three variable repeats) haplotype, and this combination was a significant risk factor for coronary thrombosis among Finnish men who suffered sudden death AMI, coronary thrombosis, or died of noncardiac causes *(31)*. The odds ratio was highest among young men (odds ratio 9.2, 95% CI: 2.4–35.0). Meisel et al. found no difference in the incidence of the 5-C allele between CAD and control groups *(32)*. However when 269 patients undergoing percutaneous transluminal coronary angioplasty were examined, the presence of the −5C allele was associated with a higher incidence of 30-d adverse events. Interestingly, there was no difference among the 103 patients who underwent directional athrectomy and 278 where a stent was placed. It is unclear why the percutaneous transluminal coronary angioplasty (PTCA) group differed, considering all of the procedures have risks for thrombosis and restenosis.

A promising new polymorphic marker is GP VI, which is important in the activation of phospholipase Cγ2. A change in nucleotide 13254 of a thymidine to a cytosine results in the substitution of a serine for a proline. The allele frequency of the 13254C allele is 16%. In a study of AMI patients, the overall odds ratio for the presence of the CC genotype was not significant vs controls. However, in various subgroups, the odds ratio was 4.52 (95% CI: 1.23–16.6) and 6.48 (95% CI: 1.47–28.5) for women and patients ≥60 yr *(33)*. The mechanism of this interaction remains to be determined.

Although the role of platelet in thrombosis is undisputed, whether or not platelet polymorphism is an important risk factor for CAD remains to be determined in larger studies. Many of these markers have been discovered only within the last 5 yr. These preliminary studies suggest that the effect of polymorphism is likely to be secondary, rather than primary.

BIOCHEMICAL FACTORS

Lipoprotein Lipase

The lipoprotein lipase *(LPL)* gene is found on chromosome 8p33 and contains 10 exons spanning 30 kilobases. This gene produces a 475 amino acid protein that is posttranslationally modified to a signal peptide and the 448 amino acid mature enzyme that has a molecular weight of about 60 kDa. *LPL* is anchored to the vascular endothelium and removes lipids from the circulation by hydrolyzing triglycerides present in chylomicrons and very low density lipoproteins. Familial *LPL* deficiency causes marked chylomicronemia and premature atherosclerosis, but is relatively rare. There are at least four polymorphic variants of the *LPL* gene that have a more subtle effect on plasma lipid concentrations and cardiovascular risk. If these polymorphisms are associated with a reduced activity of *LPL*, they may be genetic risk factors for atherosclerosis.

Two of the most widely studied polymorphism to lipoprotein lipase are the restriction fragment length polymorphic sites *Hin*dIII and *Pvu*II, located on introns 8 and 6, respectively. The *Hin*dIII site results in a thymine→guanosine substitution and has an allele frequency (presence of the restriction site, H$^+$) of roughly 70%. The *Pvu*II site results in a cytosine to thymine substitution and has an allele frequency (P$^+$) of about 45%. Given the importance of lipoprotein lipase to lipid metabolism, attempts have been made to correlate the presence of these polymorphisms to lipid levels. Gerdes et al. showed that subjects with the H$^+$H$^+$ genotype had higher triglyceride (mean = 125 mg/dL) and lower high-density lipoprotein (HDL) cholesterol concentrations (mean = 49 mg/dL) than those with the H$^-$H$^-$ genotype (110 and 53 mg/dL, respectively) *(34)*. Larson et al. put enrolled subjects on the same low-fat, low-cholesterol and high-carbohydrate and high-fiber diets prior to lipid testing, and found no difference in *Hin*dIII genotypes for triglycerides and HDL cholesterol *(35)*. The total and low-density lipoprotein (LDL) cholesterol, however, was increased for women in the H$^+$H$^+$ group. Other investigators found similar results for triglycerides for the *Pvu*II polymorphism (158 for P$^-$P$^-$ vs 213 mg/dL for P$^+$P$^+$) *(36)*.

The presence of the H$^+$ allele is associated with a higher frequency of coronary disease. When comparing *Hin*dIIII polymorphism to the number of disease coronary arteries, the H$^+$H$^+$ genotype had a higher incidence of multivessel disease (odds ratio: 4.4, 95% CI: 1.73–11.33) than the combined H$^+$H$^-$ and H$^-$H$^-$ genotypes among Italians patients surviving AMI *(37)*. Because the H$^+$ allele has the higher prevalence, the presence of the H$^-$ variant would be interpreted to offer a protective effect toward CAD. Similar but less dramatic results were obtained for the *Pvu*II polymorphism where the P$^+$P$^+$ genotype had an odds ratio of 1.73 (95% CI: 1.03–2.89) vs the P$^-$P$^-$ genotype *(36)*. Studies examining the risk of particular H and P genotypes with CADs are being initiated. In one study, the H$^+$H$^+$ genotypes was significantly associated with an odds ratio of 2.0 (95% CI: 1.11–3.70) vs the H$^-$H$^-$ genotype in 725 patients undergoing angioplasty for ACS and 168 control subjects with normal coronary arteries *(38)*. This same study produced a trend for the P$^+$P$^+$ vs the P$^-$P$^-$ genotypes, but results did not reach significance (odds ratio: 1.39, 95% CI: 0.84–2.28).

Another widely studied polymorphism in lipoprotein lipase is the point mutation of a cytosine for a guanosine in nucleotide 447 of exon 9, resulting in the substitution of serine for a permature termination codon. The termination polymorphism can be detected with *Mnl*I and has an allele frequency of about 5%. The presence of the stop mutation phenotype (GG) appears to offer a protective effect toward CAD through the lowering of triglyceride and raising the HDL cholesterol concentrations *(39)*. The CAD incidence of the heterozygous (GC) and stop polymorphism (GG) was lower than for the wild-type (CC) phenotype (odds ratio: 0.38, 95% CI: 0.19–0.81) among 189 Japanese subjects. In contrast, a European study of 125 subjects showed no difference in C477G polymorphism between these CAD and control groups *(40)*. Clearly the number of subjects is too low at this time to make any definitive conclusions about the C477G polymorphism for lipoprotein lipase.

A single nucleotide substitution at nucleotide 9 of exon 2 produces an amino acid change from aspartic acid to asparagine. This polymorphism can be detected using the restriction endonuclease *Bcl*I. The allele frequency is rather low at about 1–5% *(40)*. For this reason, this polymorphism has not yet been widely examined in population studies.

Another A→G SNP has been identified in nucleotide 291 of exon 6 resulting in the substitution of an asparagine for a serine. The allele frequency of the Asn291Ser substitution is about 2.5%. Preliminary studies have suggested that the heterozygous carriers had increased triglycerides and decreased HDL cholesterol, and a predisposition toward ischemic heart disease in women (odds ratio: 1.89, CI: 1.19–3.01) *(41)*.

Apolipoprotein E Genotypes

The apoproteins are the protein components of lipoproteins. There are five major apoproteins, labeled A–C, apo E, and apo (a), with subclasses that exist for many of these. Apoproteins function to activate enzymes in lipoprotein metabolism, maintain the structural integrity of the lipoprotein complex, and facilitate the uptake of lipoproteins into cells through surface receptors. Apo E is a 34-kDa glycoprotein found in all major lipoproteins except LDL. Apo E plays an important role in the transportation and metabolism of triglycerides, chylomicrons, and very low density lipoprotein (VLDL) remnants. There are three major isoforms of Apo E, designated as E2, E3, and E4, and are encoded by the *apo E* gene, located on chromosome 19, to produce the ε2, ε3, and ε4 alleles. The ε2 contains a cysteine in amino residues 112 and 158, the ε3 contains a cysteine and arginine in these positions, and the ε4 contains an arginine in both locations. The presence of the ε4 genotype is associated with the presence of Alzheimer's disease *(42)*. The frequency of the ε2 allele is greatly dependent on the population. In one study of southern Europeans, it was 8%, that of ε3 about 83%, and that of ε4 about 9% *(43)*. The frequency of the ε4 allele is higher among African blacks.

Studies have shown that individuals with the ε2 alleles have the lowest LDL concentration and highest apo E, while those with the ε4 alleles have the reverse. It is possible that the apo E4 protein binds to the LDL receptor, thereby interfering with the clearance of LDL from the circulation. Because LDL is recognized as a risk factor for CAD, studies have been conducted to determine if apo E genotypes are linked. A meta-analysis conducted by Wilson et al. combined the results of nine published observational studies in men (*n* = 1971 cases) and four studies (*n* = 181 cases) in women *(44)*. The presence of the ε4 allele and presence of CAD produced an odds ratio of 1.38 (95% CI: 1.22–1.57) and 1.26 (1.13–1.41), respectively. In contrast, Frikke-Schmidt et al. found that the ε4 genotype was significantly associated with CHD for men (*n* = 693 cases) but not women (*n* = 247 cases) *(45)*.

Polymorphisms in other parts of the *apo* E gene have been identified, that is, within the promoter region. These include a A→T change at position –491, C→T change at position –427, and a G→T change at –219 *(46)*. In a study of 1245 AMI cases and controls, the –219T polymorphism was associated with increased risk for AMI (odds ratio: 1.29, 95% CI: 1.09–1.52). This polymorphism was not linked with the other polymorphisms in the promoter gene or with the ε alleles.

Methylene Tetrahydrofolate Reductase (MTHFR)

Homocysteine is formed from the metabolism of methionine, as shown in Fig. 7. Homocysteine is metabolized back to methionine with vitamin B_6, B_{12}, and folate as cofactors, or transsulfurated to cysteine. High concentrations of homocysteine have been implicated as a risk factor for a number of diseases such as peripheral vascular disease, stroke, and CAD. A meta-analysis was conducted examining the relationship of plasma homocys-

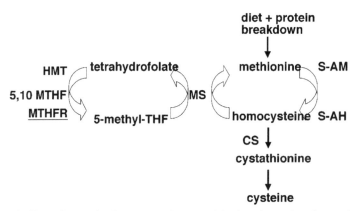

Fig. 7. Metabolic pathway for homocysteine. Methionine from the diet and metabolism of proteins is converted to *S*-adensylmethionine (S-AM), *S*-adenosylhomocysteine (S-AH), and then to homocysteine. With 5-methyltetrahydrofolate (5-THF) as a substrate, homocysteine is then remethylated back to methionine and tetrahydrofolate by methionine synthase (MS). Using vitamins B_6 and B_2 as cofactors, respectively, THF is remethylated to 5-THF by serine–glycine hydroxymethyltransferase (HMT) and methylenetrahydrofolate reductase (MTHFR), respectively. Polymorphisms in the *MTHFR* gene are the subject of many clinical investigations. In an alternate pathway, homocysteine is also converted to cystathionine by cystathionine β-synthase (CS) and then to cysteine.

teine and development of CAD *(47)*. Of 14 case-control studies involving more than 4700 patients, the odds ratio for development of CAD was 1.7 (95% CI: 1.5–1.9). Clinical trials are being conducted to determine if lowering homocysteine concentrations will result in a reduced risk for CAD. Commercial assays for homocysteine are available and are routinely used in clinical practice. The upper limit of the normal range for homocysteine in plasma is 15 µmol/L. However, a lower concentration that is within the normal range, for example, 12 µmol/L, may be a more appropriate limit for low or no disease risk.

A major cause of hyperhomocysteinemia is dietary deficiency of vitamins B_6, B_{12}, and folate. As such, the United States has recently introduced folate fortification in grain in an attempt to reduce the prevalence of dietary-induced hyperhomocysteinemia. Folate supplementation is inexpensive and has no side effects. The genetic basis of hyperhomocysteinemia has been known for many years, and was the principal basis behind the hypothesis that abnormal homocysteine metabolism led to premature atherothrombotic events. Rare causes of homocystinuria include genetic deficiencies of methionine synthase and cystathionine β-synthase, important enzymes in the degradation of homocysteine. Pathologic changes within the coronary and cerebral arteries in children with congenital homocystinuria, that is, intimal damage, hyperplasia of smooth muscles, lipoprotein aggregates, and so forth are identical to that found in adult atherosclerotic plaques.

A severe deficiency in MTHFR can also cause hyperhomocysteinemia and homocystinuria. MTHFR is a homodimer of 77-kDa subunits and is a key enzyme in the folate cycle that generates 5-methyltetrahydrofolate, the substrate for methionine synthase (Fig. 7). The severe MTHFR deficiency is rare, with only a few dozen cases described worldwide. At least 18 different point mutations have been demonstrated to produce these severe forms of MTFHR deficiency.

There are five common polymorphisms in MTHFR. The most common and widely studied of these is a cytosine to thymine substitution in nucleotide 677 of exon 4. This polymorphism has an allele frequency of about 35% and homozygosity frequencies of 10–15%. The homozygous genotype is associated with <20% of the normal MTHFR activity and thermolability in lymphocyte extracts resulting in low plasma folate concentrations and a mild hyperhomocysteinemia. In the study of Dunn et al., subjects under 50 yr old had a mean homocysteine concentration that varied from 15.8 and 15.9 for the homozygote wild-type and heterozygote, which increased to 21.4 µmol/L for the homozygous C677T variant ($p < 0.0001$) *(48)*.

There have been many studies that have attempted to correlate MTHFR polymorphism to CAD, with conflicting results. A meta-analysis of 10 studies on 5644 patients produced an odds ratio of 1.30 (95% CI: 1.11–1.52) for CAD and the presence of the 677T variant *(5)*. However, a major limitation in these studies is the failure to factor in plasma folate as a confounding variable. It may be possible that a reduced MTHFR activity can be compensated by the presence of a high plasma folate level potentially normalizing the homocysteine concentration.

Angiotensin Converting Enzyme (ACE)

ACE is a critical enzyme in the renin–angiotensin–aldosterone (RAA) axis. Under the action of renin, angiotensinogen is first degraded to the decapeptide angiotensin I and then to the octapeptide angiotensin II by ACE. Angiotensin II is further degraded into a heptapeptide, angiotensin III, by angiotensinase. When there are periods of blood and fluid loss, the RAA axis is essential in maintaining blood pressure by stimulating vasoconstriction (via angiotensin II), sodium plasma volume retention, and potassium loss, and inactivating bradykinin (vasodilator). Prolonged stimulation of the RAA axis leads to cardiovascular remodeling and has been implicated in the pathogenesis of neointimal hyperplasia. The use of ACE inhibitors has been shown to reduce atherosclerosis in animal models *(49)*.

There is a common polymorphism in the *ACE* gene in intron 16 involving the insertion (I) or deletion (D) of a 287-bp *alu* repeat sequence. The allele frequency for the insertion is 45%. The concentration of plasma ACE is increased in patients with the DD vs the II genotypes (e.g., 494 vs 299 ng/mL, respectively) *(50)*. The first study that correlated the presence of the DD genotype to ACS was published in 1992 on 1343 cases and controls *(51)*. Subsequently, a meta-analysis was conducted combining the results of 15 studies on 8873 cases and controls *(52)*. The cumulative meta-analysis produced an odds ratio of 1.26 (95% CI: 1.15–1.39) for the DD allele.

The accuracy of these early studies was questioned by Shanmugan et al., who showed that the D allele is preferentially amplified in heterozygote subjects *(53)*. These investigators suggested the use of primers that specifically recognize the insertion-specific sequence. More recent articles that have used the preferred primers have not demonstrated a relationship between ACE polymorphism and presence of CAD *(54)*.

Given the role of the RAA axis on stimulating the growth of smooth muscles, ACE polymorphisms have been examined as a contributor to restenosis after angioplasty *(55)*. These authors suggest that the pathophysiology of post-PTCA restenosis is related to smooth muscle cell migration and remodeling rather than proliferation. In contrast, stent placement may be more related to the growth effects of ACE. The study of Amant et al.

showed an inverse relationship between the number of D alleles present and the minimum lumen diameter at 6 mo after successful stent implantation *(56)*. The follow-up to these observations was a therapeutic drug trial where these investigators examined the success of ACE inhibitors on the restenosis rate in a randomized double-blind placebo-controlled trial *(57)*. To their surprise, they showed that the restenosis rate was not reduced by ACE inhibitor treatment, but in fact was exaggerated. Others have shown no association with ACE DD genotype and stent placement with regard to 1-yr outcomes *(58)*. The precise role of ACE polymorphism for ACS remains unclear at this time.

Because the RAA system is important in the pathophysiology of congestive heart failure (CHF), the effect of ACE polymorphisms has also been studied to determine if there is a correlation to CHF. Like results for CAD, the studies conducted to date are conflicting. Candy et al. correlated ACE genotypes with left ventricular systolic performance as measured by ejection fraction using both echocardiography and radionuclide ventriculography *(59)*. McNamara reported higher survival rates for CHF patients who were not treated with β-blockers *(60)*. However, Montgomery was unable to find an association of ACE polymorphism in 99 patients with idiopathic dilated cariomyopathy *(61)*. One explanation for the lack of an association between the DD polymorphism was suggested by Spruth et al. *(62)*, who found no difference in mRNA expression between the DD, ID, and II genotypes. Finding genetic markers for patients with CHF may be more difficult than for patients with ACS because there may be more heterogeneity in the pathophysiology of CHF.

A polymorphism also exists in the gene for angiotensin receptor type 1, where there is a change from an adenine in nucleotide 1166 to a cytosine. This mutation may be linked to increased prevalence of hypertension and coronary vasoconstriction. A early study suggested that this polymorphism was linked to the ACE D/I polymorphism, that is, the combination of the DD and 1166CC phenotype produced a significant association for AMI (odds ratio: 3.95 95% CI: 1.26–12.4) *(63)*. This association has not been confirmed in more recent studies *(64)*. In a study in which angiotensin II was given to volunteers, investigators concluded that the A1166C polymorphism does not have an effect on the actions of angiotensin II *(65)*.

β-Blockers

Cardiac inotropy and chronotropy are modulated in part by β_1 and β_2-adrenergic receptors expressed in the human heart. Patients with heart failure have an overstimulation of neurohormones such as the catecholamines, resulting in a down-regulation of the β-receptors. The use of β-blocker therapy improves clinical symptoms and cardiac output by slowing the heart rate and improving the rhythm. Under a situation of increased RAA axis stimulation, polymorphisms in the β-receptors may predispose an individual to the development of heart failure.

There are many polymorphisms in the β_1 receptor gene that encodes for a 478-amino-acid protein. Many of these polymorphisms, however, are silent and thus their significance in development of CHF can be questioned *(66)*. Two of these polymorphisms have been studied with regard to idiopathic dilated cardiomyopathy. One involves nucleotide 145, in which there is a change from an adenine to a guanosine resulting in the substitution of serine for a glycine. The other is at nucleotide 1165, where there is a change from a guanine to a cytosine resulting in a arginine to glycine substitution. The allele frequencies for the 145G and 1165C are 15% and 25%, respectively. These polymorphisms were studied in a cohort of patients with CHF. In a study of 821 cases in controls, the 1165G polymorphism was not associated with idiopathic dilated cardiomyopathy *(67)*. In another study, Borjesson et al. found the 49G allele frequency was higher than for the 49S allele *(68)*. These investigators also reported significant differences in survival rates with the mutation (odds ratio: 2.34, 95% CI: 1.30–4.20). The amino- (N)-terminal sequence where the 49S mutation resides may be important to fold the receptor within the membrane, while not being the target for receptor activation. These observations may help explain why some individuals respond to β-blockade while others do not. Prospective pharmacogenomic trials for different $β_1$ and $β_2$ blockers will be the next logical step in this area.

Three common polymorphism in the $β_2$ receptor are in amino acid position 16 substituting an arginine for a glucine, position 27 substituting a glutamine for a glutamic acid, and 164 substituting an arginine for an isoleucine. The allele frequencies for the respective polymorphisms are 61%, 43%, and 2%. The polymorphism in positions 16 and 27 have different susceptibilities to agonist-induced down-regulation. The 164 polymorphism exhibits a decreased affinity for $β_2$-adrenogeric angonists, and an uncoupling of receptors from the G_s protein. In volunteer subjects, the increase in heart rate and systolic blood pressure among those with the Thr164Ile polymorphism was less than for the wild-type *(69)*. In a study of 471 case and controls, Liggett et al. found no difference in the allele frequencies for CHF patients and controls *(70)*. However, when the 1-yr outcomes were compared, patients with the 164 ile polymorphism had a higher death risk rate and need for cardiac transplantation than CHF patients with the wild-type mutation.

SUMMARY

Although many of these genes demonstrate a significant correlation with polymorphisms and the incidence of CAD or heart failure, the degree of risk is not particularly high in any case (odds ratio typically between 1 and 2). Most investigators agree that the pathogenesis of these diseases is too complex and diverse to be explained on the basis of a single gene mutation. Discrepancies in results of individual studies may be the result of inadequate numbers of subjects enrolled or heterogeneity in the sex and/or racial make of the population studied. However, several studies have shown that the presence of some mutations is linked to others and their effect on disease progression may be additive. Unfortunately, all of the studies published to date involve only a handful of gene mutations on a limited number of subjects enrolled. The costs for performing the DNA analysis prohibits the analysis for more than just of few of these genes at any given time. This chapter discussed only a minority of the polymorphisms that are known to exist among the various proteins and factors known to participate in the disease. However, the technology for detecting gene mutations is changing with the development of reusable microarrays or "gene chips." In the very near future, it will become practical to examine 50 or 100 genes following a single amplification of DNA from the same individual. Polymorphisms that are not correlated to CAD alone may be important when used in combination with other factors.

Genes that have been initially targeted are those proteins known to participate in the pathophysiology of cardiac diseases. Given that none of these factors studied to date have produced particularly high odds ratios (i.e., they are typically <2.0), it may be appropriate for future studies to concentration on the effect of polymorphisms in the success of therapy, both pharmacologic and percutaneous. This justifies the current interest in the genes that modify platelet function, ACE inhibitors, and β-blockers. Perhaps the work should be further focused in therapies where there is variability in response and/or success. A specific polymorphism may be an important factor in the lack of success in some instances.

ABBREVIATIONS

ACE, Angiotensin converting enzyme; ACS, acute coronary syndromes; AMI; acute myocardial infarction; APC, activated protein C; apo, apoprotein; CAD, coronary artery disease; CHF, congestive heart failure; CI, confidence interval; GP, glycoprotein; HDL and LDL, high- and low-density lipoprotein; HPA-3, human platelet alloantigen-3; LPL, lipoprotein lipase; MTHFR, methylene tetrahydrofolate reductase; NCEP, National Cholesterol Education Program; PAI-1, plasminogen activator inhibitor-1; PCI, percutaneous coronary intervention; PTCA, percutaneous transluminal coronary angioplasty; RAA, renin–angiotensin–aldosterone; SNPs, single nucleotide polymorphisms; tPA, tissue plasminogen activator.

REFERENCES

1. Expert Panel on Detection, Evaluation, and Treatment of High Blood Cholesterol in Adults. Executive Summary of the Third Report of the) Expert Panel on Detection, Evaluation, National Cholesterol Education Program (NCEP and Treatment of High Blood Cholesterol in Adults (Adult Treatment Panel III). JAMA 2001;285:2486–2497.
2. Pepe G, Rickards O, Vanegas OC, et al. Prevalence of Factor V Leiden mutation in non-European populations. Thromb Haemost 1997;77:329–331.
3. Ridker PM, Hennekens CH, Lindpaintner K, Stampfer MJ, Eiseberg PR, Miletich JP. Mutation in the gene coding for coagulation factor V and the risk of myocardial infarction, stroke, and venous thrombosis in apparently healthy men. N Engl J Med 1995;332:912–917.
4. Bauer KA. The thrombophilias: well-defined risk factors with uncertain therapeutic implications (review). Ann Intern Med 2001;135:367–373.
5. Ridker PM, Hennekens CH, Miletich JP. G20210A mutation in prothrombin gene and risk of myocardial infarction, stroke, and venous thrombosis in a large cohort of US men. Circulation 2000;99:999–1004.
6. Wu AHB, Tsongalis GJ. Correlation of selected single nucleotide polymorphisms of coagulation factors to risk for cardiovascular disease. Am J Cardiol 2001;87:1361–1366.
7. Martinelli I, Bucciarelli P, Margaglione M, DeStefano V, Castaman G, Pier Mannuccio M. The risk of venous thromboembolism in family members with mutations in the genes of factor V or prothrombin or both. Br J Haematol 2000;111:1223–1229.
8. Meade TW, Mellows S, Brozovic M, et al. Haemostatic function and ischaemic heart disease: principal results of the Northwick Park Heart Study. Lancet 1986;2:533–537.
9. Girelli D, Russo C, Ferraresi P, et al. Polymorphisms in the Factor VII gene and the risk of myocardial infarction in patients with coronary artery disease. N Engl J Med 2000;343:774–780.
10. Fellowes AP, Brennan SO, George PM. Identification and characterization of five new fibrinogen gene polymorphisms. Ann NY Acad Sci 2001;936:536–541.

11. Green FR. Fibrinogen polymorphisms and atherothrombotic disease. Ann NY Acad Sci 2001; 936:549–559.

12. Doggen CJM, Bertina RM, Cats VM, Rosendaal FR. Fibrinogen polymorphisms are not associated with the risk of myocardial infarction. Br J Haematol 2000;110:935–938.

13. Ridker PM, Vaughan DE, Stampfer MJ, Manson JE, Hennekens CH. Endogenous tissue-type plasminogen activator and risk of myocardial infarction. Lancet 1993;341:1165–1168.

14. Juhan-Vague I, Pyke SD, Alessi MC, Jespersen J, Haverkate F, Thompson SG. Fibrinolytic factors and the risk of myocardial infarction or sudden death in patients with angina pectoris. ECAT Study Group. European Concerted Action on Thrombosis and Disabilities. Circulation 1996;94:2057–2063.

15. Ye S, Green FR, Scarabin PY, et al. The 4G/5G genetic polymorphism in the promoter of the plasminogen activator-1 (PAI-1) gene is associated with differences in plasma PAI-1 activity but not with risk of myocardial infarction in the ECTIM study. Thromb Haemost 1995;74:837–841.

16. Iacoviello L, Burzotta F, Di Castelnuovo A, et al. The 4G/5G polymorphism of PAI-1 promoter gene and the risk of myocardial infarction: a meta analysis. Thromb Haemost 1998; 80:1029–1030.

17. Ossei-Gerning N, Mansfield MW, Stickland MH, Wilson IJ, Grant P. Plasminogen activator inhibitor-1 promoter 4G/5G genotype and plasma levels in relation to a history of myocardial infarction in patients characterized by coronary angiography. Arterioscl Thromb Vasc Biol 1997;17:33–37.

18. Mizuno K, Satomura K, Miyamoto A, et al. Angioscopic evaluation of coronary-artery thrombi in acute coronary syndromes. N Engl J Med 1992;326:287–291.

19. George JN. Platelets. Lancet 2000;355:1531–1541.

20. Weiss EJ, Bray PF, Tayback M, et al. A polymorphism of a platelet glycoprotein receptor as an inherited risk factor for coronary thrombosis. N Engl J Med 1996;334:1090–1094.

21. Ridker PM, Hennekens CH, Schmitz C, Stampfer MJ, Lindpaintner K. PI[A1/A2] polymorphism of platelet glycoprotein IIIa and risks of myocardial infarction, stroke, and venous thrombosis. Lancet 1997;349:385–388.

22. Laule M, Cascorbi I, Stangl V, et al. A1/A2 polymorphism of glycoprotein IIIa and association with excess procedural risk for coronary catheter interventions: a case-controlled study. Lancet 1999;353:708–712.

23. Kastrati A, Koch W, Gawaz M, et al. P1A polymorphism of glycoprotein IIIa and risk of adverse events after coronary stent placement. J Am Coll Cardiol 2000;36:84–89.

24. Bottiger C, Kastrati A, Koch W, et al. Polymorphism of platelet glycoprotein IIb and risk of thrombosis and restenosis after coronary stent placement. Am J Cardiol 1999;84:987–991.

25. Kunicki TJ, Kritzig M, Annis DS, Nugent DJ. Hereditary variation in platelet integrin $\alpha2\beta1$ density is associated with two silent polymorphism in the $\alpha2$ gene coding sequence. Blood 1997;89:1939–1943.

26. Santoso S, Kunicki TJ, Kroll H, Haberbosch W, Gardemann A. Association of the platelet glycoprotein Ia C_{807} T gene polymorphism with nonfatal myocardial infarction in younger patients. Blood 1000;93:2449–2453.

27. Von Beckerath N, Koch W, Mehilli J, Bottiger C, Schomig A, Kasatrati A. Glycoprotein Ia gene C807T polymorphism and risk for major adverse cardiac events within the first 30 days after coronary artery stenting. Blood 2000;95:3297–3301.

28. Kroll H, Gardemann A, Fechter A, Haberbosch W, Santoso S. The impact of the glycoprotein Ia collagen receptor subunit A_{1648}G gene polymorphism on coronary artery disease and acute myocardial infarction. Thromb Haemost 2000;83:392–396.

29. Kandzari DE, Goldschmidt-Clermont PJ. Platelet polymorphisms and ischemic heart disease: moving beyond traditional risk factors. J Am Coll Cardiol 2001;38:1028–1032.

458

Wu

30. Corral J, Gonzalez-Conejero R, Lozano ML, Rivera J, Vicente V. New alleles of the platelet glycoprotein Ibα gene. Br J Haematol 1998;103:997–1003.
31. Mikkelsson J, Perola M, Penttila A, Karhunen PJ. Platelet glycoprotein Ibα HPA-2 Met/ VNTR B haplotype as a genetic predictor of myocardial infarction and sudden cardiac death. Circulation 2001;104:876–880.
32. Meisel C, Afshar-Kharghan V, Cascorbi I, et al. Role of Kozak sequence polymorphism of platelet glycoprotein Ibα as a risk factor for coronary artery disease and catheter interventions. J Am Coll Cardiol 2001;38:1023–1027.
33. Croft SA, Samani NJ, Teare MD, et al. Novel platelet membrane glycoprotein VI dimnorphism is a risk factor for myocardial infarction. Circulation 2001;104:1459–1463.
34. Gerdes C, Gerdes LU, Hansen PS, Faergeman O. Polymorphisms in the lipoprotein lipase gene and their associations with plasma lipid concentrations in 40-year old Danish men. Circulation 1995;92:1765–1769.
35. Larson I, Hoffmann MM, Ordovas JM, Schaefer EJ, Marz W, Kreuzer J. The lipoprotein lipase HindIII polymorphism: association with total cholesterol and LDL-cholesterol, but not with HDL and triglycerides in 342 females. Clin Chem 1999;45:963–968.
36. Wang XT, McCredie Rm, Wilcken DEL. Common DNA polymorphisms at the lipoprotein lipase gene: association with severity of coronary artery disease and diabetes. Circulation 1996;93:1339–1345.
37. Gambino R, Scaglione L, Alemanno N, Pagano G, Cassader M. Human lipoprotein lipase HindIII polymorphism in young patients with myocardial infarction. Metabolism 1999;48: 1157–1161.
38. Anderson JL, King GJ, Bair TL, et al. Association of lipoprotein gene polymorphisms with coronary artery disease. J Am Coll Cardiol 1999;33:1013–1020.
39. Sawano M, Watanabe Y, Ohmura H, et al. Potentially protective effects of the Ser 447-ter mutation of the lipoprotein lipase gene against the development of coronary artery disease in Japanese subjects via a beneficial lipid profile. Jpn Circ J 2001;65:310–314.
40. Raslova K, Smolkova B, Vohnout B, Gasparovic J, Frohlich JJ. Risk factors for atherosclerosis in survivors of myocardial infarction and their spouses: comparison to controls without personal and family history of atherosclerosis. Metabolism 2001;50:24–29.
41. Wittrup HH, Tybjaerg-Hansen A, Abildgaard S, Steffensen R, Schnohr P, Nordestgaard BG. A common substitution (Asn291Ser) in lipoprotein lipase is associated with increased risk of ischemic heart disease. J Clin Invest 1997;99:1606–1613.
42. Higgins GA, Large CH, Rupniak HT, Barnes JC. Apolipoprotein E and Alzheimer's disease: a review of recent studies. Pharmacol Biochem Behav 1997;56:675–685.
43. Corbo RM, Vilardo T, Ruggeri M, Gemma AT, Scacchi R. Apolipoprotein E genotype and plasma levels in coronary artery disease. A case-control study in the Italian population. Clin Biochem 1999;32:217–222.
44. Wilson PW, Schaefer EJ, Larson MG, Ordovas JM. Apolipoprotein E alleles and risk of coronary disease. A meta-analysis. Arterioscl Thromb Vasc Biol 1996;16:1250–1255.
45. Frikke-Schmidt R, Tybjaerg-Hansen A, Steffensen R, Jensen G, Nordestgaard BG. Apolipoprotein E genotype: epsilon32 women are protected while epsilon43 and epsilon44 men are susceptible to ischemic heart disease. J Am Coll Cardiol 2000;35:1192–1199.
46. Lambert JC, Brousseau T, Defosse V, et al. Independent association of an APOE gene promoter polymorphism with increased risk of myocardial infarction and decrease APOE plasma concentrations-the ECTIM study. Human Mol Genet 2000;9:57–61.
47. Boushey CJ, Beresford SA, Omen GS, Motulsky AG. A quantitative assessment of plasma homocysteine as a risk factor for vascular disease. JAMA 1995;274:1049–1057.
48. Dunn J, Title LM, Bata I, et al. Relation of a common mutation in methylenetetrahydrofolate reductase to plasma homocysteine and early onset coronary artery disease. Clin Biochem 1998;31:95–100.

49. Shuh JR, Bleh DJ, Frierdich GE, McMahon EG, Blaine EH. Differential effects of renin–angiogensin system blockade on atherogenesis in cholesterol-fed rabbits. J Clin Invest 1993; 981:1453–1458.

50. Rigat B, Hubert C, Alhenc-Gelas F, Cambien F, Corvol P, Soubrier F. An insertion/deletion polymorphism in the angiotensin I-converting enzyme gene accounting for half the variance of serum enzyme levels. J Clin Invest 1990;86:1343–1346.

51. Cambien F, Poirier O, Lecerf L, et al. Deletion polymorphism in the gene for angiotensin-converting enzyme is a potential risk factor for myocardial infarction. Nature 1992;359:641–643.

52. Samani NJ, Thompson JR, O'Toole L, Channer K, Woods KL. A meta-analysis of the association of the deletion allele of the angiotensin-converting enzyme gene with myocardial infarction. Circulation 1996;94:708–712.

53. Shanmugan V, Sell KW, Saha BK. Mistyping ACE heterozygotes. PCR Methods Appl 1993;3:120–121.

54. Rice GI, Foy CA, Grant PJ. Angiotensin converting enzyme and angiotensin II type 1-receptor gene polymorisms and risk of ischaemic heart disease. Cardiovasc Res 1999;41: 746–753.

55. Zee RYL, Fernandez-Ortiz A, Macaya C, Pintor E, Lindpaintner K, Fernandez-Cruz A. ACE D/I polymorphism and incidence of post-PTCA restenosis: a prospective, angiography-based evaluation. Hypertension 2001;37:851–855.

56. Amant C, Bauters C, Bodart JC, et al. D allele of the angiotensin I-converting enzyme is a major risk factor for resetenosis after coronary stenting. Circulation 1997;96:56–60.

57. Meurice T, Bauters C, Hermant X, et al. Effect of ACE inhibitors on angiographic restenosis after coronary stenting (PARIS): a randomised, double-blind, placebo-controlled trial. Lancet 2001;357:1321–1324.

58. Koch W, Kastrati A, Mehilli J, Bottiger C, von Beckerath N, Schomig A. Insertion/deletion polymorphis of the angiotensin I-converting enzyme gene is not associated with restenosis after coronary stent placement. Circulation 2000;102:197–202.

59. Candy GP, Skudicky D, Mueller UK, et al. Association of left ventricular systolic performance and cavity size with angiotensin-converting enzyme genotype in idiopathic dilated cardiopathy. Am J Cardiol 1999;83:740–744.

60. McNamara DM, Holubkov R, Janosko K, et al. Pharmacogenetic interactions between β-blocker therapy and the angiotensin-converting enzyme deletion polymorphism in patients with congestive heart failure. Circulation 2001;103:1644–1648.

61. Montgomery HE, Keeling PJ, Goldman JH, Humphries SE, Talmud PJ, McKenna WJ. Lack of association between the insertion/deletion polymorphism of the angiotensin-converting enzyme gene and idiopathic dilated cardiomyopathy. J Am Coll Cardiol 1995;25: 1627–1631.

62. Spruth E, Zurbrugg HR, Warnecke C, et al. Expresion of ACE mRNA in the human atrial myocardium is not dependent on left ventricular function, ACE inhibitor therapy, or the ACE I/D genotype. J Mol Med 1999;77:804–810.

63. Tiret L, Bonnardeaux A, Poirier O, et al. Synergistic effects of angiotensin-converting enzyme and angiotensin-II type 1 receptor gene polymorphisms on risk of myocardial infarction. Lancet 1994;344:910–913.

64. Batalla A, Alvarez R, Reguero JR, et al. Synergistic effect between apolipoprotein E and angiotensinogen gene polymorphisms in the risk for early myocardial infarction. Clin Chem 2000; 46:1910–1915.

65. Hilgers KF, Langenfeld MRW, Schlaich M, Veelken R, Schmieder RE. 1166 A/C polymorphism of the angiotensin II type 1 receptor gene and the response to short-term infusion of angiotensin II. Circulation 1999;100:1394–1399.

66. Podlowski S, Wenzel K, Luther HP, et al. β_1-adrenoceptor gene variations: a role in idiopathic dilated cardiomyopathy? J Mol Med 2000;78:87–93.

67. Tesson F, Charron P, Peuchmaurd M, et al. Characterization of unique genetic variant in the β_1-adrenoceptor gene and evaluation of its role in idiopathic dilated cardiomyopathy. J Mol Cell Cardiol 1999;31:1025–1032.
68. Borjesson M, Magnusson Y, Hjalmarson A, Andersson B. A novel polymorphism in the gene coding for the beta$_1$-adrenergic receptor associated with survival in patients with heart failure. Eur Heart J 2000;21:1853-1858.
69. Brodde OE, Rainer B, Tellkamp R, Radke J, Stefan D, Insel PA. Blunted cardiac responses to receptor activation in subjects with Thr164Ile β_2-adrenoceptors. Circulation 2001;103: 1048–1050.
70. Liggett SB, Wagoner LE, Craft LL, et al. The Ile164 β2-adrenergic receptor polymorphism adversely affects the outcome of congestive heart failure. J Clin Invest 1998;102:1534–1539.

Index